MONITORING ENVIRONMENTAL MATERIALS
AND SPECIMEN BANKING

Commission of the
European Communities
Environment and Consumer
Protection Service Brussels

Federal Ministry for Research
and Technology Bonn
Federal Environmental Agency
Berlin (West)

United States
Environmental Protection
Agency
Washington D. C.

INTERNATIONAL WORKSHOP
ON MONITORING ENVIRONMENTAL MATERIALS
AND SPECIMEN BANKING

Berlin (West)

October, 23rd - 28th 1978

PATRONAGE

E. PAETZOLD

Senator for Health and Environmental Protection

MONITORING ENVIRONMENTAL MATERIALS AND SPECIMEN BANKING

Proceedings of the International Workshop,
Berlin (West), 23-28 October 1978

Edited by

N.-P. LUEPKE

Institute of Pharmacology and Toxicology,
University of Muenster

1979

MARTINUS NIJHOFF PUBLISHERS

THE HAGUE/BOSTON/LONDON

The distribution of this book is handled by the following team:

for the United States and Canada

Kluwer Boston, Inc.
160 Old Derby Street
Hingham, MA 02043
USA

for all other countries

Kluwer Academic Publishers Group
Distribution Center
P.O. Box 322
3300 AH Dordrecht
The Netherlands

ISBN 90-247-2303-5

LEGAL NOTICE

Neither the Commission of the European Communities or any person acting on behalf of the Commission is responsible for the use which might be made of the following information.

PRINTED IN BELGIUM

Commission of the
European Communities
Environment and Consumer
Protection Service Brussels

Federal Ministry for Research
and Technology Bonn
Federal Environmental Agency
Berlin (West)

United States
Environmental Protection
Agency
Washington D. C.

INTERNATIONAL WORKSHOP
ON MONITORING ENVIRONMENTAL MATERIALS
AND SPECIMEN BANKING

Berlin (West)

October, 23rd - 28th 1978

ORGANIZING COMMITTEE

CHAIRMEN

H. v. LERSNER
Federal Environmental Agency

M. CARPENTIER
Commission of the European Communities

D. S. BARTH
U. S. Environmental Protection Agency

VICE CHAIRMEN

D. A. FLEMER
U. S. Environmental Protection Agency

F. SCHMIDT – BLEEK
Federal Environmental Agency

J. SMEETS
Commission of the European Communities

COORDINATOR and Responsible for Final Report

N. - P. LUEPKE
Institute of Pharmacology and Toxicology
University of Muenster
Federal Republic of Germany

RAPPORTEURS

C. PRIES
The Netherlands

D. K. PHELPS
L. C. RANIERE
United States of America

P. MUELLER
Federal Republic of Germany

SCIENTIFIC SECRETARIAT

R. AMAVIS
Commission of the European Communities

H. D. SCHENKE
Federal Environmental Agency

LOCAL SECRETARIAT

Ch. MORAWA
R. LAZARUS
Federal Environmental Agency

According to the recommendations made during the International Workshop on ‚The use of biological specimens for the assessment of human exposure to the environmental pollutants' which was held in April 1977 in Luxembourg, this International Workshop on ‚Monitoring environmental materials and specimen banking' under special considerations of aquatic and terrestrial ecosystems was arranged to be held from 23rd till 28th October 1978 in Berlin (meetingplace: Deutscher Reichstag). A joint sponsorship by the Commission of the European Communities, Brussels, the Federal Ministry for Research and Technology, Bonn, in connection with the Federal Environmental Agency, Berlin, the U. S. Environmental Protection Agency, Washington, D. C., and the patronage by the Senator for Health and Environmental Protection, Berlin, are greatfully acknowledged.

ORGANIZING COMMITTEE

EDITORIAL NOTE

For the preparation of this Workshop, a number of background contributions have been requested by the Organizing Commitee. These have been used by the rapporteurs:

P. MUELLER
D. K. PHELPS
C. PRIES
L. C. RANIERE

and the coordinator:

N. - P. LUEPKE

to prepare a draft report which has been used as the basic discussion document during the Workshop.

Both the final approved general report and the background documents are published in these proceedings.

N. - P. LUEPKE

PREFACE

Ever since the industrial revolution, large numbers of environmentally hazardous materials are introduced into the global environment annually; a list of all substances which are at present regarded as environmentally hazardous might contain thousands of compounds, and new substances are still being added. Several major activities are necessary of adequately ensure the protection of human health and the environment from the often subtle effects of these materials. These activities include toxicological and ecological research, control technology development, the promulgation of regulatory guidelines and standards, and the monitoring of environmental materials and specimen banking. **In the absence of effective monitoring environmental materials and specimen banking, the detection of serious environmental contamination from pollutants may occur only after critical damage has been done.**

Environmental problems are independent of national boundaries and international collaborative programmes should be encouraged. Sponsoring organisations and other international and national bodies should encourage monitoring and specimen bank programmes and develop harmonised systems for data acquisition and evaluation. **An international pilot programme of monitoring and specimen banking is needed and is technically feasible.**

The conclusions and recommendations, for both implementation and research, should be of interest to other international and national bodies in addition to the three organisation sponsoring this International Workshop. Nevertheless this joint sponsorship should help to assure that the resulting conclusions and recommendations will have a worldwide audience and that effective coordination of existing programmes will be possible.

The commitment of governments is, of course, necessary for such implementation. Hopefully the scientific papers, the published proceedings, and the continuing support and interactions of the participants, will ensure that the concerned governments will be provided with adequate informations on which to determine appropriate commitments to the establishment of both global and national montoring and specimen banking programmes.

N. - P. LUEPKE

CONTENTS

X

WORKING PAPERS SUBMITTED FOR THE WORKSHOP

XII

FINAL REPORT

CONCLUSIONS AND RECOMMENDATIONS

General Aspects

1. The participants recommend the establishment of systems for the monitoring of the actual environmental exposure to substances which have, or may have, adverse effects on the environment.

2. The participants recommend the establishment of environmental specimen banks which are important in analyzing trends in exposure to previously unrecognized pollutants or pollutants for which analytical techniques may at present be inadequate.

3. Pilot specimen banks should be established as soon as possible in order to study the problems of organizing long time storage in banking programs.

4. In order to ensure the efficient and economical operation of specimen banks, sample collection, storage, analysis and quality control of data should be centrally located or at least co-ordinated for each program and the number of storage sites and analytical laboratories kept to a minimum.

5. A banking system for living tissue (clone bank) should be established in order to be able to recognize the adaptation processes of species to changing environmental exposure.

6. The above activities should be harmonized internationally as much as possible. They should utilize the resources and experience of closely related programs which already exist, e. g. the U. S. - German Environmental Tissue Bank Program, the U. S. Pesticide Monitoring Program and the Mussel Watch Program.

7. In addition to scientific, technical and monetary factors, legal and ethical considerations must be taken into account when planning monitoring and banking programs.

Ecological Aspects

8. The ecological characteristic of collection areas should be carefully selected so as to allow extrapolation of results and observations to larger regions.

9. The environmental samples selected should take account of aquatic (limnic and marine), terrestrial, and urbanic ecosystems.

Selection of Specimens

10. The species selected for specimen banking programs should have regard to likely monitoring programs; they will depend upon the specific objectives and design of the program considered. The species selection is to be planned in consultation with analytical chemists, biologists, pathologists, toxicologist, physiologists, ecologists, statisticians, and others concerned, in order to ensure adequate design, sampling, and analytical methodology. The selection of specimen types is made according to general and specific criteria (see tables 1 to 5).

11. A number of plant species are discussed and recommended for monitoring environmental materials and specimen banking (see Tables 6 to 7).

12. Invertebrates discussed and recommended for monitoring and banking in the terrestrial compartment are honey bee, carabid and earthworm (see tables 8 to 9); regarding the aquatic compartment a lot of biological specimens are discussed and selection criteria developed (see tables 10 to 11).

13. The restricting factor in the selection of birds and mammals is their sufficient availability (see tables 12 to 13). Out of a multitude of birds species suitable for a monitoring and banking program, starlings (Sturnus vulgaris) and ducks (Anas platyrhynchos or Anas rubripes) are particularly recommended (see table 12). The samples which can be taken for banking purposes from fairly large birds and mammals include gonads (testis/ovary), thyroid, adrenal glands, bone, adipose tissue, blood, kidney, liver, lung, muscle (skeletal), spleen, and in particular, feathers, thymus, and bursa of fabricius from birds as well as from mammals teeth, lens, hair, and brain (see table 14).

14. The qualitative and quantitative monitoring of aero plankton as well as its long time storage in a specimen bank would be desirable.

15. Analytical quality control is essential. A reliable system of analytical quality control calls for the use of well trained and experienced analytical personnel, interlaboratory quality control programs for participating laboratories, the use of two or more independent analytical methods and the use of certified reference materials for the validation of analytical techniques.

16. In considering pollutants to be monitored, priorities should be established on the basis of current and predicted exposure, the size of populations at risk and the severity of effects.

17. After definition of chemical categories, a list of high-priority categories and chemical pollutants as candidates for inclusion in an environmental monitoring programme was established. The methodology used considered bioaccumulation, environmental persistence and chronic toxicity (incl. mutagenicity, teratogenicity, carcinogenicity etc.) as equally important criteria, and acute toxicity as being less important (see table 15).

18. Careful consideration should be given to the relationship between environmental exposure and the concentrations in indicator specimens. ‚Normal' concentrations and those associated with specific adverse effects should also be taken into account. This will assist in data evaluation and, where necessary, the initiation of appropriate action.

19. A monitoring and specimen banking program should take into consideration any pre-screening or other data available on new chemicals or other new technological developments.

Table 1

GENERAL CRITERIA FOR
SELECTION OF SPECIES/ENVIRONMENTAL COMPARTMENTS, MONITORING OF POPULATIONS IN THE WILD (NOT LISTED IN ORDER OF PRIORITY)

1. **Food Chain – Trophic Relationships**
    Food web relationships and dynamics
    Diet

2. **Adequate Information Base (biological, physiological, etc.)**

3. **Population Characteristics**
    Abundance
    Distribution (international)
    Habitat
    Longevity (life span allow sampling of more than one year class including some long-
            lived species)
    Population Trend Data
    Population Genetics
    Sensitive Annual Cycles or Life Stages
    Life Table Functions

4. **Physiological Characteristics**
    Should not regulate against uptake
    Turnover rate commensurate with desired integration time-length of measurement
    Not significantly alter ingested pollutants (monitor for biochemical effects)
    Not contain large amounts of tissue elements which interfere with analyses
    Nutritional status
    Accumulation of pollutants without mortality

5. **Evident Importance to the Environment and Man**
        Health Effects
        Economic
        Sociological — Political
        Esthetic (conservation)
        As Food for man or other resource
        Consument of similar pattern as humans

6. **Pharmacokinetics (any pollutant)**
        Metabolism of toxic substances
        Entry, transport, fate, effects

7. **Pollutant — Organism — Ecosystem — Relationships**
        Should continously monitor
        Mobility, action radius, minimum evasion
        Likelihood of exposure

8. **Collection Criteria**
        Costs and maintenance
        Adequate body size
        Abundant
        Easy to collect and to prepare
        Collect in consistent or standard manner
        Easy to sex
        Taxonomic identification easy to do
        Require minimum of dissection and preparation
        Sampling (scale, level of resolution)
        Representativeness

9. **Experimental Tests**
        Dose-response effect relationships
        Suitability for laboratory and field experimentation
        Integration of information with field data

10. **Integration with other National or International Species Usages**

11. **Specimen Bank Objectives as well as Effects Monitoring Objectives**

Table 2

GENERIC CONSIDERATIONS FOR THE SELECTION OF PLANTS, INVERTEBRATE ANIMALS AND VERTEBRATES FOR MONITORING ENVIRONMENTAL MATERIALS AND SPECIMEN BANKING

I   **Perceived Importance to Man and the Environment**
        Health Effects
        Economics
        Sociological
        Political
        Aesthetic — Conservation
        Food for Man

II   **Population Characteristics**
>Abundance
>Distribution
>Trophic Level

III   **Individual Characteristics**
>Ease of Identification
>Well Characterized Taxonomically
>Longevity
>Metabolism and Pollutant Accumulation Characteristics
>Sensitivity to Biological Effects
>Annual Cycle Characteristics — Stage of Life Cycle
>Genetics

IV   **Other Considerations**
>Adequate Information Base
>Logistic and Organizational
>Collection Criteria
>Costs
>Amenability to Experimental Evaluation

Table 3

SPECIFIC CRITERIA FOR THE SELECTION OF PLANT SPECIES FOR MONITORING ENVIRONMENTAL MATERIALS AND SPECIMEN BANKING

I.   ADEQUATE INFORMATION BASE CONCERNING

   A. **Response to specific pollutant insult via previously developed dose-response curves**
    1. Symptomatic response
      a) acute
      b) chronic
    2. Asymptomatic response, i. e., invisible or hidden injury*
      a)   Physiological changes, morphological changes with no measurable yield effects
      b)   Physiological changes that result in yield effects that are measurable

   B. **Response to pollutant combinations via previously developed dose-response curves**
    1. Symptomatic response
      a)   less than additive
      b)   additive
      c)   synergistic
    2. Asymptomatic response, i. e., invisible or hidden injury*
      a)   Physiological changes, morphological changes with no measurable yield effects
      b)   Physiological changes that result in yield effects that are measurable

C. **Ability of the plant species to accumulate the various pollutants to be monitored**
   1. Gaseous form uptake
      a)   Levels of metabolic utilization and ability to identify as external constituent
      b)   Levels of toxicity and ability to idetify in residuals following toxicity
   2. Surface depositions
      a)   migration into plant system
      b)   residuals on surfach
   3. Soil-root uptake interactions and efficiency of subsequent accumulation in plant organs or tissues

II.   FOOD CHAIN – TROPHIC RELATIONSHIPS

III.   POPULATION CHARACTERISTICS

A. **Abundance**

B. **Distribution**
   1. International
   2. National
   3. Regional

C. **Site specifications**

D. **Longevity**
   1. Annuals – genetic stability
   2. Perennials
      a)   woody plants
      b)   overwintering as root or similar organ

E. **Population genetics**

F. **Sensitive annual stages**

IV.   PHYSIOLOGICAL CHARACTERISTICS

A. **Able to express sensitivity and/or accumulate over wind range of environmental limitations including nutritional requirements**

B. **Well understood relationship between pollutant accumulations and mortality**

C. **Mechanism of entry transport, and fate well understood**

D. **Ease in identification**

* Invisible or hidden injury = injury to the organism that results in a reduction of growth or yield without the expression of any other visible symptom.

Table 4

SPECIFIC CRITERIA FOR THE SELECTION OF INVERTE-
BRATE ANIMALS FOR MONITORING ENVIRON-
MENTAL MATERIALS AND SPECIMEN BANKING

I.   System Characteristics
   A. Representative of critical component, functions, and processes
   B. Degree of data extrapolation: laboratory to field, season-to-season, comparability of sites, etc.

II. Population Characteristics
   A. Abundance and expendability
   B. Wide distribution
   C. Population trends
   D. Trophic level
   E. Migration pattern
   F. Life table functions
   G. Population stability monitoring

III. Individual Characteristics
   A. Ease of identification (well defined taxonomy)
   B. Ability to age, class, and sex
   C. Body size
   D. Longevity
   E. Diet and habitat
   F. Accumulation of compounds of interest
   G. Sensitivity to biological effects
   H. Exposure to pollutants
   I. Annual cycle characteristics – stages of the life cycle
   J. Genetics (active-homozygous for exposure)
   K. Intermediary metabolism allows adequate monitoring

IV. Logistical – Organizational – Other
   A. Costs (time, $, personnel) and maintenance
   B. Collecting, preparation, packaging, and transportation in a consistent, standardized manner
   C. Scale and resolution of sampling programme

V.   Adequate Abiotic and Biotic Information Base
   A. Land use, air and water quality data, and climatological data should be available relative to the species
   B. Baseline data on physiology, reproduction, life table information, susceptibility to disease, parasite burdens and pollutant concentrations. Must be able to integrate this information with other monitoring systems. Analysis and evaluation of the combined material is desirable.

Table 5

SPECIFIC CRITERIA FOR SELECTION OF VERTEBRATES FOR MONITORING ENVIRONMENTAL MATERIALS AND SPECIMEN BANKING

	Passive Monitoring		Active Monitoring*		Specimen Banking
	Trend	Effect	Trend	Effect	
I. Population Characteristics					
A. Abundance and expendability	MB	MB			MB
B. Ease of propagation			M	M	
C. Wide distribution	MB	MB			MB
D. Population trends (known or possible to determine)		MB			MB
E. Trophic level	MB	MB	M	M	MB
F. Migration patterns	MB	MB	M	M	MB
G. Life table functions	MB	MB			MB
II. Individual Characteristics					
A. Ease of identification (well-defined taxonomy)	MB	MB	M	M	MB
B. Ability to age-class and sex	MB	MB	M	M	MB
C. Body size	MB		M	M	MB
D. Longevity	MB	MB			MB
E. Diet and habitat	MB	MB	M	M	MB
F. Exposure to pollutants	MB	MB	M	M	MB
G. Metabolism/accumulation of compounds of interest	MB	MB	M	M	MB
H. Sensitivity to biological effects of pollutants		MB		M	
I. Annual cycle characteristics/stage of life cycle	MB	MB	M	M	MB
J. Representative of ecosystem components	MB	MB			MB
K. Genetics	MB	MB	M	M	MB
L. Suitability for laboratory and field experimentation	MB	MB	M	M	MB
III. Logistical/Organization Characteristics					
A. Costs for collection and maintainance	MB	MB	M	M	MB
B. Ease of collecting, preparing, packaging, and transporting in a consistent, standardized manner	MB	MB	M	M	MB
IV. Supplemental Information Base					
A. Baseline data on physiology, reproduction, susceptibility to disease, parasite burdens, pollutant concentrations and dose-effect relationships	MB	MB	M	M	MB
B. Information on other national and international programmes (so they can be integrated)	MB	MB	M	M	MB
C. Land use and climatology data	MB	MB	M	M	MB

*   apparently not feasible to use birds for experimental exposure
M = mammals
B = birds

Table 6

LIST OF PLANT SPECIES DISCUSSED FOR MONITORING ENVIRONMENTAL MATERIALS AND SPECIMEN BANKING IN TERRESTRIAL ECOSYSTEMS

Lichens

Peltigera rufescens
Cladonia rangiformis
Stereocaulon nanodes
Umbilicaria spec.
Lecanora spec.
Hypogymnia physodes
Evernia prunastri
Parmelia furfuracea

Moss

Sphagnum spec.
Hylocomium splendens
Rhytidiadelphus spec.
Bryum argenteum
Hypnum cupressiforme
Tortula muralis
Grimmia pulvinata
Brachythecium rutabulum

Grass culture technique

Lolium multiflorum

Other (higher) plant species

Aesculus hippocastanum
Tilia spec.
Acer spec.
Platanus spec.
Sambucus nigra
Syringia vulgaris
Solidago spec.
Taraxacum spec.
Plantago media
Beta vulgaris
Lactuca sativa
Solanum tuberosum
Brassica oleracea
Spinacia oleracea
Phaseolus vulgaris
Taxus baccata
Picea omorica
Picea abies
Pinus silvestris
Avena spec. (sativa, fatua)
Triticum spec.
Hordeum spec.
Poa annua
Nicotiana tabaccum
Glycine soja
Populus spec.
Larix spec.
Daucus carota

Table 7

PLANT SPECIES RECOMMENDED FOR MONITORING ENVIRONMENTAL MATERIALS AND SPECIMEN BANKING

	SO_x		O_3		F		PAN		NO_x		Heavy Metals	
	Accum.	Symp.	Accum.	Symp.	Accum.	Symp.	Accum.	Symp.	Accum.	Symp.	Accum.	Symp.
Active												
Trend	1-7	1-9	—	1-7	1-5	1-6	—	1-5	—	1-7	1-5	—
Effect	1-7	1-9	—	1-7	1-5	1-6	—	1-5	—	1-7	1-5	—
Passive												
Trend	1-4,7	1-4,7	—	1,5	1,4,5	1,4,5	—	3,4,5	—	1,2,5	1,3,5	—
Effect	1-4,7	1-4,7	—	1,5	1,4,5	1,4,5	—	3,4,5	—	1,2,5	1,3,5	—
Banking	1,2,3,6,7		NA*		1-5		NA*		NA*		1-5	

SO_x	O_3	F	PAN	NO_x	Heavy Metals
1 Lichens**	1 Tobacco	1 Lichens**	1 Alfalfa	1 Larch	1 Pinus
2 Annual Rye-grass	2 Pine	2 Gladiolus	2 Bean	2 Picea	2 Oats
3 Pine	3 Bean	3 Corn	3 Annual Rye-grass	3 Oats	3 Annual Rye-grass
4 Poplar Familiy	4 Oats	4 Poplar Family	4 Dandelion	4 Bean	4 Poa
5 Bean	5 Grape	5 Pine	5 Pinus	5 Sunflower	5 Lichens**
6 Alfalfa	6 Radish	6 Apricot		6 Radish	
7 Moss	7 Tomato			7 Soybean	
8 Radish					
9 Soybean					

*   NA = not applicable; Symptoms record, photographs only

**   species by source/region/area etc., (native vs. exotic)

Table 8

LIST OF INVERTEBRATE ANIMALS DISCUSSED FOR MONITORING ENVIRONMENTAL MATERIALS AND SPECIMEN BANKING IN TERRESTRIAL ECOSYSTEMS

Oligochaeta

Collembola

Nematoda

Carabidea   Abax ater
Carabus coriaceus
Carabus auratus
Pterostichus vulgaris

Saltatoria   Chorthippus bruneus

Julidae   Schizophyllum sabulosum

Gastropoda   Cepaea hortensis
Cepaea nemoralis

Coleoptera   Galeruca tanaceti
Agelastica alni
Melolontha melolontha
Leptimotarsa docemlin.

Lepidoptera   Melanargia galathea
Pararge aegeria
Brenthis ino
Biston betularia

Hymenoptera   Apis mellifica

Table 9

INVERTEBRATE SPECIES RECOMMENDED FOR MONITO-
RING ENVIRONMENTAL MATERIALS AND
SPECIMEN BANKING

Criteria Species	System Characteristics	Population Characteristics	Individual Characteristics	Logistical Organization	Adequate Information Base	Effects, Trends, Banks	Active / Passive	Summation
Pollinators a) Managed Honeybees	3	3	3	3	3	3	3	21
b) Native Bees, Flies Beetles	2	2	1	2	2	2	2	13
Pest Population Regulation a) Carabids	3	3	3	3	2	3	1	18
b) Spiders	3	3	2	2	1	2	1	14
Detritus Processors a) Drosophila	1	2	2	2	1	1	2	11
b) Earth Worm	3	3	2	3	3	3	3	20
c) Isopods/Millipedes	3	2	2	2	2	2	2	15
d) Ants (mount)	2	3	2	3	2	1	1	14

1 = poor
2 = adequate
3 = very good

Table 10

LIST OF CRITERIA FOR SELECTION OF SPECIMENS FOR MONITORING ENVIRONMENTAL MATERIALS AND SPECIMEN BANKING IN AQUATIC ECOSYSTEMS (NOT LISTED IN ORDER OF PRIORITY)

1. Importance to man
2. Position of the species in the food chain
3. Abundance
4. Distribution
5. Collection costs and maintenance
6. Availability
7. Mobility and action radius
8. Habitat
9. Physiology
10. Accumulation of pollutant without mortality
11. Should be sedentary in order to show levels of pollutants representative of the area under study
12. Longevity (life span should allow sampling of more than one year class)
13. Adequace of size
14. Hardy enough to survive laboratory bioassay
15. Be able to tolerate brackish water
16. Should not regulate against uptake of the pollutant
17. Should have a turnover rate commensurate with the desired integration time-length of measurement
18. Should continously monitor
19. Not significantly alter ingested pollutant to form not attibutable to original pollutants
20. Not contain large amounts of tissue elements which interfere with the analyses
21. Require minimum of dissection and other preparation for analyses
22. Remain within a limited geographic range during the period of monitoring
23. Not ingest amounts of sediments sufficient to invalidate measurement of pollutants in water
24. Be easy to collect (e. g. without boat or special equipment)
25. Be easy to prepare for shipment to analytical laboratories with minimum of contamination for handling
26. Should be collected in consistent or standard manner
27. Sex of individual specimens
28. Ideally should have a previous history of use in field monitoring and in laboratory response studies.

Table 11

LIST·OF BIOLOGICAL SPECIMENS DISCUSSED FOR MONITORING ENVIRONMENTAL MATERIALS AND SPECIMEN BANKING IN AQUATIC ECOSYSTEMS

Macroalgae

brown algae	Fucus serratus

Bivalve Molluscs

blue mussel	Mytilus edulis
cong. mussel	Mytilus californianus
oyster	Ostrea equistris
oyster	Crassostrea virginica
freshw. mussel	Dreissena polymorpha
surf clam	Spisula solidissima
ocean quahog	Arctica islandica

Fish

grey mullet	Mugil cephalus
deepsea bathyal	Antimora rostrata
carp	Cyprinus carpio
buttfish	Pleuronectes spec.
jap. ricefish	Orizias latipes
salmon	Salmo gairdneri
pike	Esox lucius
dogfish	Squalus acanthius

Table 12

LIST OF BIRDS DISCUSSED FOR MONITORING ENVIRON-
MENTAL MATERIALS AND SPECIMEN BANKING

starling	Sturnus vulgaris
ducks	Anas platyrhynochos
	Anas rubripes
bald eagles	Haliaeetus leucucephalus
cormorant	Phalacrocorax carbo
little tern	Sterna albifrons
oyster catcher	Haematopus ostralegus
peregrine	Falco peregrinus
buzzard	Buteo buteo
raven	Corvus corax
herring gull	Larus argentatus
robin	Turdud migratorius
mourning dove	Zenaidura macroura
house sparrow	Passer domesticus
rock dove	Columba livia

Table 13

LIST OF MAMMALIAN SPECIES DISCUSSED FOR MONITO-
RING ENVIRONMENTAL MATERIALS AND SPECIMEN BAN-
KING IN TERRESTRIAL ECOSYSTEMS

house mouse	Mus musculus
deer mouse group	Peromyscus spec.
rat group	Rattus rattus
	Rattus norwegicus
muskrat	Ondatra zibethica
cottontail rabbit	Sylvilagus spec.
striped skunk	Mephitis mephitis
deer group	Odocoileus spec.
big brown bat	Eptesicus fuscus
red fox	Vulpes vulpes
pine vole	Pitymys spec.
prairie vole	Microtus spec.
common shrew	Sorex araneus
pygmy shrew	Sorex minutus
whitetoothed shr.	Crocidura russula

Table 14

DISSECTION OF VERTEBRATE ANIMALS

If organisms are small, the whole body should be preserved. If large, the organs known to be useful for residue analysis and/or which it is believed will be useful in the future, could be stored; these are listed in the table below (B = bird, M = mammal).

Tissues	Vertebrate Group	Specific Regions or Parts to be banked
Gonads (Testes/ovary)	MB	
Thyroid	MB	
Adrenal gland	MB	
Bone	MB	left
Tooth	M	tibia
Lens	M	first molar
Adipose tissue	MB	left
Blood	MB	renal fat capsule
Hair	M	minimum of 100 ml
		clippings from middorsum, between scapulae
Feathers	B	primary and secondary wing feathers
Brain	M	left half of midsagittally sectioned brain
Kidney	MB	
Liver	MB	left median globe, min. of 100 g
Lung	MB	transverse slab left lung
Muscle (skeletal)	MB	left thigh, minimum of 100 g
Spleen	MB	distal half, minimum of 100g
Thymus	B	
Bursa fabricii	B	

Table 15

LIST OF CHEMICAL POLLUTANT CATEGORIES RANKED AC-
CORDING HIGH-PRIORITY FOR CONSIDERATION IN AN
ENVIRONMENTAL MONITORING PROGRAMME:

A.   **Aliphatic and Alicyclic Compounds**
    a) Haloalkanes, Haloalkenes
    b) Carboxylic Acids, Anhydrides, Ketones, Peroxides and Salts
    c) Haloethers
    d) Haloketones
    e) Esters and Lactones

B.   **Aromatic Compounds**
    a) Polycyclic Aromatic Hydrocarbons (PAH)
    b) Aromatic Nitrogen Compounds (Amines)
    c) Aromatic Compounds with Aliphatic Side Chains
    d) Halophenols and related Compounds
    e) Nitrophenols

C.   **Heterocyclic Compounds**

D.   **Inorganic Substances and Organometallic Compounds**

I. INTRODUCTION

I. 1. TERMINOLOGY AND DEFINITIONS

The terms used in this report take careful account of the terminology and definitions accepted and used on a worldwide scale. Nevertheless it was found necessary to adopt a few specific terms and definitions.

The following terms with their definitions are used in the present report and were used during the International Workshop on Monitoring Environmental Materials and Specimen Banking.

Ecosystem

An ecosystem is an adaptive subsystem of the biosphere, composed of both abiotic and biotic elements and characterized by the possibility of self-regulation; they include terrestrial, freshwater marine and urban ecosystems.

Area System

An area system refers to areas of distribution of a population, in some cases extending over various ecosystems.

Chemical Pollutant

A chemical pollutant is a chemical substance (inorganic or organic) inserted in ecosystems which cause adverse effects, e. g. disturbance, damage or even fatality to the system or for single elements of it. The same chemical could have also beneficial effects in other circumstances. Physical agents, e. g. heat, are considered only insofar here as they modify the effect of chemical pollutants. Chemical pollutants are frequently anthropogenic but sometimes are also natural, or both.

Environmental Materials

Environmental materials include any specimens or other samples representative of an ecosystem. This document deals mainly with biological specimens.

Indicator Specimen

An indicator specimen is that which is representative of the state of an ecosystem or compartments of an ecosystem, as regards accumulation or other effects.

Monitoring

The systematic determination of pollutant levels and/or effects in environmental materials as a function of time and space. From the ecological point of view ‚active‘ and ‚passive‘ monitoring may be distinguished: ‚active monitoring‘ relates to the determination of field conditions by means of the exposure of laboratory cultured organisms to these conditions.
‚Passive monitoring‘ relates to the determination of field conditions by means of the exposure of wild living organisms.

Specimen Banking

The systematic collection and storage of samples with minimal changes for deferred examination (analysis or other evaluation). The examination is generally deferred for a period of years, or even decades, following collection, so that samples can then be studied in relation to newer knowledge, including improved methods.

Effects

Any measurable changes which results from exposure to pollutants. In the present report an effect is termed ,adverse' if there is any impairment of functional capacity, such as a decrease in ability to compensate for additional influences, or a decrease in ability to maintain equilibrium, or an increase in susceptibility to other environmental influences.

I. 2. OBJECTIVES OF THE WORKSHOP AND THE FINAL DOCUMENT

Ever since the industrial revolution, man has been subjecting the Earth's biosphere to an increasing variety of chemical insults. Some, such as naturally occurring toxic elements and compounds, have reentered the environment through industrial processes at rates much greater than those of natural degradation of removal from the biosphere; other hazardous pollutants with molecular structures never before encountered by living organisms may be synthesized. In most industrialized nations, environmental problems associated with these pollutants were initially conceived as disturbing but unavoidable penalties of a rapidly expanding economy and technologically advanced society. However in the last decade, increasing attention, has been focused on the occurrence and effects of pollutants in the environment. Refinements in analytical techniques have resulted in the discovery that many substances are more widely distributed than previously reported. Serious accidents which have involved exposure to acutely toxic materials have resulted in a public demand for more effective governmental control and industrial mitigation. Furthermore, recent toxicological research has increased public awareness of the subtle, chronic effects of many common chemical substances which are routinely released into the environment. A list of all substances which are at present regarded as environmentally hazardous might contain thousands of compounds; and new compounds are still being added. In order to adequately ensure the protection of human health and the environment from the often subtle effects of these materials, several major actions are required.
These include toxicological research, the development of control technology, regulatory guidelines and standards promulgation, and monitoring of environmental materials and specimen banking. This is extremely important because without effective monitoring of environmental materials and specimen banking, the detection of serious environmental contamination from pollutants may occur only after critical damage has been done.

The objectives of this workshop are to:

— assess types of pollutants for which monitoring environmental materials and specimen banking is of importance and utility;

— assess types of environmental materials best amenable for monitoring environmental materials and specimen banking;

- examine the technical feasibility of such programmes and draw up recommendations for their implementations;

- draw up recommendations regarding further research and development requirements.

The objectives for the final report are to identify:

- the reasons for monitoring environmental materials and specimen banking;

- a practical framework, including cost estimation, for monitoring environmental materials and specimen banking;

- the state-of-the-art of monitoring environmental materials and specimen banking;

- ethical and legal considerations on monitoring environmental materials and specimen banking;

- recommendations regarding further research and development requirements.

It is expected, that the International Workshop and the final document will provide the governments with considerable information.

I. 3. MONITORING ENVIRONMENTAL MATERIALS

Systematic sampling and prompt analysis of environmental materials can help greatly in understanding the relationships of exposure to pollution and environmental hazards. It is envisaged that ‚**Monitoring Environmental Materials**' might jointly contribute:

- information regarding the integrated past and recent exposure of ecosystems or part of the ecosystem to certain pollutants. This information is important for the determination of trends of pollutant levels in environmental materials, for the development of adequate criteria (dose-effect relationships) and for the definition of quality guides, objectives and standards for pollutants;

- to an evaluation of the effectiveness of existing guides, standards and control measures on changing pollutant burdens;

- detection of populations at risk before serious effects occur;

- determining the presence and extend of hazards from environmental exposure to pollutants;

- correlating levels of pollutants in the environment with sources of contamination;

- building-up of a data bank with comparable results;

- for establishing priorities as regards research.

I. 4. SPECIMEN BANKING

‚**Specimen banking**' means the systematic collection and storage with minimal alterations of samples for deferred examination, analysis and evaluation; these activities will usually be deferred for a period of years of decades following collection, permitting reinvestigation of materials from the past using newer techniques which are not at present available. A combination of monitoring and banking programmes may be often possible.

It is envisaged that ‚Specimen Banking' might jointly contribute to the same objections as stated in section I. 3. – ‚Monitoring Environmental Materials'. Regarding ‚**Specimen Banking**' specifically:

— analysis of stored specimens may facilitate the determination of base-line trends and potential hazards of new and previously unrecognized exposures to different substances in the environment;

— analysis of stored specimens for substances just recognized as pollutants and therefore previously not determined;

— retrospective analysis may contribute to knowledge of relationships between chemicals and effects including possible antagonistic or synergistic effects;

— retrospective dose estimates for chronic disturbances, damages or other adverse effects with long latent periods;

— analysis may be deferred until better information becomes available regarding the most appropriate materials to analyse for specific chemicals;

— analysis may be deferred until analytical methods or better methods become available;

— subsequent analysis comparison with previous analytical data. Chemical analytical and sampling techniques are continuously improving with more sensitive methods, improved instrumentation and better quality control.

II. SELECTION OF POLLUTANTS AND POLLUTANT CATEGORIES OF INTEREST FOR MONITORING ENVIRONMENTAL MATERIALS

A chemical pollutant is a chemical substance (inorganic or organic) inserted in ecosystems which cause adverse effects, e. g. disturbance, damage or even fatality to the system or for single elements of it. The same chemical could have also beneficial effects in other circumstances. Physical agents, e. g. heat, are considered only insofar here as they modify the effect of chemical pollutants. Chemical pollutants are frequently anthropogenic but sometimes are also natural, or both.

During the International Workshop held 1977 in Luxembourg the environmental pollutants were categorized in the following three broad classifications:

a)   Inorganic substances (including organometallic compounds)
b)   Organo-halogenated compounds
c)   Other organic compounds.

For the purpose of detailed discussions during the International Workshop and regarding present and potential environmental pollutants these categories have been further subdivided as follows (not listed in priority):

a)   **inorganic substances**

As, Be, Cd, Co, Cr, F, Hg, Mo, Mn, Ni, Pb, Pd, Se, Sn, Tl, V, Zn,
Methyl-Hg, other organo-metallic compounds (Pb, Sn)

b)   **organo-halogenated compounds**

organochlorine pesticides (incl. phenoxy herbicides and halogenated phenols) and metabolites
polychlorinated and polybrominated biphenyls and metabolites
halogenated dioxins and related compounds
halogenated solvents
propellants (esp. fluorinated)

c)   **other organic compounds**

aliphatic and aromatic hydrocarbons (incl. substituted)
polycyclic hydrocarbons
aliphatic and aromatic amino- and nitro-derivatives
nitroso-compounds
alcohols, glycols, ethers, ketones, aldehydes, acids and amides
phenols and derivatives
organo phosphorus esters
phthalate esters
mycotoxins and antibiotics
anabolic and hormonal substances
plastic monomers.

The focus of interest in Monitoring Environmental Materials relates primarily to chemical pollutants effecting important biological processes, species and ecosystems related to the ,welfare' of man. Explicitly to be excluded are direct human health considerations and traditional ,non-chemical' pollutants including radionuclides. It is, however, important that a protocol for monitoring environmental pollution provides sufficient flexibility to include any new pollutant groupings or other specific categories as may be required in the future. But the intensive consideration of radionuclides in other national and international programmes is reason for initial exclusion.

Pollutants can be categorized by a systematic ranking regarding

    a)   their chemical and/or physical properties
    b)   the ecological and/or ecophysiological relevance
    c)   the biological and/or toxicological efficacy.

It is widely accepted that prioritization criteria for pollutants must include the following factors ,variously weighed or arrayed'

    (1) toxicity
    (2) persistence
    (3) movement
    (4) bioaccumulation
    (5) degradation
    (6) transformation
        (,toxification')
    (7) pollutant sources and distribution

The major concern in developing a systematic approach is the need to accomodate, as yet, unknown pollutants which may be identified in the future. It is also essential that consideration be given to metabolites and other degradation products of ,primary' pollutants which will be initially addressed.

One approach to narrowing the very broad concept of ,toxicology' is to make the distinction between toxic and hazardous pollutants. In this context **toxic** refers to any in all living material whereas **hazardous** pollutants by definition have a direct bearing on human health or welfare.

During this International Workshop on Monitoring Environmental Materials and Specimen Banking it was suggested and considered to develop a more detailed categorization of organic compounds and to establish a list of high-priority categories and substances as candidates for inclusion in an environmental monitoring programme. It was suggested and considered practical to rely heavily on the Mitre-Corporation Report entitled ,Base line plan for design of a hazardous substance monitoring programme'.

The development of categories for organic compounds was based on functional groups; the arrangement of organic compounds by functional groups is a valid approach, because, due to common structural features, compounds within a category will display marked similarities in their solubilities, chemical reactivities and biological manifestations. The following table contains a list of all organic categories developed in the a. m. study.

Table 1 Categories of Organic Compounds

1. Aliphatic and Alicyclic Compounds

    A. Alkanes
    B. Alkenes
    C. Alkynes
    D. Alcolhols and Glycols
    E. Ethers
    F. Aldehydes
    G. Ketones
    H. Carboxylic Acids, Anhydrides, Ketenes, Peroxides and Salts
    I. Esters and Lactones
    J. Epoxides
    K. Aliphatic and Alicyclic Halogen Compounds
       1. Haloalkanes, Haloalkenes, and Haloalkynes
       2. Haloalcohols and Haloglycols
       3. Haloethers
       4. Haloaldehydes
       5. Haloketones
       6. Halocarboxylic Acids, Haloanhydrides, Halosalts and Haloacidhalides
       7. Haloesters
       8. Haloamines
       9. Haloamides
       10. Haloepoxides
       11. Halothio Compounds
       12. Halonitriles
    L. Aliphatic Nitrogen Compounds
       1. Amines and Hydroxylamines
       2. Amides, Imides, Hydrazides, Hydrazines and Hydrazones
       3. Nitriles, Oximes and Lactams
       4. Azo Compounds
       5. Nitrosamines
       6. Ureas
       7. Imines
       8. Nitro Compounds
       9. Carbamates (Urethanes)
    M. Aliphatic Sulfur Compounds
       1. Thiols (Mercaptans) and Sulfides
       2. Thiocarbonyls, Thioamides and Thioimides
       3. Sulfones, Sulfoxides, Sulfonic Acids and Sulfenes
       4. Sulfenamides
       5. Dithiocarbamates, Thiocarbamates and Salts

2. Aromatic Compounds

    A. Hydrocarbons
       1. Monocyclic
       2. Polycyclic
    B. Phenols
    C. Esters
    D. Aldehydes
    E. Ketones
    F. Carboxylic Acids, Anhydrides, Peroxides, and Salts
    G. Ethers
    H. Aromatic Halogen Compounds
       1. Ring Halocompounds
       2. Side Chain Halocompounds
       3. Halophenols and Related Compounds
       4. Haloaldehydes
       5. Halocarboxylic Acids, Haloanhydrides, Halosalts and Haloacidhalides
       6. Haloethers

      7. Haloketones
      8. Haloamines
      9. Halonitro Compounds
     10. Halonitriles

I.   Aromatic Nitrogen Compounds
      1. Amines
      2. Anilides, Imides, Hydrazides and Amides
      3. Nitriles and Oximes
      4. Azo Compounds
      5. Nitrosamines
      6. Nitro and Nitroso Compounds
      7. Carbamates
      8. Ureas
      9. Imines
     10. Nitrophenols
     11. Isocyanates

J.   Aromatic Sulfur Compounds
      1. Thiols and Sulfides
      2. Thiocarbamates
      3. Sulfones, Sulfoxides, Sulfonic Acids and Salts
      4. Sulfenamides

K.   Aromatic Compounds with Aliphatic Side Chains

3. Heterocyclic Compounds

A.   Heterocyclic Nitrogen Compounds
      1. Unsym./Sym./Triazines, Diazines and Related Compounds
      2. Pyridines, Piperidines, Piperazines and Acridines
      3. Pyrroles and Pyrrolidines
      4. Indoles
      5. Quinolines
      6. Imidazoles
      7. Benzothiazoles
      8. Morpholines
      9. Aziridines
     10. Azafluorenes
     11. Carbazoles
     12. Salts
     13. Nitrogen and Halogen

B.   Heterocyclic Oxygen Compounds
      1. Furans
      2. Morpholines
      3. Xanthenes
      4. Dioxanes

C.   Heterocyclic Sulfur Compounds
      1. Thiophenes
      2. Benzothiazoles
      3. Imidazoles

4. Organophosphorus Compounds

A.   Phosphates and Related Compounds
B.   Phosphonates and Related Compounds
C.   Phosphines and Related Compounds
D.   Phosphorus – Halogen Compounds
E.   Oxyazaphosphorines
F.   Phosphine Oxides
G.   Phosphorus – Nitrogen Compounds
H.   Phosphorus – Sulfur Compounds

5. Organometallic Compounds

After the chemical categories were defined, several lists of potentially hazardous materials were selected and than sorted into the a. m. categories; a total of 702 compounds were sorted in this manner. The following lists were integrated in the a. m. report:

a) Hazardous Substances List
U. S. EPA, 1975 (306 substances)

b) Toxic Pollutants in Point Source Water Effluent Discharge
List of 120 chemicals and categories from Section 307 (a) under the Federal Water Pollution Control Act.

c) Scoring of Organic Air Compounds, June 1976 MITRE, MTR - 6248
List of 337 chemicals and categories.

d) Final Report of NSF Workshop Panel to Select Organic Compounds Hazardous to the Environment, April 1975
List of 80 chemicals and categories.

e) Potential Industrial Carcinogens and Mutagens
List of 88 chemicals compiled by the National Center for Toxicological Research.

f) Occupational Carcinogens for Potential Regulatory Action
List of 116 chemicals and categories.

g) Chemicals Tested or Scheduled for Testing at the Fish-Pesticide Research Laboratory, Department of Interior
List consists of 174 toxic chemicals.

h) Substances with Chronic Effects other than Mutagenicity, Carcinogenicity, or Teratogenicity; A Subfile of the NIOSH Registry.
Criteria Documents prepared or Planned by NIOSH, February 24, 1977
List of 127 chemicals and categories.

i) Suspected Carcinogens; A Subfile of the NIOSH Registry
List of 1.900 chemicals and categories.

j) Suspected Mutagens; A Subfile of the NIOSH Registry
List of approximately 100 chemicals and categories.

k) The Ecological Impact of Synthetic Organic Compounds on Estuarine Ecosystems, September 1976, EPA-600/3-76-075
List of 9 chemicals.

l) Threshold Limit Values for Chemical Substances and Physical Agents in the Workroom Environment with Intended Changes for 1976, American Conference of Government Industrial Hygienists
List of approximately 570 chemicals and categories.

m) National Occupational Hazard Survey (1972 - 1974)
List of the top 500 hazards.

n) Chemicals Being Tested for Carcinogenicity by the Bioassay Program, DCCP, National Cancer Institute 1977
List of 372 chemicals.

o) EPA/Office of Toxic Substances List of Priority Toxic Chemicals, 1977
List of 162 chemicals.

p)   A Study of Industrial Data on Candidate Chemicals for Testing, EPA contract 86-01-4109, November 1976
     List of 650 chemicals and categories.

q)   General List of Problem Substances, Environmental Contaminants Committee, Ottawa, Ontario, Canada, 1977
     List of 160 chemicals and categories.

r)   Preliminary List U. S. Toxic Substances Control Act (TSCA)
     330 chemicals and chemical categories.

s)   Multimedia Environmental Goals (MEG) list U. S. EPA
     620 compounds and chemical categories.

After the chemical categories were defined, the a. m. list of potentially hazardous materials were selected and integrated, a list of high-priority categories and substances as candidates for inclusion in an environmental monitoring programme was established.
Of the categories into which the chemical compounds were organized, thirteen were identified as preliminary candidates for a monitoring programme. The methodology used considered bioaccumulation, environmental persistence and chronic toxicity (incl. mutagenicity, teratogenicity, carcinogenicity etc.) as equally important criteria, and acute toxicity as being less important.

The following chemical categories were ranked according to high-priority for consideration in a monitoring programme:

A)   Aliphatic and Alicyclic Compounds

     1 K 1   Haloalkanes, Haloalkenes
     1 K 10 Carboxylic Acid, Anhydrides, Ketones, Peroxides and Salts
     1 K 3   Haloethers
     1 K 5   Haloketones
     1 I   Esters and Lactones

B)   Aromatic Compounds

     2 H 3   Halophenols and related Compounds
     2 I 10 Nitrophenols
     2 K   Aromatic Compounds with Aliphatic Side Chains
     2 I 1   Aromatic Nitrogen Compounds (Amines)
     2 A 2   Polycyclic Aromatic Hydrocarbons (PAH)

C)   Organometallic Compounds

D)   Heterocyclic Compounds

     3 A 9   Azaridines

E)   Inorganic Substances (including organo-metallic compounds)

III. SELECTION OF ENVIRONMENTAL MATERIALS RELATED TO ECOSYSTEMS AND POLLUTANTS OR POLLUTANT CATEGORIES

III. 1. GENERAL ASPECTS

The scientific, technical and logistical problems, associated with development of an international monitoring programme of biological sampling and specimen banking are generally recognized as being exceedingly profound and complex. The systems ecologists, the toxicologists, the physiologists, the pathologists, molecular biologists, analytical chemists and other participating scientific disciplines all have differing perspectives to bring to bear. Thus, the essential multidisciplinary nature of environmental monitoring and specimen banking will require maximum understanding, considerable forbearance and some compromise among contributing disciplines.

The objectives of any valid and useful large scale monitoring network should include the identification of temporal and geographic trends in the distribution of pollutants, as well as their potential effects upon man, his resources and the environment. Both ,active' or ,experimental' (i. e., experimental or controlled exposures) and ,passive' or ,field' (i. e., observations and measurements under field conditions) monitoring programs are thus required. These methods, wisely employed, can help mankind avoid adverse and possibly irreversible impacts from toxic chemicals and other hazardous pollutants.

However, it must be considered, that a great number of substances, which will be immediately metabolized in organisms, cannot be recorded or at least only with difficulty with such an ecological monitoring program.

Long term data sets are necessary for determining the anthropogenic contribution to observed environmental changes over broad geographical areas. Furthermore, an ecologically oriented framework for monitoring is required, especially in the passive sampling mode, so that information concerning community structure and function can be used in the interpretation of data obtained through the observation and measurement of ,indicator species'.
Finally, the implementation of a national or international environmental monitoring network will require a substantial level of effort in terms of both money and manpower. To be cost effective, such a program will need careful consideration at all levels of planning and review, and an equally well-planned system of quality assurance.

III. 2. REVIEW OF PAST AND CURRENT PROGRAMMES

III. 2. 1. Terrestrial Ecosystem

An important step toward the establishment of a global monitoring system is the national screening analyses of chlorinated hydrocarbons or heavy metals in starlings, ducks, woodcocks, predatory birds and other terrestrial as well as aquatic species carried out in different regions of the U. S. A.
Another promising attempt in achieving international biological monitoring was performed in the years 1966 to 1976 by member nations of the OECD, regarding mainly aquatic but also some terrestrial wildliving species as in indicators for the contamination level of organochlorine pesticides

(OCP) and mercury. The main objective of the study was to establish the levels of pesticide contamination in selected species, sampled at prearranged times in a prescribed manner in areas believed to be free of pesticide contamination arising from any local usage of OCP. The earlier study in 1966/1967 had demonstrated the occurence of certain types of pesticide residues in several species of wildlife in areas where pesticide usage was unknown, but no attempt was made to compare the analytical abilities of the laboratories involved. The second study thus included a program of analysis of different types of samples exchanged among the participating laboratories. The results indicate the degree of background contamination of the environment, as exemplified by the species selected, which were the starling, pike, marine mussel, and dogfish. The range of variation of residues among individuals of a natural population is much larger than that due to analytical error or to differences among laboratories.

The third OECD stude (1969 - 71) included analysis for OCP polychlorinated biphenyls and mercury; appropriate exchange samples were circulated. The wildlife samples, both freshwater and marine, included fish and fish-eating birds. Whereas the second study had been confined to areas believed to be uncontaminated by direct application or disposal of pesticides, study evaluated both uncontaminated and contaminated areas in order to establish differences, if any, in contamination levels. Measurements of eggshell thickness of certain species of birds also made in an attempt to correlate these with organochlorine residue levels. In all, 26 laboratories in 12 countries took part in this third study.

In discussions between members of a U. S. working group and representatives of the Federal Republic of Germany it became apparent that these two countries have historically approached the subject of environmental monitoring from two very different perspectives but that recently there has been a convergence of thinking which may provide for a very useful combination. In Germany there appears to have been a concentration upon monitoring for increased body burdens of specific industrial source materials and their effects upon particular species; basically an autecological approach (cf. Schönbeck, H. and H. van Haut 1971: Measurement of Air pollutants by means of vegetation. Bioindicators of landscape deterioration, Prague, 30 - 38.

Guderian, R. 1977: Air Pollution. Phytotoxicity of Acidic Gases and its Signifiance in Air Pollution Control. Springer, Heidelberg.

Steubing, L. 1979: Monitoring aerial inorganic pollutants by plant indicator specimens. Int. Workshop on Monitoring Environmental Materials and Specimen Banking, in press.

Müller, P. 1978: Urbane Ökosysteme. Forschung im Bereich Umweltgrundsatzangelegenheiten. Bundesministerium des Innern, pp. 303, Bonn).

In the United States there seems to have been a greater emphasis on monitoring for natural trends in both abiotic and biotic parameters and their implications to ecosystem structure and function with concern about man's influence more or less appended to the whole. Now we detect a sudden convergence of thinking by both Germans (cf. Ellenberg, H., Fränzle, O. and Müller, P. 1978: Oekosystemforschung im Hinblick auf Umweltpolitik und Entwicklungsplanung. Bundesministerium des Innern, pp. 143, Bonn.

Drescher-Kaden, U. 1979: Advantages and problems of using wildliving animal species as indicators for environmental pollution, Int. Workshop on Monitoring Environmental Materials and Specimen Banking. In press) and Americans (Botkin, D. et al. 1978: A Pilot Program for Long-Term observation and Study of Ecosystems in the United States. In Report of a Second Conference on Long-Term Ecological Measurements sponsored by the National Science Foundation) in which there is a perceived need for carefully managed national and international monitoring networks, organized within an ecosystematic framework to investigate both long term trends in natural ecological processes and the deviations from these trends as influenced by human activities.

Consequently, our efforts have been directed toward the establishment of criteria for the selection of ecological components to be monitored within an **ecosystematic** framework. This ecosystematic framework provides a context for the interpretation of both anthropogenic and natural trends in hazardous residuals and biological disturbances.

Although an international monitoring network was a major consideration in the development of criteria, the actual selection of organisms often focussed upon North American species with similar European ecological equivalents.

III. 2. 2.   Aquatic Ecosystem

Prior to 1965 there were no comprehensive formal monitoring programmes for contaminants in aquatic ecosystems. Nevertheless numerous individual studies before and since that date have contributed greatly to our understanding of relationships between ecosystems, pollutants and biological system.

Macroalgae — Fucus serratus — is the only macroalga that is currently being used as a biological monitor of sorts. A single large collection was made in 1971. The alga is processed and samples are distributed internationally as a basis for intercalibrating methods of paricipating laboratories using radionuclides as the naturally-induced contaminant of interest. This programme is succesful. The use of this biological group is urged for consideration in the future specimen banking.

Bivalve (Marine) Molluscs — Bivalve molluscs are employed biological monitors in a formal nationwide (U. S.) programme sponsored by the U. S. Environmental Protection Agency. The programme was initiated in 1976. **Mytilus edulis,** the blue mussel; **M. californianus,** a congeneric species of Mytilus; and the oysters, **Ostrea equistris** and **Crassostrea virginica** were chosen as biological monitors or ‚sentinal‘ organisms. This monitoring programme is called ‚Mussel Watch‘.

Each of one hundred and seven coastal stations in the U. S. A. are sampled annually for 25 kilograms of animals. Tissues are analyzed for residues of chlorinated and petroleum hydrocarbons, heavy metals and transuranics. Representative samples from each site are examined histopathologically.

Results to date indicate areas of heavy concentration of chlorinated hydrocarbons; but no apparent differences in heavy metal levels between stations located on the open coastline. However, latitudinal differences in heavy metal residues analyzed in the surf clam, **Spisula solidisima,** and the ocean quahog, **Arctica islandica** have been described. Lower levels were found in specimens from the more southern portions of their ranges. Both animals are marine bivalve species which are found offshore. Higher levels in the more northerly specimens is related to heavy metals emanating from the highly polluted Hudson River. Oysters from the upper reaches of an estuary in Long Island Sound were found to have significantly higher levels of cadmium, silver, copper, zinc, nickel and manganese than other samples. Other workers have reported similar metal elevations in bivalve molluscs as from upper estuarine areas that coincide with high population centers and concentrations of industrial activity. The use of the bivalve molluscs has proven to be very effective to date.

Fish — Freshwater — There are now 117 sampling stations which comprise a part of the National Pesticide Monitoring Programme approximately half of these are sampled in alternate years. This programme was initiated in 1964 to monitor levels and trends of selected environmental contaminants. The initial programme appeared to be limited to pesticides using three species of fish collected from 50 stations.

By 1970 residue analyses was extended to include polychlorinated biphenyls as well as organochlorine insecticides and the number of stations was expanded to 100.

Mercury was included in residue analysis during 1969 through 1973. Lead, arsenic, selenium, and cadmium were added to the analytical list from 1971 through 1973. Metal analyses were apparently dropped from the programme after 1973, and current emphasis appears to be focused on pesticides.

Fish — Marine — It was identified a series of references to residue analyses conducted on finfish within NOAA. However, these references encompass a series of discrete studies and investigations. Emphasis in the abovenoted works appears to have been placed on a survey of metal levels in tissue residues from fish collected from different trophic levels (apex predators, herbivorous forms, and fish intermediate within the food chain) as well as geographic areas to approach the general question of whether or not heavy metals are a ,problem' in finfish. The answer based on these efforts appears to be ,no'; heavy metals do not appear to be a general problem in finfish.

There appears to have been no formal programme, using a single or limited number of finfish, collected systematically over time from a geographically comprehensive series of established stations for purposes of biological monitoring carried out in the marine environment. The use of finfish for biological trend monitoring in the sense of the work reported for freshwater fish remains to be seriously addressed in the marine environment.

Work on the coastal finfish, grey mullet (**Mugil cephalus L.**) indicates that the species holds promise as for use as a biological monitor. It has been shown experimentally concentrate pesticides such as methoxychlor and mirex. It is ubiquitous between the latitudes of 42° N and 42° S. It feeds at the sediment/water interface on detrital particles and ingests some sediments. Some pollutants are concentrated in sediments and organic debris (detritus).

The potential of deep sea organisms for future use as biological monitors for some pollutants was discussed. However, no systematic monitoring effort that employs deep sea forms for trend monitoring has been or is underway.

However, analyses of a series of deep sea bathyal fish, including **Antimora rostrata**, detected the presence of dieldrin, DDD, DDT, and aldrin, however endrin, heptachlor, heptachlor epoxide, lindane and mirex were below the level of detection. It was suggested that **A. rostrata** may serve as a baseline for future monitoring of those organochlorines that were below the level of detection in the analyses referred to above. Another observation, is that **A. rostrata**, the bathyal demersal fish, was found to have an order of magnitude greater residue of DDT in livers than was detected in various epipelagic oceanic fishes.

A series of discrete analyses indicates that heavy metals are not noticeably high in any tissue residues from most truly deep oceanic fish species.

Birds — There is a report on a current monitoring programme for residues of persistent compounds in ducks, the mallard **(Anas platyrynchos)** and the black duck **(A. rubripes)** which together are found throughout the contiguous U. S.

Two hundred and thirty-five samples are collected once every third year. The programme was initiated in 1965 and has continued since that date. Samples are analyzed for organochlorines and heavy metals.

Summary of past and present programmes:

Prior to 1965 there were no formal monitoring programmes for contaminants in aquatic ecosystems that were comprehensive in either time or space.
Prior to and since that date there have been numerous individual studies that have contributed greatly to our understanding of relationships between ecosystems, pollutants and biological systems.
In the United States of America there are currently two formal monitoring programmes reported for aquatic ecosystems: the National Pesticide Monitoring Program, U. S. Fish and Wildlife Service; and the ‚Mussel Watch Program‘ sponsored by the U. S. Environmental Protection Agency. The former uses freshwater finfish and water fowl as biological monitors for persistent contaminants such as organochlorines and heavy metals. The latter utilizes marine bivalve molluscs as biological monitors for halogenated and petroleum hydrocarbons, heavy metals and transuranics. A third programme (1965 to 1972) also utilized a marine bivalve mollusc, to monitor levels of pesticide residues.
It was revitalized in 1977 for one year at one-half the level of effort.

III. 3. CRITERIA FOR THE SELECTION OF ECOSYSTEM COMPONENTS AND PROCESSES

Environmental monitoring is a very complex topic. Many scientists and technicians actively involved in environmental monitoring projects fail to understand the diversity of programs encompassed by the term ‚environmental monitoring‘. The authors of this paper are not entirely free of this problem. Each one of us has undoubtedly established his or her own interpretation of the types of activities which represent environmental monitoring. The criteria for the selection of organisms and soil characteristics reflect the biases of the different disciplines and experiences of the personnel involved in their development. Several types of monitoring activities, were identified and defined prior to the development of specific criteria. These monitoring activities are discussed briefly in the following section.

III. 3. 1.   Active and Passive Monitoring and Specimen Banking

There are important distictions between ‚active‘ and ‚passive‘ monitoring and the results that may be achieved by each.

Active Monitoring generally implies the intervention of a standard species (or group of species) into a variety of ecosystems or communities. The species is routinely examined for residuals of interest, of for visable signs of adverse effects (e. g., the coal miner's canary in a cage).

Passive Monitoring on the other hand implies examination of existing ecosystems (or communities) for trends in specific contaminants, or changes in functional or structural phenomena.

The active mode of monitoring presents a clear case of biotic filtering of the environmental transport media. For example, using a standard pot of annual ryegrass (**Lolium sp.**) in a variety of ecosystems provides a comparable set of measurements of atmospheric deposition of contaminants onto a standard substrate . . . the ryegrass leaves. The projection of the implications of this measurement from the ecosystems of interest to man is, however, untrustworthy. One way of avoiding this problem would require active monitoring of the accumulation of contaminants in many native species. Alternatively, native species may be examined as a community, with an emphasis on monitoring the ecological functions involved. This difference is crucial, and must be recognized, since the two approaches are best used as an **integrated pair**, not independently, with the active mode providing a measurement of buildup or recession of contaminant loading in the habitat, and the ecologically oriented, passive sampling, providing the information of community structure of function with which to provide a context for interpretation.

Both ‚effects‘ monitoring and ‚trend‘ monitoring can be accomplished by employment of either strategy. If it is desirable to determine the relative state of the environment in relation to concentrations of variety of hazardous materials, then it becomes necessary to monitor trends both in residuals and in biological effects.

For example, as part of the rationale supporting the use of vegetation as biological monitors of pollutant loading, one must consider the use of increases and/or decreases in visual symptom expression over time. Many pollutants may accumulate substantially in the tissues of biota and yet not induce visible symptoms or alterations of a physiological or morphological character. Conversely, there are several major pollutants that may cause extensive injuries to biota and yet not accumulate to any significant extent. For plants examples of the first group of pollutants include heavy metals and the latter group includes Ozone (O_3). A third group of pollutants may produce visible symptoms as well as accumulate in the affected tissues. Sulfur oxides, nitrogen oxides, and the halogen (F, Cl) affect plants in this manner.

Specimen Banking is a systematic collection and storage of samples for deferred examination, analysis and evaluation. In the past, specimen banking has been used most often for the chemical analysis of residuals in biological tissues, soil and sediment. The usual method suggested for preservation has been deep freezing.

Other approaches to specimen banking exist. For example, if specimen banking is going to be used to improve the effective information base upon which social, environmental, political and economic decisions are made, then it is wasteful to employ methods that limit the use of specimens to chemical analysis. The potential value of these tissues at little additional cost may be greatly enhanced by use of methods that will also allow histological or pathological evaluation, biochemical evaluation, etc.

Properly used, tissue banks will permit the detection of subtle biochemical or other indices that may reflect contaminants that would otherwise remain unsuspected; or would indicate the presence of transient, acute, nonpersistent contaminants; and in some cases these biological analyses may be more sensitive than direct chemical analyses.

Most importantly, histological, biochemical or other biological measures can establish or confirm the significance of tissue concentrations. Where as well-characterized, specific, quantitative relationship between the pollutant exposure and a biological response is known, the biological response may serve as a better sensor than direct assay for the pollutant.

Considering the experiences and expertises of all participants during the International Workshop on Monitoring Environmental Materials and Specimen Banking tables considering ecosystems, specimens and pollutants or pollutant categories similar to the following should be prepared, in the near future.

Selection of Indicator Specimen in Domestic and Farm Animals for Trace Elements

trace element / organ	Arsenic	Berryllium	Cadmium	Cobalt	Chromium	Fluorine	inorganic Mercury	Methylmercury	Molybdenum	Manganese	Nickel	Lead	Palladium	Selenium	Tin	Thallium	Vanadium	Zinc
Kidney			+	(+)	(+)		+	(+)			(+)	+		+		(+)		+
Liver			+	+	(+)		+	(+)	(+)			+		+				+
Muscle			o									o		o				
Brain							(+)	+										
Lung					(+)										(+)		(+)	
Spleen											(+)							+
Skin			o											(+)				
Bone			o	(+)	+					+		+			(+)	(+)		
Teeth					+				+									
Whole blood	o						(+)	+	+		(+)			+				(+)
Blood cells								+				+						(+)
Plasma					+									o				+
Milk (cow)	+								+	+	o	+		+			(+)	+
Urine	+		(+)			+	+											o
Hair, Wool, Feathers	+		o		(+)		+	+	(+)	+		+		+		(+)		+

+   Usable as monitoring organ; accumulation or indicator function proved
(+)   Advantage not proved for animals / or: of limited use
o   Unsuitable

III. 3. 2.   Terrestrial Ecosystem

III. 3. 2. 1. The Ecosystem Framework

In order to establish an effective national and international monitoring network, we have chosen to take as points of departure a recent effort towards the establishment of a United States pilot program for long-term ecological monitoring (NSF, 1979) and a recent effort in Germany (BMI, 1978). The idea behind the U. S. and German initiative is to select a minimum set of monitoring sites that would provide a representative cross section of the major ecosystems in the United States and in Germany. This monitoring network should encompass the full range of climatic condiditions, soil types, and biological communities found in such systems, thereby providing a reference framework within which ecosystem attributes might be most usefully selected for measurement and interpretation. The utility of such a framework has recently been perceived and applied in the German monitoring effort as well.

In the U. S. initiative, it was deemed appropriate to limit the choices of sites to those areas relatively undisturbed by human influence. Furthermore, the network should eventually be expanded to document ecosystems that are experiencing manmade modifications.

We believe, however, that both types of sites should be included at the outset. At a minimum, as many of the pristine sites as possible should be paired with ecologically comparable sites which have been or will soon be heavily influenced by industrial and other human activities. The U. S. initiative is almost entirely directed toward the passive monitoring of long term ecological trends in free living systems as a basis for recognizing and evaluating the significance of natural and man caused effects. The German experience, however, suggests that a strong admixture of active monitoring and passive monitoring using indicator and accumulator organisms transferred to specific locations, would be highly desirable for monitoring contaminants of potential concern. This idea may be effectively extended to the systems level by using transplants of small segments of functioning ecosystems (e. g., transplantation of a specific clone of the circumboreal quaking aspen, including the native soil profiles). We propose, then, that the active monitoring stressed in the German program be added to the passive monitoring of the U. S. program. Active monitoring data will provide a measure of trends in contaminant loading in ecosystem components and passive monitoring data will provide the structural and functional context within which the ‚signifiance‘ of these trends may be interpreted.

Some considerations for the selection of sites for a national monitoring network include:

— Sites where productive and useful short-term research has already been conducted.
— Pristine and man-influenced ecosystems where key parameters can be monitored.
— Sites representative of major ecosystems and populations.
— Sites in which active scientists have shown interest.
— Sites considered important to major ecological issues.
— Sites protected and accessible for research purposes.

Applications of these priniciples has led to 14 provisional selections for the relatively pristine sites in the United States (NSF 1979); see below.

Vegetation Types	Second-Order Ecoregions	Sites
Tundra	Tundra	Naval Arctic Research Laboratory
Boreal Forest	Subarctic	Mt. McKinley National Park
Pacific Northwest Forest	Marine	H. J. Andrews Experimental Forest
Californian Forest	Mediterranean	San Joaquin Experimental Forest
Northern Desert	Desert	Arid Lands Ecology Reserve
Southern Desert	Desert	Big Bend National Park
Rocky Mountain Forest	Steppe	Rocky Mountain Park or Fraser Experimental Forest
Shortgrass Prairie	Steppe	Central Plains Experimental Range
Tallgrass Prairie	Prairie	Konza Prairie or Wichita Wildlife Refuge
Northeastern Forest	Warm Continental	Hubbard Brook Experimental Forest or Harvard Forest
Central Forest	Hot Continental	Oak Ridge National Environmental Park, or Coweeta Experimental Forest, or Great Smoky National Park
Southeastern Forest	Subtropical	Savannah River National Environmental Research Park
Tropical	Rainforest	LaSelva Station
Tropical Savannah	Savannah	Everglades National Park

These 14 vegetation types cover more than 90 % of the total area of the United States. Selection of comparable man-influenced sites will be determined by a separate effort. Considerable care should be taken in selecting a specific site within each of these areas identified as part of the monitoring network. Within a given site the vegetation/soil/slope/altitudinal variable which most closely represents the vegetation type of interest should be identified. Within the spatial range of this variable at least five sampling stations should initially be selected. Subsequent adjustments in the number of stations would depend upon the degree of variation encountered during sampling. In order to interpret biological trends, we must know how they correlate with abiotic trends, both with respect climatic, and geochemical processes and to contaminant processes. It is not possible, in fact, to properly interpret a biological trend in response to contaminant gradients unless data on natural abiotic factors which could also bring about the response also are known. Those that seem to be generally important in all ecosystems, include (for rationale of selection, see NSF, 1979):

Physical factors:
- Meteorological functions such as short wave insolation, air temperature, precipitation, wind speed, and dew point.
- The water content of soil.
- Inorganic and organic erosion.
- Snow depth and moistur equivalence.

Chemical factors:
- Precipitation should be assayed for pH, Ca, Mg, K, Na, Cl, NH_2, NO_x, and total sulfur.
- Dry fall sedimentation (for analysis of the same elements as above).
- Soil analyses of nutrient content (Ca, Mg, K, Na, SO_2, N, C, and phosphate) should be performed on samples from major horizons in the rooting zone.
- Chemical character of soil solution in the rooting zone also should be analyzed.

At all sites certain initial conditions should be established and reevaluated periodically. As a minimum, the following steps should be taken to provide standards of reference for the appraisal of potential changes in the ecosystems of interest.

Prepare: (1) map of geological features; (2) map of physiographic and land use features; (3) map of soils and/or sediments; (4) map of vegetation; (5) comprehensive lists of species; (6) records of biotic and abiotic aspects of catastrophic events; and (7) aerial and ground benchmark photographs.

The following ecosystem survey areas (excluding marine ecosystems) for the FRG can be derived (cf. Ellenberg, Fränzle and Müller 1978):

Aguatic ecosystems
- a) Lake Constance (Bodensee)
- b) Lake Sleswig-Holstein
- c) Elbe River
- d) Rhein River

Terrestrial ecosystems
- a) Solling
- b) Alps
- c) Lüneburg Heath
- d) Jülich ‚Börde'
- e) Swabian Alps

Urban-industrial ecosystems
- a) Berlin
- b) Frankfurt
- c) Saarbrücken

These survey areas should be linked in a network of **active monitoring programs**. A survey project of free-living plant and animal species **(passive monitoring)** should register the trophic linkage between the species and see to it that the selected species or at least biologically similar population also occur in North America and if possible, in other continents.

III. 3. 2. 2 Specific Criteria for the Selection of Environmental Materials Related to Terrestrial Ecosystems.

In terrestrial ecology as in aquatic ecology, the major considerations in selecting or recommending ,sentinel' species, tissues, or other materials for the monitoring of environmental materials and specimen banking revolve around a set of broad biological problems that include but are not limited to 1) representativeness, 2) reproducibility, 3) uniformity, 4) stress tolerance, 5) comparability, and 6) relevance or signifiance. Each of these and perhaps certain other biological considerations must be addressed as ,specification criteria' along with the physical/chemical factors related to collection methods, handling, transportation, analysis, preservation, storage, and cost considerations for each of the types of data/pollutants to be monitored.

Prior to the development and compilation of new lists of considerations (criteria) for the selection of organisms and soil, each of us carefully reviewed the existing list of criteria for monitoring populations in the wild presented in the following Table.

List of Criteria (not listed in order of priority) Selection of Species/Environmental Compartments Monitoring of Populations in the Wild

1. Food Chain − Trophic Relationships
   Food web relationships and dynamics, Diet
2. Adequate Information Base (biological, physiological, etc.)
3. Population Characteristics
   Abundance
   Distribution (international)
   Habitat
   Longenity (life span allow sampling of more than one year class including some long-lived species)
   Population Trend Data
   Population Genetics
   Sensitive Annual Cycles or Life Stages
   Life Table Functions
4. Physiological Characteristics
   Should not regulate against uptake
   Turnover rate commensurate with desired integration time-length of measurement
   Not significantly alter ingested pollutants (monitor for biochemical effects)
   Not contain large amounts of tissue elements which interfere with analyses
   Nutritional status
   Accumulation of pollutant without mortality
5. Evident importance to the Environment and Man
   Health Effects
   Economic
   Sociological
   Political
   Esthetic (conservation)
   As Food for man or other resource
   Consument of similar pattern as humans
6. Pharmacokinetics (any pollutant)
   Metabolism of toxic substances
   Entry, transport, fate, effects

7. Pollutant/Organism/Ecosystem Relationships
   Should continuously monitor
   Mobility, action radius, minimum evasion
   Likelihood of exposure
8. Collection Criterea
   Costs and maintenance
   Adequate body size
   Abundant
   Easy to collect and to prepare
   Collect in consistent or standard manner
   Easy to sex
   Taxonomic identification easy to do
   Require minimum of dissection and preparation
   Sampling (scale, level of resolution)
   Representativeness
9. Experimental Tests
   Dose-response effect relationships
   Suitability for laboratory and field experimentation
   Integration of information with field data
10. Integration with other National or International Species Usages
11. Specimen Bank Objectives as well as Effects Monitoring Objectives

The criteria appeared to be generally logical and useful.

Each criterion was applicable to the selection of at least one major group of organisms. Each major group of organisms (or ecosystem compartment), however, had other special considerations which did not appear on the list. Furthermore, several criteria which might be considered important for one group (e. g., vertebrates) were not applicable for another group (e. g., plants). Furthermore, we found that these types of criteria in the selection of soil or aeroplankton components. The problems of sampling soil and aeroplankton are dissimilar to the considerations for monitoring other living systems, many of which are well-defined taxonomically and can be collected and evaluated on a species or population basis.

A number of generic considerations that are critical to the selection of all biota under consideration were nevertheless identified.

Generic Considerations for the Selection of Plants,
Invertebrate Animals and Vertebrates for Environmental Monitoring and Specimen Banking

1. Perceived Importance to Man and the Environment
   Health Effects
   Economics
   Sociological
   Political
   Aesthetic/Conservation
   Food for Man
   Surrogate for Tissue, Organism, or Committee which is perceived to be important to man and the environment
2. Population Characteristics
   Ease of Indentification/Well Characterized Taxonomically
   Longevity
   Metabolism and Pollutant Accumulation Characteristics
   Sensitivity to Biological Effects
   Annual Cycle Characteristics/Stage of Life Cycle
   Genetics
   Repestability of response under different conditions

4. Other Considerations
    Adequate Information Base
    Logistic and Organizational
    Collection Criteria
    Costs
    Amenability to Experimental Evaluation

The factors listed under ,Perceived Importance to the Environment and Man' are considered a prior justification for environmental monitoring and specimen banking. Although not listed, we recognize that ,surrogates' may exist which may not be essential or directly important to man and the environment, but which may be indicative of tissues, organisms, or communities that are important. Because the perceived importance to man and the environment is a prior consideration, it will not be discussed further.

Specific Considerations for the Monitoring of Soils

We believe that active and passive monitoring studies of soil chemical and organismal responses must be included in any effective monitoring program that is national or international in scope. Soil is the principal medium and reservoir of nutrients that promote growth and survial of plant, microbial, and animal populations in terrestrial ecosystems. Soil also is the major repository of environmental pollutants which enter the ecosystems. There is need for further research and development to maximize the potential of soils monitoring for monitoring the transport, transformation, fate, and effects of pollutants. However, soil are now known to be very sensitive to certain pollutants. For example, recent field experiments in a Montana grassland revealed that leaf litter decomposition was significantly retarded by chronic exposure to SO_2 (ten parts per hundred million) compared ton non-SO_2 treated litters.

Specific Considerations for the Selection of Plants

The following Table lists specific considerations for the selection of plant species in a large-scale monitoring system that employs both active and passive sampling modes and specimen banking.

Specific Considerations for the Selection of Plant Species as a Component of an Environmental Monitoring Program

1. Adequate information base concerning:
    Response to specific pollutant insult via previously developed dose-response curves
    a) Symptomatic response
        a. Acute
        b. Chronic
    b) Asymptomatic response, i. e., invisible or hidden injury*
        a. Physiological changes, morphological changes with no measurable yield effects
        b. Physiological changes that result in yield effects that are measurable.
    Response to pollutant combinations via previously developed dose-response curves
    a) Symptomatic response
        a. Less than additive
        b. Additive
        c. Synergistic
    b) Asymptomatic responses, i. e., invisible or hidden injury*

*   Invisible or Hidden Injury-Injury to the organism that results in a reduction of growth or yield without the expression of any other visible symptom.

a. Physiological changes, morphological changes with no measurable yield effects
b. Physiological changes that result in yield effects that are measurable
Ability of the plant species to accumulate the various pollutants to be monitored
a) Gaseous form uptake
   a. Levels of metabolic utilization and ability to identify as external constituent
   b. Levels of toxicity and ability to identify in residuals following toxicity
b) Surface depositions
   a. Migration into plant system
   b. Residuals on surface
c) Soil-root uptake interactions and efficiency of subsequent accumulation in plant organs or tissues

2. Food Chain — Trophic Relationships
3. Population Characteristics
   Abundance
   Distribution
   a) International
   b) National
   c) Regional
   Site specifications
   Longevity
   a) Annuals — genetic stability
   b) Perennials
      Woody plants
      Overwintering as root or similar organ
   Population genetics
   Sensitive annual stages
4. Physiological Characteristics
   Able to express sensitivity and/or accumulate over wind range of environmental limitations including nutritional requirements
   Well understood relationship between pollutant accumulations and mortality
   Mechanisms of entry transport, and fate well understood-metabolic
   Ease in identification

Specific Considerations for the Selection of Invertebrate Animals

The following table lists the specific considerations for selecting invertebrate organisms for environmental monitoring and specimen banking.

Specific Considerations for the Selection of Invertebrate Animals as a Component of an.Environmental Monitoring Program

1. System Characteristics
   a. Representative of critical component, functions, and processes
   b. Degree of data extrapolation: laboratory to field, season-to-season, comparability of sites, etc.
2. Population Characteristics
   a. Abundance and expendability
   b. Wide distribution
   c. Population trends
   d. Trophic level
   e. Migration pattern
   f. Life table functions
   g. Population stability monitoring
3. Individual Characteristics
   a. Ease of identification (well defined taxonomy)
   b. Ability to age, class, and sex
   c. Body size
   d. Longevity
   e. Diet and habitat
   f. Accumulation of compounds of interest
   g. Sensitivity to biological effects
   h. Exposure to pollutants
   i. Annual cycle characteristics/stages of the life cycle
   j. Genetics (active-homozygous for exposure)
   k. Intermediary metabolism allows adequate monitoring

4. Logistical/Organizational – Other
   a. Costs (time, $, personnel) and maintenance
   b. Collecting, preparation, packaging, and transportation in a consistent, standardized manner
   c. Scale and resolution of sampling program
5. Adequate Abiotic and Biotic Information Base
   a. Land use, air and water quality data, and climatological data should be available relative to the species
   b. Baseline data on physiology, reproduction, life table information, susceptibility to disease, parsite burdens and pollutant concentrations. Must be able to integrate this information with other monitoring systems. Analysis and evaluation of the combined material is desirable.

Specific Considerations for the Selection of Vertebrate Animals

Criteria for selection of specimens that are useful in monitoring and in specimen banking are shown in the following table.

	Passive Monitoring		Active Monitoring *		Specimen Banking
	Trend	Effect	Trend	Effect	
Population Characteristics					
Abundance and expendability	MB**	MB			MB
Ease of propagation			M	M	
Wide distribution	MB	MB			MB
Population trends (known or possible to determine)		MB			MB
Trophic level	MB	MB	M	M	MB
Migration patterns	MB	MB			MB
Life table functions	MB	MB			MB
Individual Characteristics					
Ease of identification (well-defined taxonomy)	MB	MB	M	M	MB
Ability to age-class and sex	MB	MB	M	M	MB
Body size	MB		M	M	MB
Longevity	MB	MB			MB
Diet and habitat	MB	MB	M	M	MB
Exposure to pollutants	MB	MB	M	M	MB
Metabolism/accumulation of compounds of interest	MB	MB	M	M	MB
Sensitivity to biological effects of pollutants		MB		M	
Annual cycle characteristics/stage of the life cycle	MB	MB	M	M	MB
Representative of ecosystem components	MB	MB			MB
Genetics	MB	MB	M	M	MB
Suitability for laboratory and field experimentation	MB	MB	M	M	MB
Logistical/Organization Characteristics					
Costs for collection and maintenance	MB	MB	M	M	MB
Ease of collecting, preparing, packaging, and transporting in a consistent, standardized manner	MB	MB	M	M	MB
Supplemental Information Base					
Baseline data on physiology, reproduction, suspectibility to disease, parasite burdens, pollutant concentrations and dose-effect relationships	MB	MB	M	M	MB
Information on other national and international programs (so they can be integrated)	MB	MB	M	M	MB
Land use and climatology data	MB	MB	M	M	MB

* apparently not feasible to use birds for experimetal exposure
** M = Mammals; B = Birds

Certain vertebrate animals will be useful in determining geographic and temporal trends in residue levels of some environmental pollutants. Whenever possible the same specimens, or others collected at the same time and place, and analyzed soon after collection should also be placed in a specimen bank for possible future analyses.

Whereas some mammals may be suitable for experimental exposure (active monitoring) in the field, it appears that birds are not generally suitable for active monitoring on natural sites. Exceptions include the monitoring of airborne pollutants, in urban ecosystems. Birds, can, however, be experimentally tested with known pollutants, and such studies have been used to determine the effects of pollutants on birds at environmentally realistic levels. Passive monitoring and field surveys are useful in determining the concentrations of pollutants in wild-living birds and thereby may be used to suggest the dietary exposures for testing.

Considerations for the Monitoring of Aeroplankton

Aeroplankton includes viruses, bacteria, protozoa and algae, pollen, and certain insects that are transported passively through the air. They are introduced into the air from many sources. Their densities, abundancies, and viability while airborne may exhibit great temporospatial variability. Viability is influenced by numerous environmental conditions such as relative humidity, temperature, light, atmospheric gaseous composition, etc.

Some aeroplankton are pathogenic agents that may affect plants and animals including man. This is of concern, in part, because some pollutants are facilitators or potentiators of infectuous disease.

The abundance and composition of aeroplankton varies greatly as a function of human activities that affect dispersion, viability, and injection rates. It would thus seem desirable to establish passive monitoring systems for aeroplankton. With the paucity of information on the distribution of kinds and numbers of airborne microorganisms in the world-atmosphere, selection of criteria species (except possibly in the case of pollen) is not recommended. Active monitoring of the effects of the gaseous composition of the atmosphere at specific locations on the survival of airborne organisms may help us to interpret the above passive measurements as well to detect previously unknown aerial pollutant materials.

Meteorological measurements must be made at the time and near the site of aerobiological sampling.

Effects monitoring of atmospheric conditions may be tested by placing bacterial aerosols with test gas mixtures in closed and stirred containers or by passing natural air or gas mixtures over microorganisms suspended on micro-threads and subsequently measuring the rate or extent of change in a characteristic of the suspended microorganisms (e. g., viability, mutations). Special methods for effects monitoring of pollen are also available.

Passive monitoring of airborne microorganisms may be performed using relatively large air volume samples in which they are either impacted directly onto culture media for subsequent enumeration and identification, or impinged into a collecting solution and the solution inoculated onto culture media. Pollen may be collected in Hirst-type traps or roto-rodtype traps for subsequent microscopic and culture processing.

There is no known simple way to passively measure the effects of a polluted atmoshere on the in situ aeroplankton although a test aerosol of microorganisms might be injected into the atmosphere and downwind surviving organisms compared to a mathematical estimation of the surviving population.

With respect to the banking of aeroplankton, we may note that while pure cultures of microorganisms have been preserved alive for extended periods of time by freeze drying, we do not know whether such is practical for mixed collections of airborne microorganisms in various states of physiological activity. Nevertheless, dried collections of microorganisms may be made from the above impinger samples and stored in vacuo indefinity. It is possible to store strained microorganisms on microscope slides. Pollen may be stored dead on microscope slides or alive by conventional palynological techniques.

III. 3. 2. 3.   Selection of Environmental Materials and Specimen Related to Terrestrial Ecosystems and Pollutants or Pollutant Categories

III. 3. 2. 3. 1. Soils

Soils and sediments tend to accumulate pollutants. They vary, however, with respect to certain physical and chemical characteristics that may alter sorption capacities for various pollutants. For example, non-polar high molecular weight organic pollutants are sorbed more strongly and in higher quantities on soils high in organic matter than on soils low in organic matter. Positively charged pollutants are sorbed in higher quantities on soils of higher cation exchange capacity (> 15 meq/100g) than on soils of less cation exchange capacity (< 5 meq/100 g). Such characteristics may provied guides for the selection of soils for monitoring. Thus, it is suggested that soils with the following physical and chemical properties should have high priority with regard to selection: pH > 6.5; organic matter > 7 %, cation exchange capacity > 15 meq/100 g; and % clay > 35 %. Furthermore, level poorlydrained soils tend to accumulate more pollutants than soils located on steep-well-drained slopes and should be selected preferrentially.

Passive Monitoring

Composite samples taken from within specific soil series should be utilized in passive monitoring systems. Appropriate presentday soil classification nomenclature should be employed. The location of sampling sites should be identified on the most recent soil maps and filed as a permanent record. For routine monitoring procedures, litter and surface soil samples (0 - 15 cm) will suffice. For passive effects monitoring, we recommend that respiration be measured in situ, using CO_2 traps in air-tight exclosures (metal or plastic cylinders, ca. 10 cm dia). These cylinders, when placed 15 -20 cm. into the mineral soil, will give a measure of total respiration per unit area of littersoil. If some litter-free cylinders are also employed, litter respiration rates can be determined by difference.

Active Monitoring

In addition to pollutant monitoring, the measurement of several soil processes are recommended. These should include decomposition, denitrification, soil nitrogen transformations, and sulfur transformations, total soil respiration, and litter respiration. It is also desirable to determine the content of certain chemicals such as soluble sugars and protein or cellulose.

Appropriate dose-response experiments would be desirable to aid interpretation of the ‚effects‘ monitoring results. Test should also be conducted to determine levels of pollutants and rates of pollutant transfer that alter the biological activity of the soil. Transfer rates to ground water and to plants is also of concern.

Specimen Banking

We recommend the banking of freeze dried soil cores and litter. The time, site, depth, and (if possible) previous history of the sample (e. g., forest cut over 20 years ago, etc.) must be specified.

Biological effects monitoring is probably not generally possible or useful with soils. Possible exceptions are fungal fruiting bodies and rhizomorphs.

III. 3. 2. 3. 2. Plants

Specific plants recommended for pollutant monitoring and specimen banking are presented in the following table. Reflected in this table is the fact that not all pollutants that are phytotoxic are accumulated by a plant during the process of stress response and the development of symptoms. In other cases, pollutant accumulation may occur without the development of evident symptoms. Thus, in some cases, symptoms only may be evaluated; in other cases, pollutant accumulation only may be measured; and in yet other instances, both may be assessed.

Plants Recommended for Monitoring and Specimen Banking

	SOx		O₃		F		PAN		NOx		Heavy Metals	
	Accum.	Symp.	Accum.	Symp.	Accum.	Symp.	Accum.	Symp.	Accum.	Symp.	Accum.	Symp.
Active	1-7	1-9	-	1-7	1-5	1-6	-	1-5	-	1-7	1-5	-
Trend	1-7	1-9	-	1-7	1-5	1-6	-	1-5	-	1-7	1-5	-
Effect	1-7	1-9	-	1-7	1-5	1-6	-	1-5	-	1-7	1-5	-
Passive	1-4,7	1-4,7	-	1,5	1,4,5	1,4,5	-	3,4,5	-	1,2,5	1,3,5	-
Trend	1-4,7	1-4,7	-	1,5	1,4,5	1,4,5	-	3,4,5	-	1,2,5	1,3,5	-
Effect	1-4,7	1-4,7	-	1,5	1,4,5	1,4,5	-	3,4,5	-	1,2,5	1,3,5	-
Banking	1,2,3,6,7		NA*		1-5		NA		NA		1-5	

SOx	O₃	F	PAN	NOx	Heavy Metals
1 Lichens**	1 Tobacco	1 Lichens	1 Alfalfa	1 Larch	1 Pinus
2 Annual Ryegrass	2 Pine	2 Gladiolus	2 Beam	2 Picea	2 Oats
3 Pine	3 Bean	3 Corn	3 Annual Ryegrass	3 Oats	3 Annual Ryegrass
4 Poplar Familiy	4 Oats	4 Poplar Familiy	4 Dandelion	4 Bean	4 Pea
5 Bean	5 Grape	5 Pine	5 Pinus	5 Sunflower	5 Lichens
6 Alfalfa	6 Radish	6 Apricot		6 Radish	
7 Moss	7 Tomato			7 Soybean	
8 Radish					
9 Soybean					

*NA   Not Applicable; Symptom records, photographs only.
**   Species by source/region/area etc., (Native vs. Exotic).

III. 3. 2. 3. 3   Invertebrate Animals

Invertebrate taxa recommended for monitoring and specimen banking are considered in the following table.

Invertebrates Recommended for Environmental Monitoring and Specimen Banking★

Functional Groups	System Characteristics	Population Characteristics	Individual Characteristics	Logistical Organization	Adequate Information Base	Effects, Trend, Banks	Active Passive
Pollinators a) Managed Honeybees	3	3	3	3	3	3	3
b) Native Bees, Flies, Beetles, Lepidoptera	2	2	1	2	2	2	2
Pest Population Regulation a) Carabids	3	3	3	3	2	3	1
b) Spiders	3	3	2	2	1	2	1
Detritus Processors a) Drosophila	1	2	2	2	1	1	2
b) Earth worm	3	3	2	3	3	3	3
c) Isopods or Millipedes	3	2	2	2	2	2	2
d) Ants (mount)	2	3	2	3	2	1	1

★ 1 = poor
   2 = adequate
   3 = very good

The actual species to be selected for a given monitoring system must be made by a qualified expert on the basis of the previously discussed selection criteria, objectives of the monitoring program, and sit-specific considerations.

Invertebrate taxa to be selected for monitoring or specimen banking should be representative of critical (key) components, functions, or processes of the ecosystems of concern. Furthermore, those groups selected should have a potential for providing information on trends or effects sooner or at lower cost than other types of specimens. Thus, phytophagous insects are not included on the table because we believe that pollutant uptake and effects will appear earlier in the plants upon which the insects feed. Thus, monitoring of these insects might not provide much information beyond that which could be derived from plants (except grashopers; cf. **Stenobothrus lineatus**).

46

Extensive review and discussion led to the rejection of many invertebrate groups as potential pollutant monitors (see below).

Rejected Invertebrates and Rationale

Protozoans
- biomass small
- no unique information
- sensitivity to micro-climate effects

Tardigrades
- biomass small
- basic information base inadequate

Nematodes
- difficult to collect
- what kind of indicators are they if at all?
- available information mainly concerns economically important species

Phytophagous Insects
- offer little or no information that could not be obtained from plants

Hymenopterous Parasites
- sampling and collection more difficult than for predators
- don't believe that much additional information except as concerns specific host-parasite interaction could be derived as compared to that from predators which are more general ,feeders'

Centipedes
- occupy the same functional component as carabids and spiders, but regulate detrital populations rather than pests and as such could be worthwhile to include, but we don't know as much about them (general information, pollution interactions, etc.) as about carabids and possibly spiders.

III. 3. 2. 3. 4 Vertebrate Animals

A primary consideration in selecting vertebrate specimens is the feasibility of obtaining them. Starlings **(Sturnus vulgaris)** and ducks **(Anas platyrhynchos** or **A. rubripes)** are included in the U. S. National Pesticide Monitoring Program; bald eagles **(Haliaeetus leucocephalus)** also are routinely analyzed for residues of pollutants. Of the specimens analyzed in this ongoing monitoring program, subsamples (starlings and duck wings from selected localities as well as bald eagles) could be placed into a specimen bank for long-term storage and possible retrospective analysis. Additional specimens of starling might be collected and prepared (i. e., labeled, weighed, packaged, etc.) for storage as whole birds. However, the numbers that would be needed (probably 8 - 10 individuals for each subsequent analysis) should be determined within reasonable limits. In addition, tests should be conducted in a pilot program to determine the feasibility of long-term preservation of dissected tissues.

Insofar as possible, the monitoring and specimen banking programs should include those species already being collected in the National Pesticide Monitoring Program. Species that were selected for that program meet many of the criteria previously outlined.

Other avian species in the United States that satisfy many of the criteria include the herring gull **(Larus argentatus)** or other locally abundant gull species, the robin **(Turdus migratorius),** and mourning dove **(Zenaidura macroura)** or house sparrow **(Passer domesticus);** both carnivores and granivores are represented here. Gulls may reflect pollutant levels in aquatic and/or terrestrial ecosystems because they feed in both. In urban areas, the rock dove **(Columba livia)** may be a good indicator of pollutant levels. Some of these species are widespread in distribution and could also be collected in Europe, or their ecological counterparts may be taken there (cf. **Turdus merula, Falco tinnunculus, Accipiter gentilis, Phasianus colchicus, Columba palumbus).**

Mammalian species that satisfy many of the above criteria include house mouse (**Mus musculus**), deer mous group (**Peromyscus** spp.), muskrat (**Ondatra zibethica**), cottontail rabbit group (**sylvilagus** spp). striped skunk (**Mephitis mephitis**), deer group (whitetail and mule, **Odocoileus** spp.), and big brown bat (**Eptisicus fuscus**). The cosmopolitan house mouse will reflect situations closely linked with human habitats, both urban and rural. The mostly granivorous **Peromyscus** spp., and the **Sylvilagus** spp., mostly foliar or flower eaters, will obtain residues of pollutants in both near-human and more remote habitats. **Ondatra** will allow monitoring the body burdens of residues *from* aquatic macrophytes. The **Odocoileus** spp., are browsing herbivores and will have long exposure histories because they are longer lived. The carnivorous **Mephitis** will obtain pollutant residues from two lower trophic levels. The insectivorous **Eptesicus fuscus** is also representative of a high trophic level, and in addition, since it is migratory, will integrate exposure over a larger geographic area. We do not know, however, how valuable these species may be in reflecting environmental levels of various pollutants because they may metabolize and excrete compounds of interest. The various species are included here because of other criteria (i. e., distribution, abundance, trophic levels, etc.).

The Germans analyzed the following species:
Crocidura and **Sorex**
Lepus europaeus
Capreolus capreolus
Vulpes vulpes

A Working group from the Museum National d'Histoire Naturelle, France, prefered:
Microtus arvalis; **Erinaceus europaeus**; **Capreolus capreolus**; **Rupicapra rupicapra**; **Vulpes vulpes**.

If organisms are small, the whole body should be preserved. If large, the organs known to be useful in the future, could be stored; these are listed in the table below.

Tissues	Vertebrate Group from which these originate★	Specific Regions or Parts to be Banked
Gonads (testes/ovary)	MB	
Thyroid	MB	
Adrenal gland	MB	Left
Bone	MB	Tibia
Tooth	M	First molar
Lens	M	Left
Adipose tissue	MB	Visceral: renal fat capsule
Blood	MB	Minimum of 100 ml
Hair	M	Clippings from middorsum, between scapulae
Feathers	B	Primary and secondary wing feathers
Brain	M	Left half of midsagittally sectioned brain
Kidney	MB	Half of the left kidney, sectioned midsagittally
Liver	MB	Tip of left median lobe; minimum of 100 g
Lung	MB	Transverse slab taken from left lung, mid-level
Muscle (skeletal)	MB	Sample from left thigh; minimum of 100 g
Spleen	MB	Distal half; minimum of 100 g
Thymus	B	One -3 lobes
Bursa of fabricius	B	

★ (B = Birds, M = Mammals)

These tissues were provisionally selected because they are known either to detoxify or to accumulate pollutants:

1. Those which detoxify and are likely to be immediately affected and /or to accumulate pollutants are the liver, kidney, and respiratory tract.

   Those useful for trend monitoring (i. e., accumulation) are:

   a. Adipose and brain — for lipophilic substances
   b. Lung — for aerially dispersed particulates
   c. Liver, kidney, hair, bone, eye, lens, muscle — for heavy metals
   d. Blood — aqueous and adipophyllis pollutants

2. Eye lenses and teeth are often useful for aging adult, long-lived mammals
3. The following are useful for effects monitoring:

   a. Thyroid gland — directly involved in metabolic responses
   b. Adrenal gland — reflects stress
   c. Blood — reflects hemopoietic and other responses to pollutant
   e. Gonads — reflect reproductive state

Because some organs in medium-sized and large mammals and birds are too large for storage whole, samples of these should be banked. Standardizstion of sampling is, therefore, necessary to avoid analytic bias due to uneven distribution of pollutants within these organs. It is worth noting that some specimens can be stored under ambient conditions: specifically hair, feathers, and teeth.

III. 3. 3.   Aquatic Ecosystem

Considerable thought was given by all contributors to the establishment of criteria for selection of biological specimens for monitoring environmental materials and specimen banking in aquatic ecosystems.

1) importance to man
2) position of the species in the food chain
3) abundance
4) distribution
5) collection costs and maintenance
6) availability
7) mobility and action radius
8) habitat
9) physiology
10) accumulation of pollutant without mortality
11) should be sedentary in order to show levels of pollutants representative of the area under study
12) longevity (life span should alow sampling of more than one year class)
13) adequacy of size
14) hardy enough to survive laboratory bioassay
15) be able to tolerate brackish water
16) should not regulate against uptake of the pollutant
17) should have a turnover rate commensurate with the desired integration time-length of measurement
18) should continuously monitor
19) not significantly alter ingested pollutants to form not attributable to original pollutants

20)   not contain large amounts of tissue elements which interfere with the analyses
21)   require minimum of dissection and other preparation for analyses
22)   remain within a limited geographic range during the period of monitoring
23)   not ingest amounts of sediments sufficient to invalidate measurement of pollutants in the water
24)   be easy to collect (e. g. without boat or special equipment)
25)   be easy to prepare for shipment to analytical laboratories with minimum of contamination for handling
26)   should be collected in a consistent or standard manner
27)   sex of individual specimens
28)   ideally should have a previous history of use in field monitoring and in laboratory response studies.

The above list represents a compendium of input from all workshop contributors. The criteria presented have been generated from different historical needs including use of algae, bivalve molluscs, fish and aquatic birds as biological monitors. In spite of the diversity of needs which generated the list, it is for the most part generally applicable and probably represents a reasonable set of criteria for application in future specimen banking activities regardless of pollutant categories or ecosystems.

Several items on the list deserve further discussion. It was recommended that item 2 (trophic position) include apex predators, herbivorous forms, and intermediate forms of finfish. Also it was noted, that due to progressive concentration of persistent pollutants through successive levels of the food chain, a chosen species food habits must be representative of the segment of that environment at which monitoring is primarily directed.

Item 11, emphasises on choosing a sedentary species. Such a choice must depend on the nature of the segment of the aquatic environment being monitored. Sedentary species might best represent physically active, rapidly changing coastal areas such as estuaries or intertidal zones. But in those areas which tend toward a more homogenous set of conditions, such as truly open ocean epipelagic zones, a wide ranging species such as the blue shark may be as appropriate an integrator of the environment as is the mussel of a coastal area. The species of choice must be a reasonably representative integrator, both with respect to habitat and the physiochemical nature of the environment.

Item 13, adequacy of size, must take into consideration, abundance as well as size. Perhaps adequacy of ‚biomass‘ should be substituted for ‚size‘ in this case. Total biomass of plankton or bacteria may be an adequate measure of ‚size‘.

Item 18, states that the species of choice should monitor continously. In temperate climates, bivalve species greatly reduce or cease pumping activity altogether at temperatures of roughly 10°C and below. Yet these molluscs hold great promise as biological monitors.

Item 22 cites the desirability of the species remaining within a geographic zone. As in the case of Item 11 above, the geographic boundary is really less important than the environmental redundancy of the area being monitored.

Item 23 recognizes the disadvantage of the presence of sediments. However, if depuration in clear seawater is a practical operation, the comparison of levels between sediment contaminated and depurated animals becomes an important data point allowing some distinction between movement of materials or particles through the environment. Absence of particulate sediments in alimentary systems is no guarantee that this is not route of entry.

With regard to (9) and (19) it was expressed about PAH: the metabolic pathway in micro-orga-nisms and animal tissues leads to epoxids, diols, phenols and quinones. The oxidation of these aromatic compounds proceeds very rapidly and there is therefore no accumulation to be observed in animal tissues.

Further it was stressed the need for collection and storage of water and sediment samples in addi-tion to biological materials in a useful specimen bank system. Due to logistic limitations arising from highly specialized space requirements for long-term storage, careful consideration should be given to the use of the biological specimen as an integrator of its environment versus the attempt to store the individual components of its environment for additional reference.

By way of illustration, we may vote thate once kepone was defined as a current problem in the James River Estuary (because of detection of the material in the then current samples of water, sediment, and biota), it was possible to go back to archived oyster samples and establish from those archived (banked) specimens the point in time at which biological contamination first oc-cured. Was it necessary in this case to have archived sediment and water samples? Would the wa-ter samples, had they existed, provide enough additional information to warrant the cost of stor-age of that material in a proper state for future analyses? Is not the fact that biological specimens may concentrate and integrate materials from the environment one of the main forces behind establishment of a specimen bank?

Further consideration was suggested of the use of biological specimens currently present in the archival museums of the world. For example there are presently 36.000.000 specimens of finfish, dating back too years in some cases, already stored in the museums of the U. S. and Canada. Mu-seum specimens were used effectively to compare mercury (Hg) levels among fish groups, with no apparent bias introduced by storage. Some other heavy metals concentrations have been demon-strated to change as a result of fixation in formalin and maintenance in alcohol. However, there are bone collections for fishes and marine mammals as well as shell collections of marine molluscs which might be of value for future analyses.

Some authors recommendations summarized:
a) in monitoring rivers, shallow lakes and coastal waters select species living both in the wa-ter and in the sediments, e. g. zoöplankton and/or phytoplankton and/or certain molluscs.
b) correlate, as possible, geochemical behaviour of mud with concentrations in the water and biological tissues at one location, to get a picture of the impact.
c) after selection of the habitat, select species for surveillance according to trophic level.

Conclusions:
Historically monitoring of both inorganic and organic contaminants in aquatic wild fowl, and ma-rine bivalves has been successfully empolyed in formal trend analysis. Several formal programmes, current as well as past, have developed an insular type of specimen banking activity. In addition to the specimen banking activities related to formal monitoring programmes. NOAA has archived some marine fish, sediment, and water samples. There are now extant in the U. S. archived samp-les of waterfowl, finfish, and molluscs.

We recommend the serious consideration of a pilot tissue specimen bank that takes advantage of one or all of the ongoing formal monitoring and tissue banking programmes extant within the par-ticipating countries.

The stronger programmes in the U. S. appear to be those that use wildfowl, freshwater finfish, and marine bivalves.

Regarding the pilot environmental specimen bank in the Federal Republic of Germany the following species were discussed: **Dreissena polymorpha, Mytilus** species, macro-algae, **pleuronectes, Cyprinus carpio,** sludge. The use of macroalgae and of the mullet as a marine finfish as well as use of open ocean fish also holds promise.

In general, the monitors of choice appear to work well with both organic and inorganic compounds.

Serious discussion must be devoted to the various zones within the aquatic ecosystems and how they relate to proximity to man's activities. Estuaries, embayments, open coastlines, offshore areas and open ocean systems generally divide out in a decreasing plane in relation to tissue residues traceable to man's activities. Should a tissue banking system be aimed at the baseline of relative cleanliness offered by the open sea, or should it rather identify and subsequently monitor areas of known contaminant impact such as esturaries and embayments. Should coastwise sampling be preferrentially initiated so that an early warning system might identify the movement of contaminants from the estuaries toward the more pristine open marine systems?

Priorities must be established for the immediate and long range goals of an international tissue banking activity.

Important criteria for the selection of specimens in a pilot monitoring and banking programme are:
— sample collection procedure available;
— sample preparation for analysis established;
— combined programmes to reduce total cost.

IV. TECHNICAL CONSIDERATIONS

IV. 1. GENERAL REMARKS

In sampling, preparation, transportation and storage of environmental materials and specimens for monitoring and banking programmes, certain strict precautions must be taken to obtain adequate information relative to the purpose of the study and the substance to be measured. Analytical chemistry begins when a sample is taken and the analyst should be fully involved from this point. Contamination of samples and loss of e. g. volatile pollutants during collection and following steps may be more of a problem in some cases than others, and specific risks of contamination and loss are described in the following.

The wide spread of reported values for both organic and inorganic substances (esp. in the ng/g level) can be derived from uncritical application of analytical techniques (s. also chapter V) as well as from ‚positive' or ‚negative' contamination.

IV. 2. COLLECTION, COLLECTION EQUIPMENT, SAMPLE PREPARATION AND TRANSPORTATION

Contamination and loss problems start with collection of environmental materials and biological specimens. Sampling in areas remote from laboratories requires certain strict precautions. Samples that have been subjected to prolonged transportation under adverse conditions may be useless and collection should therefore be restricted those samples that can be adequately preserved in the field. Speed is of the essence if one wants to minimize the errors in estimates of pollutants within organisms that are obtained in the field. No chemicals may be used to collect environmental materials and specimens. Samples should be collected in an adequate, non-contaminating manner (e. g. shocking, trawling and trapping).

Special cleaning procedures for materials and instruments used for sampling are necessary, as well as special sampling techniques to avoid contamination of the sample by pollutants from the environment during sampling. Loss of volatile compounds during sampling is a less serious problem with respect e. g. to phthalates, organophosphates, mycotoxins and antibiotics, but should be considered in monitoring other organic compounds of higher volatility. It is desirable to avoid metallic instruments in sampling environmental materials and specimens intended to be examined for inorganic pollutants. Similar considerations may be applied to knives, scissors and other instruments necessary for organ dissection. Of course there are plastic or glass knives and scissors, but using them, no guarantee is given, that they do not contaminate the sample perhaps more than the metallic instruments. The recommended procedures for obtaining samples free from contamination include the use of quartz or borosilicate glass instruments, or those made of titanium, titanium carbide, boron carbide, carbon steel or aluminium. Titanium knives have been used and resulted in no contamination except for titanium. They may be easier to use than the other types of instrument. Contamination by copper, manganese, chromium, nickel, iron, cobalt, silver, tin, antimony and tantalum have been demonstrated by several authors when using stainless steel instruments. Recently the use of lasers has been proposed for cutting biological tissues, but laser cutting might produce excessive heat at the cut surface and potential losses of volatile organic and inorganic compounds or pyrolytic changes.

For organic compounds , instruments and other materials made of organic compounds, which come into contact with the sample, must be avoided (plastic gloves should be used with caution). Studies requiring data on the distribution of a substance within a tissue would, of course, involve the preservation of the intact tissue or whole organ. Homogenization of the specimen may be employed in instances where a substance is inhomogeneously distributed or where replicate analyses are to be carried out by different labs. However, great care must be exercised with the homogenization procedures to avoid contamination. Homogenization is best carried out in some types of commercial feed mixer which automatically divides the sample, mixes, and recombines the mixed product; nevertheless avoidance of metallic instruments is difficult. Ultrasonic or brittle fracture methods may give some advantages. Also it must be ensured that any portion taken is representative of the whole. A representative sample implies that it should be homogeneous.

All specimens should be transferred to permanent storage containers as soon as possible and handled as few times as possible having in mind that each additional handling enhances the possiblility of introducing contamination.

The composite samples from each station may be shipped in the same container. Environmental materials and specimens should be handled and processed for shipment in such a manner as to avoid any contamination by pesticides, metals, or chemicals such as oil or PCB's. The samples should be delivered directly by special mobile laboratories or shipped by air to the analytical laboratories and/or storage locations.

IV. 3. CONTAINER MATERIALS

Changes in the forms and concentrations of the numerous environmentally important substances in specimens stored for extended periods may occur in several ways. Processes such as surface adsorption and sample degradation may reduce the concentrations of various components and/or produce species which may not have been present in the original sample. On the other hand, contamination from the container and evaporation of specimen fluids could lead to apparent increases in trace substance concentrations or losses in the case of volatile trace components. In addition, superimposed on these processes are the factors which will affect their rates, such as, container material, contact time and area.

There have been numerous studies performed in recent years directed toward the identification of suitable container materials and optimum storage conditions, but much of this work is contradictory. In many cases, the analytical data were invalidated because of problems not associated with the storage but with other links in the analytical chain such as sampling and procedural contamination.

It should be emphasized that the material used for containers for samples or aliquots of samples for monitoring environmental materials and specimen banking should show no interaction with the sample or parts of it.

Since organic chemicals migrate in the course of time into containers of organic material and since metal surfaces might catalyze unwanted chemical reactions in the sample, glass or glass like containers only give the needed safety to avoid loss and minimize reactions.

With respect to organic compounds of high or moderate lipophilic properties, polyethylene or even perfluoropolyethylene and similar materials are not suitable. The use of quartz or borosilicate glass seems to be the best for this purpose, although cost and methods of sealing (closure) must be considered. Nevertheless, adsorption of some compounds, e. g. phenols, on to the glass surface may occur. Gold, aluminium or other metals without catalytic properties may be appropriate, but there is no experience in this field.

With respect to inorganic substances, glass and plastic material contain easily detectable amounts of trace (and bulk) elements. In the case of plastic some of these elements are residues of polymerization catalysts. Most of these elements are leached from the surface of the containers when treated with diluted acids. Heavy metals may be removed by using complexing agents. In every case an intensive cleaning procedure is necessary before using a container. Several authors suggest cleaning methods for most trace element work, treatment of the container with hydrochloric acid (1+1), nitric acid (1+1) and ultrapure distilled water. The procedure requires several weeks. Purest materials are polytetrafluoroethylene and conventional polyethylene.

It must be mentioned, that in extreme trace element analysis terms like ‚metal free containers' or ‚washed metal free' should be avoided. At best ‚metal poor' may be used.
For practical purposes this means:

a)   testing any material contacting the specimen,
b)   having regard to the **analytical blank** in every case.
c)   treat sample containers with **same precautions** as samples.

Summarized the following container characteristics should be considered:

— minimum interaction between specimen and container
— minimum interaction between specimen and external environment
— container capable of withstanding all possible temperature changes.

IV. 4. STORAGE METHODS

Adequate storage to preserve the integrity of the samples is one of the most difficult obstacles to overcome. It is widely recognized that the storage of environmental materials and specimens is subject to a variety of uncertainties when one is considering the identity and levels of trace elements and organics. Possible approaches to short and long term tissue preservation include:

1. Chemical preservation

For example formaldehyde has been used traditionally to stabilize and preserve biological tissues chemically. This method has proved excellent for the purpose for which it was originally designed i. e. for histological examination. Chemical preservation is detrimental to sample integrity, as most organic compounds are affected by these procedures and at the present time, however, this method is not recommended for preservation prior to chemical analysis.

2. Radiation sterilization

One method which has been used to sterilize tissue samples is irradiation. For example, in the preparation of the NBS Orchard leaves; the samples were irradiated with 4.9 Mrad from a cobalt-60 source. However, one disadvantage of this technique is that high level irradiation alters the chemical structure of tissue and causes the breakdown of certain labile organic compounds, some of which may be the pollutants which are being analyzed in the monitoring and banking programmes. This method is applicable only for elemental analysis because of potential ionization damage to compounds.

3. Lyophilization (freeze drying)

It is a fact, that certain trace elements and organic compounds can be volatilized at temperatures normally used for oven drying, therefore, in order to safeguard against pollutant losses through volatilization it is possible to lyophilize the specimens. Lyophilized tissue can be maintained with a high degree of integrity for long periods at room temperature. It may be necessary to store some samples in an inert atmosphere, but transportation, shipment and distribution is facilitated and the handling for further processing is simplified. Regarding organic compounds, lyophilization is not suitable, because there is a significant loss of volatile and even moderately volatile compounds. Freeze drying may be useful for trace element specimens, though loss of highly volatile elements like mercury or organo-metal compounds seems to be possible. But there are several references which indicate that this loss from tissue samples is negligible. The procedure can be generally recommended for inorganic but not organic analysis. Precautions must be taken to avoid contamination and losses.

4. Storage of extracts

The storage of extracts may be an advantage in the case of some groups of chemical compounds; nevertheless, this results in various new contamination problems; rates and amounts of adsorption or leaching of inorganic and organic traces are higher. Further the extraction procedure may entail the loss of some polar compounds, which are not amenable to environmental monitoring at present and which are therefore of great importance for specimen banking.

5. Ashing

Low temperature ashing is a potential method for trace metal pollutants not subject to volatilization at the temperatures used, but is not applicable for organic chemicals and may present problems even for the analysis of certain elements.

6. Rapid and deep freezing

Rapid and deep freezing seems to be the most acceptable method for maintaining sample integrity and preserving the potential for contaminant investigations. Deep freezing — in general, the lower the temperature, the better — may provide satisfactory stability of the sample provided the temperature used for storage is -80° C or colder. In order to minimize migration of water within the container, fluctuations in the storage container should be avoided.

Temperatures warmer than this do not adequately protect against enzymatic degradation of the stored sample. Therefore, for routine purposes liquid nitrogen freezers are recommended which should maintain a specimen temperature of -80° C or colder, depending on their location within the freezer. However, in the deep-freezing procedure the freezing rate is still an open question and needs further basic research. Depending on the specimen to be stored, freezing rates of 1°/min. up to some 1000°/sec. (shock freezing) have been found adequate.

Temperatures of -80° C or even -196° C as well as exclusion of oxygen seem to be the methods of choice for storing tissue specimens over prolonged periods. Evaluation work on these conditions is in progress.

IV. 5. CONCLUSIONS AND RECOMMENDATIONS

In sampling, preparation, transportation and storage of environmental materials and specimens for monitoring and banking programmes certain strict precautions must be taken.
Special cleaning procedures for materials and instruments used for sampling are necessary, as well as special sampling techniques to avoid contamination of the sample and/or loss of pollutants. All specimens should be transferred to permanent storage containers as soon as possible and handled as few times as possible. The samples should be delivered directly by special mobile laboratorie or shipped by air to the analytical laboratories and/or storage locations.
Regarding the container materials the following points should be observed:

- minimum interaction between specimen and container
- minimum interaction between specimen and external environment
- container capable of withstanding all possible temperature changes
- choice of container material is dictated by the sample to be stored and the substance to be determined
- conventional polyethylene, borosilicate glass, teflon and quartz should be considered
- the cleaned container should be protected from environmental contamination (e. g. dust) before and during sample insertion
- to reduce oxidation of the sample, the container should be evacuated or filled with a high-purity inert gas

Low-temperature ashing is not advocated because of the possibility of volatile metal losses but may have certain advantages for specimens such as bone.
Chemical preservation, radiation sterilization and storage of extracts were not recommended as storage methods.

Freeze drying appears to be an excellent method for samples intended for inorganic analysis, but sample size may be limited to 25-50 g of material.
In recommending the rates of freezing, the rate of thawing should also be considered and further investigation regarding these may be needed.

It is not possible to suggest a ‚standard method‘ for storage of all kinds of specimens and related to all pollutants or pollutant categories; nevertheless, temperatures of -80° C or even -196° C as well as exclusion of oxygen seem to be the methods of choice for storing tissue specimens over prolonged period.

It is recommended that reference materials be certified at the ng/g levels for inorganic substances in matrices similar to those selected for inclusion in this monitoring and banking programme.

As specific types of specimens are identified, appropriate sampling and storage protocols will have to be developed and followed by all participants in this programme. Where these operations are performed in a less standardized manner, they should be documented in detail as to how the samples were collected and prepared for analysis and/or storage; this information to accompany all specimens collected. In addition, it was suggested to archive representative samples of the equipment used in sampling and sample preparation in order to permit later retrospective analysis of these items.

The technique of cryogenic brittle fracture appears to be an excellent method for pulverization of frozen tissues and bone prior to subsampling.

For long-term storage, losses of moisture and volatile pollutants due to container permeability must be avoided.

The permeability of container materials, at low temperatures, to gases should be more thoroughly investigated.

Further information is needed concerning the permeability to water vapour of Teflon and other container materials at low temperatures and all containers with samples placed into storage at low temperatures should first be accurately weighed.

It is recommended that a centralized approach be taken to problems of sample storage. Even small-scale sample alterations resulting from slightly different storage techniques could lead to increased variability in measured pollutant concentrations.

V. ANALYTICAL ASPECTS

V. 1. INTRODUCTION

In the analytical aspects of the subject there are general considerations and some details of extreme importance regarding the special objectives of monitoring and specimen banking. From the moment of sampling** to the final handling of the sample, precautions against contamination must be taken. Therefore it is desirable to minimize the number of steps of the procedure.

Detailed descriptions of methods are not given here. The development of techniques and the gain in accuracy and sensitivity are dynamic processes.
Analytical Chemistry publishes a comprehensive annual review supplement, devoted in alternate years to the applied aspects and to the fundamental aspects of the subject.

In monitoring aquatic ecosystems the most important matrices are:
— water, fresh and saline with low concentration of contaminants requiring careful analysis in order to obtain sufficient accuracy;
— sediment, organic and inorganic phases, with varying concentrations of contaminants;
— biological tissue, with relatively the highest levels of contamination by processes of bioaccumulation but prior to chemical analysis a clean-up or digestion of the samples is necessary*.
The efficiency of each step in the preparation of samples should be checked by model-experiments using radio-isotopes. This method has shown that freeze-drying is not efficient as had previously been thought and that considerable losses of toxic metals such as cadmium may occur. The size of sample to be analyzed and the number of specimens needed to give a sample representative of the ecosystem under consideration should be determined for each item in the program. Biological variability has to be excluded as far as possible from the analytical results, e. g. the analytical variation is the major one.

In specimen banking each sample should be divided in to a number of sub-samples. Each sub-samples taken for analysis from the bank must be discarded afterwards because thawing and freezing can influence the condition of the sample.

There is a need for the harmonization of the definitions of some of the terms used in analytical chemistry.
The workshop adhered to the definitions currently being considered by the International Union of Pure and Applied Chemistry, which are
— **Precision** (Reproducibility). The closeness of agreement between the results obtained by applying the experimental procedure several times under prescribed conditions in an interlaboratory collaborative study.
— **Accuracy.** The closeness of agreement between the true value and the mean results obtained by applying the experimental procedure a very large number of times. In practice this should involve as many results as possible, the total number being stated.

— **Limit of Detection.** The smallest concentration (or amount) of substance which can be re-

** see chapter IV under sample collection and transportation.
* see chapter IV under sample-preparation.

ported with a specified degree of certainty by a definite, complete analytical procedure.
- **Sensitivity.** The change in measured value resulting from a concentration change of one unit. These were considered specifically in relation to methods established by interlaboratory collaborative study and whilst values or limits for each were not discussed in detail the idea was put forward that in practice the assessment of precision (reproducibility) should be based on studies in which the procuct of (number of participating laboratories) times (samples examined) should be at least 30, the number of participating laboratories normally being at least six (but, in special cases only, never less than three); and the concentration range covered should be stated. It was recognized that it is not normally possible to maximize simultaneously all of the main parameters above; and that there were others which were not quantifiable (but no less important) including practicability and applicability.

V. 2.   ANALYTICAL METHODS

V. 2. 1. Methods for Toxic Elements

The importance of always considering the analytical aspects of all important steps from sampling, transportation, short or long-term storage, sample preparation, standardization and analysis, to data reduction shall be emphasized. Thus the analyst must continuously participate in all steps of the whole procedural chain, from sampling to data evaluation.

Although a number of analytical techniques for trace elements can be mentioned: atomic absorption spectrophotometry, neutron activation analysis, differential pulse stripping voltammetry, emission spectroscopy (spark-, flame- and plasma source), X-ray fluorescence spectroscopy and so on, each with their own advantages and limitations, only a few methods can be selected in a routine programme.
The selection criteria are:
- sensitivity
- accuracy
- reliability
- availability
- cost
- precision
- speed
- applicability to specific element and species
- minimal sample pretreatment
- multielement capabilities

Particularly for the determination of toxic elements in aqueous samples atomic absorption monitors for Hg are available commercially and automated voltammetric monitors for Pb, Cd, Cu and Zn in fresh and seawater have been developed recently; they allow the repeated analysis of the mentioned elements at the 0,1 μg/L level, or even lower, several times/hour in a preselected sequence during about one month, after which sevicing is needed.

Typical detection limits for the most important elements, if a specimen bank is considered, obtained with modern analytical methods are listed in Table 1. In order to reduce the possibility of systematic error, it is essential that two or more independent approaches be used unless a reference material in the matrix of interest is available for calibration. When independent methods are used, all aspects of the analytical chain should be performed independently wherever possible.

No single, specific method can be given for sample preparation, e. g. digestion, dissolution etc., for all materials, and the applicability of the various sample preparation methods must be evaluated before adoption for this type of work. In addition, the analytical procedure should include a statement concerning the format for reporting the analytical data, e. g., wet vs. dry weight basis.

Table 1
Typical relative detection limits for trace metals and other elements of environmental interest (aqueous solution for AAS and DPSV, non-interfering matrix for NAA).
Values in 10^{-6} g/kg, i. e. µg/kg

Element	AAS [1]		DPSV [2]	NAA [4]
	flame	electrothermal		
As	30	0.3	30[3]	1.0
Ba	15	1.5	–	0.1
Be	3	0.09	–	–
Ca	1.5	0.03	–	–
Cd	3	0.003	0.001	0.2
Co	15	0.15	30[3]	0.05
Cr	4.5	0.3	3	1.0
Cu	1.5	0.04	0.005	0.5
Fe	15	0.06	30	2.0
Hg	300	3.0	0.002	0.001
K	1.5	0.003	–	0.1
Mg	0.15	0.003	–	–
Mn	3	0.006	30[3]	0.5
Mo	30	0.09	100	0.3
Na	0.3	0.015	–	0.2
Ni	3	0.3	1	200
Pb	15	0.06	0.001	–
Se	150	1.5	0.05	0.02
Si	30	1.5	–	–
Sn	30	0.3	0.01	2.0
Sr	3	0.15	–	0.2
Ti	75	60	100	10
Tl	30	0.3	0.005	–
V	75	3	100	0.1
Zn	1.5	0.0015	0.05	0.1

1) Atomic absorption spectrophotometry: data from Welz, ‚Atomic Absorption spectroscopy‘, Verlag Chemie, 1976. For electrothermal AAS the values are calculated for a 50 µl sample, the graphite atomizer HGA 2100 or HGA 500 with automated sampling and instruments as PE 503 or 410; detection limit defined as three times the standard deviation of the respective noise level (IUPAC recommendation).

2) The values given for DPSV are practically evaluated determination limits, rather than computed detection limits based on the noise level. Instrumentation: PAR 174 with various mercury drop, mercury film and solid electrodes and cells (average cell volumes 20 ml).
3) Given values for direct differential pulse polarography or voltammetry, instead
4) Given values refer to a sample size of 0,5 g wet weight and a thermal neutron flux of 10^{13} $n \cdot cm^{-2} \cdot sec^{-1}$.

V. 2.2. Analytical Aspects of Halogenated Organic Compounds

There is no single system available which will screen samples for a large number of individual substances, although a number of useful multi-residue systems for analysis are available.
Organo-halogen compounds can be subdivided in several ways, according to the volatility, polar or non-polar nature and whether they are neutral, acidic or basic.
Relatively little residue data are available for volatile organo-halogenated compounds such as trichloroethane or bischloromethylether, due in part to the greater sensitivity needed for these. Such compounds have mainly been in water or aquatic systems.

Organo-halogen compounds of high polarity such as chlorophenols, choroanilines and chloroalkyl-phophates present same problems in analysis: even if they can be isolated by means of classical techniques they must be derivatised for gas chromatographic analysis, as otherwise recovery, sensitivity and reproducibility might be poor. Very polar organo-halogenated compounds to be analyzed such as trichloroacetic acid, which cannot be extracted by means of conventional solvents, can still present analytical problems, but adsorption techniques may be useful. The basic analytical technique used for the assay of most organo-halogenated compounds is gas chromatography with electron-capture detection, which is particularly sensitive to multi-halogenated substances (see Table 2). For identification of the specific residues the gas chromatograph can be coupled to a mass-spectrometer.
In routine analysis the mass-spectrometer should be equipped with a 3- or 4-channel multiple ion detector (MID).

Table 2   Detection Limits of Some Chloro-Compounds with ECD

Compound		Detection limit in pg
dichloromethane	$CH_2 Cl_2$	50
trichloromethane	$CHCl_3$	7
tetrachloromethane	CCl_4	0.002
1.1.2 trichloroethane	$CHCl_2 - CH_2 Cl$	3000
1.1.2 trichloroethene	$CCl_2 = CHCl$	50
1.1.1 trichloroethane	$CCl_3 - CH_3$	2

Although chromatographic columns, especially capillary columns, can separate a large number of substances, it is mostly essential to remove interfering co-extracted materials prior to analysis. With regard to the physical-chemical properties of the substances to be analyzed it is also an advantage to separate the halogenated compounds into some groups prior to gas chromatography. The various stages of the analysis are extraction, cleaning-up, pre-separation by GC, HPLC or co-destillation, GLC-analysis and finally (not always necessary) confirmation by MS.

62

Scheme 1

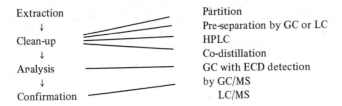

Extraction	Partition
Clean-up	Pre-separation by GC or LC
Analysis	HPLC
Confirmation	Co-distillation
	GC with ECD detection
	by GC/MS
	LC/MS

Extraction is normally carried out by partitioning into non-polar solvents in which both the halogenated compounds and lipids are very soluble. Steam distillation has been used for particular groups of compounds, but normally extraction is effected by direct partition into the solvent at room temperature or by Soxhlet or similar extractors.

The co-extracted lipids and pigments are removed either by partition between the non-polar and a polar solvent (e. g. hexane and acetonitrile) or more commonly by passing the crude extract through an adsorbent column (alumina, Florisil, charcoal) and eluting the halogenated residues with an appropriate solvent while the lipids, etc., remain on the column.

The pre-GLC separation is also performed on adsorbent columns (silica, Florisil, alumina), various solvents being used in succession to elute particular groups of substances, especially in the analysis of organochlorines. For example, hexachlorobenzene, aldrin, and PCB's can be separated from DDE, TDE, DDT, the haxachlorocyclohexanes, dieldrin and many other pesticides.

The latter group can be further subdivided if necessary. The extracts so obtained can then be injected directly into the gas chromatograph, the residues being identified by their elution times and their concentrations determined by comparison with reference standards. Different stationary phases on the GLC columns can provide variations, in retention times which assist in confirming the identity of residues. Alternative clean-up techniques have been used in some laboratories, primarily treatment with strong acids or alkalis to destroy the lipids.
Such methods result in the destruction of a few halogenated compounds, but are adequate if these particular compounds are of no interest.

Automation is not commonly used in environmental analysis, where both the nature and concentration of residues may vary very widely between samples, and in consequence the rate at which samples can be analyzed is very low, perhaps only 5 - 10 samples daily per operator.

Where the concentrations to be determined are low, as in most environmental samples, precautions must be taken to ensure that no contamination of the samples or apparatus causing interference in analysis, can arise from extraneous materials. For organochlorine compounds for example, the solvent (normally hexane) must be specially purified all adsorbents tested for freedom from electron-capturing contaminants, all glassware solvent-washed or otherwise pre-treated, and all plastic materials excluded from the entire procedure (plasticisers can interfere seriously in the analysis). In addition to EC-detection, coulometric detection may also be used for chlorinated substances. Some typical detection limits of some organo-halogen compounds are given in Table 3.

Table 3

Substance	Subtrate	Technique	Detection Limit kg/kg	
DDT and derivatives	Tissue	GLC	10^{-8}	(1 g sample)
			10^{-9}	(10 g sample)
Aldrin, Dieldrin	Water	GLC	10^{-8}	(1 litre sample)
Pentachlorophenol	Tissue	GLC	5.10^{-9}	(50 g sample)
	Water	GLC	10^{-8}	(200 ml sample)
PCB's	Tissue	GLC	2.10^{-8}	(1 g sample)
	Water	GLC	2.10^{-8}	(1 l sample)
Vinyl chloride	Food	GLC	5.10^{-8}	
	Water	GLC	5.10^{-9}	
2,4D 2,4,5-T Dichloroprop.	Grain	GLC	$2\text{-}5.10^{-8}$	
2,4 D 2,4,5-T 2,4 DB Dichloroprop. MCPA	Water	GLC	$2\text{-}25.10^{-8}$	
2,4 - D 2,4,5-T MCPA	Soil	GLC	5.10^{-9}	
TCDD	Soil, grass	GC/MS	10^{-8}	
	Fish,	GC/MS	5.10^{-9}	
	Water	GC/MS	10^{-10}	
	Milk	GC/MS	3.10^{-9}	
Chloroform	Grain	GLC	5.10^{-8}	
	Water	GLC	8.10^{-8}	
Carbon tetrachloride	Water	GLC	25.10^{-9}	
Trichloroethylene	Water	GLC	5.10^{-8}	

V.2.3 Other Organic Compounds

Many other organic compounds are of interest for ecotoxicological surveys, some of which are considered briefly below.

Generally, the basic steps in the analysis are the same as for organochlorine compounds: extraction, clean-up, pre-separation, analysis and confirmation.

Aliphatic and aromatic hydrocarbons may occur in environmental samples, the analytical approach is gas chromatography with a limit of detection varying down to 1 picogram/kg. Although for the most part chemically relatively stable substances, particularly at deep freeze storage temperatures, insufficient information is available regarding the stability of a large range of straight and branched chain aliphatic and aromatic compounds.

Polycyclic **Aromatic Hydrocarbons (PAH)**, some of which are carcinogenic to man. The most sensitive methods for the determination of the PAH are based on glass-capillary gas chromatography with flame-ionisation detector (FID). HPLC with fluorescence spectrometric detection can also be used but is less selective.

The FID has approximately the same sensitivity for all PAH compounds. Thus, the detection limit for benz(a)pyrene is about 0.2 ng.

Complete extraction is possible but samples which cannot be completely dissolved in any solvent require to be pretreated, either by digestion or by a lengthly series of extractions with different solvents.

All methods require a selective enrichment of the PAH from the material. The better the separation from other substances, the more reliable will be the quantitative aspects for a single PAH.

Nitrosamines. Analysis again involves a preliminary extraction or separation, a detection and estimation stage, followed by a confirmation of the identity of the species. The latter is of particular importance in trace nitrosamines work because of the wide variety of possible interferences and therefore calls for the use of GC - MS or the specially developed thermal energy analyser.

The initial extraction stage (steam distillation or solvent extraction) is followed by concentration into a small volume of solvent. The detection limit is about 0.1 microgram/kg. Since nitrosamines may be decomposed by light, sample and standard solutions should be stored in the dark.

V.3.   PROFILE AND FINGERPRINT METHODS

Complicated mixtures of chemicals may present great difficulty to the analyst. To follow biodegradation, bio-accumulation or the elimination of a single specific chemical may be particularly difficult. It may be possible to follow processes or changes of a profile of selected parameters which are able, to a certain extent, to characterize the mixture.

In this way, a non-specific method such as total organic carbon or total organic bound chlorine can give some overall information about the mixture. Determination of the toxicity of a sample toward a limited number of organisms may also provide a concise but useful profile. Such a procedure, now under development, may be described as ‚biological titration‘ in which the increase or decrease of acute and/or subchronic toxicity of the mixture is followed.

Fingerprint methods of analysis involve matching a pattern of responses in a chromatographic or other separatory system of detection in an extract, of the conversion products or, directly, on unknown substances. Examples include the pattern of n-alkanes from a seawater extract to characterise crude-oil contamination; or the GLC response after hydrolsysis of a glyceride mixture or the amino-acid pattern from a polypeptide. Pyrolysis followed by mass-spectrometry has been used similarly.

Pattern recognition is a much wider concept, based on general mathematical principles. It can be applied to such multiresponse analytical techniques. Kowalski and Bender have discussed the general approach to the problem of predicting an obscure property of a collection of substances from indirect measurements, for example the prediction of atomic composition from emission spectrometry; or the molecular structure from NMR spectrometry; or the reactivity of a mixed system.

Linear and non-linear mapping techniques are used, both for single and multi-source data, the former being well-established for mass, infrared, NMR and gamma spectrometry. Pattern recognition techniques have also been used for the identification of oil spills and have an obvious potential for the ‚recognition' of unkown compounds.

The fatty acid characteristics of the glycerides from natural oils have long been used as a basis for the identity and commercial quality of such oils.

Pattern recognition based on chemical constituents has also been widely used for the characterisation of distilled alcoholic beverages and various fruit products and Kowalski has attempted to classify wines according to their trace metal profiles.

Such techniques could be useful in environmental monitoring to draw attention to changes in residue patterns and the need to investigate new or unknown residues.

V. 4.   PARTLY AND FULLY AUTOMATIZED ANALYTICS

The automation of analysis is developing progressively, but for monitoring purposes is mainly confined to routine use.
- Atomic absorption spectrometry can be combined with a sample-changer and automatic injection while the computer reads the signals and prints the concentrations.
- Neutron activation analysis is automated to a very high degree: the counting of the samples and the γ - spectra evaluation is now computerized completely.
- Gas-liquid chromatography with automatic injection, sophisticated integrators or coupling to the computer gives the results directly related to the standards used in the procedure.
- Auto-analyzer equipment with sample identification and print-out of the concentrations is available.
- Mass-spectrometers, coupled to GC and a dedicated minicomputer can store mass-spectra of all components of a mixture and produce those which are of interest later. These spectra can be compared with a library of mass-spectra of Cyphernetics for identification.

At the moment only mercury monitors are commercially available. A monitor for lead, cadmium, copper and zinc for ranges down to 10^{-10} kg/kg has been developed and will be commercially available very soon.

V. 5.   STANDARDISATION AND QUALITY CONTROL

Residue analysis calls for a high degree of professional competence and experience and, since it is also expensive, should as far as possible be centralized. Steps should be taken to ensure that inter-analyst comparisons are made using certified reference materials.
Minimization of interanalyst variation coupled to proper control of instrument calibration procedures and frequent checks against standards should assure the high degree of quality control required for the specimen bank program. It may be useful to select a very precisely described method, preferably one which has been the subject of a successful collaborative analytical study using the same instrumentation, with built-in controls and using standards prepared for and distributed from a central point. With experience it should be possible to achieve a standard deviation of the

order of 10 % or even better. It is also advisable to check a routine method by another independent method from time to time. Thus, results by an AAS method could be checked by neutron-activation methods.

VI. PROGRAMME DESIGN AND ORGANIZATIONAL ASPECTS

This chapter covers the various types of programmes that can be initiated, the concepts central to the design of a programme, practical organizational aspects, and the advantages of collaborative programmes at international level.

For the pollutants and indicator specimens listed in chapter III, the monitoring of environmental materials and pilot specimen banking may be initiated immediately. For other pollutants and environmental materials, for which information is lacking further research is necessary. Both for the monitoring of environmental materials and specimen banking, design and operation will depend significantly upon the objectives, the specimens and the pollutants of concern.

Taxa selection and procedures for collecting, preserving, transporting, storing, and analyzing samples are complex decisions that depend upon the materials to be monitored and the relation of these materials to the biological populations chosen for study. Populations are dynamic entities, composed of individuals, and possessing group characteristics such as abundance, seasonal changes, movements, age structure, trophic level, genetic make-up, and rates of natality, mortality, and reproduction. Each of these characteristics as well as others affects the choice of candidate specimens. Also, subject populations must be examined with respect to the pollutant categories of interest (if identified). These considerations include: (1) the likelihood, frequency, and levels of exposure; (2) the transport, accumulation, transformation, stability, and persistence of the pollutant (s) within a population; (3) interactions which might potentiate or antagonize biological activity; and (4) sensitivity.

VI. 1. GOAL AND OBJECTIVES

The goal for environmental monitoring specimen banking is to provide information useful in the protection of living aquatic and terrestrial resources and their habitats.

The objectives for environmental monitoring

include: 1. The establishment of baselines
2. The monitoring of effects with active and passive Monitoring programmes.
3. The monitoring of trends (i. e. changes from baselines in biota and the physical environment) with active and passive Monitoring programmes. Genetic variability of wild populations and their daily and seasonal population fluctuations allow conclusions to be drawn about the quality of a particular area only if the sampling programme is structured either to assess to ,control' soures of variation.
Naturally death rates and pollutant accumulation can only indicate relative toxicity in regard to human populations and thus can only reflect a relative risk in certain sites.
4. The elucidation of movement of materials (contaminants or microconstituents) through foodchains and partitioning between the physical and biotic components of the ecosystems. Food-webs are the basic structure of energy and matter transfer in ecosystems. This is why we think that the analysis of such food-webs is necessary to the actual pollution burden and potential risk to biotic resources and for humans. But area-related analyses of food-webs — at least in the Federal Republic of Germany — have not progressed beyond their early stages. It is thus obvi-

ous that exclusive consideration of the benzpyrene content in the air without an account of its derivatives in the human food chain (e. g. smoked herring) leads to area evaluation for which ‚air' is a factor with unjustified decisiveness. This thought can be extended at least to recognize that all the substances we can measure have already been used as ‚key substances' for burdening prognoses for air and water; the obvious question about transfer of substances within food chains, however, has not even been considered. We know that the accumulation and breakdown of pollutants in individuals, populations and food chains can be accomplished in very different ways according, for example, to species, age and sex.

5. To use changes in trends or movement along specific pathways to provide an early warning or ‚red flag' that some, possibly deleterious, event has occured in the environment.

6. To use the foregiong in the regulation of use of the aquatic environment for agricultural, industrial, and domestic purposes and for waste disposal.

The objectives for specimen banking include:

1. To retain, for indefinite periods, samples of biota and the physical environment which can be used to:

   a) Measure levels of materials which are not now but may be deemed important in the future

   b) Remeasure materials now found in samples when new, more accurate, analytical tools become available

   c) Measure amounts of materials at sites or strata or in biota which are not now of concern but which may receive materials in the future

   d) Provide a historial documentation of changes in materials or microconstituents, of a toxic nature, which may be important in future litigation, legislation or regulation.

Environmental Specimen Banking Systems exist (Pilot projects) in the United States, in France and in the Federal Republic of Germany.

Oak Ridge National Laboratories, under the auspices of the U. S. Environmental Protection Agency, completed a Environmental Specimen Bank survey in 1975. This survey identified 675 environmental specimen collections maintained by various institutions or investigators throughout the United States, including the following types of materials: atmospheric, geological, human tissue, animal tissue other than human, plant tissue, water. Taxonomic collections were not included in this survey. Results of the survey indicate that very few collections are suitable for retrospective chemical analyses because of the collection, preparation and storage techniques being utilized; many of these collections were not maintained for such purposes. However, the survey alerted the scientific community to a national interest in their collections; it caused some investigators to reexamine their practices; and, since the survey data base is being maintained, the NESB offers opportunity for information exchange among scientists who may find access to specimens or data from other locations useful.

The U. S. Environmental Protection Agency and the National Bureau of Standards are working to establish a National Environmental Specimen Bank. This system is intended to provide ‚credible real time monitoring data for an environmental early warning system and well preserved and documented environmental samples for future retrospective analyses'.

In order to avoid a possible confounding factor associated with a long term trend and/or effects (monitoring) program, the maintenance of a **living specimen bank** system should also be considered.

The elimination of genetically sensitive individuals from a population tendes to simplify any given gene pool. Selection of more and more tolerant individuals follows slow increases in insult burdens. Thus, the dying off (or reduced reproductive capacities) of sensitive individuals may reduce the genetic heterogeniety within the population and errors in evaluating pollutant effects may follow. Thus, good accumulators of a specific pollutant may do so to toxic levels, die off, and no longer be available for monitoring. Thus, pollutant impact may be erroneously evaluated.

A good example of such an occurrence is the loss of sensitive ponderosa pine in the San Bernardino Mountains of Southern California. Higher levels of pollutant are currently needed to produce symptoms in the remaining population and ,impact' could be interpreted as being reduced. Such a situation is possible also in the case of eastern white pine that occurs throughout much of the northeastern United States.

A **live** clonal bank of specimens may therefore of value. This living bank would be composed of known sensitive plants clonally propagated. Individuals of differing sensitivity responses (sensitive intermediate, tolerant; low accumulators to high accumulators) should be maintained for reference into the future. Thus, present ,baselines' of genetic material may be of assistance in evaluating future burdening of the ecosystem (trends) and associated impacts (effects).

Various uses may also be made of pollen that has been naturally stored for thousands of years as compared to contemporary banking for future references. Such a natural ,banking' system may be made available through lake bottom cores, etc., for many different types of organisms.

The participants concurred that meaningful monitoring and banking must occur over time spans of at least decades; government funding/sponsorshop must therefore be projected for at least one decade.

1. The objectives of specific monitoring and speciemen banking programs will dictate the exact length of the program; some programs concerned with a site specific release of a certain material may require only a year or two, whereas the atmospheric input of a substance such as lead (Pb) will require decades to document the integrated effects at several sites.
2. In addition to the actual research must be done in regard to the efficacy of these; i. e. does storage effect the levels of a particular material in various samples?

Species, materials and pollutants to be selected for monitoring and specimen banking must be based upon criteria which are developed for specific programs or geographic areas (cf. chapter III)

1. Species should be selected on the basis criteria which include feeding types or adaptation to specific ecological niches. (ecosystemic correlations)
2. Pollutants to be monitored must be carefully considered, taking into account those that are presently known to be deleterious to biota and those deemed to be potentially harmful; areas in the U. S. where kepone and PCB's were later found had been monitored for other substances but the kepone and PCB's were not found before they had accumulated in biota to significant levels.

Monitoring of environmental materials and specimen banking may be undertaken by combining new programs with those already existing to reduce cost and increase efficiency. Subsamples from those specimens already being collected in the National Pesticide Monitoring Programs (starling and duck wings) could thereby be stored under appropriate conditions for long periods.

If additional collections are to be initiated for the purposes of the proposed monitoring and specimen banking program, there very likely will be problems in obtaining the specimens and processing them for storage. Problems will be especially significant if tissues, rather than whole bodies, are to be stored. It may not be feasible to store separately all of the tissues that may be desirable for analysis because of the amount of work required to remove, weigh, and properly package the tissues for storage in containers that are suitable for storage of tissues intended for analysis of a broad array of pollutants.

Statistical and biomathematic requirements for a valid program should be given careful consideration. Procedures used in the National Pesticide Monitoring Program and in the Organization for Economic Co-Operation and Development (OECD) program should be viewed in regard to these requirements.

The types of data being currently collected under the auspices of the National Atmospheric Deposition Program (U. S. A.) could be usefully incorporated into any environmental monitoring program that might be implemented. Participating institutions are: Science Education Advisory/ Agricultural Research, U. S. D. A.; United States Geological Survey; United States Department of Agriculture – Forest Service; United States Environmental Protection Agency.

The objectives of the program are to collect and identify the chemical constituents found in wet and dry depositions from areas typical of regions of the United States. Samples are collected weekly and analyzed at the Illinois State Water Survey Laboratory, Champaign/Urbana, Illinois, and residuals are maintained in storage at that facility for future reference banking.

Biological effects studies are also being designed in support of the project in order to utilize the collected data on an immediate use basis.

Programmes must be well organized prior to implementation. The following is a suggest outline for the specimen banking program:

1. **Administration of program; key component is the planning group:**
   a) Toxicologists
   b) Ecologists
   c) Chemists
   d) Statisticians
   e) Epidemiologist; relate distribution and abundance of materials to ‚disease syndromes'
2. **Sampling**
   a) Species determination
   b) Frequency of collection
   c) Location of sampling; stations, areas, ecosystems, strata
3. **Sample handling**
   a) Instruments; free of contaminants of significance
   b) Containers; free of contaminants;
      prevent oxidation or other changes in samples

c) Transportation; eliminate change in temperature; result in most rapid transit

4. **Sample preparation techniques**
   a) Specific protocols for organics
   b) Specific protocols for inorganics
   c) Common protocols for organics and inorganics
5. **Analytical techniques**
   a) Specific protocols for organics
   b) Specific protocols for inorganics
6. **Storage protocols**
   a) for organics
   b) for inorganics
   c) Common protocols for both organics and inorganics
   d) Periodic research (analyses) to determine if stored samples change in quality and to improve techniques
7. **Data accumulation**
   a) Storage of data
   b) Retrieval of data
   c) Multivariate analyses of data
8. **Legal significance and requirements**
9. **Decision making and data use.**

For arthropods preparation and storage procedures often incorporate one or more of the following
— Dried specimens (including lyophilization)
— chemical digestion in acid or base
— dissolution or immersion in solvent
— preservatives
— evacuated and sealed containers
— whole or partial organisms
— homogenates
— rapid freezing or
— other techniques designed to ensure that the specimen will continue to reflect the original concentrations of the substances of interest.

Drawn from work on honey bees the following recommendations are presented on obtaining, handling, and storing insect specimens prior to residue analyses for pesticides and trace elements:
— A minimum sample size of 100 gms wet weight should be obtained for pesticide determinations; 3 gms for trace element determinations.
— All insect specimens should be at the same development stage egg, larvae, pupa, or adult. For honey bees, further adult distictions include nurse bees, foragers, and guards.
— As far as feasible, all sampling, storage, and analytical apparatus should be of glass or stainless steel if the specimens are being tested for organic pesticides; but all this equipment should be of appropriate plastic such as polyethylene if inorganic compounds and trace elements are of primary interest.
— All specimens should be placed in freezer chests under dry ice as soon as they are obtained (we aspirate living bees into temporary containers) to both kill the insects and prevent decomposition.

- All specimens should be transferred to permanent storage containers as soon as possible and handled as few times as possible.
- All specimens should be kept in dark storage until analyzed at -30° C for short-term, -80° C or less for long-term.
- All equipment must be scrupulously cleaned before use. If plastic equipment must be re-used, it should be cleaned with detergent solutions, washed with reagent grade acids, and rinsed with distilled and deionized water as described by TARAS et al. (1971). All glass and metal equipment should be cleaned detergent solutions, rinsed in distilled and deionized water, then with reagent grade acetone and hexane (FDA Analytical Manual, 1975).
- Specimens intended for pesticide determinations should be stored in glass jars capped with aluminium foil; for inorganic or trace element determinations, samples should be kept in clean, sterile, plastic Whirl Paks ® (only for short-term storage).

These recommendations are intended to be illustrative and not definitive. Equipment and containers made or lined with plastics which incorporate little or no plastizers, catalysis residues, or other additives (Teflon ®, Teldar ®, or laboratory grade polyethylene) might be usable for a wide range of applications. This should be verified. Borosilicate glass and quartz should be tested further. If materials are used as surface coatings in containers, the coating must be examined periodically for peeling and cracks which could lead to contamination from the base container material.

From the scientific and experimental point of view the programme as a whole — which includes sampling, sample pretreatment, realtime monitoring, analysis and banking — may be regarded as a very difficult task. But the programme is necessary and methods for collection, preservation and storage of Environmental materials are well established and do not pose insuremountable problems. Thus, operationally specimen banking will be constrained solely that deposit selectively e. g. heavy metals and/or protect sensitive enzyme systems binding the pollutants to proteins and thus reducing their toxicity. Consequently, if the area-specific food chains are not analyzed, residue analyses with birds, game animals, or invertebrates can only show how dangerous a pollutant is for a particular species but cannot indicate the burdening of an area. Goshawks (**Accipiter gentilis**), which mostly live on rabbits in one area, must necessarily have different PCB-contents than those of a different area where their main prey is wood pigeons (**Columba palumbus**).
For short food chains continuous analyses can be carried out; for food-webs, however, they can only be done sensibly wia continuous ecosystem analysis and monitoring.
The Environmental Specimen Bank concept has to be supplemented by an ecological monitoring programme, for which only those specimens can be used that have been collected within the framework of ecosystemic complex research in representative regions of a country (cf. chapter III).

VI. 2 STATISTICAL AND BIOMATHEMATICAL REQUIREMENTS

One of the most basic and important of monitoring and banking problems is how many specimens to collect to obtain useful results. The vast body of data on important pollutants (such as metals and halogenated hydrocarbons) show that body burdens do not follow normal or Gaussian distributions and have in general a more or less pronounced positive skew. The importance of this finding must be taken into account in the design of future sampling programmes and in the interpretation of the results.

When undertaking a programme for a specific pollutant or group of pollutants, the available data should be examined to estimate the ranges of expected levels and the variability for specific population groups and systems. If this information is not available, then a sub-sampling (50 to 100 samples if the population is homogeneous) should be carried out to give a first estimate of the pollutant distribution. The data on ranges of pollutants, or the results from the sub-samples should then be discussed with a statistician. The statistician should also be given a definition of the programme aim, the parameters under consideration for the determination of the sample size etc., and how the data will be treated. Account will also have to be taken of the analytical and contamination errors as well as the biological variablity.

Descriptive statistics must include reliable measures of central tendency and of frequency distribution. In cases where data are not normally distributed and cannot be made so by transformation, measures of central tendency and of dispersion should be calculated by appropriate non-parametric means. These descriptive statistics may include, but are not limited to, arithmetic mean, geometric mean, median, maximum and minimum and dispersion (percentils, standard deviation, etc.). Some indication should be made as to the use and definition of ‚trace' amounts.

The advice of statisticians is vital for the application of correct statistical techniques to ensure the best possible interpretation of the data. The results of statistical evaluations must be assessed in conjunction with biological implications. Extrapolation beyond the range of the original data should be done with caution.

VI. 3   GENERAL GUIDELINES

Some general principles and guidelines for the design of all programmes dealing with the collection and analysis of biological specimens follow:

— studies should only be started when the overall purpose and objectives have been clearly identified, as these will determine the type of programme;

— expert statistical advice must be available from the outset to ensure that suitable statistical principles are incorporated into the design and that statistically valid methods are employed for the handling and interpretation of data;

— The biological specimens selected should be representative of the target system and body burdens of interest;

— detailed pertinent information regarding environmental conditions at collection sites recorded;

— special attention should be given to specimen collection, with respect to the use of adequately experienced and appropriately trained staff, choice of container and transport conditions;

— storage conditions for the specimen will be determined by the pollutant and type of specimens being studied;

— suitable analytical methods should be chosen and careful attention given to the availability of laboratory services;

– a protocol should exist for data analysis, evaluation, distribution and for further investigation or action if indicated.

VI. 4. RECOMMENDATIONS FOR FURTHER RESEARCH

In past monitoring programmes there were often difficulties in selecting representative indicator organisms, regions and seasons for valid interpretation; the necessity of including other biological information and a deficit in basic ecological facts finished these projects. A representation of ‚Basic Ecological Concepts' implies a thorough study of autecological, synecological and ecosystemic findings and discussions with research teams. The environmental specimen bank concept must be supplemented by an ecological monitoring programme, for which only those specimens can be used that have been collected within the framework of ecosystematic complex research in representative regions of a country.

The species for a specimen bank pilot programme should be selected with regard to existing monitoring programmes.
The options are:
– sample collection procedure known
– sample preparation for analysis known
– combined programmes reduce the total cost.

Improved interpretation and application of monitoring and retrospective biological data related to significance of altered uptake, retention and transformation rates of chemical pollutants.

Development of standard or reference measures of persistence both at individual organism and ecosystem levels. Model species and ecosystems should be established to make early work manageable.

Understanding of factors influencing process of biological availability, food conversion efficiences, transformations, retention times, trophic relationships, and altered food web dynamics.

Pharmacokinetic studies in both field and laboratory for several class compounds in a wide array of taxa. These should include comparative analyses of sensitive and resistant species.

Correlative studies between dose-response and exposure (monitoring) data to include early functional, subclinical of prepathological changes) are needed to assess significance of pollutant concentration trends.

Determine the relationship between environmental exposure and pollutant levels in accessible indicator specimens. Research is needed to determine the concentrations of critical elements within a system at which adverse effects begin to occur.

Knowledge of pollutant, chemical and biological interactions including disease predisposition and naturally occuring toxics is desirable. It is also important to elucidate the mechanisms for adaptation, resistance and limits of resiliency.

Modifiers of pollutant transport, uptake, transformation and effects need study. These includes nutritional influences, climatic stress, modes of exposure, pollutant interactions and physiological status, age and organism stage of development.

VII. COST ESTIMATION

VII. 1. MONITORING ENVIRONMENTAL MATERIALS

The actual costs for planning and implementing programmes for the collection and analysis of environmental materials will vary considerably according to the objectives and magnitude of the programmes, the country where it is carried out and the facilities available; also reading the working papers of this International Workshop on Monitoring Environmental Materials and Specimen Banking one will find a wide range in the cost for estimates for collection, storage and chemical analysis which are not always quite comparable.

Generally, the costs of monitoring programmes are depending largely on the following variables:

- according to the objectives of the programme, e. g. magnitude of programme, scope of pollutants of interest, scope of ecological characterization of the studied areas and systems; nature of the environmental specimens chosen and their locations.
- according to the geographic coverage
- according to the quantity and number of samples to be collected and analyzed,
- according to the facilities available,
- according to the availability of trending people.

Nevertheless, a discussion of some of the variables, however, may serve as a guide as to what may be expected depending on the programme undertaken.

In a programme having broad geographic coverage, one of the most costly items is collection of the samples (aquatic ecosystems for example: if the stations are some distances offshore and ocean-going vessels are needed or if the stations are inshore the amount of coast-line to be covered). The collection costs cán be reduced by assuming that local personnel at each site will collect and freight the samples to a central location. If project personnel have to be sent to the sites for collection and handling, the cost will increase considerably due to the travel involved. Nevertheless, the full costs of collecting samples vary widely between the terrestrial, freshwater and coastal and open sea environment.

Regarding open sea sampling the cost should be increased significantly. Nevertheless, joint programmes should decrease the sampling costs.

In a programme having a broad ecological characterization of collection areas and ecosystems − a necessary supporting programme in biological monitoring and banking − the costs therefore are remarkable. It was estimated that for the ecological characterization of an area system in the Federal Republic of Germany an average DM 1 Million per year and per each system (aquatic, terrestrial, urbanic) was needed.

Regarding the quantity and number of samples to be collected it was found that the costs per sample for a given area system were usually not direct proportional to the quantity and number of samples collected and stored, but regarding the analytical costs there was a proportionality.

Regarding the above mentioned points the following rough figures can give only an impression of the amounts of money involved. The costs of monitoring could be sub-divided under the following headings:

a) programme design and area characterization
b) locating, identifying and collecting samples
c) preservation, transport and storage
d) subsampling, sample preparation and analysis
e) calculating data and reporting on standard forms
f) computer punching and processing, including statistician's time
g) executive and administrative group operations and time.

Regarding the point a) it was estimated that for the programme design and for the ecological characterization of an area system in average DM 1 Million per year and per each system (aquatic, terrestrial, urbanic) (incl. ca. 45 % personnel costs) was needed.

Excluding the point a) and regarding the points b) and c) and knowing the experiences of the OECD programmes and the past and current monitoring programmes in the United States and the Federal Republic of Germany it was estimated that on therefore in average 10 % - 15 % of the other annual total costs must be spended.

Regarding the points e), f) and g) these costs amounted to a further 5 % - 10 % of the total expenditure.

Analytical costs were easier to assess, as some countries purchased service from commercial laboratories and others monitor such costs routinely. Analytical costs included staff salaries, chemicals and solvents, overheads and a fraction of the purchase price of equipment appropriately amortised. General it was estimated, that the average analytical costs are 80 % - 85 % of the total costs of the monitoring programmes.

Regarding the cost aspects of chemical analysis in the following an estimation in greater detail is given including overheads costs of instruments and laboratory operating. There will only be referred to analysis which can be done in routine; development of methods for assay of a special chemical is not included.

Trace element analysis

— Multi-element analysis with neutronactivationanalysis, detection limits in ppm, in average
  12 - 15 concentrations — DM 250/sample
— Neutronactivationanalysis with chemical separations, detection limits in ppb - range, first
  concentration — DM 150
— each further concentration in the same sample — DM 60
— Atomic absorption spectrometry analysis detection limits in ppb - range — DM 60/concentration
  in sub - ppb - range — DM 80/concentration

Organo-halogenated compounds

— Assay for pesticides and PCB — DM 300
— Determination of chlorophenols (in ppb - range) — DM 160
— Determination of chloro-parafins — DM 400

Other organic compounds

— Petroleum derivatives, hydrocarbons, fingerprints of alkanes — DM 350

— Profile of PAH, including clean-up	DM1.800
— Nitrosamines	DM 300 - 1.000

VII. 2. SPECIMEN BANKING

At the present time, it is very difficult to estimate costs of specimen banking, as the techniques solving this task are not clearly recognized. There is only little information on the cost of specimen banking except for developmental aspects and pilot bank programmes in the U.S.A. and the Federal Republic of Germany, but nevertheless, the introductory remarks made in VII. 1. Monitoring Environmental Materials are also valid in view of specimen banking.

The build-up of a research programme regarding ecological characterization of collection areas and ecosystems is also a necessary supporting programme for specimen banking. Costs of sample collection and of analysis in banked materials will be roughly the same as in monitoring programmes, but it is anticipated that a major cost for specimen bank programmes in contrast to biological monitoring will be for the storage of specimens.

Also increasing costs due to increasing sample number in the bank must be calculated. Once, at the beginning of the work, it was estimated that investments of about DM 1.5 Million must be required. But nevertheless, one of the highest parts is manpower. Thus, it is obvious that even the most sophisticated cooling system for the bank (e. g. liquid nitrogen) will not markedly increase the total annual costs as much as the steady increase of personnes costs. Another reason for the relatively high personnel costs (USA ca. 40 % - 45 %, in the Federal Republic of Germany ca 45 % - 50 % of the total costs) is also that a well trained and experienced staff has to be very carefully selected to guarantee the best possible performance of the projects as a whole.

VII. 3. CONCLUSIONS

It is thus clear that cost estimates in greater detail can be made only for very specific programmes, be it ‚monitoring environmental materials‘ or ‚specimen banking‘, in a given country.
However, one can estimate the different steps necessary to implement any programme of this nature, and the type of requirements in terms of staff, technical equipment, space facilities, administrative assistance etc. The recommendations made in chapter VI can also be used as a framework for budget items to be considered in developing a programme (e. g. quality control of analytical procedure).

International collaboration will undoubtedly be beneficial in providing a more cost effective and expeditions acquisition of high quality date for use in resolving problems of mutual interest.

Increased cost effectiveness will result, among other things, from:

— international collaboration
— combination of existing monitoring programmes and pilot specimen bank programmes
— centralized laboratory analytical services and local personnel collecting and handling samples
— standardized reference material repository
— comparability of data for expediting decisions
— avoidance of duplication in resolving research problems of common interest.

The combined costs of monitoring environmental materials and specimen banking are genrally negligible in comparison to the costs of damage associated with existing adverse effects on man and his environment caused by environmental pollution.

VIII. ETHICAL AND LEGAL CONSIDERATIONS

There are differences among various countries and sometimes between states within the same country, with respect to the regulations, customs and restrictions that must be considered in planning and implementing programmes for the collection, storage and analysis of biological specimens.

Experience with Western European and North American countries participating in the OECD studies has indicated that, in respect of data obtained from wildlife sampling and analysis, there are no problems of confidentiality. The selection of species for analysis could be limited by laws protecting wildlife, but difficulties arising from such laws are unlikely in view of the need to choose species which are abundant. However, there may be restrictions (close seasons) on the capture of some bird or fish species.

Storage of specimens within the country of origin should not present difficulties, but any requirements to transport specimens across frontiers for analysis or specimen banking may infringe laws of import and export, and of disease control enforcement.

Summarized in planning and implementing programmes for the collection, storage and analysis of biological specimens the following regulations, customs and restrictions must be considered within the borders of the **Federal Republic of Germany**:

1. Environmental research supplies the scientific findings which are indispensable as aides for decision-making and as basis for measures taken in the range of environmental policies. In particular extensive data is required on the exposure of chemicals to man and his natural environment. When compiling such data, researchers are dependent upon specimen sampling in the natural environment (for the purpose of subsequent laboratory analysis). Soil and air as well as plants and animals may be subject to such sampling (environmental sampling).

2. Under law in force there are indeed a number of regulations which empower environmental authorities or their authorized representatives to draw samples. However, all these authorizations have in common that they only allow sampling in order to check the observance of the respective environmental regulation, thus serving as control of law enforcement. Laws governing environmental protection, in turn, describe as their objective the protection of the natural environment from already recognized strains and dangers caused by certain hazardous substances. There are, however, no provisions made under existing law for the authorization to take samples for mere research purposes, i. e. for the determination of environmental strains and hazards without further legitimate purposes.

3. Therefore, environmental authorities or their authorized representatives are denied sovereign action when taking environmental samples for mere research purposes. In this respect they are governed — principally just like everyone else — by the respective regulations of civil law or public law.

3.1. The barriers imposed by private law for the drawing of environmental samples result primarily from the regulations of the law of things, in particular those of private property, and possibly those of other real rights.

3.1.1. Private property of an object entitles the owner to exclude the exertion of even the slight-
est influence on the object, i. e. to also prohibit sampling of the object, unless his claim
is barred by a law or by the rights of a third party, thus committing him to tolerance (§§
903, 1004 Civil Code of the Federal Republic of Germany). A general legal obligation of
the proprietor to tolerate environmental sampling, however, does not exist.
Particularly the public welfare-related objective of research persued when drawing environmental samples does not obligate the proprietor to tolerate sampling. Therefore, the
environmental authorities or their authorized representatives require the consent of the
proprietor when intending to transfer property of an object's sample.

3.1.2. The same applies if the drawing of samples affects (yet) other real rights besides property.
Also in these cases sampling is only permissible with the consent of the respective legal
proprietor. This should especially be observed in the case of sampling by which real rights
of usufruct (so-called servitudes) are affected, as well as in the case of sampling of animals
and other things which are governed by shooting and fishing rights and which thus are –
with the exemption of free fishing in the coastal seas – under the exclusive authority of
the respective person or body authorized to pursue hunting or fishing.

3.2. Especially those regulations dealing with the protection of the natural environment are
considered to be pertinent barriers of the public law for the drawing of environmental
samples.

3.2.1. Among them is, in particular, the Nature Conservation Law which allows sampling in especially protected parts of nature and countryside or of especially protected species of
animals and plants only in extracts.

3.2.2. With respect to the sampling of animals, those regulations resulting from the Animal Protection Law as well shooting and fishing regulations pertaining to game and fish preservation have to be observed.

3.2.3. For the drawing of water, soil and plant samples in the range of waters, the Water Supply
Law is a relevant barrier. According to it , all substantial samplings in inland waters (surface and underground waters) are principally subject to authorizations.

4. Partly divergent from the legal maxims outlined above, the following particularities are in
effect for sampling in the range of public roads, waters, the seashore as well as wood and
farmland.

4.1. If sampling in the range of public roadland impairs its public use (= road traffic), a special
license for utilization based on public law is required. If an impairment of public use does,
for once, not exist, only the approval ot the street owner under private law is needed for
sampling.

4.2. Within the range of waters the proprietor has to tolerate all uses of his waters for which
an authorization under public law has been granted or which exceptionally do not require
an authorization, unrestricted only for the drawing of aqueous samples in surface waters.
Sampling of solid matter (soil and plants), however, need not be tolerated by the proprietor within these waters. By no means does his obligation to tolerate sampling refer to

things which, without being part of the water, must be used for the purpose of sampling. Sampling conducted from the banks of a surface water and sampling of ground water on real estate is, therefore, always permissible with consent of the proprietor only.

The legal status is quite different with respect to coastal waters, where sampling is not restricted by environmental authorities or their representatives neither under public nor private law.

4.3. In the range of seastores the sampling of soil and plants to a larger extent always requires an official authorization.

4.4. In woods and farmland the drawing of certain plant samples to a small extent may be tolerated under common law.

Summarized in planning and implementing programmes for the collection, storage and analysis of biological specimens the following regulations, customs and restrictions must be considered within the borders of the **United States of America.**

1. Laws affecting various stages of sampling and archiving

1.1. Access to Samples:

Amost always, the material that you want to sample belongs to someone else. Before you proceed to take it, you need to consider (1) who it belongs to, (2) what is its value to the owner, (3) who will be helped by your taking it, (4) who will be hurt by your taking it, and (5) what are the rights of the persons and things involved. Except in rare instances[1] you safely may assume that you have no rights to the materials that you want to sample unless they are granted to you specifically by the owner.

Non-human tissue samples can become very controversial subjects of adversary proceedings and therefore the sampler should be assured that sampling itself is performed under legal circumstances. Materials sampled will be owned privately or by municipal, state, or federal government. The sampler must assure a right to enter the sampling area as well as permission to sample. Ideally both permissions should be obtained in some written form from the person, corporation, or governmental body involved. In addition, certain species are protected under law to varying extents, and appropriate licensing may be required to take them.[2] Both state and federal government concern themselves with licensing the taking of finfish, shellfish, and wildlife. No species listed on the U. S. Endangered Species list[3] may be taken for any purposes by any U. S. Department of the Interior. In general, federal involvement in various hunting and fishing licensure is indirect, regulating water quality and chemical contamination of flesh, whereas state governments issue licenses regulating amount of material which may be taken, locations and means of taking, and times during which for taking plant and animal material in normally prohibited times, amounts, or places, if the material is to be used exclusively for purposes of research or monitoring. Ordinarily such licenses are issued by the state's Department of Fish and Game or its nominal equivalent.

1/eg   (a) You own the material, (b) You are acting as an agent of a duly empowered governmental agency rightfully using its police power, or (c) no one owns the material and it is outside any governmental jurisdiction.

2/eg   The National Marine Fisheries Service in the U. S. Department of Commerce administers regulations and issues permits required by the Marine Mammal Protection Act of 1972 (16 U. S. C 1361) and the Endangered Species Act of 1973 (16 U. S. C. 1531).

3/   The Endangered Species List is updated and republished annually by the U. S. Fish and Wildlife Service in the Department of the Interior. The most recent list appeared in the Federal Register for December 11, 1978.

1. 2.   Sampling Methods:

Two concerns arise in regard to method. First, the method of obtaining samples must not be prohibited by law. For example, certain states prohibit taking of specific shellfishes by SCUBA divers. Poisoning and blasting also are usually prohibited methods of sampling – although in special circumstances where such non-discriminatory methods can be justified, state exemptions may be obtained. Other methodological prohibitions concern use of specified (or non-prohibited) firearms, net-types, gear-types, or means of transportation while sampling. Again, reasonable and justifiable exemptions from such laws or regulations may be obtained from appropriate state authorities. Such laws and regulations commonly apply to organisms of commercial or recreational importance, leaving the samplers of viruses, bacteria, protozoa, liches, and many non-flowering plants much to their own devices. In the U. S., information gained by government agents by illegal means can not be used in a court of law in a proceeding against a person from whom the data or information was taken.[4]

Second, sampling methods should be scientifically sound and thoroughly documented. This is particularly important in tissue banking because the materials archived probably will be investigated well after sampling and not by the original sampler. Thus information on sampling time, place, circumstances and method must be exact and complete for the sake of highly reliable information. Reliability is extremely important if the data obtained from banked tissues are used in formulation of public policy (laws, regulations, standards, or criteria); and doubly so if they become the subject of adversary proceedings.

1. 3.   Transport of Samples:

Transport of non-human tissue samples is usually subject to question only at international borders. National concerns about importation of disease or disease vectors and exportation of commercially valuable, rare, or endangered species are reflected in federal laws concerning transfer of animal species or agricultural materials across a national border. Such prohibitions are not always obvious to the scientist, who may well understand the problems of transporting venomous reptiles or virulent microorganisms but need think twice about the impact of certain plant imports upon agricultural economy. Arrangements for international transport of even tissues samples should be made with appropriate customs and consular officials well in advance if the speedy transport and integrity of the materials is to be assured.

Within the U. S. transport of materials also poses certain legal problems. Federal transportation regulations closely regulate shipments of materials containing potentially hazardous elements such as dry ice or liquid nitrogen.[5] Materials possessing dangerous properties such as flammability, radioactivity, virulence, toxicity, and perishability usually need be transported by road or rail and here too are subject to federal and state regulation concerning mode of transport, containment, and warning markings. Although most tissue materials do not fall into the dangerous category, their media or preservative may and such matters need to be thought through well before samples are taken and shipped.

1.4.   Legal Integrity of Samples:

If data derived from archived samples are to be useful in public policy formulation, they must be able to withstand attack in an adversary proceeding. The ‚chain of custody‘ from sampler to archivist to investigator must be unbroken in the sense that the materials can be guarenteed by all concerned to be as they are represented – in kind, amount, identity, markings,

---

[4]   The U. S. Supreme Court recently discussed the development of the rule governing use of illegally obtained evidence in U. S. v. Janis, 96 S. C. 3021 (1976).

[5]   Regulations governing shipment of hazardous materials are administered by the Materials Transportation Bureau in the U. S. Department of Transportation and are published in the Code of Federal Regulations (49 CFR §§ 170 - 189).

and condition. Thus, the sampler must be able to testify that a sample was taken as recorded (time, place, circumstances, method, etc.), marked as found, and transported by some tamper-proof method by reliable means to the archivist. The archivist in turn must be able to testify that the materials were received in sealed and unadulterated condition, were permanently marked, and were maintained intact, so were given to the investigator. So for the investigator. Although all of this may seem a bit overly legalistic, upon reflection it may be recognized as nothing more than the prudent and cautions scientist would require of materials upon which one may stake a reputation among ones' peers. The only real difference between normal scientific prudence and legalistic practice is an added stress upon written accountability. To extend an introductory remark, the law can not make good science bad, nor bad science good, but it can help to make good science better — and perhaps conversely, to make bad science obvious.

2. Laws Affecting Stages of Investigation and Communication

2. 1. Worker Protection:

Laboratories, and therefore tissue archives, really are dangerous places. They abound with sharp adged glassware, poisonous chemicals, flammables, dangerous gases and persons who, no matter how well trained, may be subject to lapses in judgement. The Occupational Safety and Health Act (OSHA) is a recent U. S. attempt to improve the safety of the workplace and its healthfulness for the worker. OSHA publishes guidelines for chemically and biologically hazardous situations which, if followed, should reduce danger to persons working in potentially hazardous situations. Occupational safety regulations cover new laboratory building construction and operation, laboratory chemical and electrical equipment standards, and many other features of importance to tissue banking and scientific investigation. Although the bench scientist may not perceive him or herself as a supervisor of personnel, this incorrect perception can be corrected quickly and unpleasantly by a lawsuit resulting from an employee grievance or, far worse, a hurt employee. A conscientious program of OSHA standards checks and worker training would not be out of place in a tissue archive laboratory.

2.2. Communication and Confidentiality:

Collegial communications common among pure research personnel become a problem the moment that data or information communicated cross the translucent and fuzzy border from pure science into the realms of proprietary information or adversary evidence. Unless you are employed in a federal laboratory, you are not required to provide information to persons whom you may not know or trust without legal process such as a subpoena. If you are employed in a federal laboratory, files and data are subject to the ‚Freedom of Information Act' which, with certain exceptions (such as draft and working papers, personnel records, or confidential trade secret data), make them public information which must be offered up to the requestor within a legally set time limit. Faced with a request for data or information from an unknown, suspect, or non-research source, you should run rather than walk to your laboratory or institutional legal counsel for assistance. Unverified data or written opinions based upon preliminary or incomplete data sets never should be communicated unless they are so identified in writing — and it is good practice to traffic only in published reports when answering written requests for information. Again, upon reflection this may be recognized as the prudent method of the cautions and conservative scientist avoiding conclusions unsupported by fact.

Confidentiality is less of an issue in non-human tissue sample archiving, research, and monitoring than it is in regard to human tissues — but there are situations in which it may arise. In matters under litigation or in dealing with samples the analysis of which could disclose proprietary information, or secrets of national security importance, the rights of other parties may supercede the right of scientific disclosure. Again, should issues of confidentiality occur spontaneously to you or be brought to your attention, seek legal counsel immediately. Such situations are highly unlikely to happen to more than one in a thousand of us — even including those of us in federal and state regulatory agencies — but in spite of the odds against an occurrence, its possibility requires some consideration.

2.3.   Disposal of Samples and Process Wastes:

All laboratory wastes are subject to the same federal and state clean air and clean water laws as are any other wastes from any other sources. Therefore, appropriate permits for discharges must be obtained from federal and state authorities. The content of tissue bank process wastes can be determined either by measurement of flows and their chemical constituents or by performing mass budget calculations on the amount of preservatives and other toxics purchased per unit time and the concentrations discharged per batch, its dilution, tec. Such information is required if waste streams are discharged from the facility into publicly owned wastewater treatment works or navigable waters of the U. S.

ANNEX I

Abstracts of Working Papers

86

H. P. BERTRAM

Institut für Pharmakologie und Toxikologie
der Westfälischen Wilhelms-Universität
Westring 12
D - 4400 Münster
Federal Republic of Germany

Monitoring inorganic pollutants in domestic and farm animals

There are two points of interest concerning the use of domestic and farm animals in monitoring pollutants in the environment:
1. In contrast to wildlife domestic animals and livestock live in a restricted area with strong relation to the environment of the human population living there
2. Regarding human exposure the remarkable role of farm animals in the food chain include the necessity of monitoring these specimens.

The ‚environmental classification' of the inorganic trace elements must be based upon aspects as essentiallity, toxicity, kinetics and extent of occurrence in environment. The nonessential and toxic elements cadmium, lead and mercury should have the highes priority. The organs recommended for monitoring and banking must have an indicator function, reflecting acute and chronic exposure. Since most trace elements are distributed inhomogeneously in organisms, accumulation compartments usable as monitoring specimens have to be selected.

The distribution patterns for the different trace elements are widely unknown; in several cases indicator function is proved, e. g. liver for Cd, inorganic Hg, Pb, Se, Co, similar to wildlife and humans. Most analytical work has done about the compartments liver, kidneys, milk (cow) and hair (wool, feathers). Among the analytical procedures of choice for determination trace element concentrations, atomic absorption spectrometry including different specific methods, and neutron activation analysis must be mentioned. The uncertainty of the analytical method depends on the element, the concentration of the element and the kind of tissue. Matrix effects may cause systematic errors, influencing the accuracy of the method.

Only with critical evaluation of the method used, analytical results may serve as basis for environmental statements.

J. J. BROMENSHENK

Department of Botany, University of Montana
Missoula, Montana 59812
U. S. A.

Monitoring Environmental Materials and Specimen Banking using terrestrial insects with particular reference to elements and pesticides.

We know very little about the effects of pollutants on insects, particulary terrestrial insects. Although a few species have been used to monitor environmental quality, the number is insignificant compared to the hundreds of thousands existent. The residue analyses, which have been performed on insects, particulary for pesticides and toxic trace elements, have used mostly honey bees and some insects of the soil/litter subsystem. The only efforts to bank terrestrial insects evident in the United States are short-term and usually consist of backlogs of specimens to be analyzed rather than specimens intended for retrospective comparisons. Museum specimens represent the only long-term storage, but the value of museum insects for residue determinations would be extremely limited and appropriate only for the most stable chemicals.

Insects are indisputably important to man. Many insect species are major or critical components of natural and cultivated ecosystems The number of insects is estimated to exceed that of all othes animals and plants combined. Studies of insect populations contribute greatly to the development of ecological concepts because of attributes such as species diversity, abundance, small size, short life cycles, and ecological importance. There is no doubt that both chronic and acute exposures to pollutants may induce responses in insect systems which in turn may have considerable impacts on communities and ecosystems, although the available literature concerning these types of interactions is very limited.

Honey bees and insects occupying higher trophic levels, such as predacious beetles, appear to be bioaccumulators and/or biomagnifiers of many contaminants. Pollutant build-up and transfer through insect food chains may be a route by which higher organisms, such as insectivores and their predators, could ingest proportionally greater amounts of harmful substances.

A scenario is proposed to use honey bees to monitor pesticides and inorganic elements and compounds. Procedures suggested include samples of adult honey bees from apiaries across the United States, cold-storage (-30°C) of bees in inert containers, and analyses for pesticides as recommended by the U. S. FDA Pesticides Analytical Manual and for trace elements via atomic absorption spetrophotometry.

Taxa selection and procedures for collecting, preserving, transporting, and analyzing samples are complex decisions which depend on the materials to be monitored and the relation of these materials to the biological organisms chosen for study. It is impossible to establish easy and indisputable study or experimental formats because of the many variables involved. The planning, organization, and execution of such a program would require, at the very least, the experience and judgement of a qualified population biologist and an analytical chemist.

Centralized, national specimen banks for insect specimens and other biological specimens, such as plants, birds, and mammals, seem to be advantageous. Cost estimates for a monitoring and banking program utilizing and development program to assess feasibility and desirability would have to be performed for most of the insect species. Initial development work has been completed for honey bees and, to some extent, for carabid beetles. These insects demonstrate considerable potential as sensitive and reliable monitors and predictors of environmental pollutants, and they are practical to monitor and to measure.

P. A. BUTLER

Branch of Ecological Monitoring, U. S. Environmental Protection Agency
Sabine Island, Gulf Breeze,
Florida, U. S. A.

Use of oysters and related molluscs as biological Monitoring of synthetic organic pollutants

This report discusses the National pesticide monitoring program in estuaries of the United States.

molluscan samples were collected monthly at about 180 stations during the period 1965 - 72. Half of these stations were monitored again in 1977. The significant findings of the programs are presented and illustrated. The coordination of the programs is described, as well as the collection and processing of samples, data, handling, and program costs.

The biology of molluscs is described as it relates to their suitability as biomonitors. Some of the details of the laboratory experiments are given to characterize the reaction of molluscs to pesticides under controlled conditions.

Despite the necessity for short-term sampling, or because of it, bivalve molluscs appear to be the most useful biomonitor for indicating the fluctuating levels of pollution by synthetic organics in the aquatic environment.

Their usefulness is a result of the combination of their ubiquity, ease in handling, sensitive physiology, position in the food web, and the large store of data describing their responses to pollution under controlled conditions in the laboratory.

B. B. COLLETTE

National Marine Fisheries
Service Systematics Laboratory
Nat. Museum of Natural History
Washington, D. C. 20560
U. S. A.

Specimen Banking Marine Organisms

Two aspects of specimen banking that can be addressed by a systematic zoologist, are: criteria for species selection; and in addition to the banking of freshly collected material the possible use of archival collections of animals maintained primarily for taxonomic study.

A primary problem in the selection of marine species for inclusion in the specimen bank is the large number of species living today. Taking finfishes alone, according to the estimates of Cohen (1970) there are about 20.000 species of fishes of which 58 % are marine species. There are many more species of marine invertebrates. Criteria must be developed to select the most useful and cost effective species among this great diversity for specimen banking. Important criteria include: importance to man; trophic position; habitat; abundance; distribution; and costs of collection and maintenance.

U. DRESCHER - KADEN

Institut für Physiologie, Physiologische Chemie und Ernährungsphysiologie, Fachbereich Tiermedizin Universität München
Veterinärstraße 13
D - 8000 München 22
Federal Republic of Germany

Advantage and problems of using wildliving animal species as indicators for environmental pollution

Various factors endanger the irritable network of relations between mankind, the abiotic environment and the manyfold forms of microorganisms, plants and animals.

Some of them are concerned with chemicals employed in industry, agriculture, forestry and other scopes of life, which penetrate the biocenose as wastes, by accident or on purpose.

The survey of long term trends and geographical differences in the pollutant level in biota beside other means of environmental monitoring is very important for an early warning system, for modelling and for prediction as well as gaining information about the behaviour of the different compounds in the biocenose. The requirement of environmental survey by means of animal indicator species is well accepted but the discussion about the facilities of realization is in full progress.

In this paper we try to cover different aspects of biological monitoring by means of terrestrial wildliving species.

1. First we discuss in general advantage and problems of monitoring concepts using wildlife compared to other environmental survey systems.

2. Taking into account our experiences derived from our pilot studies on OCP in wildlife as well as literature data we will give some suggestions for the selection of representative indicator species. These references are summarized in a catalogue of criteria for amenable species.

3. Some results of our residue studies from 1970 to 1977 will than be listed as example for the feasibility of biological monitoring using freeliving animal species as indicators.

4. Part four presents conceptional and operational aspects of biological monitoring systems applying terrestrial animal species as indicators (mainly bound for the FRG but modified feasible for other nations) including suggestions for indicator regions.

H. W. DÜRBECK

Institute for Chemistry
Institute 4: Applied Physical Chemistry
Nuclear Research Center (KFA)
P. O. Box 1913, D - 5170 Jülich
Federal Republic of Germany

Naturally Occurring Steroids and Synthetic Hormons as Sensitive Monitoring Compounds for the Suitability of Pretreatment Procedures in Specimen Banking and for the Long-Term Stability of Stored Biological Samples

It should be the scope of any specimen banking facility to provide information regarding the past and present exposures of the ecosystems to pollutant groups. Therefore representative species and specimens have to be collected, sampled and stored, which may be comparatively analyzed, if advanced analytical methods are available or if compounds, which have not been regarded dangerous today are going to be recognized as hazardous pollutants. Moreover, existing problems concerning the determination of long-term trends in environmental pollutant concentrations may be investigated and probably eliminated.

However, for the establishment of any succesfully operating banking facility many general problems have to be solved, regarding sampling, sample preparation, subsampling, contamination, storage, stability and distribution apart from additional specific aspects involved with the storage of certain pollutants or specimen groups.

The compounds to be discussed are naturally occuring steroids and synthetic hormones (anabolic drugs), which in general meet three aspects of importance for a future specimen bank program.

1. Hormonal substances and anabolic steroids are regarded to be environmental pollutants.
2. Due to their chemical structure these compounds are most suitable for monitoring the stability of a sample when pretreated for banking purposes or when stored for a long period of time.
3. Hormones are present in many of the species, which have been selected to have the highest priority for specimen banking (i. e. milk, mussels, seawage sludge). Moreover, they may be found in blood, urine, fat and muscular tissue.

R. A. DURST

Center for Analytical Chemistry
National Bureau of Standards
Gaithersburg, MD 20234
U. S. A.

Container Materials for the Preservation of Trace Substances in Environmental Materials.

The success of the National Environmental Specimen Bank will be determined inlarge part by the ability to preserve the integrity of the trace substances during long-term storage. It is widely recognized that the storage of environmental materials is subject to a variety of uncertainties when one is considering the identity and levels of trace elements and organic compounds. Changes in the forms and concentrations of the numerous environmentally important substances in specimens stored for extended periods may occur in several ways. Processes such as surface adsorption and sample degradation may reduce the concentrations of various components and/or produce species which may not have been present in the original sample. On the other hand, contamination from the container and evaporation of specimen fluids could lead to apparent increases in trace substance components. In addition, superimposed on these processes are the factors which will affect their rates, such as, container material, contact time and areas, storage temperature, pH, and initial species concentration.

All of these factors are important considerations in evaluating the suitability of various containers for long-term storage.

There have been numerous studies performed in recent years directed toward the identification of suitable container materials and optimum storage conditions, but much of this work is contradictory. In many cases, the analytical data were invalidated because of problems not associated with the storage but with other links in the analytical chain such as sampling and procedural contamination.

K. W. EBING

Biologische Bundesanstalt f. Land- und Forstwirtschaft
Institut f. Pflanzenschutzmittelforschung
Königin-Luise-Str. 19
D - 1000 Berlin 33 (Dahlem)
Federal Republic of Germany

Monitoring of plants and soil for analysis of possibly hazardous contaminants and banking of these environmental specimens

Monitoring programmes for organic chemical contaminants in plants or soil with regard to the description of the surrounding of the sampling locality and observing trends following a time course had not been conducted so far. In future, such programmes should be organized within narrow limits. It is reasonable to establish a monitoring programme and a respective small specimen banking system for a few plants (especially wheat and the grass species Lolium multiflorum) and soil, and for the halogenated compounds (non-volatile chlorinated hydrocarbons, chlorophenols, chlorophenoxyalcane carbonic acids) and slowly degradionable compounds (triazine herbicides). For heavy metal traces, monitoring is unnecessary for soils and plants, because pollution of these contaminants on that matrices depends on the distance of sample locality to the emitters and their emitting intensity. Very many papers described this data with respect to plants growing on soils. So for the most cases, heavy metal trace concentrations may be estimated by those data without further experimental work. In order to obtain best results and best cost-yield-relation sampling, description of the environment of the localities, analyzing and storage should be handled in narrow connection. The number of mixed samples to be stored for analysis should be kept small. Deep freezing to -80° C is expected to be the most favourable storage technique for the sample types considered. To realize the small monitoring sub-system proposed the costs per year will not exceed 1,75 millions DM. For investigations, selections of sample localities etc. once 1,55 millions DM must be added. A respective banking system requires about 150.000.- - DM in addition.

R. ECKARD

Institut für Pharmakologie und Toxikologie der Westfälischen Wilhelms-Universität
Westring 12
D - 4400 Münster
Federal Republic of Germany

Non-halogenated compounds in aquatic and terrestrial ecosystems

There are large gaps on our knowledge concerning the distribution patterns and residue levels of the less persistent organic compounds, viz.-phthalates, nitrosamines, organophosphate pesticides, mycotoxins and antibiotics in aquatic and terrestrial ecosystems. Data available at present is mostly confined to their occurrence in some components of the human diet. Thus, some of these organic compounds have not yet been recognized as general environmental contaminants.

Sample selection for monitoring and banking is generally limited by the markedly non-homogeneous distribution patterns of these compounds, variation in their levels of pollution and the lack of accumulating organisms for them. Nevertheless, some specimens, e. g. snails, mussels and sludge as well as wheat, grass and soil may reflect acute and/or chronic exposure to some of these less persistent pollutants.

The storage of the samples necessitates the use of glass or quartz containers rather than polyethylene or teflon ones. Rapid and deep freezing is the most appropriate method for maintaining sample integrity. Long-term storage at -20° C is not an adequate measure by itself. Temperatures of

-80° C or even -196° C as well as exclusion of oxygen seem to be necessary for long-term storage of biological specimens with regard to the less persistent pollutants. Because contamination levels of these compounds are ectremely low and usually do not exceed the ppb range and because they differ widely in their physicochemical properties, several analytical systems of very high sensitivity have to be used for monitoring, e. g. GC - MS, HPLC - (MS) and CC - GC involving a large variety of detection systems.

The centralization of the research laboratories to only a few efficient ones would serve to achieve the high quality standards which are required for real time monitoring and environmental banking.

H. EGAN

Laboratory of the Government Chemist
Cornwall House, Stamford Street
London, SE 1 9NQ
United Kingdom

Biological Specimen Collection — Analytical Aspects

Much of the practical interest in the assessment of exposure to environmental pollutants is by way of trace analysis. Analytical aspects are therefore reviewed for each of the main group of pollutants with special reference to the limits of detection, in order to provide a basis for the assessment of exposure. Whilst ‚pollution' is a relative term, it is obviously necessary if trace analysis is to be used in the foregoing manner that the limits of analytical detection should be realistic in relation to the hazard which the exposure involves: the value of analysis may vary according to whether short-term or long-term exposure is concerned. The value of the analytical approach may also vary according to the substrate chosen for axamination: specimens from human population may be less appropriate for the evaluation of risk in human exposure than samples of food, water or air provided these are taken with due regard to average (or, occasionally, extrem) conditions. The groups of pollutants considered in this way include carcinogens or potential carcinogens such as mycotoxins, polynuclear aromatic hydrocarbons and N-nitrosamine compounds, together with trace metals, synthetic-pesticide and hormone residues and antibiotics.

The long-term storage of samples for subsequent analysis, perhaps a year or a decade later, presents some difficulty although for most purposes it is doubtful whether such an exercise would be worthwhile. With the possible exception of some research aspects, the analytical methods at present available have adequate sensitivity for the practical interpretation of the levels concerned in relation to the associated exposure risk. More sensitivity methods could in some cases be of value in studies of the mechanism of toxicity: but it is doubtful whether the long-term storage of samples has a vital contribution in this field.

The general question of standardisation of analytical methods (both as a basis for the assessment of the significance of exposure to pollution and for other reasons) is briefly discussed and the importance of biological standard reference material in this field is indicated.

S. W. FOWLER

International Atomic Energy Agency
International Laboratory of Marine Radioactivity
Musee Oceanographique
Principiality of Monaco

Reasibility of using macroalgae as a reference material

An assessment of the properties of macroalgae for serving as a reference material in marine pollution monitoring studies has lead to the conclusion that these organisms should be given top priority for use in the tissue bank program. Macroalgae are considered attractive candidates for pollutant specimen banking in that they are ubiquitous, sedentary integrators of many pollutant indicators in many pollution monitoring programs. International interest in macroalgae is witnessed by the use of these organisms as reference materials for world-wide pollutant intercalibration exercises.

Widely distributed near-shore species such as the brown algae, **Fucus**, are proposed as the best group of macroalgae for use in specimen banking. The red algae would be an equally good choice for monitoring deeper, off-shore waters. Recommendations are given on sample collection, tissue preparation and homogenization techniques which aim at reducing the possibility of contamination in the resultant homogenate. The prospects of long-term storage of dry homogenate appear good in light of previous tests made with macroalgae used for radionuclide intercalibration exercises.

Assuming a small initial monetary outlay, a pilot program for monitoring macroalgae is proposed which will result in the acquisition and processing of approximately 25 samples per year. An international coordination of the project is tressed, specifically within the framework of on-going national and international pollution monitoring programs.

T. E. GILLS, H. L. ROOK

NBS
BLDG. 235, Room B - 108
Gaithersburg, MD 921 - 2166
U. S. A.

Specimen Bank Research at the National Bureau of Standards to Insure Proper Scientific Protocols for the Sampling, Storage and Analysis of Environmental Materials

In 1973, the U. S. Environmental Protection Agency conducted a review of analytical methodology used for sampling, storage and analysis of environmental samples.

The major conclusion derived from that review was that the accepted procedures were completely inadequate. Deficiencies in trace analysis methodology were further documented by analytical data obtained from a number of EPA contractor laboratories on samples of SRMs 1632, Coal and 1633, Fly Ash. Many data on these materials were in error by more than an order of magnitude. Factors such as these point to the real need for critical evaluation of sampling, storage and analysis methodology for the National Environmental Sample Bank (NESB) program. For the successful implementation of an effective banking system, rigid quality control procedures ensuring comparability and traceability of results between methods and laboratories are required. Several occasions have arisen where environmental samples of known and documented history would have been valuable in assessing changes in trace constituents for the determination of their impact on human health; however, undefined or improper sampling and storage procedures were utilized.

M. GOTO

Department of Chemistry
Gakushuin University
Toshima-Ku
Tokyo, 171
Japan

Monitoring environmental materials and specimen banking
State-of-the-Art of Japanese Experience and Knowledge

The list of toxic chemicals is being made in the Environment Agency, which will include about 5000 - 6000 chemical substances. About 2000 of them are to be selected from the standpoint of production amount, use pattern and toxicity and submitted to screening tests for environmental survey to examine degradability in the air, water and soil. Environmental survey will then be performed on highly residual compounds at fixed survey points in the country. Starting from 1974 Environment Agency is carrying out the survey on the residues of selected chemicals in water, sediments and fishes at about 50 monitoring places. The results of the survey in 1974FY, 1975FY and 1976FY will be described in this paper

The movement and transformation of chemicals in the environment is, however, extremely complicated and it is therefore very difficult to predict the kinds and levels of chemicals to be detected in the environment from the statistics of consumption of chemicals and the data of ecological profile analyes. Therefore, a great effort should also be made on characterization of hazardous compounds in environmental specimens. For this and for studying the trend of environmental contamination, the system to preserve specimens taken at fixed monitoring points for several decades should be established as soon as possible.

Survey on the residues of environmental chemicals has been performed since 1974FY mainly by the Environment Agency. Survey was conducted on 33 chemicals at the estimated cost of 60210 thousand yen (approx. US $ 300.000,–) in 1974FY, 42 chemicals at 102,470 thousand yen (approx. US $ 500.000,–) in 1975FY and 78 chemicals at 95,400 thousand yen (approx. US $ 480.000,–)in 1976FY, that is, 153 chemicals were investigated in total for 3 years by 26 Prefectural Laboratories for Pollution Studies. The chemicals selected were mainly (1) those already regulated by laws because of their toxicity, (2) those of low degradability and (3) those similar in chemical structure to substances such as PCB which has previously caused environmental pollution or their substitutes. Survey was conducted chiefly on the water and sediment, but organisms were also investigated when fishes and shellfishes were living at survey points.

P. A. GREVE

Unit for Residue Analysis, National Institute of Public Health,
Postbox 1, Bilthoven
Netherlands

Organo-halogenated compounds in aquatic ecosystems

Data from past and current monitoring programmes covering aquatic ecosystems, as well as from incidental investigations indicates that from the organo-halogenated compounds much emphasis has been laid upon the organochlorine pesticides and PCBs, which compounds habe been investigated in water, sediments and a great variety of aquatic organisms. From the other organo-halogenated compounds the volatile organochlorine solvents and the chlorophenols have been studied most extensively.

Although many organo-chlorine compounds have been identified in aquatic ecosystems, still a large gap exists between the total amount of organo-chlorine found and the amount of organo-chlorine calculated from the compounds known to occur. This fact forms an argument in favour of specimen banking, together the status-quo-ante when calamities occur.

It is suggested that in monitoring activities, as well as for specimen banking, as a minimum water samples and samples of one fish species be collected and stored. When circumstances so demand, samples of sediment and/or other aquatic organisms can be incorporated in the programmes.

For the reduction and preservation of the samples freeze-drying and storage at low temperature is suggested.

G. GRIMMER

Biochemisches Institut für Umweltcarcinogene
Sieker Landstraße 19
D - 2070 Ahrensburg
Federal Republic of Germany

Polycyclic Aromatic Hydrocarbons

There are good reasons to assume that many of the human carcinoma are initiated by environmental carcinogens as e. g. polycyclic aromatic hydrocarbons (= PAH), N-containing polycyclic aromatic amines, mycotoxines and some inorganic compounds. From this the general question arises: What is the sense of doing analytical chemistry of pollutants? The answer is, to control harmful substances in the environment and first of all to control acute and chronic toxic substances for man.

Epidemiological studies indicate that the environment significant influences the incidence of human cancer although many of the specific causal agent have yet to be identified. Two major factors are known from these epidemiological studies: inhalation of cigarette smoke and inhalation of air pollutants clearly increase the incidence of lung cancer in men. By using animal tests, it is possible to identify and characterize the carcinogens in cigarette smoke, automobile exhaust condensate or air pollutants. In these cases, the fraction of PAH account for more then the half of the carcinogenic activity of even for the total carcinogenic effect.

Since the PAH are common environmental pollutants, they are supposed to contribute to cancer in other organs too. There are many so called pollutants existing in environmental concentration without detectable effect in men. But only in the case of carcinogens as polycyclic aromatic hydrocarbons there are good reasons to assume that these are the causal agents for lung cancer in man. In 1975 more than 24.000 men died in the Federal Republic of Germany of lung cancer.

H.-J. HAPKE

Abteilung für Toxikologie
Institut für Pharmakologie der Tierärztlichen Hochschule
Bischofsholer Damm 15
D - 3000 Hannover
Federal Republic of Germany

Organo-halogenated compounds in farm and domestic animals

There are not programmes at all in the sense of an observing system. Systematic investigations with representative results are not performed till today. But there is one exception: the food control. This control is prescribed by law. The datas of the residues in food are not published in general and are varying between different analysis laboratories.

In summary the equipment of a monitoring environmental materials and specimen banking may have the following form:

— Selection of farmers, who are representative for a region;
— Collection of adipose tissue and kidney from slaughtered calfs, cows and pigs and of milk and eggs;
— First determination of HCH and PCBs in the above mentioned tissues in regional laboratories;
— Storage of the results and the remaining specimens; supervised by the Collecting and Evaluations Center of the Federal Health Office, which is already established.
   This system can be proposed (in the Federal Republic of Germany or in related Centres of other Countries).
— Current evaluation of the results (and their changes from time to time and from region to region) and redetermination of HCH and PCBs in the storage tissues in the central laboratory.

A. V. HOLDEN

Department of Agriculture and Fisheries for Scotland
Freshwater Fisheries Lab.
Faskally Pitlochry
Perthshire PH 16 5LB
United Kingdom

Monitoring environmental materials and specimen banking for organo-halogenated compounds in aquatic ecosystems

Monitoring programmes must have specific objectives, and the sampling and analytical procedures must be designed to provide data which will enable the objectives to be attained with measurable precision. Both physical and biological samples can be used, but the former will be difficult to interpret in respect of the effects of pollutant levels on aquatic life.

Biological samples must be clearly specified, and the species must be selected on the basis of abundance, easy accessibility and identification, and where possible sexing and ageing, without risk to the population sampled. Where trends in contamination level at a particular location are to be monitored, a species appropriate to that site will be sufficient, but if comparisons are to be made between locations or areas, species common to those locations or ecologically equivalent species must be selected.

Samples will represent the site of sampling at the time, and not necessarily adjacent sites or other times. If pollution is localized, other sites at short distances must be sampled to determine the extent of the polluted area, but for baseline contamination levels or low-level pollution sampling sites can be more widely spaced. In biological specimens the pollutant level may vary with season and age, and also with the external pollutant concentration. Frequent sampling may be required if the pollution level fluctuates, but even for annual sampling the specimens taken must be in the same physiological condition.

Many organochlorine compounds are not very persistent in the environment and some are not accumulated to a high degree. Others, particularly certain pesticides and high molecular weight industrial compounds such as PCHs, are persistent and concentrated in lipids from the external aqueous environment by several orders of magnitude. Only a few halogenated compounds are currently monitored, and new analytical techniques may be necessary to extend monitoring to other compounds.

The factors influencing the selection of species and tissues for monitoring purposes are discussed, but in general shoaling fish and colonial invertebrates are preferred, taking advantage of their relative abundance, accessibility and the possibilities of age and size selection to reduce the variance among individuals. Experience with the OECD monitoring programme is described and costs assessed.

W. KLEIN

Gesellschaft für Strahlen- und Umweltforschung
mbH München
Institut für Ökologische Chemie
Ingolstädter Landstr. 2
D - 8042 Neuherberg
Post Oberschleißheim
Federal Republic of Germany

Organohalogenated compounds in plants and soil

Within all organic chemicals, most extensive monitoring of organochlorine pesticides has been done for several years. An exhaustive review of this activity in several countries can not be given. Typical data for US are published in Pesticides Monitoring Journal. Results of monitoring these pesticides revealed e. g. a decline in DDT-exposure of the population. Assessment of monitoring data resulted in hazard lists: actual intake versus a. d. i. Similar data as for organoclorine pesticides are available for PCB's. For the larger number of solvents and other organohalogenated compounds, only random isolated data are available.

PCB's have been found in the flora of non-inhabited areas. Thus the occurrence of organohaloge. chemicals must be expected generally in any plants and soil.

An appropriate specimen as long-term accumulator is soil from industrial, agricultural and non-inhabited areas. A seasonal accumulator, typical for human exposure, would be food grain, and a respective high-accumulator would be carrots. Suggested specimen for wild plants could be Cladonia or large leaves or water hemlock (based on PCB). Proposed container for specimen is glass. Freeze-drying reduces residues and changes analytical recovery. Therefore portional storage of original homogenized samples is proposed.

The large number of chemical individuals requires multimatrix-multiresidue methodology. Interference of non-halogenated chemicals can be overcome by glass-capillary GLC with internal standardisation. Convenient detection and determination is by GLC/ECD. So far no certified standards and reference materials are available.

For programme design it has to be decided large number of samples and good statistical representativity versus low number of specific local samples, enabling sophisticated analysis like GC/MS confirmation and no need for expensive development of routine analytical procedure. The total national costs for a minimum programme would amount to about 500.000 DM annually.

J. L. LUDKE

Columbia National Fisheries Research Lboratory
U. S. Fish and Wildlife Service
Columbia, Mo. 65201
U. S. A.

Collection, Storage, and Analysis of Freshwater Fish for Monitoring Environmental Contaminants

The National Pesticide Monitoring Program came into being about 1964 as a cooperative effort of the federal departments making-up the membership of the Federal Committee on Pest Control. This cooperative, multi-administered program continued until the passage of the Federal Environmental Pesticide Control Act of 1972 (Public Law 92 - 516) at which time the program received legislative status under the Environmental Protection Agency.

The U. S. Fish and Wildlife Service (FWS) is responsible for the fish and wildlife subprograms of the National Pesticide Monitoring Program. The primary objecive is to ascertain on a nation-wide basis, and independent of specific treatments, the levels and trends of selected environmental contaminants in the bodies of freshwater fish, and certain bird species over a period of time.

Samples for trend monitoring should be collected at predisignated times of the year and at predesignated sampling stations located along major fresh water drainage systems. Fish collected for monitoring purposes should be chosen according to the following criteria: (1) a highly ubiquitous species representative of the most widespread geographical distribution, (2) different, but closely related species with similar in natural history and feeding habits, (3) ecological equivalents, but not necessarily closest in phylogenetic relationship.

N.-P. LÜPKE, F. SCHMIDT-BLEEK

State-of-the-art of biological specimen banking in the Federal Republic of Germany

The government of the Federal Republic of Germany have made at present investigations about the facilities and limits of banking environmental specimens, to have to decree in 10, 20 or more years reference-samples of the present time for solving a number of potential problems.

The characterization of knowledged pollutants while taking, preparation and analysis and storage of samples with deep temperatures serves as reference for the optimal treated samples for the conservation of the chemical integration of persistent residues.

For sample-species it is planned:

Human livers, fatty tissues and blood, cow milk, Mytilus spec., Dreissena polymorpha, grass cultures, wheat, soil, sludge, Cyprinus carpio and macroalgae.

About the first experiences and perceptions as well as plans for carrying on the work it will be reported.

R. MARTY, A. BOUDOU

Laboratory of Animal Ecology and Ecophysiology
Bordeaux I University
33405 Bordeaux — Talence
France

Ecological action of mercury by-products on different animal tissues

Transfer ways from the sources of pollution to man are numerous and they vary according to the environment and the pollutant. All living beings present, to various degrees, the property to accumulate in their tissues substances which are little or not at all biodegradable. Therefore in a contaminated ecosystem, there appears phenomena of pollution biological amplification as the different levels of trophic chain are gradually reached.

The increasing contamination of the environment by more and more unbiodegradable toxic products (heavy metals, organic component, pesticides, additives P. C. B., biological components) requires the presence of ecotoxicological research in order to know better, in a both fundamental and practical purpose, the answer of natural ecosystems and their adaptative capacity to the different sources of pollution.

Our group of research has been working for more than 2 years for the building up of an ecotoxicological model in freshwater environment. The main purposes we have are:

— creating a complete experimental trophic chain from the primary producers (autotroph) to the consumers of the third or fourth rank.

Clorella vulgaris → **Daphnia magna** → **Gambusia affinis**
→ **Salmo gairdneri** → **Esox lucius** ←↑

— using animal or vegetable species which are characteristic of the different trophic levels, frequent in natural environment, presenting a good genetic homogenity and compatible with a breeding or stocking in laboratory.

- controlling as many abiotic factors as possible in order to reduce ‚parasitical variabilities' and to define with precision the experimental conditions (reproductible and comparative results).
- adding a toxic product for which the quantity determination techniques permit to detect — in the environment and in the organisms — very slight concentrations approaching those which can be found in natural systems.

The pollutant we study:

- mercury by-products ($HgCI_2$, $CH_3 HgCI$) radioactives (Hg^{208}) — One ppb in water.
- studying the synergy effects, positive and negative, among the only or the different pollutants tested and the abiotic factors (for instance temperatures: 10, 18 and 26° C).
- analyzing, on the physiological and biochemical levels, the ecotoxicological incidence upon the terminal links.
- conseiving and designing, later, a complexification of these models.

F. MORIARTY

The Institute of Terrestrial Ecology
Monks Wood Experimental Station I. T. E.
Natural Environmental Research Council
Abbots Ripton, Huntingdon
England PE 17, 2LS
United Kingdom

Organo-halogenated compounds in terrestrial wildlife

We lack detailed knowledge on which to design reliable monitoring or specimen banking schemes for terrestrial animals (excluding perhaps some species of birds). Any pilot scheme will need to consider:

1) What range and types of species should be sampled.
2) What aspects of persistence we are interested in.
3) whether pollutant levels in the environment are such that organisms will or will not be appreciably affected.
4) The timing and exact types of samples to be taken.
5) How to avoid artefacts from the method of capturing specimens, minimize contamination, prevent postmortem changes, store samples, avoid interference from other compounds, and confirm analytical identifications.
6) The nature and magnitude of sampling errors.

Some of these points pose difficult technical and research problems. By comparison, estimates of cost appear to be relatively simple.

P. MÜLLER

Schwerpunkt für Biogeographie, Fachbereich 6 Geographie
Universität des Saarlandes
D - 6600 Saarbrücken
Federal Republic of Germany

Basic ecological concepts and urban ecological systems

From the scientific and experimental point of view the program ‚Monitoring Environmental Materials and Specimen Banking' as a whole — which means sampling, sample pretreatment, realtime monitoring, analysis and banking — may be regarded as a very difficult task. But methods for collection, preservation and storage of Environmental Materials are well established and do not pose insurmountable problems. International and national biological monitoring programs were performed in the years 1966 to 1976. Difficulties in selecting representative indicator organisms, regions and seasons for valid interpretation, the necessity of including other biological information and a deficit in basic ecological facts finished these projects. A representation of ‚Basic Ecological Concepts' implies a thorough study of autecological, synecological and ecosystemic findings and discussions with research teams.

Because of the specific problems in the workshop, however, I will confine myself to those whose paradigmatic consideration and methodological approach are of importance for the evaluation of landscape and urban systems.

R. K. MURTON

Institute of Terrestrial Ecology
Monks Wood Experimental Station
Abbots Ripton, Huntingdon
United Kingdom

Considerations applicable to the monitoring of organo-halogenated compounds in terrestrial wildlife especially birds

From 1962 carcases of various predatory birds found dead by members of the public have been sent, in response to advertised appeals, to Monks Wood Experimental Station, Huntingdon, England: initially the scheme was introduced by the Nature Conservancy but since 1973 it has been under the auspices of the Institute of Terrestrial Ecology.

The scheme was initially introduced to record changes in tissue levels of various organochlorine pesticides to monitor the effects of Government legislation to limit the use of these chemicals. It now represents the longest running monitoring scheme involving birds of prey, with particularly good data referring to the Kestrel, Sparrowhawk, Barn Owl and Heron.

In this contribution details of the scheme are outlined and the results discussed in terms of monitoring schemes in general. It is concluded that it is not practical to define indicator species that serve as convenient monitors of unspecified environmental pollutants. It is desirable to define in advance the objective of any programme and to select appropriate methods and species. This follows because there exist wide interspecific variations in biological response to so-called pollutants, so that any data are more likely to reflect the pecularities of a species' physiology and ecology than trends in residue levels in the environment. This paper provides some evidence for this viewpoint, and it is hoped that the topic will be elaborated in more detail at the workshop in Berlin.

J. MUSICK

Institute of Marine Science
Gloucester Point
VA 23062
U. S. A.

The Role of Deep-Sea Organisms in Monitoring Environmental Xenobiotics

Deep-sea ecosystems can provide valuable baseline information about the extent of the world-wide distribution of xenobiotics. For some xenobiotics such as trace metals the deep-ocean may presently provide a baseline relatively uneffected by man. For other xenobiotics such as DDT and PCB's the deep-ocean can provide an index of atmospheric and oceanic processes of degradation and accumulation. Deep-ocean sediments may be the ultimate depository for such halogenated hydrocarbons.

C. E. NASH

Oceanic Institute
Waimanalo, Hawaii 96795
U. S. A.

The grey mullet (Mugil cephalus L.) as a marine bio-indicator

The grey mullet, **Mugil cephalus**, has unique qualities which make it potentially useful as a bio-indicator of the aquatic environment. The fish has a worldwide geographic distribution from the temperate to the tropic zones and is common to most coastal waters. It is a euryhaline species spending most of its life history in estuaries and brackishwater areas, migrating annually to sea to spawn. It is a detritus and algae feeder, also consuming particulate matter in the substrate.
Adult fish, about 1 kg in weight, are captured in many coastal fisheries providing, for the most part, the only available animal protein for the subsistence of the coastal populations. It can be captured easily by gillnet. In addition to man, predators of the adults are the higher carnivorous fishes and some marine mammals; and the juveniles make up an important part of the diet of the wading birds and fishes in the estuarine ecosystem.
The fish is farmed extensively because of its high tolerance to wide ranges of temperature (3 - 36°C) and salinity (0 - 75°/oo), and its affinity for schooling which permits intensive stocking. Its flesh is of high quality.

H. M. OHLENDORF

U. S. Fish & Wildlife Service
Patuxent Wildlife Research Center
Laurel, MD 20811
U. S. A.

Archiving Wildlife Specimens for Future Analysis

Duck wings and starlings are analyzed for organochlorines and selected heavy metals in the National Pesticide Monitoring Program. In other wildlife research projects conducted by the Patuxent Wildlife Research Center, specimens of many other species have been analyzed to determine geographic species, or temporal difference in residue concentrations. Examples include bald eagles, certain New Jersey salt marsh fauna, and the eggs of eagles, ducks, ospreys, brown pelicans, and wading birds.

Specimens usually have been archived as frozen samples so they could be reanalyzed when newer contaminants were discovered or analytical procedures were improved. The procedures used in banking these specimens have been adequate for the purposes intended. Samples should be stored at temperatures of -30° C or colder. We are now experimenting with formalin preservation of specimens and have found the method satisfactory for certain types of samples. This procedure may be more suitable and less costly than other methods of storage.

Samples usually have been collected to determine geographic patterns of residue levels in the study species, or to determine which chemicals might be associated with population declines and reproductive failure in species of concern. In some instances, the samples constitute a nation-wide collection, but more often they are taken from selected regions or localized areas. Most samples are stored frozen, both prior to analysis and after analyses are completed. Subsamples of duck wings and bald eagle carcases are the most useful and feasible avian specimens from the aquatic environment for long-term storage in locations other than the Patuxent Center.

J. PEARCE

U. S. Department of Commerce
National Oceanic and Atmospheric Administration
National Marine Fisheries Service
Northeast Fisheries Center
Sandy Hook Laboratory
Highlands, New Jersey 07732
U. S. A.

Trace Metals in Living Marine Resources Taken from North Atlantic Waters

It is assumed that tissue banks as well as other facilities for the retention of physical samples, including both water and sediments, will become increasingly important as mankind releases additional contaminants to the marine environment. It is obvious that consideralbe forethought should be given so that limited storage space can be most effectively used. Personnel within the Northeast Fisheries Center have anticipated that it would be impossible to retain samples of each species and circumscribed geographic area. It is important, however, to provide storage for long-term holdings of certain key species as well as physical samples from key environments. It is hoped that the results of the workshop on tissue banks will bring to the attention of the world the need for tissue banks as well, as provide information on the most appropriate ways for handling and storing tissues for long periods of time. Techniques such as freeze drying should be examined. Also, collection and storage procedures should be evaluated and recommendations made in regard to the most efficient way to hold tissues without contamination. For many of the contaminants now of interest to mankind the analyses must be performed at the parts per billion level. Certain contaminants may only exist at the parts per trillion level in certain instances and yet some limited information indicates that such contaminants may have an effect at these low levels.

O. RAVERA

Department of Physical and Natural Sciences
C. C. R. – EURATOM
21020 – Ispra (Varese)
Italy

Pollution in freshwater communities

The advantages and disadvantages of grouping pollutants into categories has been discussed and the relationship between the structure of a toxic substance and its biological effects illustrated. In spite of the difficulty of generalizing this relationship, its importance is evident because on this basis it is possible to predict the biological effects of new substances before they are tested. Because communities and populations of animals and plants are protected aganist pollution, but not the single individual, the effects at the community and population level have been illustrated. The importance of genetic damage has also been evaluated. The value of laboratory experiments and the difficulties involved in extrapolating their results to the natural environment have been discussed.

Some methods of biological control and their advantages and disadvantages have been listed. The need for a strategy for obtaining satisfactory information on polluted environments without adopting too heavy programme of chemical and biological analyses has been emphasized.

A comparison between the evaluation of the risk in the radioprotection field and in that for non-radioactive pollutants has been made. Some examples of the evaluation of risk concerning lake eutrophication have been given to illustrate the practical advantages of applying this fundamental concept. The most important types of risk from pollution have been listed.

H. H. REICHENBACH-KLINKE

Institut für Zoologie und Hydrobiologie der Technischen Universität München
Kaulbachstr. 37
D - 8000 München 22
Federal Republic of Germany

Aspects of pollutants or pollutant categories to other aquatic wildlife

The role of fish in the monitoring and banking of environmental materials is characterized as member of the food chain beginning in water and ending in man. On the other hand fish gives a picture of the present ecological situation in water. If we are comparing the fish with other materials in our environment several factors must be a knowledged: the fish must taken from water with special quality, it must be conserved or fixed after standardized methods and it must be a species comparable to related forms. Experiences have shown that kidney and liver are those fish organs with the greatest accumulation of heavy metals. It therefore seems best for the banking to use these organs.

M. STOEPPLER

Institut für Chemie der Kernforschungsanlage Jülich
GmbH
Inst. 4: Angewandte Physikalische Chemie
Postfach 1913
D - 5170 Jülich
Federal Republic of Germany

Choice of species, sampling and sample pretreatment for subsequent analysis and banking or marine organisms useful for Hg, Pb and Cd monitoring

The continuous transport of man made and natural amounts of toxic heavy metals and its compounds into the aquatic and marine environment makes real time monitoring and also banking of selected species necessary.

Since the total aquatic and marine load of Hg and Ce is much higher than man's contributions, for Cd only regional problems exist. For Hg also general health risks have to be considered. They are due to the biotransformation of less toxic Hg compounds into the highly toxic methylmercury, predominantly accumulated in the aquatic and marine food chain. Production and wasting of Pb by far exceeds natural sources. Though this seems only moderately reflected in the marine food chain, data from Pb accumulating tissue may contribute to a better understanding of biogeochemical phenomena.

In order to monitor particular as well as general impacts on marine and estuarine ecosystems, a balanced selection of monitoring species to distinguish between contributions of toxic metal levels from the dissolved state, from particulate matter and from food chain stages should consist of a bivalve, and algae and a teleost, non migratory fish, with a possibly later extension to a mollusc and a pelagic prey fish.

Sampling and sample preparation for marine species needs proper procedures. Dissecting, homogenizing, deep freezing down to 77° K, and packaging for subsequent analysis and/or banking should be performed in mobile units having all the necessary equipment to reduce the contamination level drastically.

For data normalization a meaningful weight basis is unavoidable and may be realized by e. g. the simultaneous use of an actual weight and a dry weight after freeze or oven drying.

The preparation of composite and single samples after shock freezing should result in sample aliquots of about 2 g fresh weight adding to a total sample amount of about 1 kg for subsequent trace analysis and banking.

Within the frame of the whole program very sophisticated and also independent analytical methods are required. For this purpose further detailed methodological evaluation and optimalization is necessary.

L. STEUBING

Institut für Pflanzenökologie
Heinrich-Buff-Ring 38
D - 6300 Lahn-Giessen
Federal Republic of Germany

Monitoring aerial inorganic pollutants by plant indicator specimens
Regional survey of different immission types by plants

The importance of monitoring by plants is that only with the aid of organisms it is possible to receive information on the effect of immissions. Contrary to this, physical chemical analyses only allow to collect information on the concentrations of special pollution components. Generally all mentioned groups of plants include useful indicator specimens for monitoring. To evaluate possible injury in the future on the vegetation, with which the food chain begins and at the end of which there is the human being, we need more multifactorial research experiments under (internationally) standardized conditions thereby results are more comparable together.

W. R. WOLF

Nutrient Composition Laboratory, Nutrition Institute,
Science and Education Administration, Federal Research,
U. S. Department of Agriculture,
Beltsville, Maryland 20705
U. S. A.

Specimen Banking of Food Samples for Long-term Monitoring of Nutrient Trace Elements

There is a growing need for more accurate and precise assessment and long-term monitoring of the nutrient content of the U. S. diet. Significant changes in the American dietary consumption have occured and continue to occur. In order to assess the magnitude, extent and trend of these changes regarding nutrient content of the diet, a long-term monitoring system must be established and maintained. Of necessity in this monitoring system is the collection and storage of representative samples to be used as a base line for future comparison. The recent establishment of a National Environmental Specimen Bank for assessment of pollutants and environmental materials is compatible with the needs for long-term nutrient monitoring. The recognition of beneficial aspects of certain of the trace elements at low levels of intake and the harmful effects of these same elements at higher levels require very precise definition of the actual levels in the diet. Analytical technology and knowledge and feasibility for obtaining proper storage conditions for monitoring trace element content of U. S. diets are good. Cooperative programs in long-term monitoring of both nutrient and trace pollutant elements will be of great and necessary benefit to both areas.

ANNEX II

Working Papers submitted for the Workshop

108

WORKING PAPERS SUBMITTED FOR THE WORKSHOP

110

MONITORING INORGANIC POLLUTANTS IN DOMESTIC
AND FARM ANIMALS

Dr. H.P. Bertram
Institute of Pharmacology and Toxicology
University of Muenster, Federal Republic of
Germany

Contents

1. Considerations on using domestic and farm animals in environmental monitoring

Environmental monitoring should be performed under the aspect of general
influence of pollutants on man. The aquatic and terrestrial ecosystem have
to be controlled as much as possible. In addition to the problems of concentration and accumulation trends of pollutants in the environment,
questions concerning "direct" exposure of man have to be answered with
highest priority, pointing out possible health hazards. Legal consequences for protection and safety of man may derive from the informations thus obtained.

In contrast to wildlife, domestic and farm animals live in a restricted
area with the possibility of supervising the environmental conditions.
Thus domestic animals and livestock can be considered as indicator species for a specific area with strong relation to the population living
there.

Another important point is the role of farm animals in the food chain. Informations on the amount of environmental contaminants in human nutrition are indispensable for the estimation of daily intake.

2. Reasons for Interest or Concern

2.1. Classification and priorities of inorganic pollutants

As suggested in the Information Note Oct. 77 the pollutant category "Inorganic substances" is defined here as the following group of trace elements (including some organometallic compounds):

As, Be, Cd, Co, Cr, F, Hg, Mo, Mn, Ni, Pb, Pd, Se, Sn, Tl, V, Zn

As a consequence of increasing industrialization small quantities of these trace elements are continuously being injected into the environment.

For the classification of the above specified elements according to their priority in environmental significance the following aspects must be taken into consideration:

a) Division in essential and nonessential trace elements. Until now the following of the listened elements are proved to be essential for man:

Cr, Co, F, Mn, Mo, Ni, Se, Sn, V, Zn

Nonessential and toxic in relatively low concentrations are

As, Cd, Pb, Hg

b) Acute and chronic toxicity. Essential trace elements become toxic too when entering an organism in large amounts. Cancerogenic elements should have a high rank of priority, also if this attribute is not exactly proved: Some nickel- and arseniccompounds and hexavalent chromium.

c) Kinetics in animal and man: Absorption, excretion; especially accumulation in specific body compartments. Elements with long biological half times require special control: the extrem long half time of cadmium needs carefully conducted epidemiologic analyses, thus having highest priority in environmental control.

d) Extent of occurence in environment, by industrial use or other sources. Some of the enumerated elements are widespread in the aquatic and terrestrial ecosystem. Metals of limited use like thallium or palladium are only of regional interest.
Furthermore decreasing industrial use (as for Arsenic) or replacement by less toxic compounds (as for methylmercury) have to be considered.

2.2. Pathways of the specified inorganics for human exposure

As mentioned in chapter 1 the most important pathway for human exposure beside direct industrial contamination is the entrance of trace elements in human nutrition of animal origin. It is remarkable that concentrations of trace elements tend to be higher than in foods from plants and that furthermore the availability of metals for absorption from the

small intestine is greater.
For environmental monitoring of farm animals the chain

    soil - plant - animal - human nutrition

is of great importance.
Granzing animals may derive their minerals not only from a variety of
plants, but may ingest directly considerable amounts of soil. The interrelations soil - plant - animal are complex. Soil or plant factors
may occur as deficiencies or excess of trace elements in farm elements.
Seasonal variation in the chemical composition of plants and difference
in elemental composition of the morphological parts of a plant are known.
Indicator or accumulator plants are well recognized, e.g. for selenium,
cobalt, fluorine. So deficiency- or toxicity-diseases in farm animals
occur, combined with low or high content of the specified trace element in specimen obtained from these animals.

Atmospheric pollution may constitute a further significant source of
elements with long-term dangers to human health. The deposition of lead
on soil and plants along highways with decreasing concentration on
greater distance is known, thus entering the food chain. Trace-element
food additives (e.g. for protection of Se- or Mn-deficiency) must be
considered too.
Since man is partially a secondary or tertiary consumer, his chances of
accumulation some elements being present in food from farm animals may
be reduced.

An important consequence of the discussed points is the necessity of analyzing the food of farm animals and correlate the values with those obtained from the organ specimen.

2.3. Metabolic, environmental and toxicological characteristics and
     assessment of current levels of trace elements in domestic and
     farm animals

Only the points of possible environmental significance concerning this
heading shall be listened in this chapter. Selection of indicator specimen resulting from specific organ distribution is given in chapter 3.1.
The following domestic and farm animals has been considered:

pigs, cows, calves, sheep (lambs, ewes), poultry (chicks, turkeys), goats,
horses, in some cases dogs, cats, rabbits.
The reported values for trace element concentration in animal tissues
are selected critically from the literature. As pointed out in chapter
4, analytical difficulties, contamination problems etc. might have led
to erroneous results in some cases. +

2.3.1. Arsenic

The trivalent As-compounds are in vivo transformed to the much less toxic
pentavalent form.
There is no evidence of accumulation in any internal organ or tissue;

+) All concentrations given in this chapter are of unaffected areas, thus
    indicating the "normal" range.

in man hair, nails and skin contain the highest arsenic levels. For
domestic and farm animals no systematic studies of As levels in tissues have appeared.

         meat (pork, beef, lamb)   0,10 µg/g wet weight
         muscle (turkey)   0,03
         liver (turkey)   0,04

         milk (cow)   0,03 - 0,06 µg/g

It must be noted, that organic pentavalent arsenic compounds as arsa-
nilic acid or substituted phenylarsonic acids are used as growth stimulants for pigs and poultry, thus influencing the As levels of tissues.

2.3.2 Cadmium

Cadmium enters the environment through its increasing industrial use,
zinc refineries etc.
It is toxic to virtually every system in the animal body. When accumulation increases more than metallothionein-bound fraction, Cd is bound
to other proteins and symptoms of toxicity appear.
Unfortunately just for this highly toxic element some reported concentration values seem to be in error. The use of modern analytical technique leads not automatically to accurate results. Flameless atomic absorption spectrometry as method of choice in cadmium trace determination
will often yield too high values, due to numerous interferences.
The distribution in animal tissues is similar to human pattern:
the highest Cd level appear in the kidneys, followed by the liver. Kidney and liver accumulation was shown in sheep, dogs, pigs.

         kidneys (sheep, beef, lamb) 0,04 - 4,42 µg/g wet w.
         liver (sheep, beef, lamb)   0,09 - 1,69
         muscles (beef, chick, pork) 0,01 - 0,10
         brain (lamb)   0,03
         wool, hair (calves)   0,74 - 0,94

         milk (cow)   1,5 - 37 µg/l

2.3.3 Cobalt

Cobalt has a low order of toxicity in all species including man. Because
of occurence of cobalt deficiency deseases in farm animals (Grand Traverse desease; Enzootic marasmus) the addition of a small proportion of
cobalt salts or ores to pastures is widely practiced. The highest Co concentrations are found in kidneys, liver and bones with relatively small
differences among species (man, pig, dog, chick, cattle, rabbit).

         liver (sheep)   0,15 µg/g dry weight
         kidney (sheep)   0,23
         spleen (sheep)   0,09

         milk (cow)   0,4 - 1,1 µg/l

2.3.4 Chromium

The hexavalent form is much more toxic than the trivalent; chronic exposure to chromate dust has been correlated with increased incidence of

lung cancer.
In man there is no special concentration in any tissue; the Cr level
decline with age except in the lungs.

muscle (beef, pork, lamb, chick)	0,02 - 0,26 µg/g wet w.
kidney (beef, pork, lamb)	0,01 - 0,18
liver (beef, lamb)	0,03 - 0,24
milk (cow)	8 - 13 ng/g

2.3.5 Fluorine

Fluorosis appears when maximum of urinary fluoride excretion is reached,
that cannot be surpassed. Deposition of retained F in soft tissues
occures as soon as the skeleton is saturated.
Accumulation tissues are only bones and teeth. Normal skeleton concentration of fluorine in adult farm animals, not unduly exposed are:

$$300 - 600 \text{ µg/g}$$

Toxic thresholds for bone F concentration in sheep, cattle and swine are
given with 2000 - 5000 µg/g.

liver (sheep, cows)	2 - 4 µg/g dry weight
kidney (sheep, cows)	4 - 5
whole blood (cows)	less than 0,1 µg/g
milk (cow)	1 - 2 µg/g

2.3.6 Mercury incl. Methylmercury

The extent of use of mercury in industry led to a widespread distribution.
In agriculture methylmercury compounds are used for seed treatment. Alkyl
derivatives of Hg are more toxic than most other chemical forms and can
enter the food chain (fish) through the activity of microorganisms with
the ability to methylate the mercury present in industrial wastes. Animal body has only an extremely limited capacity to convert inorganic
forms of Hg.
The different distribution pattern of inorganic and methylmercury compounds
is most important for brain Hg content: After administration of inorganic
Hg only little penetrates to the brain, but once mercury has entered, turnover is very slow. Methylmercury compounds are much better absorbed,
retained, more firmly bound and induce higher CNS-level, but still being
relatively slow. Higher concentrations after methylmercury exposure than
in brain were found in liver and kidneys (cats, dogs, pigs, calves).
The target organs of toxicity of inorganic mercury are liver, kidneys
and intestinal tract. Alkyl derivatives cause toxic neuroencephalopathy
with involvement of the cerebral and cerebellar cortex nerve cells.
In man highest concentrations are found in skin, nails, hair, teeth,
which acquire Hg easily from the environment. Of particular interest
is the high mercury content in the thyroid and pituitary gland (together with accumulation of selenium in a ratio 1 : 1, a possible auto-
protective effect, since Se can be considered as Hg-inactivator). Among
the other organs the kidneys contain most Hg.
The form, in which mercury is present in organs shows differences; varying amounts of methylmercury were found: maximum relative fraction of
methylmercury (65 - 97 % of total Hg) were detected in pork chops,

hog liver and brain, lowest relative fractions in kidneys and liver.
A decrease in the mercury content of foods of animal origin was
found in countries, in which methoxyethylmercury was substituted for
methylmercury:

Sweden:		1975	1968	
	pork chop	o,o3	o,o1	µg Hg/g
	liver pig	o,o6	o,o25	
	liver ox	o,o15	o,oo5	

2.3.7 Molybdenum

Molybdenum toxicity depends on age, species, amount and chemical form
of ingested Mo, content of inorganic sulfate, total sulfur, proteins,
zinc or lead in diet.
An important role plays the physiological antagonism Mo/Cu. Critical
Cu/Mo ratio in animal feeds is 2,o; lowering leads to copper deficiency
in animals. Low Mo concentration in diet may result in accumulation of
Cu in tissues with signs of chronic copper poisoning. These relationship was shown for sheep and cattle, but not for pigs.
Tolerance to Mo toxicity varies with species:

cattle < sheep < poultry < horses, pigs

Species differences of Mo-content in tissues appear to be small, and
there is only little accumulation in any particular organ. In sheep
and cattle more than half the body molybdenum is present in the skeleton, next largest in skin, wool and muscles. Liver contains only about
2 % of the total.

liver (chicks)	3,6	µg/g dry weight
kidney (chicks)	4,4	
wool (sheep)	o,o3 - o,58	µg/g
milk (cow)	18 - 12o	µg/l
milk (ewe)	< 1o	µg/l

2.3.8 Manganese

Animal tissues play only a subordinate role in manganese supply of man.
Moreover Mn has a low toxicity for mammals.
In organism it is found in higher concentration in organs rich in mito-
chondria. Beside liver and kidneys, bones show enrichment. The highest
manganese concentration was found in the retina.
Average concentrations for a range of animal species:

liver	2,5	µg/g wet weight
kidneys	1,2	
muscle	o,18	
brain	o,4o	
spleen	o,4o	
hair	o,8o	
bones	3,3	
milk (cow)	2o - 5o µg/l	

2.3.9 Nickel

Toxicity of nickel is only of interest, when industrial exposure to dusts occur. Environmental monitoring may therefore be limited to such areas (Similar considerations can be applied to several of the above enumerated trace elements as Tl, Pd, Be etc.).
Some nickel compounds such as nickel carbonyl may induce pulmonary cancer.
Nickel shows no particular concentration in any known tissue or organ.

milk (cow)   3,8 ± o,3 µg/l

Comparison of reported serum nickel levels:

man	1,1 - 4,6 µg/l
horses	1,3 - 2,5
cattle	1,7 - 4,4
dogs	1,8 - 4,2
goats	2,7 - 4,4
cats	1,5 - 6,4
pigs	4,2 - 5,6
rabbits	6,5 - 14,o

2.3.1o Lead incl. Alkyl lead compounds

Most of "natural" level of lead in air comes from the exhaust fumes of cars burning petrol containing alkyl lead additives. This oxidizing process of corse yields inorganic lead, which is spread out in all ecosystems. The tetraalkyl lead compounds though more toxic play only a limited role in the environment.
In chronic lead intoxication neurological defects, renal tubular dysfunction, and anemia are typical signs.
Absorption and retention of ingested lead is greatly affected by the dietary levels of other elements (Ca, P, Fe, Cu, Zn).
The pattern of tissue distribution in farm animals is similar to man, and the concentrations are of the same order as found for humans.
Highest concentrations are found in bones, serving as deep compartment for lead; lowest in muscles.

liver (calves, cows, heifers)	0,2 - 1,9 µg/g wet weight
brain	0,3
kidneys	1,4
muscles	0,02
milk (cow)	0,02 - 0,04 µg/g

Blood lead levels in farm animals seem to be a little lower than in man:

sheep	0,14 ± 0,o1 µg/ml
cattle	0,13 ± 0,o1
upper limit for "normal" range in man:	0,4 - 0,5 µg/ml

2.3.11 Palladium

Palladium and platinum are receiving increasing attention because of their many uses as industrial catalysts. Environmental monitoring may be

118

limited to specific areas.
About tissue distribution or indicator specimen less or nothing is
known.

2.3.12 Selenium

As mentioned above, due to concentration in soil and plants, in farm
animals excess (Alkali desease; blind staggers) and deficiency diseases
(white muscle disease; stiff lamb disease) are possible. The absorption
rate depends from the chemical forms and amounts of the element ingested
just as for arsenic or mercury. Elemental Se and selenides show low,
venites and selenates higher absorption. The strong tendency of selenium to complex with heavy metals involve reducing Se toxicity when
diet contains heavy metals as well as a protective effect against the
toxic properties of cadmium, mercury or arsenic.
In contrast to early experiments selenium is now recognized as a cancer-
protecting element.
Highest selenium concentrations are usually found in liver and kidneys,
much lower levels in muscles, bones and blood. Red cells contain more
Se than plasma (chick, man).

kidneys (pig, cattle, sheep)	11,5 µg/g dry weight
liver	1,8
muscles	o,5
spleen	1,3
lung	1,1
whole blood (sheep)	0,04 - 0,2o µg/ml
" " (cows)	0,08
" " (chicks)	o,1o
hair (cattle)	1 - 4 µg/g
similar: feathers (chicks)	
milk (cow)	3 - 1o ng/ml

2.3.13 Tin

Humans and animals are extremely tolerant of tin (poor absorption). Only
very few human Sn-poisonings from canned or other food packed in uncovered
tin plate are reported.
Average concentrations in human and animal tissues incl. milk:

o,5 - 4,o µg/g dry weight

Some remarks point out, that bones and lungs contain little more tin than
other tissues.

2.3.14 Thallium

As mentioned above, monitoring thallium concentration is of limited interest. Effluence from mineral processing and use as rodenticide will not
lead to a global contamination of the environment.
Little is known on distribution pattern in animals. Signs for bone accumulation and higher concentration in kidneys and hair are reported.

2.3.15 Vanadium

The relatively great toxicity of vanadium is affected by the diet composition, as mentioned for most other trace elements.
A vanadate/chromate antagonism seems to be of interest.
Data of animal tissues are rare and discordant. Early investigations
gave a range of< o,o2 - o,3 µg/g with consistently higher levels in
lungs. Recent results are much lower (see chapter 4):

liver (calves)	2,4 - 1o ng/g wet weight
milk (cow)	o,o7 - o,11 ng/g

2.3.16 Zinc

Zinc is relatively nontoxic for mammals. Pigs, sheep, cattle (and man)
exhibit considerable tolerance to high zinc intakes, depending greatly
on the nature of the diet (important: Cu/Zn ratio).
Richest dietary sources for man are oysters (may contain more than
1ooo µg/g). Muscle meat range before vegetables. But chronic toxicity
from dietary intake is an unlikely hazard to man. Treatment over
long periods with high zinc administration may interfere with cobalt
and iron metabolism. Increased zinc intake may be desirable; e.g. it
will reduce the tendency to accumulate cadmium (competitive binding to
proteins like metallothionein).
Acute zinc intoxication may in most cases be caused by the cadmium, that
is almost always present as a zinc contaminant.
In contrast zinc deficiencies in man and animals are described in numerous cases.
Species differences in tissue concentration are small. Highest zinc concentration in living tissue is found in the choroid of the eye (zinc
function unknown):

sheep	25o - 44o µg/g
cattle	14o - 25o
dogs	several 1ooo

High Zn levels appear in prostate and semen. A substantial portion of total
body zinc is present in hair (wool).
Blood cell fraction contains more zinc than plasma.

kidneys (pigs, beef, lambs)	6 - 55 µg/g wet weight
liver (pigs, beef, lambs)	34 - 76
brain (lambs)	1o
muscle (pigs, beef, lambs, chicks)	6 - 7o
spleen (pigs)	28
skin (chicks)	o,4
whole blood (rabbits)	2,5 µg/ml
plasma (pigs)	o,6
" (sheep)	o,5 - o,9
erythrocytes (goose)	6,5 µg/g
(rabbits, dogs)	9
hair (cattle)	115 - 135 µg/g

milk (cows, goats, ewes)   2 - 7 µg/ml

3. Considerations for sample selection, collection, containment and storage

3.1. Selection of specimens

The review in chapter 2.3 has pointed out, that most trace elements are distributed inhomogeneous in organism. Organs with the highest trace element contant are not automatically usable as environmental indicator system. The concentration of the specific pollutant in an indicator specimen has to reflect acute or chronic exposure.
Under these aspects the following farm animal specimen are proposed:

Arsenic:

Levels of As in hair may reflect arsenic exposure. Milk of cows grazing in As contaminated areas showed a significant increase from normal 0,03 - 0,06 to 1,5 µg/g. In man total urinary arsenic excretion provides a useful index of exposure.

Cadmium:

Cd levels in kidneys and liver reflect cadmium intakes over a wide range (sheep, dogs, pigs). In mice a positive correlation between urinary excretion and body burden was found.

Cobalt:

In diagnosing cobalt deficiency in ruminants liver is used.

Chromium:

In man liver and kidneys reflect regional differences in environmental Cr intakes. Hair provides a useful index of the Cr status. Whole blood is not a good indicator since blood chromium is not in equilibrium with tissue stores.

Fluorine:

Plasma fluoride level changes rapidly as response to changes in fluoride intake, but it seems usable only for short-term changes because of rapid returning to normal concentration as consequence of rapid loss to urine and skeleton. Diurnal variation in plasma F level are reported for sheep, dogs etc.
Bone fluor content is independent of day to day variation in intake. For sheep and cattle a positive correlation between urinary fluoride level and F ingestion was shown. As sources for urinary fluoride release from the skeleton as well as the food and water supply may be considered. Thus high urinary levels can reflect current ingestion or previous exposure to high intakes.
In farm animals diagnosis of fluorosis is based upon analysis of plasma urine, bones, teeth and diet. Moreover bone alkaline phosphatase activity is measured. This seems an important point of view. In some cases chemical analysis alone may be not sufficient for monitoring purposes. Specific enzyme analyses may complete the control (see Lead).

Mercury:

In every case separate analyses of organic and inorganic mercury are useful to make exact environmental mercury statement.
In man hair, urine, blood and saliva are used as diagnostic procedures. But there are some limitations: hair is unusable as indicator for metallic mercury exposure.
Blood values reflect mainly recent exposure and are not useful as indicators of accumulations in critical organs if the exposure varies. Blood/brain and blood/kidneys ratios are not constant, but change with time after an exposure or during a series of exposures. In chicks liver and kidneys reflected Hg intake.
Accumulation compartments for methylmercury compounds useful as indicator systems, are above all the blood cells, or though less reliable, whole blood. CNS and hair specimens may be used too.

Molybdenum:

Response of the tissues in dietary molybdenum is greatly influenced by dietary sulfate levels.
Content of Mo in the liver is only useful, if dietary sulfur and protein status are also known.
Whole blood relect Mo ingestion (sheep). More than 7o % of blood Mo are present in red cells.
Milk molybdenum levels are susceptible to changes in Mo exposure. In cow's milk all Mo is bound to xanthin oxidase, thus xanthin oxidase activity of such milk is proportional to its molybdenum content.

Manganese:

Manganese concentration in bones can be raised or lowered by varying the Mn intakes of the animal (calves, rabbits, pigs, chicks). The manganese level in wool (lambs) and feathers (pullets) varies significantly with Mn exposure, whereas cattle hair seems to be no good indicator.
Milk responds rapidly with changes in dietary manganese.

Nickel:

In several farm animals the nickel content of some tissues seems to be higher than in man.
In calves kidneys and spleen are probably useful as indicator systems.
Milk showed no response on varying nickel exposure.

Lead:

All tissues seem to reflect lead exposure except the muscles. Especially bones, liver, kidneys and hair are useful indicator specimens.

Since lead readily passes the mammary barrier, milk can serve as indicator too. Lead content of whole blood is of use only in combination with measurement of δ-aminolevulinic acid (ALA) in urine and, more sensitive: determination of erythrocyte δ-aminolevulinic acid dehydratase (ALAD).

Selenium:

Selenium concentrations in tissues reflect the level of environmental
Se over a wide range. In pigs a highly significant linear correlation of o,95 between selenium exposure and tissue Se was found. In
poultry and chicks liver and kidneys responded to all dietary selenium
supplementation. Muscles showed no response.
Blood selenium response was demonstrated for chicks, sheeps, cows. Hair
of cattle is a useful indicator of both Se deficiency and Se toxicity:

unaffected areas: 1 -   4 µg/g
seleniferous range: lo - 3o µg/g

Similar relations were shown for feathers of chicks.
Selenium concentrations in milk (cow) varies with Se intake, reflecting
the Se status of the soils and pastures of the areas:

normal range: 3 -   lo ng/ml
high-Se rural areas: 16o - 127o ng/ml

As indicated for lead and molybdenum, measurement of enzyme activities
may give further informations: the activity of the selenoprotein
glutathione peroxidase (GSH-Px) (highest acitivity in liver) drops significantly when Se in diet is restricted (lambs, chicks).

Zinc:

Most rapid accumulation and turnover of retained zinc occurs in the pancreas, liver, kidneys and spleen.
Zinc levels of milk reflect both low and high zinc intake.
In pigs, cattle and goats hair was proved to be a good indicator of
Zn exposure, but must be used with caution: individual variability is
very high; variations with age and part of body, and seasonal differences
has been reported.
Plasma zinc changes significantly with high or low zinc exposure as demonstrated in cats, rabbits, pigs, sheep, cattle, lambs, goats. But
numerous alterations of plasma zinc not influenced by Zn exposure have
been observed in farm animals as well as in man. Various disease
states, stress situations, diurnal variations etc. must be taken into
consideration.

The preceding considerations about selection of indicator specimens
in farm animals are summarized in the table.

Selection of Indicator Specimen in Domestic and Farm Animals for Trace Elements

trace element / organ	Arsenic	Berryllium	Cadmium	Cobalt	Chromium	Fluorine	inorganic Mercury	Methylmercury	Molyb-denum	Manganese	Nickel	Lead	Palladium	Selenium	Tin	Thallium	Vanadium	Zinc
Kidney			+	(+)	(+)		+	(+)			(+)	+		+		(+)		+
Liver			+	+	(+)		+	(+)	(+)			+		+				+
Muscle			o									o		o				
Brain							(+)	+										
Lung					(+)										(+)		(+)	
Spleen											(+)							+
Skin			o											(+)				
Bone			o	(+)	+					+		+			(+)	(+)	'	
Teeth					+				+									
Whole blood	o						(+)	+	+		(+)			+				(+)
Blood cells								+				+						(+)
Plasma					+							o						+
Milk (cow)	+								+	+	o	+		+			(+)	+
Urine	+		(+)		+	+												o
Hair, Wool, Feathers	+		o		(+)		+	+	(+)	+		+		+		(+)		+

+   Usable as monitoring organ; accumulation or indicator function proved
(+)   Advantage not proved for animals / or: of limited use
o   Unsuitable

3.2 Problems of precautions and collection; requirements for containers

Environmental monitoring organic and inorganic pollutants involves in
most cases determination of concentrations in the ppb or subppb range.
It is evident that normal cleaning procedures or precautions are insufficient.
The wide spread of reported values for trace elements in the ng/g level
(Co, Ni, Cr, Mn, Cd, Se etc.) can be derived from uncritical application of analytical techniques as well as from "positive" or "negative"
contamination.
Contamination problems start with collection of biological samples. It
is almost impossible to avoid metallic instruments in sampling tissue
specimens. Trace element contamination introduced in blood samples by
disposable needles may be of the same order as these elements are
present in blood (Ni, Co, Cr, Mn). Higher concentrated trace elements
(Cu, Fe, Zn) are not affected by these contamination sources. Similar
considerations may be applied to knifes, scissors and other instruments
necessary for organ dissection. Of course there are plastic or glass
knifes and scissors. But using them, no guarantee is given, that they
do not contaminate the sample perhaps more than the metallic instruments.
If a trace element is not distributed uniformly in organism or single
organ, the additional problem of cross-contamination must be considered.
Recently the use of laser has been proposed for cutting biological tissues.

Next problem appears, when the specimen must be stored. Glass and plastic
material contain easily detectable amounts of trace (and bulk) elements.
In the case of plastics some of these elements are residues of polymerization catalysts.
Most of these elements are leached from the surface of the containers
when treated with diluted acids. Heavy metals may be removed by using
complexing agents.
In every case an intensive cleaning procedure is necessary before using
a container. Several authors suggest as cleaning method for most trace
element work, treatment of the container with hydrochloric acid (1+1)
and ultrapure distilled water.
The procedure needs several weeks.
Purest materials are polytetrafluoroethylene and conventional polyethylene.
It must be mentioned, that in extreme trace element analysis terms like
"metal free containers" or "washed metal free" should be avoided. At
best "metal poor" may be used.
For practical purposes this means: a) testing any material contacting
the specimen, b) having regard to the analytical blank in every case.

Storage of liquid samples results in various new contamination problems.
Rates and amounts of adsorption or leaching of trace elements are
higher. Changing the pH of the solution may have contrary effects.
Therefore a drying step should be enforced after collection.
Lyophilization may be useful for trace element specimens, though loss
of highly volatile elements like mercury or organic metal compounds
seems possible. But there are several references which indicate that
this loss from tissue samples is neglectible.
Inhomogeneous organs have to be homogenized before storage. Avoidance of

metallic instruments is difficult. Perhaps ultrasonic methods give
some advantages.
Deep freezing seems to be the method of choice for storing tissue
specimens over prolonged periods. Some trace elements may change the
chemical form when quick-frozen and stored in a frozen state, but
whole element content will remain constant.
Plasma and blood samples should be quickly frozen too. Returning to
room temperature again, the denaturated proteins fail to dissolve. As
our laboratory practice with these specimens has shown, these sediments contain considerable amounts of the polyvalent trace element
ions. Thus the whole specimen has to be homogenized and used for
analysis.

4. Analytical procedures

4.1. Analytical methods of choice for trace elements in biological
specimens

For determination of trace elements in biological specimens, a number
of methods are well established, described and applicated in various
biological matrices.
A potential danger may result from the further development of automation in analytical systems, perhaps resulting in a "black box", which
works up a specimen filled in, to a lot of printed numbers, and no one
knows what happens inside.An important aspect just in environmental
control and trace analysis is the continuous requirement of special
trained scientists, able to look critically at the method used, to
find possible error sources. The task of the analyst is not to produce hundreds of values, or determine twenty-five elements in five
minutes, but to give exact results with proved accuracy.

4.1.1. Atomic Absorption Spectrometry (AAS)

This widely used method is applicable to the determination of nearly all the above listened trace elements (except fluorine). Detection
limits had been lowered to the ng and sub-ng range by development
of flameless methods allowing in many cases the determination without
preconcentration.
The graphite furnace seems to have advantages, though the process of
ashing and atomizing are not yet fully understood, thus involving
possible errors. Background correctors (deuterium continuum, or
halogen lamps) are often used uncritically. In cases of volatile elements (particular importance: cadmium) the low maximum ashing temperature (Cd 3oo° C) yields high unspecific absorption due to undestruc-
ted organic components or high inorganic salt concentration. Direct
Cd determination in matrices with high lipid content (brain, adipose
tissue, milk, oils, fat) using graphite furnace seems not possible until now. Separation of cadmium from the matrix has to be performed before analysis. As own investigations proved, background corrector is
not able to eliminate unspecific absorption when determining Cd in
the mentioned matrices directly, even after considerable dilution. This
systematic error source is based on the specific structural composition
of the background. Recently a method using the Zeeman effect was appli-

cated to this problem.
Because of very low detection limit, zinc traces should be determined by
flame AAS; contamination problems using flameless method for zinc
measurement require extreme precautions.
Arsenic and selenium traces may be determined by flameless AAS after transformation to their hydrides from an acid digest with sodium borohydride.
For mercury the cold vapor method gives the lowest detection limit.

4.1.2 Neutron Activation Analysis (NAA)

Neutron activation analysis like AAS range among the most sensitive analytical techniques known for trace element determination.
Comparison of the two methods points out advantages and disadvantages:

AAS: slightly more precise than NAA;
faster, if only 1 element has to be analysed;
no nuclear irradiation necessary.

NAA: multi-element analysis faster than with AAS;
contamination problems less;
matrix effects possible more important;
in many cases nuclear reactions involve isotopes
of low gamma energies, thus requiring separation;
more expensive.

Example for applicated NAA: in a 4-day-scheme a multielement determination
including Hg, Se, As, Cd, Co, Cr, Mo, Sn, Zn has been reported.

4.1.3 Isotope Dilution Spark Source Mass Spectrometry (ID-SSMS)

SSMS can detect all elements at detection limits down to the ng/g range.
Isotope dilution technique can in theory be applied to any element having
two or more stable isotopes.
With the combination ID-SSMS simultaneous measurement of Cd, Pb, Hg, Mo,
Ni, Se, Tl, Zn, Pd, Sn in a single organic sample has been reported.
The similar method Isotope Dilution Thermal Source Mass Spectrometry
(ID-TSMS) shows better precision, but the number of elements is limited.

4.1.4 Electrochemical methods

These methods are specific and sensitive and allow simultaneous determination of a number of metals. Organic sample preparation involves some
difficulties. Determination of Cd, Pb, Ni, Cd, Zn in biological material
is described by Differential Anodic Stripping Voltammetry (DASV) and
Pulse Polarography.

4.1.5 Other methods

There are some other methods to determine trace elements in biological
matrices, but with limited application.
X-Ray Fluorescence Analysis (XRF) was applied to the determination of
F, V, Mn, Cr, Co, Ni, Zn, Pb.
Beryllium in tissue samples was determined by Fluorescene Spectrometry;

but this methods lack selectivity.
At the lo ppb level As and Ni were measured by Molecular Absorption
Spectrometry. This method too shows interferences with other trace
metals.

4.1.6 Special problems

As mentioned earlier, it is important in some cases to determine the
different chemical forms of the trace element present in tissues.

Mercury:

Determination of alkyl mercury compounds can be performed by gas liquid chromatography after separation from the organic matrix. Methods
of choice for total Hg are NAA and flameless AAS (cold vapor method).
Moreover these two techniques allow to differentiate between inorganic and organic mercury in tissues: For AAS the sample is treated
with cysteine before reduction to elemental Hg with stannous chloride.
Without cysteine, alkyl- and alkoxy alkylmercury salts are not reduced
and inorganic Hg can be determined separately. In NAA procedure the
organomercurials can be extracted by a benzene-cysteine separation.
Measuring the whole sample yields total Hg.

Chromium:

On account of the higher toxicity of hexavalent chromium and its possible role in ling cancer, it would be of interest to state the Cr(III)
/Cr(VI) ratio in environmental specimens. A possibility is the treatment of the sample with different complexing agents and extract tri-
and hexavalent chromium separately. Determination may be performed by
flameless AAS.

Arsenic:

In flameless AAS hydride method trivalent arsenic can be reduced to
arsine separately. Another part of the same specimen may yield total
arsenic by a different reduction procedure, thus being able to cal-
culate the amount of pentavalent form from the difference.

4.2 Pretreatment requirements

The above mentioned problems of trace element contamination led to the
necessity of avoiding too much "chemistry" and handling in sample preparation. Modern analytical methods allow the direct determination of
some trace metals. Nevertheless most determinations require sample
preparation. All work should be done in rooms without any exposed parts.
"Clean benches" allow to work in filtered air, thus diminishing
contamination.
The reported "normal" range for many trace elements in tissues was progressively lowered as techniques were being improved.
Sample pretreatment procedures:

    Preconcentration: ion exchange; solvent extraction; electro-
                            deposition.

Ashing: Procedures for decomposition of organic or biological
samples have to avoid loss of volatile elements (Hg,
Cd, Se, As etc.). There are several methods yielding
a ready dissolution:
a) Wet ashing (nitric acid/sulfuric acid/perchloric acid),
   for volatile elements under reflux. No complete mine-
   ralization.
b) Low temperature ashing with atomic oxygen or micro-
   waves.
c) Burning with oxygen in a closed quartz-system, cooling
   with liquid nitrogen and dissolution in acids. No loss
   of volatile elements; best decomposition or organic
   materials including lipids and oils.

Elements causing problems under most conditions are: Hg, Sn, Se, Pb, As.

4.3. Precision and accuracy

The uncertainty of the listed analytical methods are 2 - lo %, depending
from the element and the concentration in tissues.
For critical evaluation of the analytical method used, standard reference
materials are necessary. Unfortunately there are only few standards of
animal origin usable as reference material for trace elements. The only
tissue is the NBS bovine liver.
If similar matrices are not available, accuracy can be checked by:
recovery experiments; standard addition; interlaboratroy studies (different analytical methods, different instruments, different analysts):
some results of previous interlaboratory studies showed tremendous
variations. In many cases the precision of the analytical values was
sufficient, but the final result was far away from the accurate concentration, pointing out systematic errors.
More intensive co-operation of the analytical institutes should be
managed.

5. References

1. André, T., S. Ullberg, G. Wingvist: The Accumulation and Retention of Thallium in Tissues of the Mouse; Acta pharmacol. toxicol. 16, 229-234 (196o)

2. Friberg, L., J. Vostal (eds.): Mercury in the Environment; CRC Press, Cleveland 1972.

3. Friberg, L., M. Piscator, G. F. Nordberg, T. Kjellström: Cadmium in the Environment; CRC Press, Cleveland 1974.

4. Gills, T.E., H.L. Rook, P.D. La Fleur (eds.): Evaluation and Research of Methodology for the National Environmental Specimen Bank; U.S. Environmental Protection Agency, Research Triangle Park, 1978.

5. Guenter, W., D.B. Bragg: Response of Broiler Chick to Dietary selenium; Poultry Science 56, 2o31-2o38 (1977).

6. Guthrie, B.E.: Chromium, Manganese, Copper, Zinc and Cadmium Content of New Zealand Foods; New Zealand Med. J. 82, 418-424 (1975).

7. Hammer, D.J., J.F. Finklea, P.H.Hendricks, C.M. Shy, J.M. Horton: Hair trace metals levels and environmental exposure; Amer. J. Epidemiol. 93, 84 (1971).

8. Healy, W.B., W.J. McCabe, G.F. Wilson: Ingested soil as a source of microelements for grazing animals; New Zealand J. Agr. Res. 13, 5o3-521 (197o).

9. Hislop, J.S., A. Parker: The Use of Laser for Cutting Bone Samples Prior to Chemical Analysis; Analyst 98, 694 (1973).

1o. Horvath, D.J.: Trace Elements and Health; in: P.M. Newberne (ed.): Trace Substances and Health, Part I; Marcel Dekker, New York 1976.

11. La Fleur, P.D. (ed.): Accuracy in Trace Analysis: Sampling, Sample Handling, Analysis; Vol. I, II; NBS Special Publication 422; U.S. Department of Commerce, Washington 1976.

12. Louria, D.B., M.M. Joselow, A.A. Browder: The Human Toxicity of Certain Trace Elements; Ann.Int.Med. 76, 3o7-319 (1972).

13. Maienthal, E.J., D.A. Becker: A Survey of Current Literature on Sampling, Sample Handling and Long Term Storage for Environmental Materials; NBS Technical Note 929; U.S. Department of Commerce, Washington 1976.

14. Movradineanu, R. (ed.): Procedures Used at the National Bureau of Standards to Determine Selected Trace Elements in Biological and Botanical Materials; NBS Special Publication 492; U.S. Department of Commerce, Washington 1977.

130

15. Muth, H., W.H. Allaway: The relationship of white muscle disease to the distribution of naturally occuring selenium; J. Amer. Vet. Med. Assoc. 142, 1383 (1963).

16. Oehme, F.W.: Veterinary Toxicology: The Epidemiology of Poisonings in Domestic Animals; Clin. Tox. 1o, 1-21 (1977).

17. Reinhold, J.G.: Trace Elements - A Selective Survey; Clin. Chem. 21, 476-5oo (1975).

18. Schlettwein-Gsell, D., S. Mommsen-Straub: Spurenelemente in Lebensmitteln; Hans Huber, Bern, 1973.

19. Tölg, G.: Extreme Trace Analysis of the Elements, I; Talanta 19, 1489-1521 (1972).

2o. Underwood, E.J.: Trace Elements in Human and Animal Nutrition, 4th ed.; Academic Press, New York, 1977.

21. Westöö, G.: Methylmercury compounds in animal foods; in: M.W. Miller, G.C. Berg (eds.): Chemical fallout; Charles C. Thomas, Springfield, Ill., 1969.

22. Williams, J.S.: Seasonal trends of minerals and proteins in prairie grasses; J. Range Management 6. 1oo-1o8 (1953).

23. Zitko, V., W.V. Carson, W.G. Carson: Thallium: Occurence in the Environment and Toxicity to Fish; Bull. Environm. Contam. Toxicol. 13, 23-3o (1975).

6. Summary

There are two points of interest concerning the use of domestic and farm animals in monitoring pollutants in the environment:
1. In contrast to wildlife domestic animals and livestock live in a restricted area with strong relation to the environment of the human population living there.
2. Regarding human exposure the remarkable role of farm animals in the food chain include the necessity of monitoring these specimens.
The "environmental classification" of the inorganic trace elements must be based upon aspects as essentiallity, toxicity, kinetics and extend of occurrence in environment. The nonessential and toxic elements cadmium, lead and mercury should have the highest priority. The organs recommended for monitoring and banking must have an indicator function, reflecting acute and chronic exposure. Since most trace elements are distributed inhomogeneously in organism, accumulation compartments usable as monitoring specimens have to be selected.
The distribution patterns for the different trace elements are widely unknown; in several cases indicator function is proved, e.g. liver for Cd, inorganic Hg, Pb, Se, Co, similar to wildlife and humans.
Most analytical work has done about the compartments liver, kidneys, milk (cow) and hair (wool, feathers).
Among the analytical procedures of choice for determination trace element

concentrations, atomic absorption spectrometry including different specific methods, and neutron activation analysis must be mentioned. The uncertainty of the analytical method depends on the element, the concentration of the element and the kind of tissue. Matrix effects may cause systematic errors, influencing the accuracy of the method.
Only with critical evaluation of the method used, analytical results may
serve as basis for environmental statements.

MONITORING ENVIRONMENTAL MATERIALS AND SPECIMEN BANKING
USING TERRESTRIAL INSECTS WITH PARTICULAR REFERENCE TO
INORGANIC SUBSTANCES AND PESTICIDES

Jerry J. Bromenshenk
Department of Botany
University of Montana
Missoula, Montana 59812
U.S.A.

Summary

Although a few species of terrestrial insects have been used to monitor
environmental quality, the number is insignificant compared to the hundreds of thousands existent. In the United States, the only specimen banking of insects is short-term and usually consists of backlogs of specimens to be analyzed rather than specimens intended for retrospective comparisons. Museum specimens represent the only long-term storage, but the
value of museum insects for residue determinations would be extremely
limited and only appropriate for the most stable chemicals.

Insects are indisputably important to man. Many insects species are major
or critical components of natural and cultivated ecosystems. Studies of
insect populations contribute greatly to the development of ecological
concepts because of attributes such as species diversity, abundance,
small size, short life cycles, and ecological importance. Both chronic
and acute exposures to pollutants may induce responses in insect systems
which in turn may have considerable impacts on communities and ecosystems.

Honey bees and many insects occupying higher trophic levels, such as predaceous beetles, appear to be bioaccumulators and/or biomagnifiers of many
contaminants. Pollutant build-up and transfer through insect food chains
may be a route by which higher organisms, primarily insectivores and carnivores, could ingest proportionally greater amounts of harmful substances.

Taxa selection and procedures for collecting, preserving, transporting,
storing,and analyzing samples are complex decisions which depend on the
materials to be monitored and the relation of these materials to be biological populations chosen for study. It is impossible to establish easy or
indisputable study or experimental formats because of the many variables
involved. The planning, organization, and execution of such a program
would require, at the very least, the experience and judgement of a qualified population entomologist, an analytical chemist, and a biostatistician.
Nevertheless, three functional groups (pollinators, regulators of pest
populations, and detritus processors) of terrestrial insects and other invertebrates were identified as particularly well suited for environmental
monitoring and specimen banking. Also, guidelines were developed regarding
the above procedures.

Centralized, national specimen banks for insect specimens and other biological materials, such as plants, birds, and mammals, seem to have advantages. Cost estimates for a monitoring and banking program utilizing
insects can be made for monitoring of pollution levels and banking but
are difficult to make for the monitoring of biological responses to pollutants.

Introduction

Insects are indisputably important in relation to ecosystems and to mankind.
The total number of insects is estimated to exceed that of all other animals and plants combined. Beneficial insects pollinate plants, consume
or parasitize harmful insects, improve soil, control weeds, produce useful products such as honey and silk, or provide other services "helpful"
to man. Harmful insects parasitize humans, transmit disease-producing
organisms, or compete with us for resources.

Insects, like other organisms, respond to the abiotic and biotic pressures
of their environments. These attributes of the environment together with
the genetic composition of individuals in a population determine their
presence, abundance, and evolution in any given ecosystem or area system.
The abiotic factors would include chemical pollutants, which by definition
are inimical agents introduced into ecosystems.

Considerable information exists concerning chemical, metabolic, toxicological, and other characteristics of many major organic and inorganic pollutants in relation to plants and vertebrate animals. Much less is known
about the effects of these same pollutants on most invertebrates; although many species of aquatic invertebrates have been studied with respect to noxious chemicals and other perturbations; e.g., thermal pollution. With respect to the terrestrial invertebrates, the insects and mites
have received and presumably will continue to receive scrutiny as regards
insecticides-materials that kill insects by their chemical action. In
addition, the use of pesticides to control populations of insects has
resulted in environmental contamination by persistant chemicals such as
DDT and related compounds.

Effects of chemical pollutants often are examined either in terms of harm
to human health or in terms of harm to ecosystems. The Committee for the
Working Conference on Principles of Protocols for Evaluating Chemicals in
the Environment (National Agency of Sciences, 1975) commented that subtle
effects of chemicals on human health may appear to be a superfluous concern compared to more immediate worldwide problems such as epidemic disease and starvation. The well-being of plants and animals may seem to be
an even less important consideration than human health. However, the committee voiced the opinion that "... it seems prudent to increase our understanding of chemical effects on populations and ecosystems in order to
guard against the possibility that unforeseen changes may have serious impacts on species of central importance in the natural and cultivated ecosystems upon which we depend".

The general public tends to view terrestrial insects mainly as pests. As
such, these insects often are thought of strictly in terms of a need to
control. If chemical pollutants poison or in some other way injure populations of insects, this might be interpreted as a desirable effect.

But this would be an overly simplified conclusion. Insects as a whole do more good than harm. For example, pollinating insects contribute directly or indirectly to as much as one-third of the food supply of the populace of the United States (McGregor, 1976). In uncultivated areas insects are necessary for the pollination of most soilholding and soil-enriching plants (Bohart, 1952) as well as forbs of grasslands and shrubs and herbs of temperate forests and deserts (Baker and Hurd, 1968). As another example, predaceous and parasitic insects are important and in many cases key regulators of pest insect populations. Many insect regulators occur naturally; others are introduced, manipulated, or modified by man. Harm to pollinators, predators, or parasites could have far reaching consequences to ecosystems such as serious reductions in pollination efficacy or in the ability to keep pest populations in check. Each insect population affects to some degree the ecosystem in which it is found. Some of the effects are small, others significant, and a few crucial to ecosystems.

Traditionally, mankind has regarded a few insects as beneficial, classified many others as harmful (termed pests), and ignored the rest. But, an insect is a pest because we call it one. Insect pests utilize materials of interest to man. Designations of beneficial, harmful, or pest generally have no ecological validity.

However, we number our arthropod enemies in the thousands of species (Sabrosky, 1952). In 1971, there were more than 9oo registered pesticides in the United States and an annual production of more than 1.1 billion pounds (USDA, 1972). A significant proportion of these pesticides were insecticides. Considering the magnitude of the effort and of the monetary expenditures put forth to control undesirable insects, it is amazing that we still know so little concerning the effects of chemical pollutants other than insecticides on populations of these organisms. Also, it is surprising that many environmental impact assessments conducted in the United States have totally ignored terrestrial insects (Bromenshenk, 1978a).

Past and current programs

Terrestrial insects occasionally have been used for the monitoring of the levels of chemical pollutants and their effects in ecosystems. Tissue residue analyses for pesticides and serval inorganic chemicals have been performed employing honey bees, fruit flies, insects of the soil/litter subsystem, and a few other species. But, the number of insects species that have been examined is insignificant compared to the hundreds of thousands and possibly millions of species that exist worldwide.

In the United States, terrestrial insects have just begun to be recognized as suitable environmental monitors; whereas the banking of terrestrial insects specimens for deferred chemical analyses seems to be non-existent. Specimens are preserved by some laboratories for short periods - a few hours, days, months, or occasionally years. Usually, these samples are accumulated for analytical runs or are held for further analyses. Occasionally, specimens may be stored for limited periods for retrospective comprisons with previous analytical data or until tests of appropriate analytical procedures have been conducted. In a few site-specific environmental impact assessment, samples from baseline collections were retained and compared with post-development samples.

Literature searches and my own correspondence revealed no records of existing regional, national, or international specimen banks incorporating
terrestrial invertebrates with the exception of a bank in Germany containing earthworms and carabid beetles (Dr. Paul Müller, Universität des
Saarlandes, Federal Republic of Germany, personal communication).

Taxanomic reference collections are a form of specimen bank and many contain large numbers of insects. However, most of the entomological specimens
have been dried, pinned, or kept in preservative fluids such as formalin
or alcohol. Their value in retrospective analyses would be limited because of the loss of any but the most stable chemicals from the insect
tissues and by a lack of descriptive information concerning collection,
handling, and storage procedures. Also, many of the current analytical
methods for chemical residues in biological tissues require relatively
large quantities of tissue material relative to the size of many insects.
This would necessitate the pooling of many specimens for analysis, unless
the insect specimens were very large. Many museums curators would not
be willing to supply large numbers of specimens for destructive sampling
and analysis procedures.

Van Hook and Huber (1976) conducted a survey which identified 657 extant
specimen and data collections in the United States containing atmospheric,
water, geological, microbiological, plant, and animal materials. They found
that, for the most part, these materials are not appropriate for retrospective chemical analyses because of the sampling, handling, and storage
techniques being utilized. Van Hook and Huber concluded that their survey
served to alert the scientific community to a national interest in their
collections, caused some respondents to re-evaluate their collection and
storage procedures, and facilitated information exchange among investigators concerning access to specimens and data.

Similarly, during my conversations with entomologists and analytical chemists across the United States, I discovered considerable interest in the
establishment of environmental monitoring and specimen banking programs
utilizing insects. Some investigators, especially those involved in
assessing pesticides, expressed a sense of frustration that such a program was not already in existence and volunteered to proved information
and assistance that would contribute to the development of such a program.

Rationale and Literature Review

Environmental disturbances associated with the application of pesticides
and with persistant pesticide residues remaining in ecosystems are undesirable. Hazards to non-target organisms including beneficial insects,
wildlife, and man have prompted concern and a multitude of research efforts.
Substances with a recognized or demonstrated value as biocides generally
have been characterized in terms of chemical formulation, toxicity to insects and mammals, usages, dose-responses, applications, and harzards.
For most insecticides, the mode of action and metabolism is at least partially understood, although there are surprising information gaps concerning the toxicology of some widely used pesticides.

It would be impossible to summarize the available pesticide literature
within a few paragraphs. Thomson (1975) periodically publishes guides
to all of the agricultural chemical produced in the United States.

These guides contain information concerning usages, toxicities, application rates, pests controlled, and precautions. Also, there are many review papers and books on insecticides, their action, and metabolism (e.g. O'Brien 1967; Ymamoto, 197o; Narahashi, 1971). The most comprehensive and current information about effects of pesticides on non-target insects focuses on the honey bee - Apis mellifera L.

Poisoning by insecticides affects bees, the honey and wax that they produce, and plant pollination. This is a major problem in the United States and any country with a highly developed agriculture (McGregor, 1976). Because of this situation, hundreds of pesticides have been tested as sprays or dusts for their toxicity to bees. Atkins et al.(1973) listed 399 pesticides and concluded that 2o percent are highly toxic, 15 percent moderately toxic, and 65 percent relatively nontoxic or at least nontoxic to bees. Similarly, Atkins et al. (1976) ranked 197 pesticides according to toxicity to bees. Johansen (1969) summarized insecticide hazards to wild or native bees. He found many to be more susceptible to poisoning than honey bees. Moffet et al. (1972) found that some herbicides previously classified as harmless by short-term cage tests or the application of dust formulations were highly toxic when tested by other methods. They concluded that predictions of toxic doses may be unreliable because toxicity may vary according to the methods of application and other factors.

The presence of an insecticide or other toxic chemicals on or in the bodies of dead or dying bees often is used to identify the agent or source of harm. In order to isolate these causes of bee death, analytical methods have been developed for both qualitative and quantitative determinations of insecticide residues in bees. Unfortunately, no federal laboratory in the United States routinely analyses bee specimens for all pesticide residues; although many federal, state, university, and commercial laboratories in the United States can determine if residues of pesticides occur in or on bees. Several USDA Bee Research Laboratories, a few university laboratories, and the EPA Biological Investigations Laboratory, Beltsville, Maryland, frequently perform analyses of bees, and thereby they maintain sophisticated methods and produce reliable results.

Honey bees have been used as indicators of environmental pollution by insecticides since the late nineteenth century, when scientists first began to look for the causes of regional, catastrophic bee deaths. In most cases, the bees had been exposed to inorganic insecticides such as arsenic, fluoride, mercury, and sulfur compounds. However, unexpected occasional bee losses occurred in areas where no insecticide had been used. Yet, the bees seemed to have been poisoned. Environmental monitoring and residue analyses revealed that arsenic, mercury, lead, sulfur, and other materials were being released as industrial wastes in quantities sufficient to kill bees (see reviews by Bromenshenk, 1978b; Debackere, 1972; Steche, 1975; Lillie, 1972).

Pesticides are a specific category of pollutants. The bee losses experienced in the late 18oo's were just one indication of the potential severity of effects of several other common chemical substances being released into the environment. Today, a list of the chemical pollutants suspected of being hazardous to the environment would include many thousands of chemicals and there is concern not only about acute effects but also about more subtle, chronic effects.

Since the early 197o's researchers in the United States and Europe have been exploring the possiblity of using honey bees as one of the organisms with which to monitor various chemical pollutants (Bromenshenk, 1976, 1978a, b, c, d; Toshkov et al., 1974; Tong et al., 1975; Hakonson and Bostick, 1976; DeJong and Morse, 1977; Bromenshenk and Carlson, 1975).

Honey bees have highly evolved, complex foraging patterns. They have specialized body parts for carrying nectar and numerous, branched hairs which rake in pollen. While foraging, honey bees cover tremendous dis- tances. During foraging flights, they are likely to collect, carry back, and store any chemical substance that settles on the bees themselves, on the surfaces of plants, or which is absorbed in water or adsorbed on nectar of honey. Eventually, any pollutant brought back to the hive and stored with food supplies is consumed. Besides ingesting these chemi- cals, honey bees may inhale harmful gases, mists, and fine dusts through the twenty respiratory passages which open directly to the air. Conse- quently, impurities tend to concentrate on or in the bodies of bees. In general, the leves of contaminants on or in bees exceed that in air, pol- len, flowers, nectar, or water (Maurizio, 1956; Bromenshenk, 1978b).

This gathering of noxious substances takes its toll, and honey bees appear to be more susceptible to harm by many toxic substances than domestic ani- mals and humans (Lillie, 1972). Less obvious injury to bees may include shortened life-spans, slow but steadily diminishing populations, disrupted foraging behavior, genetic mutations and aberrations, teratologies, re- duced egg laying or viability, and behavioral modifications such as toxi- cant avoidance, disorientation, and memory loss (reviewed by Bromenshenk and Carlson, 1975).

Honey bees and the materials that they gather (pollen and honey) have been used to determine the distribution and magnitude of a variety of contami- nants, including more than 4o trace and major elements. Among these are copper, zinc, phosphorous, cadmium, lead, arsenic, fluoride, and sulfur. Scientists at Los Alamos Scientific Laboratory have found that bees accu- mulate radioactive substances leaking from waste disposal areas (Hakoson and Bostick, 1976), while my own work revealed that honey bees pick up trace elements, pesticides, and radioactive materials ranging from beryl- lium, which occurs naturally in the atmosphere, to materials from atmos- pheric weapons tests (Bromenshenk, 1976, 1978a, 1978d).

A few terrestrial insects other than bees have been studied with respect to monitoring pollutants, particularly air pollutants. Groups of insects that have been investigated consist mainly of insects and other inverte- brates of the soil/litter subsystem, phytophagous insects of forests, and flies, especially house flies (Musca domestica) and fruit flies (Dro- sophila spp.).

Air pollutants reported to have significant effects on terrestrial ento- mological systems include liquid, solid, and gaseous materials, such as sulfur and nitrous oxides, ozone, hydrocarbons, fluorocarbons, smog, dusts, acid mists, major and trace elements. These contaminants may enter the bodies of insects through ingestion, respiration, or penetration through the cuticle. Chemical pollutants may act directly on insects or indirectly through alterations in food and habitat resources. Principal observed effects include mortalities of sensitive species, proliferation of pest insects (possible because of imbalances caused by predisposition of a host weakened by pollution stress to insect attack or by poisoning of predators and/or parasites which keep pest populations in check), and depressed abundance of saprophagous and predaceous insects. Non-lethal effects observed were similar to those for honey bees described earlier in this paper.

Insects of the higher trophic levels, especially pollinators and the predatory beetles, often displayed biomagnification of a variety of materials. Both bioaccumulation and biomagnification have been reported to occur in insect food chains (Carlson and Dewey, 1971; Dewey, 1972; Maurer, 1974; Watson et al., 1976; Giles et al., 1973; Rolfe et al., 1974; Munshower, 1972).

Most investigations of the effects of air pollutants in terrestrial insect systems, reported in the more than 2oo references that I examined, dealt with changes in population dynamics (abundance, distribution, etc.) associated with impacts from easily identifiable pollutant sources such as smelters, coal-fired power plants, and automobile exhausts.

The effects of toxic air pollutants often are similar to those of pesticides. The reader is referred to the discussions in the books by P.W. Price (1975); Clark et al., (1967); Metcalf and Luckmann (1975), which concentrate on the ecological implications of pest management programs.

By far, insecticides including chlorinated hydrocarbons, organophosphates, carbamates, cyclodenes, nicotinoids, rotenoids, pyrethoids, hexachlorocyclo-hexanes, fluorine compounds, arsenicale and various other compounds have received the most attention concerning adverse effects in terrestrial insect populations. Impacts of inorganic air pollutants such as compounds of arsenic, fluorine, sulfur, and nitrogen on a few species of insects have been examined with sufficient detail to provide predictions of some of the types of perturbations expected to occur and estimates of dose-responses with at least a partial understanding of the physiological mechanisms involved.

However, for most terrestrial insects and for categories or organic chemical pollutants other than insecticides, little or no effort has been made towards chemical monitoring or elucidating consequences of exposure. There are occasional reports concerning individual chemicals in relation to one or more species of insect - usually conducted in a laboratory setting and on a one time basis. These disparate studies do not constitute adequate data bases for predicting or assessing environmental disturbances.

However, there can no longer be any doubt that both chronic and acute pollution may induce serious perturbations in insect systems. Chemical pollutants may induce changes in entomological systems at all levels of organizations from the biochemical to the ecosystem. The effects of environmental contaminants may include direct effects such as insect mortalities as well as indirect effects such as altered food supplies. Furthermore, effects may demonstrate reciprocity. For example, zootoxic and phytotoxic substances may alter insect/plant interfaces by acting on the insect through the host plant or the host plant through the insect.

To date, most studies have attempted to identify easily observable events rather than to establish dose -responses, understand the physiological or ecological mechanisms involved, or monitor the levels of contaminants in insects. Much of the pertinent literature has been summarized by Haegle, 1973; Ciesla, 1975; Hay, 1975; Watson et al, 1976; Lilli, 1972; Debackere, 1972; Steche, 1975; Bromenshenk and Carlson, 1975; Bromenshenk, 1976, 1978a, 1978b, 1978c; Bromenshenk and Gordon, 1978; Ginevan and Lane, 1978).

The development of resistance in insect populations to a toxin is a phenomenon that seldom has been examined or reported in studies of air pollution exposures. This is discussed in connection with sulfur dioxide fumigation experiments using Drosophila melanogaster (Ginevan and Lane, 1978). However, by contrast, in 1967, 224 species of insects and acarines were known to have developed resistance to several categories of insecticides (Brown, 1968).

Exposure to humans

Insects may constitute pathways for exposure of humans to pollutants. Korschgen (197o) found from 2.5 to 31 times the average dieldrin and aldrin residues in Poecilus beetles (predatory) as compared to soil and vegetation levels. Korschgen noted that the levels of insecticide residues in Poecilus beetles constituted a potentially lethal dose in 1.09 meals to young quail, which fed mainly on insects. Thiele (1977) reviewed the literature on animals that feed on ground-dwelling beetles. He concluded that: (1) Hedgehogs and shrews probably consume large numbers of carabids; (2) beetles form the staple diet of mouse-eared bats; (3) mice may consume considerable quantities of ground-dwelling beetles; (4) virtually every species of bird consumes carabids; (5) carabids and grasshoppers constitute a major part of the diet of the little owl (Athene noctua), and (6) frogs and toads catch large numbers of highly active and nimble beetles. Several authors have reported that trace elements or pesticides often occurred in the highest concentration in predatory insects such as ants or carabid beetles (Dewey, 1972; Watson et al., 1976; Korschegan, 197o; Humphrey and Dahm, 1976). Also, insect pollinators appear to be biocollectors of several environmental pollutants (Dewey, 1972; Bromenshenk, 1978b). Unless insects receive lethal doses of a pollutant and are thereby removed from food chains, birds and animals feeding on insects may ingest proportionally higher levels of toxic chemicals than strictly herbivorous species. Conceivably, humans consuming insectivorous or partially insectivorous wild animals or birds could be exposed to elevated levels of toxic or harmful materials. However, wild animals and birds are not a major part of the diet of Europeans and North Americans.

There is a very slight chance of pollutants reaching humans through honey. Honey usually contains only minute or trace amounts of pesticides and toxic elements (Crane, 1975; Tong et al., 1975; Gilbert and Lisk,1978; Toshkov et al., 1974). In addition, the per capita consumption of honey is generally low in the United States, and most marketed honeys are blends of honeys obtained from any different areas. There is the remote possibility that a person who uses only honey as a sweetener, who obtains honey from an individual beekeeper, who in turn harvests honey from an area exposed to a source of toxic or carcinogenic contaminants, might ingest harmful levels of pollutants.

Pollen taken from bee colonies is consumed by some people as a protein supplement. Pollen is more likely to contain higher levels of many pollutants than honey (Bromenshenk, 1978a). For example, microencapsulated insecticides which are sprayed or drift onto floral parts may become mixed with pollen and may be inadvertently collected and stored by honey bees (Burgett and Fisher, 1978).

Sample Selection

The selection of biological specimens for the monitoring of environmental materials and specimen banking is a difficult and complex task. Discussions by the Terrestrial Workshop Groups at the International Workshop on Monitoring Environmental Materials and Specimen Banking, Berlin (West) October 23-28, 1978 and at the following workshop held in Washington D.C., December 9-1o, 1978 revolved around establishing lists of considerations or criteria based on broad biological concerns, availability of adequate information bases, and overall suitability of indicator specimens.

Table 1 presents a list of considerations developed by the invertebrate work group at Washington D.C. and reflects considerable thought by many participants at each of the workshops. The list borrows heavily for organization, wording, and concepts from the efforts of other work groups, especially the Washington D.C. vertebrate group. The items are not prioritized and are not thought to be definitive, but rather serve to point out major considerations.

Any selection of specimens for programs of environmental monitoring and specimen banking is influenced by perceived importance to the environment and man including economic, sociological, political, recreational, life support and other factors. However, an indicator specimen may be important in its own right if it serves as a surrogate for important constituents of the environment or of man.

Given that ecosystems or area systems are the basic units of interest, it seems prudent to first select candidates indicative of critical (key) components, functions, or processes of these systems, keeping in mind the goals and objectives of the monitoring and/or banking programs.

Ecosystems or area systems include man-made (e.g. urban) and man-influenced units; the latter ranging from severely impacted (industrial zones) to relatively undisturbed (natural or "pristine"). Presumably, a comprehensive environmental assessment program could contain sites from any or all of these systems. This introduces issues with respect to the selection of sites, site characteristics with reference to any indicator specimens chosen, and obvious constraints such as to which specimens occur at the sites.

Also, individual characteristics of organisms must be taken into account. For example, the organism chosen should be easy to identify and sex, sufficient in body size for residue analysis (insect specimen may be pooled for analyses but minute insects still are impractical), long enough lived to insure exposure to pollutants, and fit other considerations listed in Table 1. Perhaps the most important criteria is the availability of a workable amount of information about the biology of the organism.

This is needed to intelligently evaluate suitability.

Table 1: Selection considerations for Specimens [*]

1. System Characteristics

   - representative of critical(key) component, functions, and processes
   - degree of ability to extrapolate data: laboratory to field, season-to-season, comparability of sites, etc.

2. Population Characteristics

   - abundant and expendable
   - wide distribution
   - population trends (known or possible to differentiate)
   - trophic level (position in food chain)
   - migration pattern (extent, timing)
   - population stability monitoring (feasible)

3. Individual Characteristics

   - ease of identification (well defined taxonomy)
   - ability to age, class, and sex
   - body size (adequate)
   - longevity (sufficiently long-lived)
   - diet and habitat (preference well known)
   - accumulation of compounds of interest
   - sensitivity to biological effects
   - exposure to pollutants
   - annual cycle characteristics/stages of the life cycle/sensitive periods
   - genetics (homozygous for active monitoring)
   - intermediatary metabolism allows adequate monitoring

4. Logistical/organizational - other

   - coasts (time, $, personnel) and maintenance
   - collecting, preparation, packaging, and transportation in a consistent, standardized manner
   - scale and resolution of sampling program

5. Adequate abiotic and biotic information base

   - land use, air and water quality data, and climatological data should be available relative to the species
   - baseline data on physiology, reproduction, life table information, susceptibility to disease, parasite burdens and pollutant concentrations and dose-responses. Must be able to integrate this information with other local, regional, or national monitoring systems.

[*] List compiled by A.P. Watson, B.W. Cornaby, and J.J. Bromenshenk

Populations are dynamic entities, composed of individuals, and possessing group characteristics such as abundance, seasonal changes, movements, age structure, trophic level, genetic make-up, and rates of natality, mortality, and reproduction. Each of these characteristics as well as others affects the choice of candidate specimens. Also, subject populations must be examined with respect to the pollutant categories of interest (if identified). These considerations include: (1) The availability of contaminants

in terms of likelihood, frequency, and levels of exposure; (2) the transport, accumulation, transformation, stability, and persistence of the
pollutant(s) within a population; (3) interactions which might potentiate or antagonize biological activity; and (4) sensitivity to effects.

Logistical and organizational problems further complicate the decision
process as does the need for supplementary abiotic and biotic information
bases.

Since indicator specimens are to be utilized in programs of environmental
monitoring and specimen banking, problems of data analysis and interpretation must be considered. The major problem becomes one of sorting out the
"signal", or pollutant effect, from the "noise" or intrinsic population
variability introduced by the number of individual and population characteristics, abiotic factors such as climate, soil, and temperature, sensitivity or different species or organisms, and fluctuations in the environmental behaviour of pollutants.
It is not surprising that the Working Committee on Principles of Protocols
for Evaluating Chemicals in the Environment (1975) concluded that these
sources of variability negated the possiblity of setting out easy and indisputable experimental and/or study formats. They did note that measuring
the prevailing chemical loading was much easier than quantifying response
or biological performance of a population to that burden.

It seems appropriate that the final selection of indicator specimens should
be performed on an ad hoc basis by experts.

In keeping with this philosophy, the invertebrate work group at Washington
D.C., developed the following matrix to evaluate invertebrate candidates
thought to be indicative of critical functional groups:

Table 2: Invertebrate Criteria Matrix
Fitness Rating: (1)=Poor, (2)=Adequate, (3)=Very Good
(Developed by A.P.Watson,B.W.Cornaby, and J.J. Bromenshenk)

Functional Groups	System Characteristics	Population Characteristics	Individual Characteristics	Logistical Organization	Adequate Information Base	Effects & Trends Monitoring/Banks	Active-Passive Monitoring
Pollinators							
a) Managed Honeybees	3	3	3	3	3	3	3
b) Native bees, flies, beetles	2	2	1	2	2	2	2
Pest Population Regulation							
a) Carabids	3	3	3	3	2	3	1
b) Spiders	3	3	2	2	1	2	1
Detritus Processors							
a) Drosophila	1	2	2	2	1	1	2
b) Earth worm	3	3	2	3	3	3	3
c) Isopods or Millipedes	3	2	2	2	2	2	2
d) Ants (mound)	2	3	2	3	2	1	1

The rationale for selecting pollinators and regulators of pest insect populations was discussed in preceeding sections of this paper. The use of indicators from soil/litter/detritus systems and their importance to resource partitioning has been reviewed by Cornaby (1977).

Trend monitoring refers to pollutant levels; effects monitoring to biological response. Active monitoring utilizes stadardized test organisms (e.g., homozygous) placed at test sites; passive monitoring utilizes in situ "wild" organisms.

The following discussions focus on experimental and study formats for trend monitoring and specimen banking. Sine effects monitoring could involve responses of any or all levels of animal organization, it is impossible to address specific considerations here and as such they will be treated in a generalized manner.

Sample collection and handling

With appropriate modifications, standard sampling techniques such as sweeping, vacuuming, pit-fall trapping, soil and litter cores, and other methods normally used in population studies of insects can be utilized for environmental monitoring and to obtain specimens for banking. As far as possible, anticipated categories of chemicals to be examined by residue analysis, physical and chemical characteristics of the pollutant in question, and the presence or absence of a known or suspected pollution source, should always be considered. If residue analyses are to be conducted, utmost care must be exercised to avoid contamination or loss of the substances or elements of interest during sampling and subsequent handling.

A carefully planned and organized approach is essential. Based on personal experience, the design of any environmental monitoring and/or specimen banking program utilizing insects would require, at the very least, the interaction of an entomologist with a broad background in ecology and population studies, a skilled analytical chemist qualified to perform organic and inorganic analyses of biological specimens, and a competent biostatistician. This should avoid repetition of many common mistakes evident in some of the available literature. For example, entomologists tend to kill and preserve insects in an manner appropriate for systematics studies, e.g., alcohol or formalin preservatives, cyanide killing jars, dried and pinned specimens. They freely sort specimens with their bare hands and may use dirty (from a chemist's perspective) or rusty equipment. On the other hand, chemists often are concerned only with sample preparation and analytical determinations in the laboratory and as such are not fully aware of problems introduced during sampling, pretreatment, handling, or storage which might invalidate analytical results.

An entomologist may be aware of the complexities of the population dynamics and responses of insects, but the input of a biostatistician usually is necessary to establish adequate sampling procedures in order to adress problems of representativeness, sufficient sample size, and the ability to interpret data with respect to effects monitoring, trend monitoring, or deferred chemical analyses and evaluation. Not only are experienced and qualified investigators from several disciplines needed to design a program of environmental monitoring and specimen banking, but it is essential that they should work in concert to assure data quality and credibility.

Many of the dificiencies of large, multi-disciplinary programs are a result of inadequate information exchange among the principal investigators.

Samples to be utilized for monitoring of pollutant levels and/or specimen banking require specialized handling. Lykken (1963) stated that after gross samples have been collected, certain fundamental principles and procedures must be followed in selection of subsamples, cleaning procedures (if appropriate, and preparation for storage and/or analysis).Homogenous subsamples usually must be separated from the gross samples with a procedures of mixing, subdividing, and systematically reducing the sample. Although Lykken's review dealt with crop sample collection and preparation, he provided useful guidelines and pointed out common procedural errors which apply to other biological specimens.

Preparation and storage procedures often incorporate one or more of the following: (1) Dried specimens (including lyophilization), (2) chemical digestion in acid or base, (3) dissolution or immersion in solvent, (4) preservatives, (5) evacuated and sealed containers, (6) whole or partial organisms, (7) homogenates, (8) rapid freezing, or (9) other techniques designed to ensure that the specimen will continue to reflect the original concentrations of the substances of interest. Prior to analyses, requirements for sample treatment depend on the anticipated analysis of the samples and the use of the data. For example, honey bees are good scavengers of particulate pollutants which adhere to the branched hairs of the body and legs. Cleaning or washing would alter determinations of these materials on bees. On the other hand, if chemical residues within the tissues of insects living in soil were of interest, then one would attempt to remove soil particles clinging to the exoskeleton. Similarly, if organs rather than whole insects are to be used, care must be exercised to avoid contamination from materials in or on the rest of the body.

I have sampled honey bees and analyzed them for pesticides, trace elements, and radionuclides. Personnel at the USDA Bee Research Laboratories, the EPA Biological Investigations Laboratory, Battelle Pacific Northwest Laboratories, and several universities have provided me with invaluable assistance and guidance on sampling, handling processing, storage, and analytical procedures. Based on my own experience using honey bees the following recommendations are presented on obtaining, handling, and storing insect specimens prior to residue analyses for pesticides and trace elements:

(1) A minimum sample size of loo gms wet weight should be obtained for pesticide determinations; 3 gms for trace element determination.
(2) All insect specimens should be at the same development stage-egg, larvae, pupa, or adult. For honey bees, further adult distinctions includé nurse bees, foragers, and guards.
(3) As far as feasible, all sampling, storage, and analytical apparatus should be of glass or stainless steel if the specimens are being tested for organic pesticides; but all this equipment should be of appropriate plastic such as polyethylene if inorganic compounds and trace elements are of primary interest.
(4) All specimens should be placed in freezer chests under dry ice as soon as they are obtained (we aspirate living bees into temporary containers) no both kill the insects and prevent decomposition.

(5) All specimens should be transferred to permanent storage
containers as soon as possible and handled as few times as
possible.
(6) All specimens should be kept in dark storage until analyzed
at -3o° C for short-term, -8o° C or less for long-term.
(7) All equipment must be scrupulously cleaned before use. If plastic equipment must be re-used, it should be cleaned with detergent solutions, washed with reagent grade acids, and rinsed
with distilled and deionized water as described by Taras et al.
(1971). All glass and metal equipment should be cleaned with
detergent solutions, rinsed in distilled and deionized water,
then with reagent grade acetone and hexane (FDA Analytical Manual, 1975).
(8) Specimens intended for pesticide determinations should be stored
in glass jars capped with aluminium foil; for inorganic or trace
element determinations, samples should be kept in clean, sterile,
plastic Whirl Paks ® (only for short-term storage).

These recommendations are intended to be illustrative and not definitive.
Equipment and containers made or lined with plastics which incorporate
little or no plastizers, catalysis residues, or other additives
(Teflon ®, Teldar ®, or laboratory grade polyethylene) (Lewis, 1977)
might be usable for a wide range of applications. This should be verified.
Borosilicate glass and quartz should be tested further. If materials are
used as surface coatings in containers, the coating must be examined periodically for peeling and cracks which could lead to contamination from
the base container material.

Since most biological specimens decompose rapidly, freezing seems to be
the best method of preservation for most purposes. Lyophilization may be
appropriate for some usages, but it is not generally recommended due to
loss of substances through volatilization. Kawar et al. (1973) reviewed
pesticide stability in cold-stored plant parts, soils, dairy products,
and extractives solutions. Stability was affected by storage temperature,
pesticide species, substrate, duration of storage, interferences, and the
use of desiccants. However, these authors, and others with whom I have discussed this problem, generally concur that storage for no more than one
month at temperatures below -1o° C (preferably colder) probably would not
greatly affect the concentrations or most pesticides, inorganic elements
and compounds, or enzyme activity (used to test for the presence of some
pesticides). Storage at these temperatures for longer periods may be feasible, although -8o° C or lower will be preferred, but stability still
should be monitored. Chemical stability of stored samples should be verified by the use of fortified samples or extracts prepared at the time
of sampling, and handled and stored under the same conditions. Problems
that may occur during processing or storage include: (1) Chemical absorption onto or leaching from the container walls; (2) chemical loss or degradation due to heat, light, moisture, drying, oxidizing, or volatilizing;
(3) decomposition of the specimen, and (4) metabolic changes due to biological activity.

Short-term storage (days, weeks, months) generally may not require as
rigid procedures and elaborate validations of storage stability as long-
term storage (years, decades, centuries). However, many investigations

fail to consider this problem adequately, even for short-term storage, and simply assume short-term stability.

Frozen specimens can be shipped if packed with liquid nitrogen or dry ice (about ten pounds/day of travel) and should always be sent during the first part of a week and after holidays to avoid delays in transport and delivery caused by weekends and holidays. Note: Federal Air Transport Regulations prohibit shipments containing dry ince or liquid nitrogen.

Analytical procedures and considerations

To obtain a truly representative sample, experiments must be fully-designed before the first sample is obtained from populations in the field.

As noted before, individual, population, pollutant, and site characteristics all interact in a dynamic framework and each of these characteristics introduces intrinsic variability. Thus, the value of each sample is limited to the extent that it is representative of the set (populatio, ecosystem, etc.) from which it was obtained. The problems are separating the "signal" from the "noise" and obtaining results which are statistically and biologically reliable, significant, and interpretable. In addition, for determinations of the levels of pollutants in biological tissues, procedural sources of error introduced during collection, handling, storage, and treatment of samples must be adequately addressed to assure valid results.

Many endogenous and exogenous substances, both natural and man-made, may cause chemical determinations to indicate either smaller or larger amounts of the constituent of interest than was present originally. Substrate artifacts may give the same or similar response as the compound or element sought; such confusion is introduced in some pesticide determinations by the presence of plastic residues. Environmental contaminants or those introduced during sampling, handling, and preparation can lead to erroneous results. The analyte may be endogenous to the specimen. For example, because of the high background sulfur levels in proteins of insect tissues, it is virtually impossible to evaluate shifts in total sulfur due to sulfur oxide stress unless isotopic forms of chemical species of sulfur are determined. Validation procedures and the participation of an experienced and perceptive analytical chemist are needed.

Smart (1976) suggests two ways of testing the efficacy of an analytical method: (1) Adding a known amount of the contaminant to a large, homogenous sample which is then subsampled and preferably sent to collaborators to be analyzed, and (2) spiking (fortification), in which each collaborator is asked to add a known amount of a prepared standard chemical (analyte) to their own samples of the subject matrix or specimen and obtaining recovery figures. The analytical methodology most frequently used for analysis of pesticides in insects follows that outlined in the FDA Analytical Manual for Chlorinated Insecticides (DDT, DDE, DDD), Phosphate Insecticides (malathion, parathion), and Carbamate Insecticides (sevin, carbofuran). All methods are reported to be sensitive to o.ol ppm. Screening is done via gas chromatography, thin layer chromatography, and gas chromatography in conjunction with mass spectrometry. New methods are being developed and others constantly improved.

R.J. Barker, USDA Bee Research Laboratory, Tuscon, Arizona, has developed methods of conducting acetylcholinesterase enzyme activity determinations on the brains or heads of as few as five bees. This is a useful procedure since some pesticides and elements are known to inhibit enzyme action.

Although colorimetric measurements of elements such as arsenic have been used for years because of low cost and simplicity, specific ion probes, atomic absorption spectrometric analysis, and other methods are replacing many of the older procedures. Neutron activation analysis has the advantage of being essentially nondestructive but requires a neutron flux source such as a nuclear reactor. Specific isolation techniques like field desorption mass spectrometriy are beginning to be used, but at present these methods are too sophisticated or costly for general usage.

Chemical analytical procedures which differ from one another in sample preparation, extraction, cleanup, and determinations provide further assurances of quality of results.

As analytical methods and quality control are improved, the need for standards, quality control, and inter-laboratory checks become even more important. Although U.S. National Bureau of Standards (NBS) currently provides two organic reference materials (orchard leaves and bovine liver), no insect or invertebrate standard exists. If insects are to be seriously considered as environmental monitors and for use in specimen banking, standards, checks, and inter-laboratory collaborations are essential.

Program design

Program design parameters depend on the specimen or specimens selected, the pollutants of interest, and the magnitude of the endeavor. As stressed in other portions of this paper, the problem is extremely complex; it would be absurd to attempt to completely outline procedures for adequate population sampling which incorporate site considerations, populations characteristics and the biological effects and interactions of the substances of concern. T.R.E. Southwood (1975) published a 391-page monograph on ecological methods with particular reference to the study of insect populations. His paper included discussions of planning and field work, statistical aspects, sampling (sample unit, selection, size, number of samples, pattern of sampling, timing of sampling), mathematical models, population characteristics, and data interpretation. Ultimately, results must be subjected to statistical analyses, and the design of the program must be adequate to the needs of the anticipated mathematical treatments.

Obviously, from a statistical standpoint, the specimen or specimens chosen should be widespread in distribution, common enough to provide adequate numbers for sampling, practical to measure and monitor, susceptible or exposed to pollutants, and reliable indicators of pollution impacts. The complexity of the problem necessitates a preliminary research and development program, feasibility tests, and preferably a multi-disciplinary effort.

The magnitude of a monitoring and banking program could be as limited as a few site specific studies or as large as worldwide. Overly restrictive programs probably are of little use, especially if baselines are to be established.

In the United States fossil-fueled industrial developments are burgeoning in previously unexploited areas such as the coal-rich Northern Great Plains and acid rains continue to spread westward from the northeast (Likens, 1976). Also, new types of insecticides such as synthetic hormones and microencapsulated formulations are just beginning to be used on more than a limited scale. Thus, it would be especially valuable to obtain not only of insects but of other biological organisms from those ecosystems in the United States that are still relatively free from man's influence and to bank these specimens before conditions are altered any further. Indeally, specimens not only from sites in relatively pristine ecosystems but also from severely impacted areas such as near the Four Corners Power Plant complex in New Mexico or those agricultural areas of California with a long history of frequent and heavy insecticides application would be included for comparative purposes.

Any sample utilized in a monitoring or banking program must be adequately described or else the sample has little or no value. Descriptive information should include not only date collected, location, species, and collector, but also relevant information concerning the site, ecosystem and populations (ecotype, habitat, communities, trophic level, age structure, etc.), known or suspected exposures to the pollutants to be monitored, and procedures of sample collection, handling, preparation, and storage. Essentially the whole history of sample, including the "chain of custody" and analytical results of any determinations should be recorded in order to assess the validity of chemical recovery tests.

Data logs, format sheeets, and permanent identification tags to accompany the specimen from the time of collection until final disposal should be developed and used.
Data storage, interpretation, and retrieval probably would be best accomplished by entering and filing all relevant data on computer deck cards or tapes.

Organizational aspects

As mentioned before, the only on-going programs of environmental monitoring and specimen banking using terrestrial insects with the exception of a program in the Federal Republic of Germany, are individual efforts by researchers in Europe and the United States. The expertise of scientists who have performed these studies would be invaluable in establishing national or international programs and their collaboration could eliminate a great amount of research and development efforts. A few national environmental monitoring and banking programs using bird and mollusc tissues are in existence. The protocols developed for these materials would probably be applicable to many aspects of an insect program.

A centralized approach not only for coordinating all specimens, analysis, storage, and data control but also to coordinate insects and other biological specimens would seem to be the most efficient approach and also the best safeguard for quality control. Due to shipping problems, a centralized approach to banking has draw-backs, and a joint European-United States program might be less cumbersome if a central bank were initiated for each continent. There would be good reason to divide the storage facilities of any bank into two locations to lessen the chance of loss in case of some calamity such as fire.

Coordinated international programs would greatly increase the value and usefulness of programs to monitor environmental materials and specimen banking. It would appear that this conference and the supporting agencies would be a logical first choice for coordinating and implementing these programs. Private contractors might be utilized, but the regulatory agencies whose responsibilities encompass all aspects of the effects of chemicals in the environment should exercise at least partial involvement. In the specific case of honey bees, the American and European Divisions of the Bee Research Association might be appropriate coordinators, although they are research oriented.

The need for quality control, reference standards, field and laboratory training, standardized forms, and good program design cannot be over emphasized. Cooperative efforts are a means of ensuring reproducible results; if a method gives good results in joint effort studies, then the procedures are considered to have passed the most stringent tests that usually can be devised.

Legal considerations

In the United States there are fewer restrictions concerning the collecting, transporting, storing, and utilizing of insect specimens than for birds or higher animals. Afew species of butterflies appear on the En dangered Species list and special permits would be required to obtain these insects. Usually wild populations of insects are not thought of as being owned by someone else. Colonies of honey bees and populations of other insects such as ladybird beetles introduced to control aphids are regarded as having owners who place a value on their insects, have rights to the insects, and could be adversely affected by sampling or collecting.

Generally, access to insects for sampling is not a matter of obtaining permission from an owner but rather is a matter of receiving permission to enter an area and to conduct collecting activities.

Since most terrestrial insects have no stated recreational or commercial value (except as pests), few laws and regulations apply directly to the standard method of obtaining them. However, legal problems could arise indirectly from situations such as a horse or a cow breaking a leg in a pitfall trap. The use of poisoned baits might be prohibited in some circumstances, but one probably would refrain from using poisons on any specimen used in a banking program because of the insertion of an extraneous chemical into the specimen.

Transportation of living insect specimens across local, state, and international boundaries is subject to several regulations and laws primarily because of concerns about importing diseases or pest insects. Dead, preserved, or dried specimens fall outside of the restrictions and precautions for transportation and handling of materials and their derivatives for importation into the United States. However, since customs inspection is required, a courtesy permit from the United States Department of Agriculture, Animal and Health Inspection Service, Hyattsville, Maryland 2o782, should be obtained to facilitate passage through customs to avoid delays which might damage perishable specimens. The request for the permit(s) should include what is being importet, when it is expected to arrive, at at what port of entry, and by what mode of transportation or carrier. Exportation of insect materials, provided they are not living, from the United States and Europe, probably would not entail any legal problems, although it is possible that some countries might have regulations that would pertain.

Laws and regulations pertaining to worker protection, human safety during specimen transport, and disposal of specimens and process wastes must be observed.

Finally, as pointed out in the working paper submitted to the International Workshop by Prager and Flemer, 1978, environmental materials may become part of adversary proceedings. Therefore written permits, good records, and documentation of"chain of custody" are necessary if the data derived from the program is to be useful in this context. Also, certain rights and obligations pertain to the communication and confidentiality of information, especially as regards proprietary information or adversary evidence.

Cost estimation

Although the topic outline for this paper indicated that overall estimated costs for "monitoring environmental materials" and "specimen banking" were essential, it seems premature to make such an assessment with much validity. First, the specimens chosen, the pollutants of interest, and the magnitude of the program will all affect the overall cost. If the insects to be used have not been used in this context previously, as is the case with the overwhelming majority of species, a research and development program must be initiated. On the other hand, if insects such as honey bees, carabid beetles, or flies are utilized, the costs would not be as great because much of the preliminary development work has been completed by individual studies. Finally, if insect specimens are incorporated into a program that involves other samples of terrestrial and aquatic ecosystems, all coordinated via a centralized approach, many of the costs such as overhead, personnel, laboratory equipment, and storage would be apportioned to all specimens and as such many of the costs would be proportionally reduced.

For illustrative purposes, the following scenario (Table 3) is presented in which honey bees are to be the specimen used for trend monitoring and banking, pesticides and trace elements (and other inorganic compounds) the area to be sampled. All samples would be stored at -3o°C or lower, the bank size comparable to the existing bank of the U.S. EPA's Environmental Health, Pesticides Division for human tissues, milk, and blood serum (1o.ooo specimens, minimum 2-3 gm/sample), and all facilities would be independent of any previously establishment.

This scenario envisions a self-contained operational unit. A specimen bank reliant on several contractors or institutions for sampling, handling, processing, analyzing, or storing specimens would have increased problems of quality control, accontability, and credibility. However, costs could be reduced by utilizing on site personnel and possibly by contracting chemical analyses other than those for which the facility was equipped to do routinely.

Costs for an effects monitoring program, either as active or as a passive

TABLE 3

ESTIMATED BUDGET

INSECT SPECIMEN BANK

ALL FIGURES IN 1978 DOLLARS

SALARIES AND WAGES (12-month FTE)

Director/Entomologist	$20,000
Analytical Chemist	18,000
Laboratory Computer Technician I	10,000
Field Technician II	12,000
Field Technician I	8,000
Secretary	8,000
TOTAL SALARIES AND WAGES	$76,000
Fringe Benefits (17% of Salaries and Wages)	11,560

TRAVEL AND FIELD EXPENSES

Workshops, Collaborators, etc.	$ 2,500
Field Collections (80,000 miles @ $.15/mile)	12,000
Vehicle (four-wheel drive pickup; rental @ $200/mo)	2,400
Per Diem (2 technicians, $35/day, 22 days/mo, 8 mo)	12,320
TOTAL TRAVEL AND FIELD	$29,220

EQUIPMENT AND SUPPLIES

Office (typewriters, desks, files, forms)	$ 7,500
Laboratory	
Carbon Rod Atomic Absorption Spectrophotometer	14,000
Gas Chromatography	10,000
Thin Layer Chromatography	1,000
Mass Spectrometry	20,000
Expendable (shipping, glassware, chemicals, etc.)	9,000
TOTAL EQUIPMENT	$54,000

STORAGE FACILITIES

Freezers (8'x 10', dual control, dual unit, walk-in, -30°F, -34°C)	$10,000
Power Plant (30 KW/diesel)	5,000
TOTAL STORAGE FACILITIES	$15,000

COMPUTER TIME ($250/hour) $ 3,500

OVERHEAD (50% total salaries and wages) $36,480

GRAND TOTAL $225,760

Lab Equipment
straight line depreciation, 10-year life
$5,400/year

Office Equipment
straight line depreciation, 15-year life
$500/year

Freezer
straight line depreciation, 50-year life
$200/year

Power Plant
75-year life
cost/year is negligible

	$ 76,000
	11,560
	29,220
	5,400
	500
	36,480
	200
	3,500
$162,860	Annual Cost of Operation

	$ 7,500
	54,000
	10,000
	5,000
$76,000	Initial Cost of Operation

152

monitoring, would depend on several factors, including the geographic
scope of the project, the temporal period, the environmental components
and pollutants of interest, the responses to be measured and the level
of biological organization at which they are measured, and the resolution
required. These costs are governed by operational goals and the magnitude, scale, or scope of the work and the costs could range from thousands to millions of dollars.

Acknowledgements

For their thoughtful contributions, I am indebted to Dr. Annetta P.
Watson, Oak Ridge National Laboratory; to Dr. Barney W. Cornaby, Battelle
Columbus Laboratories, and to Dr. Paul Müller, Universität des Saarlandes.

References

Atkins, E.L., Jr., E.A. Greywood, and R.L. Macdonald, 1973: Toxicity of
Pesticides and Other Agricultural Chemicals to Honey Bees. University
of California, Division of Agricultural Sciences Leaflet 2287.

Atkins, E.L., L.D. Anderson, D. Kellum, and K.W. Neuman, 1976: Protecting
Honey Bees from Pesticides. University of California, Division of Agricultural Sciences Leaflet 2283, 15 pp.

Baker, H.G. and P.D. Hurd, Jr., 1968: Intrafloral ecology. Ann. Rev. Ent.
13 : 385-414.

Bohart, G.E.,1952: Pollination by native insects. U.S. Department of Agriculture Yearbook 1952: 1o7-121.

Bromenshenk, J.J. 1978a: Investigation of the impact of coal-fired power
plant emissions upon insects: Section 5, Entomolgical studies in the
vicinity of Colstrip, Nontan; Section 14, Entomolgical studies at the
zonal air pollution system. In: The Bioenvironmental Impact of a Coal-
Fired Power Plant. Third Interim Report, Colstrip, Montana. E.M. Preston
and R.A. Lewis, Eds. U.S. Environmental Protection Agency, Corvallis,
Oregon. EPA-6oo/3-76-o13.

Bromenshenk, J.J. 1978b: Yet another job for busy bees. The Sciences, July
and August Special Issue. The New York Academy of Sciences, New York,
New York. pp. 12-15.

Bromenshenk, J.J. 1978c: Honeybees as indicators of pollution impact from
the Colstrip power plants (Section 6); Effects of low level SO_2 on insects
(Section 18). In: The Bioenvironmental Impact of a Coal-Fired Power Plant.
Fourth Interim Report, Colstrip, Montana. E.M. Preston, Ed. U.S. Environmental Protection Agency, Corvallis, Oregon. 98 pp. (in press).

Bromenshenk, J.J. 1976: Investigations of the effects of coal-fired power
plant emissions upon insects, report of progress (Section 7). In: The Bioenvironmental Impact of a Coal-Fired Power Plant. Second Interim Report,
Colstrip, Montana. R.A. Lewis, N.R. Glass, and A.S. Lefohn, Eds. U.S. Environmental Protection Agency, Corvallis, Oregon. EPA-6oo/3-76-o13.

Bromenshenk, J.J. and C.E. Carlson, 1975: Impact on insect pollinators. In: Air Pollution and Metropolitan Woody Vegetation. W.B. Smith and L.S. Dochinger, Eds. Yale University Printing Service, New Haven, Connecticut. pp. 26-28.

Bromenshenk, J.J. and C.C. Gordon, 1978: Terrestrial insects sense air pollutants, pp. 66-7o. In: bnference Proceedings, 4th Joint Conference on Sensing of Environmental Pollutants, New Orleans, Louisiana, November 6-11, 1977. American Chemical Society. Washington, D.C. 945 pp.

Brown, A.W.A. 1968. Insecticide Resistance Comes of Age, Bull. of the Entomol. Soc. Am. 14: 3-9.

Burgett, M. and G. Fisher, 1977: The Contamination of Foraging Honey Bees and Pollen with Penncap-M. Am. Bee Jor. 117(1o): 626-627.

Carlson, C.E. and J.E. Dewey, 1971: Environmental Pollution by Fluorides in Flathead National Forest and Glacier National Park. USDA Forest Service, Northern Region, Division of State and Private Forestry, Forest Insect and Disease Branch. 57 pp.

Ciesla, W.M. 1975: The role of air pollution in predisposing trees to insect attack. In: Air Pollution and Insects. C.E. Carlson, moderator. Proceedings of the Joint Meeting Twenty-sixth Annual Western Forest Insect Work Conference and Twenty-second Annual Western International Forest Disease Work Conference. Intermountain Forest and Range Experiment Station, USDA Forest Service, Ogden, Utah, and Northern Forest Research Center, Canadian Forestry Service, Edmonton, Alberta. pp. 86-96.

Clark, L.R., P.W. Geier, R.D. Hughes, and R.R. Morris, 1967: The Ecology of Insect Populations in Theory and Practice. Methuen and Co., Ltd. London, England 232 pp.

Cornaby, B.W., 1977: Saprophagous Organisms and Problems in Applied Resource Partitioning. In:The role of Arthropods in Forest Ecosystems, W.V. Mattson, ed. Springer Verlag, New York. pp. 96-1o1.

Crane, E. (Ed.), 1975: Honey, A Comprehensive Survey. Crane, Russack, and Company, Inc.,New York, New York.

Debackere, M., 1972: Industriele luchtvervuiling en bijenteelt. (Industrial pollution and apiculture). Vlaams Imkersblad. 2(6): 145-55.

DeJong, D., R.A. Morse, W.H. Gutenmann, and D.J. Lisk, 1977: Selenium in pollen gathered by bees foraging on fly ash-grown plants. Bull. Environ. Contam. and Tox. 18(4): 442-444.

Dewey, 1972: Accumulation of Fluorides by insects near an emission source in western Montana. Environ. Ent. 2(2): 179-182.

FDA, 1975: USDA Pesticide Analytical Manual (McMahon, B.M., Ed.). U.S. Department of Health, Education and Welfare. Washington, D.C.

Gilbert, M.D. and D.J. Lisk, 1978: Honey as an environmental indicator of radionuclid contamination. Bull. Environ. Contam. and Tox. ooo7-4861/ oo19-oo32: 32-34.

Giles, F.R., S.G. Middleton, and J.G. Grau, 1973: Evidence for the accumulation of atmospheric lead by insects in areas of high traffic density. Environ. Ent. 292o: 229-3oo.

Ginevan, M.E. and D.D. Lane, 1978: Effects of Sulfur Dioxide in Air on the Fruit Fly, Drosophila melanogaster. Environmental Sci. and Tech. 12(7): 828-831.

Heagle, A.S., 1973: Interactions between air pollutants and plant parasites. Ann. Rev. Phytophath. 11: 365-388.

Hakonson and K.V. Bostick, 1976: The availability of environmental radioactivity to honey bee colonies at Los Alamos. J. Environ. Qual. 5(3): 3o7-31o.

Hay, C.J., 1975: Arthropod stress. In: Air Pollution and Metropolitan Woody Vegetation. W.H. Smith and L.S. Dochinger (Eds.). Yale University Printing Service, New Haven, CT. pp. 33-34.

Humphrey, B.J. and P.A. Dahm, 1976: Chlorinated hydrocarbon insecticide residue in Carabidae and the toxicity of dieldrin to Pterostichus chalcites (Coleoptera, Carabidae). Environ. Ent. 5: 729-734.

Johansen, C.A., 1969: The Bee Poisoning Hazard from Pesticides. Wash. Agr. Exp. Sta. Bull. 7o9. 14 pp.

Kawar, N.S., G.C. de Batista, and F.A. Gunther, 1973: Pesticide stability in cold-stored plant parts, soils, and dairy products, and in cold-stored extractives. Residue Reviews 48: 45-78.

Korschgen, L.J., 197o: Soil-food-chain-pesticide wildlife relationships in aldrin-treated fields. J. Wildlife Manage. 34(1): 186-199.

Lewis, R.G., 1977: Determination of arsenic and arsenicals in foods and other biological materials. Residue Reviews 68: 123-149.

Likens, G.E., 1976: Acid Precipitation. American Chemical Society. C&EN Special Report, Nov. 22: 29-44.

Lillie, R.J., 1972:'Air Pollutants Affecting the Performance of Domestic Animals, A Literature Review. USDA, ARS, Agr. Handbook No. 38o. 1o9 pp.

Lykken, L., 1963: Important considerations in collecting and preparing crop samples for residue analysis. Residue Reviews 3: 19-34.

Maurer, R., 1974: Die Vielfalt der Käfer- und Spinnenfauna des Wiesenbodens im Einflußbereich von Verkehrsimmissionen. Oecologia (Berl.) 14: 327-351.

Maurizio, A., 1956: Bienen-Vergiftungen mit Fluorhaltigen Industrieabgasen in der Schweiz. XVI Int. Beekeep. Congr. Prelim. Sci. Meet. p. 314.

McGregor, S.E., 1976: Insect Pollination of Cultivated Crop Plants. Agr. Handbook No 496, USDA ARS. Washington, D.C. 411 pp.

Metcalf, R.L. and W.H.Luckmann, 1975: Introduction to Insect Pest Management. John Wiley and Sons, New York, 587 pp.

Moffett, J.O., H.L. Morton, and R.H.MacDonald, 1972: Toxicity of some herbicidal sprays to honey bees. J. Econ. Ent. 65: 32-36.

Munshower, F.F., 1972: Cadmium Compartmentation and Cycling in a Grassland Ecosystem in the Deer Lodge Valley, Montana. Ph.D. Dissertation. University of Montana, Missoula, Montana. 1o5 pp.

Van Hook, R.I. and E.E. Huber, 1976: National Environmental Specimen Bank Survey, U.S. EPA. Office or Research and Monitoring, Washington, D.C. EPA-6oo/1-76-oo6. 2o7 pp.

Watson, A.P., R.I. Van Hook, D.T. Jackson, and D.E. Reichle, 1976: Impact of a Lead Mining-Smelting Complex on the Forest-Floor Litter Arthropod Fauna in the New Lead Belt Region of Southeast Missouri. Oak Ridge National Laboratory. Environmental Sciences Division Publication No.881. Oak Ridge, Tennessee. 159 pp.

Yamamoto, I., 197o: Mode of Action of Pyrethroids, Nicotinoids, and Rotenoids. A. Rev. Ent. 15: 257-272.

USE OF OYSTERS AND RELATED MOLLUSCS AS BIOLOGICAL MONITORS OF SYNTHETIC ORGANIC POLLUTANTS

Philip A. Butler
Branch of Ecological Monitoring
U.S. Environmental Protection Agency
Sabine Island, Gulf Breeze, Florida
United States of America

Molluscs as Biomonitors

The former U.S. Bureau of Commercial Fisheries initiated in 1965 a program to monitor estuarine shellfish populations for residues of organo-chloride pesticides. The program was the logical sequitur of ten years of laboratory studies which had demonstrated the reaction of oysters and other molluscs to pesticides and had shown the significance of pesticide residue data in molluscs. During the decade before 1965, there had been numerous reports of fish-kills and increased mortality in other non-target animals as a result of pesticide applications. It seemed inevitable that persistent pesticides applied on forests and farm lands would drain eventually into the coastal zone but there were few data to document where and how much.

The Bureau entered into formal and informal agreements with university State, and Federal laboratories with marine facilities which agreed to collect monthly samples of any of ten estuarine bivalves, depending on their availability. Replicate samples of 15 mature molluscs were homogenized, desiccated, and sent to a central laboratory for residue analysis. About 18o permanent stations were selected in 15 States on both coasts, but not all stations were monitored for the entire 7 years of the program which was terminated in 1972. Approximately 8,1oo analyses were completed and the data showed that DDT was essentially ubiquitous. Dieldrin was the second most commonly detected pesticide; residues of endrin, mirex, toxaphene, and polychlorinated biphenyls were detected only occasionally.

Several important findings were made which were due in part to the frequency of sampling and to the long period during which the program was conducted. Perhaps the most important was that pesticide residues in shellfish, an important element in man's diet, were not large enough to suggest a human health problem. It was also apparent in most areas, if extrapolation from laboratory experimental data is justified, that the residues were not physiologically dangerous to the bivalves themselves.

The data demonstrated the seasonal aspects of pesticide pollution in the estuary with residues usually peaking in the late spring months at the height of the fresh water run-off. It was possible to show in several areas the sequence of agricultural applications of pesticides and high residue levels in molluscs of the associated drainage basin.

A critical review of the DDT residue data in oysters from ten North Carolina stations in the period 1967 through 1971 showed the importance of continuity in a monitoring program in determining trends in pollution levels. About 11o analyses were made annually and it was found that the number of samples containing more than 1o g/kg of DDT (the detection level) declined steadily from about 85 percent in 1967 to less than 25 percent in 1971. These data reflect the general decline in DDT usage after 1968.

A final important contribution of this program resulted from the banking of split samples from Chesapeake Bay oysters collected prior to 1972. Retrospective analyses of these oysters in 1977 by the cooperating laboratory in Virginia demonstrated that high residues of kepone had been present in 1971 at a time when the chemical company, the sole cource of kepone, claimed it had not been discharging this waste into the James River.

The U.S. Environmental Protection Agency, heir to the monitoring programs formerly conducted by the Bureau of Commercial Fisheries, undertook a program early in 1977 to monitor again about half of the 1965-72 stations to determine whether any further trends in pollution levels were apparent after the five- to seven-year lapse. The orgininal cooperating laboratories agreed to participate in collecting bevalves in those stations where pesticides had been found consistently a decade earlier. Methods similar to those previously used were followed, but the samples were screened for the other chemical classes of pesticides in addition to the organochloride group originally monitored.

Only a single pre-spawning sample was collected at each station since the earlier program had shown that pesticide residues were typically highest during this period. The results were striking. DDT was detected in only two of th 87 estuaries monitored again. In the earlier program, samples from 22 of these estuaries had had a 1oo persent incidence of DDT residues. These data indicate that, for all practical purposes, DDT has disapeared from the estuarine water column. It should be noted, however, that some resevoirs of this persistent chemical remain and continue to be recycled in the food web. Juvenile fish, monitored in the 1972-76 period, were still accumulating DDT residues. This suggests a continuing partition of the chemical between bottom deposits and the biota.

(Figure 1)

Rationale

The above discussion of the findings of the earlier use of molluscs as biomonitors amply supports their value in monitoring programs. Their trophic position, e.e., filter-feeders, and their tendency to accumulate synthetic organic compounds as well as trace elements make them unique tools for the environmentalist. In estuaries, inevitably sinks for persistent chemicals that are transported in run-off waters, molluscan tissue residues accurately document the fluctuating patterns of pollution. There are ample data reflecting their value as biomonitors in fresh water and the marine environment as well.

The importance of drainage basins in transporting both soluble and insoluble chemical pollutants, the persistence and lipophilic nature of many ot these compounds, and the processes of both bio- and trophic accumulation, all of these factors contribute to the potential incorpora-

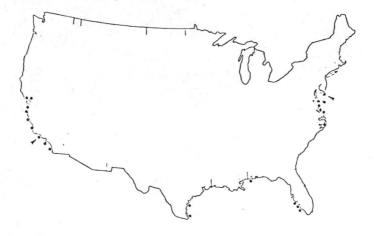

Figure 1. Molloscs as biomonitors. The diagram shows
the location [●] of the 22 estuaries in which loo percent
of the bivalve samples monitored in the 1965-72 period
contained detectable residues of DDT.
DDT was detected in only two estuaries [◄] when the
stations were monitored again in 1977.

ration of pollutants in the food that man harvests from the sea. Molluscs, in general, are probably the best indicators of chemical pollution available in the aquatic environment.

Although there has been a significant decline in the number of persistent pesticides used in recent years, there were more than 33,ooo formulations on the United States market in 1978; about half of these were registered as insecticides. And although the number of registered products has declined slightly in the past few years of record, the production of all classes of pesticides increased about 35 percent between 1971 and 1975. The persistence, mobility, and toxicity of these compounds warrant a continuing assessment of their presence in non-target sectors of the biota and environment.

Sample Selection and Storage

In the early 196o's there was an increasing awareness of the dangers of pesticides to non-target animals. There had been numerous incidents of increased mortalities of marsh fish and invertebrates following the use of pesticides to control noxious insects. There was an obvious need to discover the extent to which agricultural chemicals were eroding from farmlands and being transported, in solution or adsorbed on particulate matter, down to the estuaries. There was evidence, too, that industrial wastes containing pesticides were being discharged into river drainage systems. A monitoring program was needed to address these specific problems rather than, for example, gather baseline data from a statistically randomized series of samples.

The seasonal aspects of pesticidal applications implied the probability of a similar seasonality in pesticide pollution so that a relatively continuous monitoring device was needed. Analyses of river samples had demonstrated the difficulties in detecting the usually low levels of pesticides when present in the water, and it was apparent that an automated mechanical monitoring device would be impractical. Some substrate was required that would remove pesticides at low concentrations from ambient water, accumulate them, purge itself when the pollution ceased, and which was essentially ubiquitous. The oyster and some related molluscs filled these needs to perfection

Perhaps the most important aspect of oysters as biomonitors is that there exists so much information about their reactions to pesticides and other contaminants under controlled laboratory conditions. The effects of pesticides on growth, and rates of accumulation and purging in oysters are known for more than two hundred contaminants. These data make it possible to interpret the significance of some of the residues   identified in monitored oysters. The oyster and other molluscs have the ability to accumulate pollutants in their tissues to levels thousands of times greater than in ambient water. For example, the uptake of DDT by oysters exposed to different amounts under laboratory conditions is shown in Table 1.

A mature oyster filters about loo gallons of water daily during its normal activity so that it serves to integrate or composite a relatively large sample within a short time. The daily transport of so much water in the oyster's gill system apparently facilitates the rapid partitioning of tissue residues back into cleaner ambient water.

Table 1. Uptake of DDT by eastern oysters maintained in flowing seawater. Exposure period 7-15 days in different tests.

DDT Concentration in water	Residue in oyster	Biological magnification
ug/kg	ug/kg	(x1000)
lo.o	15o.o	15
1.o	3o.o	3o
o.1	7.o	7o
o.o1	o.72	7o
o.ooo1	o.o7	o
control	o.o6	

Table 2. Average uptake and loss of a mixture of seven chlorinated pesticides by aquatic molluscs.

Bioassay animal	Magnification in 5 days	Percent loss in 7 days
Soft clam	3ooo	75
Eastern oyster	12oo	5o
Marsh clam	7oo	5o
Asiatic clam	6oo	3o
Hard clam	5oo	75

Molluscs' low position in the trophic web and their sedentary habit contribute to the general uniformity of pollutant residues in different individuals of a localized population.

The rate of residue loss varies in different species of molluscs and, since oysters are not usually available in the more brackish or more saline areas of the estuary, studies have been made to determine uptake and purging rates on other molluscs that might be utilized. Under similar laboratory test conditions, the soft clam, Mya arenaria, proved to be the most efficient or sensitive in storing organochlorine residues. The other molluscs tested, in order of decreasing sensitivity, were: the eastern oyster, Crassostrea virginica; the marsh clam, Rangia cuneata; the freshwater Asiatic clam, Corbicula manillensis; and the quahog or hard clam, Mercenaria mercenaria. These relationships, together with the rate of purging when the animals were held in clean, flowing seawater for a week are shown in Table 2.

The suitability of oysters as biomonitors in enhanced by the fact that they can tolerate waters of varying salinity and can be transplanted easily from one salinity zone to another and held in suspended trays if, for example, a point-source of pollution is being sought. In one instance, trays of oysters were placed in different tributaries of a marsh drainage system where the bottoms were too soft for them to grow naturally. After a lo-day period, analyses of the oysters made it possible, because of the magnitude of the residues, to locate the particular factory outfall responsible for polluting the area.

Other advantages of molluscs as biomonitors include the fact that they are sedentary and indicate pollution levels in a precise area. They are easily collected and handled. Not having internal skeletons, they are easily homogenized and small enough so that many individuals can be composited for analysis to yield a picture of average pollution levels in a restricted area.

The chief disadvantage in using molluscs for monitoring is the rapidity with which they purge themselves of residues in the absence of continuing pollution in the ambient water. Estuarine pollution is frequently intermittent and may fluctuate widely depending on the season and the amount of freswater run-off. Molluscs need to be sampled at no more than 3o-day intervals to obtain a realistic pollution picture at a specified station, and this imposes a great deal of field effort as well as considerable analytical capacity. A second but minor disadvantage, if the researcher is aware of it, is the seasonal loss of lipophilic residues. Such residues tend to be localized in the gonads and consequently are lost to a large extent during the spawning season when the gametes are discharged from the animal.

Sample processing

The method of choice for preserving aquatic samples is to freeze them quickly and keep them frozen until analyzed. When the number of samples is large and the shipping distances are great, the opportunity for losing refrigerated shipments may become a serious handicap to the continuity of the monitoring data. In retrospect, it seems that the success of our molluscan monitoring program was due in large measure to the development of methods for preserving the tissues so they could be shipped dry and unrefrigerated. There were several liquid preservatives that could have been used but that, again, would have invited problems of breakage and the resultant loss of samples.

In the origninal mulluscan program, the homogenized tissues of 15 pooled individuals were mixed with a desiccant made of sodium sulfate and microfine silica. In proportions of about three of desiccant to one of tissue, this mixture becomes a dry, free-flowing powder. Such dried preparations of molluscs spiked organochloride pesticides have a shelf life of at least 3o days without loss of residues. Samples could be wrapped in aluminium foil and sent by ordinary mail to the analytical laboratory. There is no objection to freezing such desiccated samples, however, and 15 molluscs provide adequate tissue mass for replicate analyses as well as for banking and future retrospective analyses.

More recently the preparation and shipping of molluscan and fish monitoring samples has been greatly simplified by the development of unbreakable vials of methylpentene plastic. This material does not deteriorate or adulterate samples preserved with methyl alcohol, and the vials can be autoclaved for re-use. The vials are constructed to fit an electric blender, so it is possible to homogenize,preserve, and ship the sample without changing the container. This not only facilitates handling but also lessens the chances for sample contamination. From 5 to 5o grams of tissue are homogenized in the vial, weighed, and then mixed with an approximately equal amount of reagent grade methanol. These preparations may be stored without refrigeration for a month or more but they are not suitable for permanent storage because of the potential for volatilization of the contents through loosened caps. Sub-zero refrigeration remains as the most suitable method for banking permanent samples despite the inherent dangers from power shortages.

Organizational aspects

It was apparent that the effectiveness of the 1965 nation-wide molluscan monitoring program would be largely dependent on the continuity of the monthly sampling. Obviously,many people would be required if the 18o major estuaries were to be sampled adequately. Fortunately, many estuarine molluscs are commercially important and under the management of the individual States. As a result, in each area there is a cadre of specialists who are not only interested in marine pollution but also have the knowledge and equipment necessary to collect shellfish samples. These agencies were interested in having the local monitoring data for their own managments programs and they cooperated willingly in collecting samples on a timely basis and processing them for shipment to the analytical laboratory.

The successful conduct of the program hinged on the central coordinating office which prepared detailed protocols so that all samples would be processed similarly in the field. Field collection stations were supplied with identical sets of processing equipment, and the necessary chemicals were purchased in large batches for uniformity. The close contact of the coordinating office with the single analytical laboratory which initially analyzed all samples made it possible to detect and correct quickly any problems in the field processing of samples. From time to time as improvements were made in the technical handling of the samples, new protocols were distributed uniformly to the field stations by the coordinating office.

Uniformity in analytical methodology was initially ensured in the program by having all samples analyzed by the same team of chemists. This became impractical when the sample load was greatly increased at the wish of several of the cooperating agencies. To counteract the possible development of differences in chemical methodologies in different laboratories, a manual was prepared which prescribed name-brands of equipment and chemicals, and gave the detailed analytical procedures. The State chemists came to the central laboratory where they spent a work-week to familiarize themselves with the "standard" methodology. After they returned to their respective laboratories, the first few field collections were split and analyses were made by both the field and central laboratories. Excellent comparability in data was obtained and thereafter, 6 of the 15 field stations submitted only monthly data reports to the coordinating office. The orderly flow of raw data from field stations and the chemistry laboratory to the coordinating office made possible its rapid transfer to coded forms and punch cards for storage and retrieval. About one hundred analyses were processed monthly, and copies of the data forms were returned to the sample collection agency within two months of the field collection time. We believe that this rapid feedback was an important factor in enlisting continued support from the field agencies. On several occasions, this early reporting of the results made it possible to resample quickly stations where the data indicated special pollution problems might exist.

The experience gained on the several monitoring programs in which we have participated, both on the local, national, and international scene, has shown the essential nature of close coordination for any marked degree of success in achieving program objectives. The usefulness of monitoring data is directly proportional to its comparability with similar data generated at other times or in other places. Even presumably small variations in sample collection and preparation protocols may cause significant differences in the analytical results. In one instance, the substitution of clams for mussels during the summer months in one estuary made it appear that the DDT pollution had terminated when, in fact, the negative data resulted from the clams' insensitivity to this pesticide when it is present at low levels in the ambient water. Detailed sample collection and preparation protocols become increasingly important as the number of samples in a program increases.

Cost estimates

There are so many variables entering into the costs of a monitoring program that it is not possible to give any usefully predictive figures. A discussion of some of these variables, however, may serve as a guide as to what may be expected depending on the program undertaken.

In a program having broad geographic coverage, the most costly item is collection of the samples. This is especially true if the stations are some distance offshore. Our ocean fish monitoring program were especially fortunate in that another agency was operating exploratory fishing boats in the areas of geographic interest and was willing to supply fish samples without cost to us. Daily operating costs for these ocean-going vessels amount to thousands of dollars and their use would be impractical if monitoring were the sole objective. There are disadvantages, however, in such "piggy-back" operations since the monitoring agency has little or no control over vessel schedules.

Even at inshore stations, the advantages of a cooperative effort with a local agency are obvious. Local personnel are not only familiar with the geography but also usually have the necessary collecting equipment so that there can be substantial savings in both time and money. Sample collection costs are minimized in estuarine monitoring programs because of the relatively short distances involved and the fact that smaller boats can be used. In general, we found that the costs per sample for a given agency were usually inversely proportional to the number of samples collected. During a six-year period in our molluscan program, we calculated the average collection cost of the 6,600 samples was between 80 and 100 dollars. The chief variable involved was the amount of coastline covered. In New Jersey, for example, there was a single estuary with stations located along 32 miles of coastline. In California, there were numerous estuaries along about 1,000 miles of coast.

During the early stages of the molluscan program, several of the cooperating State agencies indicated they would like to have data from more sites than our analytical laboratory was equipped to handle. Consequently, we investigated the costs for establishing a one-man pesticides analytical laboratory with the basic equipment including a gas chromatograph and the chemical supplies for one year. The cost was about $20,000 in annual salary. Finally, the analytical costs are usually inversely related to the number of analyses performed, as is also true of the sample collecting costs. This, of course, is a strong point in favor of centralization of analytical effort in a wide-spread monitoring program. Such centralization also fosters a strong quality control program.

Not related to the analytical costs of the samples is the added expense of providing for the permanent storage of replicate or split samples. Today, there is a clear mandate for the archiving of representative samples from environmental monitoring programs so that retrospective analyses will be possible at some future date. Such storage costs will vary widely, but we are currently paying $15.00 per cubic foot of frozen fish samples, per annum.

Summary

This report discusses the National pesticide monitoring program in estuaries of the United States. Molluscan samples were collected monthly at about 180 stations during the period 1965-72. Half of these stations were monitored again in 1977. The significant findings of the programs are presented and illustrated. The coordination of the program is described, as well as the collection and processing of samples, data, handling, and program costs.

The biology of molluscs is described as it relates to their suitability as biomonitors. Some of the details of the laboratory experiments are given to characterize the reaction of molluscs to pesticides under controlled conditions.

Despite the necessity for short-term sampling, or because of it, bivalve molluscs appear to be the most useful biomonitor for indicating the fluctuating levels of pollution by synthetic organics in the aquatic environment. Their usefulness is a result of the combination of their ubiquity, ease in handling, sensitive physiology, position in the food web, and the large store of data describing their responses to pollution under controlled conditions in the laboratory.

SPECIMEN BANKING MARINE ORGANISMS

Bruce B. Collette
National Marine Fisheries Service Systematics Laboratory
National Museum of Natural History,
Washington, D.C. 2o56o
U.S.A.

Two aspects of specimen banking that can be addressed by a systematic zoologist, are: criteria for species selection; and in addition to the banking of freshly collected material the possible use of archival collections of animals maintained primarily for taxonomic study.

Criteria for Species Selection

A primary problem in the selection of marine species for inclusion in the specimen bank is the large number of species living today. Taking finfishes alone, according to the estimates of Cohen (197o) there are about 2o,ooo species of fishes of which 58 % are marine species. There are many more species of marine invertebrates. Criteria must be developed to select the most useful and cost effective species among this great diversity for specimen banking. Important criteria include: importance to man; trophic position; habitat; abundance; distribution; and costs of collection and maintenance.

Importance to man. It seems logical to select species that are important to man, particularly as food directly or indirectly through meal being fed to livestock and poultry. Species should be selected from three groups: commercial species harvested for food such as herrings (Clupeidae), cods (Gadidae), salmons (Salmonidae) and tunas (Scombridae) among finfishes; shrimps (Penaeidae and Pandalidae), oysters (Ostreidae), mussels (Mytilidae), clams (Veneridae and Myidae), and squids among shell fishes; species of importance to recreational fisheries such as salmons (Oncorhynchus), striped bass (Morone saxatilis), bluefish (Pomatomus saltatrix), and billfishes (Istiophoridae); and species utilized for meal, oil, or petfood such as menhadens (Brevoortia), Peruvian anchoveta (Cetengraulis mysticetus), and krill (Euphausia superba).

Trophic position. Species should be selected from several different trophic levels.; microfilter feeders such as clams, oysters, and mussels; planktivores such as herrings and anchovies (Engraulidae); carnivores such as salmons, tunas, bluefish, and striped bass; and high level carivores such as billfishes, sharks, porpoises, and whales. Larger numbers of specimens of small species from lower trophic levels carnivores need to be banked because multiple samples can be taken from each specimen.

Habitat. Species should be selected from different habitats, both stressed and unstressed: estuaries, rocky shores, sand beaches, mud bottoms, coral reefs, epipelagic, and deep sea. Samples should come from polar, temperate, and tropical waters.

Abundance. To facilitate collecting adequate samples,both now and in the future, it is important to select abundant species rather than rare species.

Distribution. To facilitate comparisons between different parts of the world, it is desirable to select some wide-spread species such as the blue-fish (Pomatomus saltatrix), tunas (Thunnus and Katsuwonus), and billfishes (Makaira and Istiophorus).

Costs of collection and maintenance. To keep costs down to an accep-table level, it is necessary to select species that are easily sampled (abundant commercial and recreational species for example). Species should be large enough to provide enough tissue for replicate sampling and yet small enough to enable storing a reasonable sample of indivi-duals from many localities. Accurate identifications are vital to the success of the banking program.

We can conclude that the highest level priority should be given to banking widespread, abundant, medium-sized species that enter man's food chain through commercial and recreational fisheries and through use as food for livestock.

Specimen Storage

There are two different ways to go about storage of specimens. One is to select the best method(s), agree on criteria for species selection, and begin to store material now. This has the advantage of banking the most important material under a standard set of collection and storage techniques thereby facilitating analysis. Freezing is probably the best overall technique but the costs of collecting, transporting, and long-term maintenance of frozen material will be high. Suggestions have been made in the past to store some frozen material in Antarctica which insures permanence but makes access difficult. Other techniques include ashing which saves space but loses or alters some compounds and freeze-drying which also saves space and requires little energy after ini-tial processing.
Another approach is to concentrate on development of appropriate tech-niques to utilize small samples of material already present in the archival museums of the world. Considering finfishes in museum collec-tions in the United States and Canada, there are 36,000,000 specimens already stored and easily retrievable by taxonomic group (Collette and Lachner, 1976). Mercury concentrations have been compared in recently collected and historical material from museums of epipelagic top level predators (tuna and swordfish, Miller et al., 1972) and benthopelagic fishes (Barber et al., 1972) and no changes in mercury level were found to have taken place during storage. However, Gibbs et al. (1974) found changes in other heavy metal concentrations in midwater fishes, which they attributed to fixation in formalin and maintenance in alcohol. Spe-cimens that have been collected for taxonomic and zoogeographic studies may not provide adequate material for additional purposes. Removal of tissues for testing purposes may be difficult both because of the time and effort involved and because of the resulting damage to archival mate-rial . Balanced against the foregoing shortcomings is an enormous base of samples dating back, for some species, over loo years that should be used whenever possible.
For fishes and marine mammals, there are also archival bone collections

and most mollusk collections consist largely of dry shells. Appropriate techniques need to be developed to analyze small samples of bone and shell to take advantage of collections of calcified tissue. Bones and shells have usually not been previously treated with chemicals. Museum collections of fish bones are not nearly as extensive as are the collections of material stored in alcohol.

Literature Cited

Barber, Richard T., Aiyasami Vijayakumar, and Ford A. Cross. 1972: Mercury concentrations in recent and ninety-year old benthopelagic fish. Science 178: 636-639.

Cohen, Daniel M. 1970: How many Recent fishes are there? Proc. Calif. Acad. Sci., 4th ser., 38: 341-345.

Collette, Bruce B. and Ernest A. Lachner. 1976: Fish collections in the United States and Canada. Copeia 1976: 625-642.

Gibbs, Robert H., E. Jarosewich, and Herbert L. Windom. 1974: Heavy metal concentrations in museum fish specimens: Effects of preservatives and time. Science 184: 475-477.

Miller, G.E., P.M. Grant, R. Kishore, F.J. Steinkruger, F.S. Rowland, and V.P. Guinn. 1972: Mercury concentrations in museum specimens of tuna and swordfish. Science 184: 1121-1122.

ADVANTAGE AND PROBLEMS OF USING WILDLIVING
ANIMAL SPECIES AS INDICATORS FOR ENVIRON-
MENTAL POLLUTION (HERE ESP. TERRESTRIAL
ECOSYSTEMS)

U. Drescher-Kaden:
Institut für Physiologie, Physiologische Chemie und
Ernährungsphysiologie im Fachbereich Tiermedizin der
Universität München

Introduction

Various factors endanger the irritable network of relations between mankind,
the abiotic environment and the manyfold forms of microorganisms, plants
and animals. Some of them are concerned with chemicals used in industry,
agriculture, forestry and other scopes of life., which penetrate the biocenose as wastes, by accident or on purpose. The survey of long term trends
and geographical differences in the pollutant level in biota beside other
means of environmental monitoring is very important for an early warning
system, for modelling and for prediction as well as gaining information
about the behaviour of the differents substances in the biocenose.

The demand for environmental survey by means of animal indicator species
is well accepted but the discussion about the facilities of realization
is in full progress.

An important step towards the aim - a global monitoring system by wildlife
control - are the national screening analyses of chlorinated hydrocarbons
or heavy metals in starlings, ducks, woodcocks, predatory birds and other
terrestrial as well as aquatic species carried out in different regions
of the U.S.A.

Another promising attempt in achieving international biological monitoring
was performed since 1966 by member nations of the OECD, regarding mainly
aquatic but also some terrestrial wildliving species as indicators for the
contamination level of CCP and mercury.
The final report has been presented on the last OECD-meeting Dec. 1978 indicating that the project has proved the feasibility of international monitoring by wildlife apart of difficulties in the financial support, in
selecting representative widely distributed organisms, regions and seasons
for valid interpretation. The need for including other biological data has
also been shown. Therefore the present project has been stopped and new
concepts based on the information of the former are now in discussion.

In the GFR to date more than 9o % of projects are restricted to aquatic
systems. But just in a country with so divergent regions as to geography,
landuse, vegetation one should consider the investigation of the contamination level in different geographic areas by means of terrestric fauna.

Division scheme

In this paper we try to cover different aspects of biological monitoring
by means of terrestrial wildliving species.

1. First we descuss in general advantage and problem of monitoring
   concepts using wildlife compared to other environmental survey
   systems.
2. Considering the experiences gained from our former pilot studies
   on OCP in wildlife as well as literature data we will give some
   suggestions for the selection of representative indicator species.
   These references are summarized in a catalogue of criteria for
   amenable species.
3. Some results of our residue studies from 197o to 1977 will than be
   listed as example for the feasibility of biological monitoring
   using freeliving animal species as indicators.
4. Part four presents conceptional and operational aspects of biological monitoring systems applying terrestrial animal species as indicators (mainly bound for the GFR but modified feasible for other
   nations) including suggestions for indicator regions.
5. Although the actual costs for planning and implementing programs
   for the collection and analysis of indicator organisms will vary
   considerably according to the objectives and magnitude of program
   we will give some estimations.
6. As proposal for international residue data collection bound for
   computerizing data a form sheet is attached, we have employed
   during our studies in order to gain as much information as possible.

Part 1

While in most cases of environmental control it is impossible to consider
the whole ecosystem the investigator is restricted to some components of
the toal as indicators susceptible to exposure.
The techniques employed depend on a series of criteria e.g. whether the
impact is concerned to structure and/or functioning of the ecosystems,
whether the pollutant is transported by abiotic (water, air, soil) or
biotic systems (microorganisms, flora, fauna) and whether it causes bio-
depression, biostimulation or no effect, discerning direct and/or indirect hazards.
In respect to its special transportation mechanisms, metabolic characteristics and susceptibility to stress e.g. exposure to pollutants, the
food web has to be regarded as a separate system. Concerning its direct
and indirect relation to mankind it seems in some ways superior as indicator for pollution than abiotic systems. Taking humans as part of the
food chain there is a need for epidemiological studies in the environment. As indicated by the substantial increased level of some persistent
pesticides in animal tissue compared to other transportation media our
knowledge about carry over (e.g. time lag to the distribution in other
media, retention, cumulation, metabolization, excretion) is still frag-
mentary.
As it is impossible to study all problems with humans one has to perform

etiological studies drawing conclusions from laboratory experiments with animals as models.

Some disadvantages using animals as indicators for pollution have to be mentioned. Apart from laboratory trials with confined conditions animals in epidemiological studies react mainly to the total multifactorial impact. It is difficult to discern the susceptibility to special noxious factors from other detrimental hazards.
There are also problems with sample selection and collection. Additional we are encountered with a series of difficulties concerning analytical procedures. Comparing freeliving to experimental or domestic animals as for their indicator function we must consider both advantages and disadvantages. The choice depends on the special problem under investigation.

With experimental or domestic animals kept in optimal health and nutritional status under controlled environmental conditions the direct effect of pesticides can be evaluated.
As domestic stock is breeded for optimal performance and maximum production, and as we have no close related experimental species for most freeliving species the results of contamination studies and survey projects can only be transferred with reservation to wildlife.

In the contrary, feeliving animals in their natural habitat - not only confronted with single or multiple pollutants but also suffering from other factors as climate, stress, food restriction, infestation - can demonstrate the effective hazard of environmental chemicals to organisms additional stressed from other factors out of human control.
Keeping no waiting terms they are directly exposed to environmental hazards compared to domestic animals and man. We cannot control them in their habitat regarding food and managing conditions.
While domestic stock nowadays is fed with mixtures of food components showing different contamination levels harvested from distant located regions (therefore extreme levels being diluted by components with lower values) and in some countries - e.g. in the GFR since 1975 - governed by maximum pesticide tolerances in feedstuff, freeliving animals are influenced by the special conditions of their habitat with its food and water supply.
They give evidence not only of global contamination but above all of local exposure.
Additional in some countries they are still confronted with environmental chemicals off limit in food and feedstuff. They can also better serve as part of an early warning system in representative habitats apart of their survey being precondition for national protection activities.
Possible troubles emerging with the use of wildliving species as indicator organisms culminate in four topics related to the program designed.

a) Difficulties with sample collection
b) Difficulties with observations and measurements of animals in their
   natural habitat
c) Scarce knowledge about most freeliving species referring to biology,
   ecology, behaviour, stress susceptibility
d) Problems arousing in laboratory study (feeding trials concerning aspects of toxicology, residue accumulation and metabolism).

Although wildliving animals can be considered as good indicator organisms for environmental pollution most of attempts to include them into biological monitoring to date are unsatisfactory.

Applying wildlife as indicator for exposure/effect relationships we can use several techniques:

1. Residue evaluation of pollutants in animals of different regions in succeeding years.
2. Investigating the effect of environmental chemicals upon the indi-viduum regarding condition criteria (body weight, fat depots, vita-min storage, eggshell thickness), reproductive rate, growth crite-ria, morphological and histological changes in organs and tissues, enzymes, hormons ...
3. Studying the effect of environmental chemicals upon the population (dynamics, density and distribution pattern)
4. Investigation of the changing nutrition supply and pattern due to the employment of environmental chemicals (herbicides, insecticides, fungicides, rodenticids or fertilizers ...)

The critical evaluation of the pollutant impact on wildliving animal spe-cies requires data from all research directions. E.g. a valid interpreta-tion of residue monitoring demands additional information about toxico-logy, metabolism, ecology of the selected indicator species in defined ha-bitats.

Due to our residue studies about OCP in freeliving fauna we will try to elucidate some problems to assess the species suitable for indicator function.

Part 2

The residue values of OCP in freeliving animals of different habitat in the GFR vary over a large range due to a series of criteria.

a) Specimen

The selection of suitable specimens for residue analysis in wild animals has to be well considered regarding the type of pollutant and the availa-bility of tissue.
For OCP-analysis we comprised when possible two matrices - liver and adi-pose tissue.
Adipose tissue shows better the situation of chronic contamination while in the liver the acute exposure caused by uptake of contaminated food or mobilization of fat-reserves containing pesticide residues can be evalu-ated.
As animals due to their nutritional status not always possess fat-reserves the investigator has to restrict to special seasons or - with more ana-lytical efforts - measure the residue level in muscle fat (showing mostly comparable pattern to adipose tissue). But it is not reliable to replace missing fat data by liver fat data, as both matrices have divergent pes-ticide pattern and contamination levels.
Although eggs of wildliving birds are not always from everywhere and eve-ry bird species available they are of great value to demonstrate the contamination level of the parent birds and to give some explanation for lacking breeding success.
Our studies about the residue level in eggs of raptor birds and goosander suggest that there are not only differences in the residue concentration

between different clutches but among eggs of the same nest.

Physiological and health status, age, sex

Most of the animals sampled for our monitoring program were killed for
analysis in order to obtain values from fresh samples destined to human
use and which seemed to tolerate the measured residue values. Sometimes
we also got animals found dead the cause of death being obscure or due to
parasitic infestation, so we could compare these two groups. The residue
values in the two groups varied over a large range. But at least in herbi-
virous animals there seem to be no significant relation between the residue level and the physiological and health status. Otherwise it cannot be
denied that animals with a certain degree of contamination are more susceptible to stress (food restriction, parasites ...).Unlike herbivora some carnivora found dead showed extreme elevated residue levels that could have
caused death.
Otherwise we found also in living raptors killed for anlysis comparable
high concentrations.
As to date we have neither toxicological nor accumulation studies with
freeliving carnivorres we can only presume such relations. Same the
correlation between high residue values and eggshell thinning and fragili-
ty causing low breeding success can only be demonstrated with some bird
species and single pesticides. Though feedings trials demonstrated to some
extent differences in the residue accumulation due to the sex of the experimental animal other factors of the natural habitat seem to be of more
influence than sex on the residue level of freeliving animals. In many
species to process of pesticide bioaccumulation reaches a plateau before
the animals are grown up. Therefore the observed differences in the mean
residue level of juvenile versus adult individual showed only tendencies
and no statistical significance. In field studies we must assume that
other factors superpose this relation.
Already fetuses of red- and roe deer exhibited traces of OCP in their liver. In two cases when mother and fawn were killed at the same time we
observed corresponding contamination levels.

Species differences

Comparing mean values exhibit species-differences in the residue level
but most differences can be attributed to different feeding type, habitat selection,metabolic size and physiological peculiarities.

Feeding type (herbivor, carnivor, insectivor, omnivor)

Regarding the residue level and pesticide pattern we can divide groups
of animals with different feeding habits and digestive properties.
Herbivora as primary consuments have much lower contamination levels of
persistent pesticides than carnivora and insectivora. This can be stated
for larger herbivora mammals like roe deer, red deer, chamois and hares
destined for human consumption but also in small animals like mice and
squirrel. Unlike herbivora the carnivora of different body size have not
only accumulated greater amounts of pesticides but still have some compounds in their tissue not allowed in the GFR since some years.
One of the assumptions for an national or international monitoring system
based on wildlife is the distribution and abundance of the selected indicator species. But sometimes it is difficult to get enough individuals
from one region. Looking for amenable species we have to deliber if and

to what extent we can substitute one species by another. So it is hardly possible to obtain hares from the alpine regions with little forestry and agriculture, while other species from these areas are not accessible in other habitats. For another example we have to test other representatives of carnivora like marten or ermine regarding indicator quality because foxes are frequently not available due to rabies control as well as raptor birds due to protection.

Beside from ecophysiological criteria we have to evaluate, to what degree the residue level differs between species of similar feeding type in the same habitat.

Regarding samples from red deer and chamois - inhabiting comparable home-range and showing similar feeding habits - we got no statistical divergent residue values.

On the other hand it seems not applicable to choose in one region hares in the other habitat rabbits as indicator species as the latter retain higher HCB-values and still dieldrine in their tissue.

We have to deal with similar problems in herbivore birds. Due to feeding habits and habitat preferences we find in pheasants and partridges more HCB than in gallinous species living in woods like the mountain cock or black grouse, exhibiting more DDE-residues.

Among carnivores it depends on the spectrum of prey whether residues of the one or another pesticide are prevalent. So in the eggs and liver of barn owls we analyzed lower levels of HCB than in the tawny owl. This was also stated by other investigators e.g. Baum et al. (1975) who discovered that raptor birds with herbivorous prey like the buzzard have lower pesticide residues than these with carnivorous prey as goshawk, peregrine falcon and sparrowhawk.

Analogue we found in the latter more DDE than in goshawk and buzzard.

Preculiarities of metabolism

Although living in the same habitat and preferring similar nutritional pattern the residue values in chamois seem not to be representative for marmots. In the latter species we found almost for every OCP higher levels than in the ruminants suggesting that these deviations could be due to peculiarities in fat mobilization and metabolism during hibernation stress.

Collection season

In order to observe trends of pollution in wildlife during succeeding years it is also indispensable to compare material derived from the same season. As example the lindane residue level in wild ruminants from the same habitat - exhibiting no differences due to species - shows annual variations with elevated values in summer.

Habitat

It must be emphasized that material from venison shops is not fit for estabishing trend analysis though it is of interest in the scope of food control. Apart of a considerable share imported from states of the eastern bloc the game is collected from a variety of habitats with different vegetation and land use. On the other hand to accomplish indicator functions the animals need not necessarily be game. Among 4o investigated freeliving species were only 11 game species.

In order to sustain trend survey of pollution over a range of years the samples have to be taken from the same habitat. By this the number of comparable individuals from one species is further diminuished.
Otherwise in order to compare the pollution level in wildlife from diffe- rent geographic regions it is of extreme importance to have an exact knowledge about the landuse and vegetation in the collection area. For instance it is insufficient for valid interpretation to compare greater areas such as Bavaria to Hessia or surrounding of Munich to Frankfurt because the samples of hares derived from 5 adjacent areas around Munich showed as high variations as we got by the comparison of one bavarian ha- bitat with one area of the Ruhrgebiet.
In order to establish a reliable monitoring system the different survey areas in the GFR have to be classified according landuse, vegetation, distance from settling regions and other criteria.

Migratory birds, a special indicator for habitat control

Migratory birds can be considered as indicators in special respect because of their residue level representing the pollution not only in their native but also in the foreign countries they migrate to.

As example we collected woodcocks during springtime in two different re- gions of the GFR. Though they showed different lindan and heptachlorepo- xide levels their contamination level was in the "normal range" of other comparable species living at the same collection site. Unlike these data the contamination with DDE was far higher as we have measured in other nonmigratory species from the same area and season, indicating that they could have been exposed to this compound in the country they migrated to in winter.
During summer the DDE-level seems to become diluted by additional fat accumulation as the animals killed in autumn on their return to the polluted winter habitats contain much lower DDE-residues.

Part 2: Catalogue of criteria

As explained before we are encountered with a series of preliminaries to select representative species just regarding residue-analyses. Additional the investigator has to consider ecological, physiological, hehaviour and technical criteria.

1: Environmental chemicals:

  a) The species to select should react to the noxious agents but with- out mortality within a certain range of contamination.

  b) The time lag from exposure to accumulation should be characteristic.

  c) Special features of accumulation and metabolization of the noxious chemicals are of interest and should be known.

2. Distribution and abundance of the species:

  As the monitoring system is bound for nationwide survey the indicator species should be distributed in all screening regions resp. comparable species available.

As the residue level varies over a large range the species in one survey area must be so abundant that the collection of enough samples per area and season representative data for trend interpretation.

Causes for these variations may be age, sex, reproductive stages, situation of pesticide accumulation and different pesticide application in the special area. Therefore enough animals should be available to select individuums of special characteristics.

3. Availability of population trend data:

As for regarding exposure/effect relationships as well as securing sufficient material for residue analysis, data about decline, increase or no alteration of population density in a given biotope must be available.

4. Background information:

The selection of representative indicator species is also based on information about popultion dynamics, ecology, physiology.

5. Defined body resp. metabolic body size:

a) in respect to sample collection:
The individuum should be large enough as to provide sufficient material for residue analysis and to avoid pooling.

b) The animals should be of proper size to provide favourable relations between food requirement and metabolism.

6. Nutritional status:

Beside of it must be guarantied that the nutritional status of the animals allows deposit-fat sampling in the collection season.

7. Action radius:

The action radius should not be too narrow or too wide as to draw conclusions about the contamination of a certain area. For carnivorous animals one has to put other standards then for herbivores or for birds other than for mammals.

8. Home range:

Apart from migratory species used for special informations the indicator species should reflect the situation of the local habitat and doesn't tend to migrate due to food supply.

9. Position of the species in the food chain:

For biological monitoring the investigator has not only to decide, whether to take an animal high positioned in the food chain (carnivor or insectivor) or in lower positions (herbivores) but also to consider the type of specialization (generalist or specialist) regarding food habits. It depends on the program focused on. (e.g. specialists are far more dependent on the changes of food supply and will show respective population trends. Generalists can evade to other food components).

1o. Relations to mankind:

    a) regarded as food
    b) in respect being food consument of similar pattern as humans
    c) in respect to toxicological model studies

11. Facilities of differential diagnoses:

    Many reactions of the animals are not direct related to pollution
    but account for other adverse factors like infestation or food
    restriction. For this reason one should select species sufficient
    investigated as for applying differentail diagnoses.

12. Feasibility of laboratory tests or relations to experimental animal
    species:

    Valid interpretation of monitoring residue data require studies
    of the dose/accumulation/effect relationships in the assigned
    indicator species.

Regarding the criteria listed before the selection of species amenable for
use as indicator species will be very difficult. From the one or another
reason most animal species are not suitable as indicators. E.g. on
account of securing enough material raptor birds are only appropriate
to a certain degree. Meeting most of the above cited criteria we have to
choose more than one species per region to establish a reliable monitoring system.
In part 4 we will give some suggestions for suitable indicator species.

Part 3

The investigation of about 2ooo samples from 4o freeliving species in
the GFR during the period 197o-1977 indicates following results:

All samples investigated up to now contained total residues of OCP above
detection limit. Even in animals living in alpine regions considered as
local nonpolluted we sometimes measured considerable amounts of residues.
These findings suggest a cooperation of residue analysts with other scientific research branches as meterology, geology, water research ....

All over the investigation period HCB and lindane remained the most abundant residues in all species studied.
Dividing our investigation into the periods 197o-1973 and 1975-1977 the
increase of PCB's is the most striking figure not only in carnivores but
also in herbivores.
Due to the habitat and feeding type of the species the abundance of dieldrine, a-HCH and H-epoxide varies to a great extent. But in general it is
to state that dieldrine and H-epoxide became less important for the herbivores (with some exceptions) whereas these compounds are still abundant
in carnivores. Though DDT was replaced by other pesticides during the last
years DDE remained still present in most samples. Clordane, oxychlordane,
Endrine and a-Endosulfan are randomly found or only of local importance.
Beside of differences in the distribution of some substances due to the
feeding type and collection site the abundance of compounds as H- epoxide
was often greater in liver than in adipose tissue.

While the level of OCP residues in most herbivores (with some exceptions
reviewed below) remained within the tolerance limit the liver fat, adipose tissue and eggs of raptors contained often high levels esp. of HCB,
H-epoxide, DDE, Dieldrine and PCB's. Otherwise in some herbivorous birds
the HCB-level is also far above the tolerance limit while in ruminants it
is very low.

Due to the landuse in the collection site some pesticides were prevalent
in the examined species. For instance in areas with intensive forestry
red deer and chamois contained higher levels of lindane than in recreation areas and little forestry.
In the same way the variable level of some pesticide residues in the liver
of hares derived from various collection sites of the GFR indicate differences in land use. While the DDE-concentrations remain similar in all
regions - illustrating global contamination - the residues of lindane, H-
epoxide and sometimes PCB's or HCB varied in some areas showing local influence of land use e.g. industry and agriculture.

Apart of differences in the residue level due to the collection site the
the residue values from single species varied to a great extent presenting also extremes in animals stated as clinical healthy. Only in some
cases high pesticide levels were correlated to poor condition.
Reviewing results of Conrad (1977) in the GFR significant negative correlations between eggshell thickness and DDE-content of raptor eggs were
evident in sparrow hawk, goshawk and barn owl (tyto alba), while relations
to the PCB level were obvious in sparrow hawk and goshawk.

Apart of differences in the degree of contamination in the same species from
different habitats or of animals from the same site but divergent feeding
habits we can state some changes in the residue level of freeliving animals during successive years in the GFR.
Taking hares as indicators the level of HCB and dieldrine decreasing, the
former reaching a lower plateau the latter declining to zero. While the
DDE-level remains about the same range the concentration of lindane seems
to increase. From 197o we observe inclining PCB concentrations the values
from 1977 indicating a possible plateau. In other species - provided that
we were able to collect enough specimens - we could observe corresponding
trends.

But due to the high variations - including extreme values - and unfortunately often low numbers of individuals we are only abel to illustrate
tendencies.

Based on sufficient animal numbers of the representative species it is
feasible to conduct a reliable biological monitoring.

Part 4

The existance of a functional national biological monitoring is precondition for establishing international or global systems. As shown before
the environmental impact on biota demands multidisciplinary cooperative
study.

Schematic we can list several topics which contribute from different points
of view to the understanding of the relations between environmental influ-

ences and the reaction of the fauna also to meet the dangers.
The priority of the different research branches depends not at last
on the interests and the facilities of the single countries according to geographic, topographic, vegetation, fauna, economic, politic
and population density criteria.

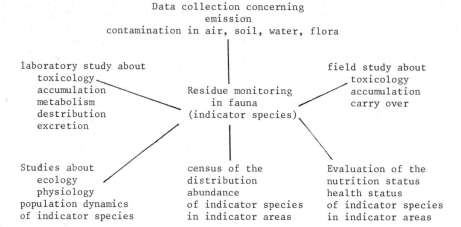

The problem exposure - fauna can be approached from every direction listed
obove. But as it is impossible to start with all problems at the same time
we need concept a smaller program - such as residue monitoring - to be
extended by time.

In the following paragraph we would like to demonstrate some operational
aspects giving guidelines and recommendations for residue monitoring in
the GFR:

Subject: Monitoring residues in prepresentative freeliving animal species
from different regions

Aim: Establishment of a functioning national survey system using only
few indicator species under the angle of view to extend the project including additional data to improve the information gained
by residue analyses.

Duration: For evaluation of the actual situation in different collection
sites   1 year
For evalution of trends   at least   3 years

Preliminaries

a) First it has to be clarified if this survey work can be done on a voluntary basis or has to be demanded and supported by national governments.

b) It has also to be considered if this project can be performed by one
analytical institution or if the work has to be distributed among several laboratories.

Pilot studies indicate, that a functioning and reliable monitoring system needs directions and financial support. As this project involves a lot of workers and material effort to date no single institution or analytical laboratory could manage these investigations with all its coordination, administration and evaluation beside other routine work.
According to the divergent procedures one institution is overtaxed by sample collection combined with analysis, evaluation, collecting additonal data and interpretation.

From this reason we have to detail:
a) Projection, coordination and evaluation committee
b) Institutions engaged with sample collection
c) Laboratories for residue analysis
d) Institutions dealing with additional data collection
   often combined with b) e.g. game biologists.

Prework

1) Establishment of a coordination committee constituted by representatives from different disciplines.

2) Appointing of an administrator working only within this project (e.g. a game biologist).

Competence of 1 and 2

a) Selection of environmental chemicals of interest for investigation. Due to the past experiences the main interest will be directed still to the OCP, PCB, Hg, Pb (refer to the last EG-workshop).

b) Selection of the indicator species referring to the catalogue of part 2. With regard to the GFR following species could be taken into closer consideration:

	Herbivor	Carnivor
Mammals	hare, roe deer	fox, marten
Birds terr.	pheasant, blackbird	buzzard
aquat.	duck species	(goosander)

c) Selection of specimens regarding a) Considering OCP:

mammals	liver, adipose tissue or muscle fat
birds	liver, fat eggs
small animals	whole carcass

d) Selection of interesting monitoring regions according to: 1. Bundesländer
   2. land use:
   protection or recreation areas
   mainly agriculture
   intensive forestry
   intensive industry
   within settlements
   3. additional criteria as comparability of collection sites regarding vegetation, meteorological and topograpical criteria

   4. Collection and analytical facilities

    5. Abundance and easy approach to the selected indicator species
       comp. b

e) Determination of the collection and investigation period:
  except of egg collection: we would suggest autumn

f) Selection of the participating institutions:

    1) regarding collection and additional data sampling

      Suggestion: Game biology, Zoology, Ornithology, Veterinary,
                Hunters depending on the species of interest

    2) regarding residue analysis:

      Suggestion: Institions for food-, feedstuff control, Vete-
                rinary, depending on technical facilities, storage,
                comparable methods controlled by enquetes.

Organization by 1 and 2

1. Literature data collection
2. Meetings for discussion of a-f
3. Material collection
4. Additional investigations
5. Residue Analysis
6. Material storage and distribution for 5
7. Administration (mainly 2)
8. Financial transactions

Main work

1. Performance of sample collection

   a) Measurements of the collection site: weight, sex and - when possible -
     age determination; census of condition

   b) Collection-protocol

   c) Collection for residue analysis

   d) Collection for differential diagnosis (nutrition and health status)

   e) Conservation (ice, formol) and storage till distribution

   f) Transportation to the investigation sites (by car or post)

Facilities: For sample collection of indicator species like hares, foxes,
pheasants the investigator could attend battues otherwise one has to
rely to the accurate work of confidential hunters (roe deer, buzzard,
goosander and other game species) or prepara ters and ornitologists who
should be equipped with devices for measurements, protocol, collection,
conservation, storage and mailing. This proceeding demands an intensi-
tive information and training of the coworkers.

2. Performance of investigation

   a) fat analysis

   b) residue analysis

c) parasitus consus or pathological survey of suspicies samples

d) additional data

3. Evaluation and interpretation of the data

a) residue analyses

b) additional data and differential diagnoses

c) total interpretation including literature data

Facilities: All information should be collected and all analytical results reported in a uniform and standardized manner (comp. part 6) as for computing and collection in a data bank.

Part 5   Cost estimations

Though the actual costs will vary considerable we try to give some informations about the cost shares.

In respect to the outlined programm the division of costs into personal, material, travels, meetings, chemicals is not favourable.

a) Costs during preliminary work

1. Administrator and scientific supervisor: full time job
   about 5o ooo DM/year (also involved in b)

2. Travelling costs for the administrator: a year ticket for
   every region of the GFR about 5 ooo/year

3. Daily allowances and travelling expenses for the administrator:
   depending on the amount of travels

4. General costs for administration:
   including secretary (no full time job), typewriter, pocket computer,
   writing materials, telephone, mailing devices, photocopies, photos,
   financial management ...

5. Literature collection and evaluation

6. Expenditure compensation for the consulting and organizing committee
   about 5 scientists occasional involved

7. Meetings including travelling costs and daily allowances for the
   consulting committee.

Concerning point 3 to 7 close cost estimations depend on the designed program: estimation could vary between 2o ooo - 3o ooo DM/year.

b) Costs during main work

Based on the assumption that lo hares, lo pheasants, lo foxes or marten or buzzards from 5 regions of different landuse in 8 Bundesländer of the GFR have to be collected for residue analysis the number of individuals per year in the GFR amounts to 12oo. (As OCP are analyzed in liver and depot fat, Hg in liver and Cd in the kidney the total number of specimens amount 48oo). Additional data and differential diagnoses have to be derived from 12oo animals.

1. Adminstrator comp. a 1

2. Travelling costs and expenditure compensation for the collecting staff depending on the persons involved:
   a) hunters or:
   b) the administrator himself and technical staff (students, only engaged for some weeks) or:
   c) Scientists as game biologists or veterinarian also involved in additional data collection or diagnosis work

3. When occasion arises: Costs for buying the game samples

4. Devices for material collection
   a) vials
   b) protocols and writing material
   c) weighing devices and preparation devices
   d) transportation devices like cooling bag
   e) chemicals like formaline, dry ice or thermoelements
   f) refrigerator for storage
   g) mailing or transportation costs (by post or car)

The estimated expenses for point 2 to 4 amount approximately depending in persons involved and equipment 2o ooo/year

5. Residue analyses under the premission that loo % will be supported: 36o ooo DM/year : the actual costs are higher

6. Differential diagnosis and additional data (in some cases combined with 2 c) about 5o ooo DM/year (loo % have to be supported)

7. Data evaluation and interpretation

8. General expenses comp. a 4

Part 6

Biological Monitoring using freeliving indicators species

Form sheet destined for computer evaluation of pesticide residue data (here:OCP) in wildliving animal indicator species of the GFR

oooooo = unknown   code number = defined

classification of the sampled individuum	A	Species
	B	Fauna Class
	C	Feeding type Carnivor Herbivor Omnivor Insectivor specialist generalist
	D	Analysis protocol number
	E	Sampling protocol number
	F	Date
description of the collection site	G	Collection site
	H	Land use unknown mingled agriculture forestry of G industry settlement recreation
	I	Vegetation type of G
	K	Additional contamination data air water soil plants available of G
data about the indicator individuum	L	Age of the indicator animal
	M	Sex of the indicator animal
	N	Body weight
	O	General nutritional stage
	P	Marrow fat index
	Q	Vitamin A storage in the liver or other criteria
	R	Egg shell thickness
	S	Health stage parasites infestation
data about residue analysis	U	Specimen for analysis liver fat eggs muscle ...
	V	Organ or tissue weight
	W	Fat content of the organ or tissue
	X	Applied Method extraction clean up gaschromat. data
	Y	Residue data (ppm/freshweight or ppm/fat or ppm/dry weight) HCB αHCH Lindane ß HCH γHCH Heptachlore H-epoxide Aldrine+Dieldrine p,p-DDE p,p-DDD p,p-DDT and isomers PCB's other compounds

NATURALLY OCCURRING STEROIDS AND SYNTHETIC HORMONES AS
SENSITIVE MONITORING COMPOUNDS FOR THE SUITABILITY OF
PRETREATMENT PROCEDURES IN SPECIMEN BANKING AND FOR THE
LONG-TERM STABILITY OF STORED BIOLOGICAL SAMPLES

Dr. H.W. Dürbeck
Institute for Chemistry
Institute 4: Applied Physical Chemistry
Nuclear Research Center (KFA)
P.O. Box 1913
D-517o Jülich
Federal Republic of Germany

Introduction

It should be the scope of any specimen banking facility to provide information regarding the past and present exposures of the ecosystems to
pollutants or pollutant groups. Therefore representative species and
specimens have to be collected, sampled and stored, which may be comparatively analysed, if advanced analytical methods are available or
if compounds, which have not been regarded dangerous today are going
to be recognised as hazardous pollutants. Moreover, existing problems
concerning the determination of long-term trends in environmental pollutant concentrations may be investigated and probably eliminated.

However, for the establishment of any successfully operating banking
facility many general problems have to be solved, regarding sampling,
sample preparation, subsampling, contamination, storage, stability
and distribution apart from additonal specific aspects involved with
the storage of certain pollutants or specimen groups.

It is the aim of this paper to discuss briefly some of these problems
and to suggest possible ways of solutions which, however, have still
to be investigated experimentally in most cases. In General the paper
follows the sequence of topical headings outlined in the recommendations
for preparing this working paper.

The compounds to be discussed are naturally occuring steroids and synthetic hormones (anabolic drugs), which in general meet three aspects
of importance for a future specimen bank problem.

1. Hormonal substances and anabolic steroids are regarded to be
   environmental pollutants (cf. chapter II).

2. Due to their chemical structure these compounds are most suitable for monitoring the stability of a sample when pretreated
   for banking purposes or when stored for a long period of time.

3. Hormones are present in many of the species, which have been
   selected to have the highest priority for specimen banking

(i.e. milk, mussels, seawage sludge). Moreover, they may be found
in blood, urine, fat and muscular tissue.

I. Review of Past and Current Programs

According to our knowledge the only systematic program concerning the
determination of synthetic steroids in various biological samples
is carried out in the Institute for Applied Physical Chemistry of the
Nuclear Research Center (KFA) in Juelich. This program was started
about 3 years ago and covers the real-time monitoring of synthetic
steroids and naturally occuring androgens in blood, meat and urine
as well as preliminary studies of sample pretreatment, sample storage
and sample stability. Details of this program will be discussed in the
chapters to follow.

II. Rationale for Interest or Concern

Naturally occuring androgens and synthetic anabolic steroids are well-
known to stimulate the biosynthesis of proteins (1). Although the
mechanism of this biochemical activity has not been completely understood, these compounds are frequently used to improve the physical
performance and to accelerate the production of muscular tissue. According to these effects at least three areas of application have to be
mentioned:

- as therapeutical drugs and supporting adjuvants for the
  therapy of various diseases with protein deficiencies (2-6),

- as food additives in animal feeding to improve the nitrogen
  balance and to accelerate the rate of growth of slaughter cattle
  (7,8),

- as doping agents in several branches of sports to achieve
  gain in muscular strength and size (9-14).

From their chemical structure (cf. fig. 1) it is evident that synthetic anabolic steroids may be classified as less musculinizing substitutes for the naturally occuring androgens. The active principles
- known so far - may be summarized in the following items:

- 17β-hydroxy group (generally)
- 5α -configuration for saturated Ring A steroids
- 17α-alkylgroup for oral administration

- Depot effect.

- 17β-hydroxy group conjugated with long chain fatty acids
  or aromatic carboxylic acids.

The search for anabolic compounds with a negligible androgenic component has produced some loo or 2oo different drugs (15), which
are commercially available and which are widely used. However, these
are all still afflicted with the undesirable androgenic effect, which
is more or less pronounced depending on structural details. Furthermore cases of liver damage after the administration of massive doses
have been reported (16-18) and even small quantities administrated
over a long period of time may cause an irreversible change in voice
pitch (19,2o). It's for these reasons that synthetic steroids are

186

Androstane Group

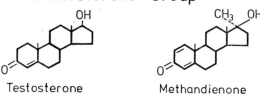

Anabolex   Ermalone

Testosterone Group

Testosterone   Methandienone

Oestrane Group

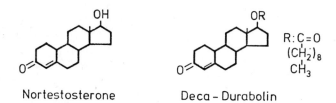

$$R:C=O$$
$$(CH_2)_8$$
$$CH_3$$

Nortestosterone   Deca - Durabolin

Figure 1. Classification of synthetic anabolic steroids
and some typical representatives.

controlled drugs.

Nevertheless very little is known about metabolism, actual toxicity, excretion rate and total amount of excretion. From our experiments some recent findings of pharmacokinetic and metabolic studies may be summarized as follows:

1) for orally applicable compounds the rate of metabolism seems to be more rapid than their excretion. Therefore, the application may be detected only via the metabolites.

2) For the compounds investigated these metabolites are totally excreted within a few days after the last drug administration.

3) However, for methandienone and related drugs, only 5 % of the administrated compound are recovered in form of the major metabolites. The fate of the remaining 95 % is unknown. Accumulation in fat, liver, kidney and muscular tissues may be a possibly reason for this observation.

The environmental exposure to man and the ecosystems is estimated to proceed via the food-chain slaughter cattle-man. Although the use of such drugs for nutrition purposes is strictly prohibited in most countries of the western hemisphere, many cases of abuse have been reported. Since reliable data about this abuse are not available, current levels of environmental exposure may not be given.

Apart from this environmental significance the discussed compounds are generally most suitable for monitoring the stability of biological samples to be stored in an environmental specimen bank. It was shown in extended experiments, that most of the compounds investigated undergo degradation (dehydroxylation), when the sample or matrix is treated in an unsuitable manner.Due to this situation, selected steroid compounds (natural and sythetic) may be used as sensitive monitors for the stability of specimens during the pretreatment procedure of the storage period.

Especially form this point of view some generally applicable aspects of monitoring and banking biological samples will be discussed in a condensed manner, the basic tropics being based on own experimental results. The matrices suitable in this context should be blood (whole blood, serum, plasma), urine, muscular and fat tissue, liver, kidney, milk and possibly seawage sludge.

Considerations for sample selection, collection, containment, shipment, and storage.

Considering the facts and aspects outlined before, the selection of samples to be stored should be orientated to acute problems, which are closely related to the environmental exposure to toxic substances such as polychlorinated hydrocarbons, polychlorinated biphenyls, polycyclic aromatic hydrocarbons and most of the compounds listed in the recommendations for preparing this working paper. Naturally occuring steroids and synthetic hormones, whereever present, may in addition be regarded as reference materials for such samples, in which the speciation of a pollutant is of significant importance. It may be expected that in a biological sample in which the steroid pattern remains constant during all pretreatmant procedures the pollutants of interest will keep unchanged concerning their quantity and their chemical structure.

For the long-term storage of a biological specimen many pretreatment procedures have to be considered, the most important ones (including significant side problems) are listed in the following scheme. This scheme includes specimen procurement, processing, storage and distribution. Furthermore a system of record-keeping and quality control must exist within this frame work.

Therefore, in a pilot phase basic studies concerning the following detailed items have to be performed with maximum care.

1. Studies on the "chemical stability" of specimens or tissues
   1.1. after sampling
   1.2. after transport to the specimen bank
   1.3. after processing or clean-up
   1.4. during the storage period under different conditions
        (cf. 2) within constant time intervals.

These studies may be carried out by recording the analytical "fingerprint" of different compounds (steroids as representatives for labile compounds, PAH's as examples for stable compounds).

2. Evaluation of storage conditions, which guarantee maximum stability of the chemical and biological information.
   2.1.   during sample preparation
   2.1.1. Without any preliminary clean-up
   2.1.2. homogenisation and subsampling under inert gas
          atmosphere at different temperatures
   2.1.3. γ-ray sterilisation or chemical conservation
   2.1.4. freeze-drying under different conditions
   2.1.5. shock freezing
   2.1.6. deep-freezing under temperature controlled conditions

   2.2.   during specimen storage
   2.2.1. at different temperatures (-4°C, -2o°C, -8o°C, -19o°C)
   2.2.2. in different containers
   2.2.3. in inert gas atmosphere

   2.3.   during the thawing period
   2.3.1. moderate thawing under temperature controlled conditions
   2.3.2. rapid thawing (microwave heating)

3. Studies on suitable containers

   3.1. mechanical stability at low temperatures
   3.2. studies on gas permeability
   3.3. embrittling of plastic materials
   3.4. chemical resistance

4. Studies on contamination problems
   4.1. during sampling, transport, processing, storage and further
        distribution by container materials or additives (plastisizers,
        catalysts).

From these problems generally to be considered a few aspects have been extensively studied in context with the Environmental Specimen Bank Program sponsored by the Federal Ministry of Research and Technology (BMFT) and by the Federal Environmental Agency (Umweltbundesamt):

- container material
- storage procedures for "short-term" monitoring environmental materials
- "long-term" specimen banking

Keeping in mind that only organic pollutants are considered in this paper, biological specimens are best sampled, stored, transported and distributed in glass vessels or appropriate size.For short-term storage (i.e. 24 hours) temperatures of -4°C may be recommended and should be perferred to a temperature of -2o°C, which seems to be the worst temperature at all. It was shown that at this temperature the cell-skeleton is going to break up, thus favouring an increased enzyme activity.

For long-term storage (i.e. for banking purposes) deep-freezing and freezing-drying are the most accepted methods. Deep-freezing, in many cases, guarantees satisfactory stability of the sample provided the temperature used for storage is - 8o°C or colder. Temperatures warmer than this do not adequately protect against enzymatic degradation of the stored sample. Therefore, for routine purposes liquid nitrogen freezers are recommended which should maintain a specimen temperature of -1oo°C or colder, depending on their location within the freezer.

However, in the deep-freezing procedure the freezing rate is still an open question and needs further basic research. Depending on the specimen to be stored, freezing rates of 1°/min up to some 1ooo°/sec. (shock-freezing) have been found adequate.

Freeze drying, in general, seems to be advantageous over deep-freezing. The samples can be stored in normal glass containers and kept at room temperature. Transportation, shipment and distribution is facilitated and the handling for further processing is simplified.

However, according to our experimental results, the freeze-drying procedure itself needs further intensive basic research, since the fingerprint of the reference steroids does not remain unchanged during this pretreatment process. On the other hand, it may be predicted that by applying strictly controlled low-temperature and vacuum conditions, this method can be satisfactorily developed so that even as labile compounds as steroids do not change their chemical structure. For further stability of the freeze-dried specimen it is recommended to store the sample with a vaccum sealed inside.

IV. Analytical Procedures

To obtain a scientifically sound basis for the analysis of naturally occurring steroids and synthetic hormones, within the last few years in our institute some generally applicable analytical methods have been developed using HPLC, GLC and capillary GC/MS as basic instrumental techniques (21-23).

A major part of this development has been dedicated to systematical

studies to obtain the highest degree of accuracy, precision, specificity and reproducibility. In general, this may be accomplished by
intercomparing the obtained results with the findings of other reliable laboratories or by applying different and idependent analytical
methods to the same analytical problem, to exclude sources of systematical errors. According to these essential principles of modern analytical chemistry at least two methods are to be applied which finally
are expected to yield consistent and corresponding results. Keeping
these essential aspects and remarks in mind a generally applicable
scheme for the determination of steroids in different matrices and
different binding states is illustrated in fig. 2 and 3. It is the
aim of this paper to emphasize crucial points of the experimental
performance rather than to repeat known and published procedures of
steroid analysis.

Clean-up

The samples (Fluids, solid specimens, homogenized specimens, freeze-
dried or deep-freezed samples) are stored in glass vessels. The un-
conjugated steroids are removed from the sample by extracting with
CH_2CI_2 and the organic phase is cleaned-up according to the procedure
recently published in detail (21,24). For conjugated compounds (Glu-
coronides, sulphates) enzymatic hydrolysis with "Helix pomatia" or
β-glucoronidase/arylsulphatase is recommended (25).

Contamination

It is obvious that all chemicals used during the clean-up procedure
are of the highest obtainable purity and that they have been checked
for their suitability. In general this is indispensable for organic
solvents which are usually contaminated with phthalates and silicones.

Moreover, in the drying procedure which is essential for the derivatisation to follow the normally applied inorganics, such as anhy-
drous Na_2SO_4 or $MgSO_4$ are absolutely unsuitable due to their high
content of phthalates and other plastizisers. Thus, filtration through
a soft paper filter is to be preferred for the removal of adherent
water droplets followed by a prolonged vacuum evaporation under ambient
and strictly controlled temperature conditions.

Derivatisation

The derivatisation of the steroid extracts, i.e. silylation and (or)
methoximation with additional chemicals and their impurities involved,
has been extensively tried to become a negligible part of the total
clean-up procedure. However, for steroids with polar substituents and
for their detection with GLC or GC/MS derivatisation is still the method
of choice, since the resolving ability of the chromatographic columns
and the sensitivity of the detecting systems is markedly increased.

According to detailed preliminary experiments on the silylation of
sterically hindered hydroxy groups in steroids a mixture of N-methyl-
N-trimethylsilyltrifluoroacetamide (MSTFA) and trimethylchlorosilane
(TMCS) (1o:1) in pyridine is recommended, which guarantees total derivatisation. This reagent is added to the dry sample extract and kept
at room temperature for approximately 3o min. Without further treat-

ment the solution is than ready for gas chromatorgraphy.

Instrumental Points

From the instrumental methods applied, for routine purposes HPLC and
GLC - with packed or capillary columns - are employed predominantly
as screeining procedures, while capillary GC/MS is mainly used for the
elucidation of unknown metabolite structures or in cases of uncertainty.
Since details of these measurements as well as their operating conditions
have been published elsewhere (21-23), for GLC and GC/MS only two
points of general importance have to be emphasized here:
- The inertness of the chromatrographic columns and
- the interface for the GC/MS coupling of glass capillary columns.

Both aspects have been thoroughly investigated in our institute and the
results obtained have been published recently (26,27).

Sensitivity

GLC with packed columns of different polarity as well as HPLC and
capillary GC/MS are capable of detecting about 5 ng of each steroid
compound (RSD + 8 %) (21), which is equivalent to a concentration
down to 1o μg/l in the samples examined. The sensitivity may be increased by at least a factor of 1o by GC/MS with single ion-monitoring.
Moreover, the determination byGLC has been totally automated by apply -
ing autosampling and data processing devices, thus providing a simple
and time saving screening procedure. The time for the total analysis
including the clean-up procedure amounts then to about 3 hours.

V. Program Design

Within the general framework outlined in chapter II, it is intended
to perform the sampling, real-time monitoring, analysis and storage
of three - probably four - matrices in the pilot phase of the specimen
bank program, i.e.: blood, urine, mucular and fat tissue and probably
seawage sludge. With these matrices optimal conditions for the long-
term stability (quantity and chemical structure) of organic pollutants
shall be developed, using steroids and polycyclic aromatic hydrocarbons as reference materials. It is intended to record the chromatographic fingerprints of the compounds in question throughout all necessary pretreatment procedures and to optimize the techniques, whenever
alterations in the chromatographic pattern are observed. The results
obtained will be made available in form of preliminary reports or
publications as particular contribution to the pilot specimen bank
program.

Apart from this basic research program which is regarded as most important for all participants of a pilot program a real-time monitoring
program concerning the fluxes of synthetic hormones and their metabolites in the food-chain animal- food/livestock/man shall be performed.
Moreover, the real-time monitoring of PAH's in the matrices listed above
is intended. In this context the aspects of significant population
groups, of suitable ecosystems, of samples and their appropriate environment should be considered by other experts, that we hope to find among
the participants of the Berlin-Workshop.

192

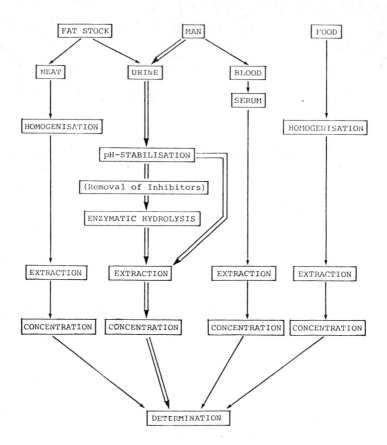

Figure 2. Schematic diagram for the steroid clean-up procedure in different matrix types.

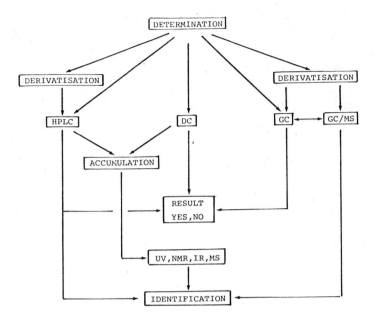

Figure 3. Schematic diagram for the determination of steroids
in sample extracts by different instrumental methods.

194

In general, the basic research program should be accompanied by statistical investigations and by a data storage program. Due to the fact, that most of the analytical informations are primarily obtained in form of digital signals, a data storage on a disc or a magnetic tape is envisaged, which may then be further processed by our IBM-computing system. In the case of chromatographic methods involved, retention times, peak areas, the type of integration and further parameters of interest could be stored, thus offering simple possibilities of calculating quantities and concentrations or identifying chemical structures. Moreover, data comparison and statistical evaluations could be performed, provided the appropriate software is available.

VI. Organizational Aspects

From the scientific and experimental point of view the program as a whole - which means sampling, sample pretreatment, real-time monitoring, analysis and banking - may be regarded as a very difficult task and should therefore be carried out only be well-trained and experienced staff. Moreover, a clear instruction and a precise documentation of all data needed is mandatory. It should also be emphasized that the detailed performance of all necessary sub-procedures or programs should be developed by the cooperation of experts from different scientific branches, i. e. biology, medicine, analytical and physical chemistry, biochemistry, electronics, mathematics and cryogenics.

Being aware that the success of an environmental specimen bank is mainly determined by these aspects, first approaches for an interdisciplinary cooperation have been initiated. On the other hand, to our opinion it is absolutely necessary that the banking facility is centralized to one selected location. Though this centralization may cause additional shipment and distribution problems, it offers the ideal opportunity to have the pilot bank research program performed under identical conditions.

VII. Cost Estimates

A preliminary cost estimation for the "Real-Time Monitoring" and "Operating a Pilot Specimen Bank" was recently prepared for the Federal Ministry of Research and Technology. Since this calculation is based on the present available instrumentation and technical staff, only additional costs for operating a specimen bank were taken into account. The cost estimation given below may be understood in the same context. However, to addresses only to the particular compounds and aspects discussed in this paper and covers the real-time monitoring of four selected matrices, the sampling, sample preparation (clean-up), analysis and banking.

Cost Estimates [+] per Annum for a Sub-program "Hormonal Compounds and Polycyclic Aromatic Hydrocarbons" in the Frame of a "Pilot Specimen Bank Program"

[+] Approximate current market prices. Excludes building costs, building and equipment maintenance.

Initial investments

Liquid-nitrogen refrigerator	3o.ooo,--
Freeze-dryer	65.ooo,--
	95.ooo,--
	=========

Current Costs

Salaries (Scientists, technical staff)	24o.ooo,--
Travelling costs	15.ooo,--
Collection and transport of samples	2o.ooo,--
Chemicals, reference materials, solvents etc.	25.ooo,--
Storage	
Liquid nitrogen cooling	3o.ooo,--
Variety of glass bottles, shipping boxes and containers	1o.ooo,--
Analysis	
Analytical equipment (GC, HPLC, GC/MS, balance, micro- wave equipment)	4o.ooo,--
Data processing (Software development)	2o.ooo,--
	4oo.ooo,-- DM
	=========

From these roughly calculated figures it can be seen that more
than the half of the annual amount must be spent for salaries. On the
other hand the estimation for the technical staff (two man years) is
the absolute minimum to perform the designed program or even parts
of it. Moreover, it is obvious from these data that the banking facility has to be centralized to one location to keep the salaries as
low as possible. Finally, it can be expected that the cost ratio
salaries/equipment will not markedly change, if the establishment
of a larger-scale specimen bank is intended.

References

1) Kochakian, C.D. and Murlin, J.R.: The effect of male hormone on
   the protein and energy metabolismn of castrate dogs.
   J.Nutr. 1o, 437 (1935).

2) Bierich, J.R.: Die klinische Anwendung anabolischer Steroide.
   Mschr. Kinderheilk. 114, 444 (1966).

3) Littmann, K.P.: Was is gesichert in der Therapie mit anabolen
   Steroiden?. Internist 14, 621-63o (1973).

4) Charash, L.: Anabolic steroids in the management of muscular dystrophy. Pediatrics 36, 4o2-4o5 (1965).

5) Faludi, G., Dykyj, R., Chayes, Z.W. and Nodine, J.H.: Anabolic steroids in muscular, neurologic and hematologic disorders. J. Amer. med. Wom. Ass. 23, 346-351 (1968).

6) Kley, H.K. and Krueskemper, H.L.:Androgene-Biochemie, Wirkungsweise, therapeutische Anwendung. Med. Klinik 68, 295 (1973).

7) Glimp, H.A. and Cundiff, L.V.: Effects of oral melengestrol acetate and a testosterone-diethylstilbestrol implant, breed and age on growth and carcass traits of beef heifers. J. Anim. Sci. 32, 957-961 (1971).

8) Bidner, T.D., Merkel, R.A. and Miller, E.R.: Effect of a combination of diethylstilbestrol and methyltestosterone on performance, carcass traits,serum and muscle characteristics of pigs. J. Anim. Sci. 35, 525-533 (1972).

9) Mader, A.: Anabolika im Hochleistungssport. Leistungssport 7, 136-147 (1977).

1o) Freed, D., Banks, A.J. and Langson, P.: Anabolic steroids in athletics. Brit. Med. J. 3, 761 (1972).

11) Hervey, G.R.: Are Athletes wrong about anabolic steroids? Brit. J. Sports Med. 9, 74 (1975).

12) Imhoff, P.: Anabole Steroide und Sport. Schweiz. Z. Sportmed. 18, 19-85 (197o).

13) Johnson, L.C. and O'Shea, J.B.: Anabolic steroid: effects on strength develpment. Science 164, 957-959 (1969).

14) Ryan, A.J., Athletics, in Anabolic-Androgenic Steroids, C.D. Kochakian, ed., (Springer Verlag, Berlin-Heidelberg-New York, 1976).

15) Ippen, H.: Index Pharacorum, p. 24o ff (Georg Thieme Verlag, Stuttgart, 197o).

16) Meadows, A.T., Naiman, J.L. and Valdesdapena, M.: Hepatoma associated with androgen therapy for aplastic anemia. J. Pediat. 84, 1o9-11o (1974).

17) Henderson, J.T., Richmond, J. and Sumerling, M.D.: Androgenanabolic steroid therapy and hepatocellular carcinoma. Lancet, 1973 I, 934.

18) Farrell, G.C., Uren, R.F., Perkins, K.W., Joshua, D.E., Baird, P.J. and Kronenberg, H.: Androgen-induced hepatoma. Lancet 1975 I, 43o-431.

19) Arndt, H.J.: Stimmstörungen nach Behandlung mit androgenen und anabolen Hormonen. Münch. med. Wschr. 116, 1715 (1974).

2o) Schäfer, E.L. and Buchholz, R.: Fehler und Gefahren der Hormontherapie. (Georg Thieme Verlag, Stuttgart, 1974).

21) Dürbeck, H.W., Büker, I., Scheulen, B. and Telin, B.: GC and capillary gc/ms-determination of synthetic anabolic steroids. J. Chromatogr. (1978) in press.

22) Dürbeck, H.W., Frischkorn, C.G.B. and Frischkorn, H.E.: Untersuchungen zum Stoffwechselverhalten des Dianabol. Ein Beitrag zur Bestimmung von Anabolika. Dtsch. Zeitschr. f. Sportm. 29, 97-1o3 (1978)

23) Frischkorn, C.G.B. and Frischkorn, H.E.: Investigations on anabolic drug abuse in athletics and cattle feeding. II. Specific determination of the anabolic drug dianabol in urine in nanogram-amounts. J. Chromatogr. 151, 331-338 (1978).

24) Dürbeck, H.W., Frischkorn, C.G.B., Büker, I., Scheulen, B. and Telin, B.: The Determination of anabolic steroids in human body fluids, Proceedings of the 9th Materials Research Symposium, National Bureau of Standards, Washington, D.C. Io.-13. April 1978 (in press).

25) Frischkorn, C.G.B. and Ohst, I.: Rückstandsuntersuchungen an Lebensmitteln, I. Mitt.: Enzymatische Kurzhydrolyse von Steroidkonjugaten zur Bestimmung anaboler Steroide bei Schlachtvieh. Z. Lebensmittel-Unters. Forsch. (1978) in press.

26) Dürbeck, H.W., Büker, I. and Leymann, W.: Ein neues Interface für die GC/MS-Kopplung von Glaskapillarsäulen. Chromatographia 11, 295-3oo (1978).

27) Dürbeck, H.W., Büker, I. and Leymann, W.: Ein modifiziertes Interface für die GC/MS-Kopplung von Glaskapillarsäulen. Chromatographia (1978) in press.

CONTAINER MATERIALS FOR THE PRESERVATION
OF TRACE SUBSTANCES IN ENVIRONMENTAL SPECIMENS

Richard A. Durst
Center for Analytical Chemistry
National Bureau of Standards
Washington, D.C. 2o234

Introduction

The success fo the National Environmental Specimen Bank (1) will be determined in large part by the ability to preserve the integrity of the trace
substances during long-term storage. It is widely recognized that the storage of environmental materials is subject to a variety of undertainties
when one is considering the identity and levels of trace elements and organic compounds.
Changes in the forms and concentrations of the numerous environmentally important substances in specimens stored for extended periods may occur in
several ways. Processes such as surface adsorption and sample degradation
may reduce the concentrations of various components and/or produce species
which may not have been present in the original sample. On the other hand,
contamination from the container and evaporation of specimen fluids could
lead to apparent increases in trace substance concentrations or losses in
the case of volatile trace components. In addition, superimposed on these
processes are the factors which will affect their rates, such as, container material, contact time and area, storage temperature, pH, and initial
species concentration. All of these factors are important considerations
in evaluating the suitability of various containers for long-term storage.

There have been numerous studies performed in recent years directed toward the identification of suitable container materials and optimum storage conditions, but much of this work is contradictory (2). In many
cases, the analytical data were invalidated because of problems not
associated with the storage but with other links in the analytical chain
such as sampling and procedural contamination.

Container Materials

While certain container materials can be eliminated a priori, it is usually necessary to consider the container composition vis-a-vis the type of
sample and/or the components of interest in the sample. Accordingly, it
is unlikely that samples intended for trace organic analysis would be
stored in plastic containers or acidified water samples in glass containers if trace elements were to be determined. While these are obvious
examples of incompatible sample/container combinations, even these may
be acceptable under certain storage conditions and for special requirements.

The National Environmental Specimen Bank is somewhat unique in that both trace elements and trace organics are of environmental concern and a choice must be made as to storing the samples in a single container material suitable for both types of components or in two different container materials optimized for the components of interest. In the former case, the choices are much more limited and compromises must be made, whereas in the latter, the increased complexity of separate sampling, sample handling and storage procedures may be excessive. In the EPA/NBS Environmental Pilot Bank, this is one of the questions to be answered by careful evaluation of a variety of container materials under different cleaning procedures and storage conditions.

At NBS, most of the research to date has been concerned with trace element contamination and losses, while trace organic problems have largely been avoided by the use of carefully cleaned glass containers and immediate freezing of the samples. In a recent study (3), twelve different plastics were examined by gravimetry, isotope dilution mass spectrometry, and neutron activation analysis in order to evaluate the rate of water loss, the levels of impurities present in the plastics, and the quantities of trace elements leached from the plastics during acid cleaning.

The annual rate of water loss, based on weighings at 17 and 66 days, are given in Table 1. The polypropylene, Teflon, and conventional polyethylene have water loss rates compatible with long-term storage of aqueous samples, whereas the other plastics may be adequate for shorter storage periods (3).

Table 1. Annual Rate of Water Loss from Plastic Containers

Material	% Loss/year [1]
Polypropylene	0.04
Teflon	0.05
Conventional polyethylene	0.1
Polyvinyl chloride	0.5
Polymethylpentane	1
Polycarbonate	2

[1] Average values based on weight loss measured at 17 and 66 days

Since the closure may have been responsible for a significant portion of the water loss, these values should not be construed as permeability data but merely typical losses from these types of containers. These losses could be reduced in practice by sealing the container in a vapor barrier or storage at an ambient relative humidity comparable to that of the aqueous samples.

The concentrations of trace elements contained in the plastics were determined by neutron activation analysis (3). The ten plastics studied showed striking differences in trace element composition as illustrated in Table II for several of the elements determined.

Table II. Trace Elements in Plastics Determined by Neutron Activation
Analysis (Concentrations given in ng/g)

Element	CPE	LPE	PP	PMP	PS	PC	TFE	FEP
Na	1×10^3	15×10^3	5×10^3	2oo	2×10^3	3×10^3	16o	4oo
Al	5oo	3×10^4	6×10^4	6×10^3	5oo	3×10^3	23o	2oo
Ti		5×10^3	6×10^4	5×10^3	1×10^3			
Mn		1o	2o	1o	2o			6o
Co		4o				6		
Zn		5×10^5		3×10^4				
Br	$\geq$2o	8oo	$\geq$5	$\geq$2	$\geq$1	3×10^4		$\geq$2
Sb	5	2oo	6oo					
Au			o.1	o.6	o.04	o.03	o.4	

CPE = conventional polyethylene; LPE = linear polyethylene;
PP = polypropylene; PMP = polymethylpentane; PS = polystyrene;
PC = polycarbonate; TFE and FEB = types of Teflon

In agreement with the results of other workers, the purest materials appear
to be Teflon, PS, and CPE. Comparison of these data with those obtained in
leaching experiments indicate that the bulk of most trace element impurities
present is distributed throughout the matrix, rather than concentrated at
the surface.

The acid-leaching experiments were performed on four types of plastic using
two acids prepared from ultra-pure reagents. In this study (3), the plastic
bottles were first rinsed with distilled water to remove any surface contamination and then filled with a 1+1 mixture of ultra-pure HNO_3 or ultra-
pure HCl and ultra-pure water (4). The leaching process was allowed to
proceed for one week at room temperature (8o^{o}C for the FEP bottle) before
the analyses were performed. The results obtained by isotope dilution mass
spetrometry are given in Table III for a selected group of the impurity
elements measured.

Table III. Impurities Leached from Plastic Containers (ng/cm^2)

Element	FEP HNO_3	FEP HCl	LPE HNO_3	LPE HCl	CPE HNO_3	CPE HCl	PC HNO_3	PC HN1
PB	2	2	2	o.6	o.7	18	o.3	1o
Al	6	4	1	4	1	1o	5	3
Na	6	2	1o	6	8	42	3	8
Sn	1	1	1	<1	<o.8	<o.8	o.2	13
Cd	o.4	o.6	o.2	o.2	o.2	o.2	o.3	8
Se	o.2	o.8	o.4	o.4	3	<o.3	o.5	<o.5
Zn	4	4	8	9	2	1	o.8	-
Cu	2	6	o.4	1	2	o.7	o.8	<6
Ni	2	o.8	1.6	o.8	o.5	o.3	o.7	o.3
Fe	2o	16	3	1	3	1	3	<49
Cr	o.8	4	o.2	o.8	o.8	o.3	o.3	< 5
Mg	8	1	o.6	o.4	o.7	o.7	2	o.8

Values which are below 2 ng/cm^2 or prefixed by < are upper limits

---

The results of these experiments indicate that HNO_3 and HCl leach various elements with different efficiencies, and it is recommended that both acids, in sequence, be used for cleaning these containers (3). After cleaning, the Teflon and CPE bottles have been found to be the least contaminating. Based on experience at NBS and reports of other studies, a recommended method for cleaning plastic containers has been proposed (3):

1. Fill container with 1+1 analytical reagent grade HCl.

2. Allow to stand for one week at room temperature (8o°C for Teflon).

3. Empty and rinse with distilled water.

4. Fill with 1+1 analytical reagent grade HNO_3.

5. Repeat steps 2 and 3.

6. Fill with the purest available distilled water.

7. Allow to stand several weeks or until needed, changing water periodically to ensure continued cleaning.

8. Rinse with purest water and allow to dry in a particle- and fume-free environment.

For the storage of biological tissues and fluids, rapid freeze drying immediately after sampling has been recommended but suffers from the disadvantage that some volatile components may be lost (2). A more viable approach would appear to be the immediate freezing of the sample or sub-samples to the lowest conveniently attainable temperature. This approach serves two purposes: 1) it reduces or stops both chemical and biological processes which could result in sample changes, and 2) it reduces the mobility of sample and container components thereby lessening the possibility of contamination and/or losses due to adsorption or volatility. However, because of concentration gradients which may be produced during freeze-thaw cycles and physical changes, e.g., cell destruction, caused by freezing, it is highly recommended that all sub-sampling be performed prior to the freezing step. Unfortunately, the unavailability of clean facilities at most sampling sites usually precludes this procedure because of the probability of sample contamination during the sub-sampling. Instead, the sample, which has been frozen as rapidly to avoid component fractionation, is sub-sampled while still in the frozen state at a location which has a clean facility.

When the sample is frozen, especially at cryogenic temperatures, the reduced interaction between the sample and container permits greater flexibility in the choice of container material. However, even under these conditions it is inadvisable to store samples intended for trace organic analysis in any type of plastic container which incorporates additives such as plasticizers, organometallic or other stabilizer anti-oxidants, colorants, or any other components which may be leached or volatilized from the plastic. The only plastic which conforms to this requirement is Teflon, which, after proper cleaning, is also suitable for the storage of samples intended for trace element analysis.

Glass (quartz or Pyrex), with Teflon (or aluminium foil) lined caps, is also suitable for trace organic samples and may be satisfactory for frozen trace element samples. At the present time, the key to long-term storage appears to be storage at cryogenic temperatures to reduce reactions and interactions to a minimum. Under these conditions, both glass and Teflon appear to be suitable storage container materials.

Provisional Pilot Bank Procedure

A tentative protocol (5) has been developed for the initial sampling and storage of human liver samples in the Pilot Bank. Briefly, this protocol consists of careful sampling during autopsies using specially cleaned surgical instruments, plastic gloves, and Teflon work surfaces. The excised liver will be dissected to provide sections which will be sealed in Teflon bags and immediately frozen in liquid nitrogen. The frozen sections will be sent to NBS in special liquid nitrogen shipping containers. At NBS, they will be sub-sampled while still frozen and sealed into the storage vials. All of the sub-sampling will be performed in a biological work station located in a class-loo clean room. The storage vials will then be transferred to freezers held at -25oC and -8ooC and also liquid nitrogen freezers (vapor-phase storage) located in an adjoining class-loo clean room where they will be stored for the five-year duration of the Pilot Bank with periodic removal of selected vials for retrospective analysis.

Initially, special Teflon-sealed glass and Teflon vials will be evaluated as potential containers for the Specimen Bank. Other types of materials will be evaluated as they are identified as providing desirable storage characteristics. Both trace element and trace organic analyses will be performed during the Pilot Bank study and, on the basis of the results of these analyses, the optimum container material will be selected.

References

1. G.M. Goldstein, "Plan for a National Environmental Specimen Bank", Environmental Health Effects Research Series, EPA-6oo/1-78-o22, March 1978.

2. E.J. Maienthal and D.A. Becker, "A Survey of Current Literature on Sampling, Sample Handling, and Long Term Storage for Environmental Materials", NBS Tech. Note 929, U.S. Government Printing Office, Washington, D.C. 2o4o2, 1976.

3. J.R. Moody and R.M. Lindstrom, Anal. Chem. <u>49</u>, 2264 (1977).

4. E.C. Kuehner, R. Alvarez, P.J. Paulsen, and T.J. Murphy, Anal. Chem. <u>44</u>, 2o5o (1972).

5. E.J. Maienthal, "Development of a Preliminary Protocol for Sampling, Sample Handling and Long-Term Storage of Human Liver", in The National Environmental Specimen Bank Research Program for Sampling, Storage and Analysis, T.E. Gills, H.C. Rook, and R.A. Durst, editors, EPA Contract Report, EPA-1AG-D5-o568, (in process).

MONITORING OF PLANTS AND SOIL FOR ANALYSIS OF POSSIBLY
HAZARDOUS CONTAMINANTS AND BANKING OF THESE ENVIRONMEN-
TAL SPECIMENS

Dr. K.W. Ebing
Biologische Bundesanstalt für Land- und
Forstwirtschaft
Inst. für Pflanzenschutzmittelforschung
Königin-Luise-Straße 19
looo Berlin 33 (Dahlem)
Federal Republic of Germany

1. GENERAL REMARKS

At the "International Workshop on the Use of Biological Specimens for
the Assessment of Human Exposure to Environmental Pollutants" in Luxembourg, 18th-22nd April 1977, the delegates had recommended to work out
a proposal for monitoring and banking of non-human environmental substrates in addition to their own paper resulting from the workshop.

The following exposition serves as a discussion paper for a further workshop which is intended to fulfill the demands of the delegates in Luxembourg. These remarks of their reports which apply generally to all of
the monitoring environmental materials and specimen banking, are not
repeated here.

Plants may be contaminated by trace amounts of hazardous compounds and
elements evoked by industry, traffic, and plant protection. The contaminants enter the plants either by immission from the atmosphere or
-y uptake from the soil upon which they are cultivated. Therefore, soil
is a most important source for contaminating generations of plants and
should be monitored as well as air and water.

The different kinds of environmental contaminants cover a very broad
spectrum. For the purpose of environmental monitoring, it should be reasonable to limit analytical work on organic compounds substituted to a
higher degree with halogen, as generally the eco-toxicity increases with
increasing halogen content of the molecule. Further limitation has to
be made in that only non-volatile substances should be considered. Finally, expectancy of long-lasting existence of the contaminants in the
host matrices should be the criterion to elect for environmental analysis.

2. REVIEW OF PAST AND CURRENT PROGRAMMES

Monitoring programmes for contaminants in plant material must be considered apart from total diet or "marked basket studies", because results
from such investigations do not allow to establish relations between the
plants contaminated and the countryside from where they originate.
In some cases differentiation between meal compartments of animal or
plant origin is impossible. Comprehensive studies on such total diet
types had been conducted preferably in the United States by FDA since

at least 1961 for many years covering more than 25 cities. Likewise in Japan for several years similar investigations including preferably organo-chlorine and phosphorus ester insecticides, some chlorinated phenoxy acid type herbicides, cadmium and arsenic were carried out. Also Great Britain (since 1966), Canada (since 1969) and Switzerland (since 1956) undertook similar monitoring studies, preferably for analysis of organochlorine insecticides and sometimes phosphorus esters.

Beside such work, in many countries, especially in the Netherlands, Great Britain, Japan, Denmark, Switzerland, Austria, Sweden, Germany, Poland and presumably further countries in East Europe, analysis of food offe-red at their markets are being carried out mostly for organochlorine in-secticides and sometimes in addition to phosphorus ester insecticides, PCB and related compounds, toxic metals, dithiocarbamates etc. The re-sults obtained by these investigations are not suitable to be discussed for monitoring from the view-point of this paper, because the samples analyzed contain only one part of the plants (the edible one), and they are often mixed of material coming from both the home country and foreign sources; and mostly the latter dominates. Furthermore, in several samp-les the material has been previously processed.

In Poland in 1969 and 1971 limited studies were conducted on organochlorine residues in medicinal plants used in that country. In the Netherlands, in 1972 and 1974, berries and sepals of strawberries (together with the cor-responding soil) were analyzed for organochlorine and phosphorus ester insecticides, dithiocarbamates, captan, dichlofluanide, dicofol and BMC to evaluate any accumulation of these pesticides in plants and soil. Similar work had been done previously (1971 - 1972) in that country with dithiocarbamates, thiram, and endosulfan in lettuce.

On the other hand, no comprehensive monitoring programmes for environmen-tal contamination of plants with regard to both the description of the surrounding environment, and indicating the local distribution of the pollutants following a time course exist so far.

Some first dispositions for several pesticides monitoring programmes in the sense mentioned above do exist covering soils. In a monitoring pro-gramme for agricultural insecticides, which started in 1971 in Arizona, soil has been one (minor) of several environmental materials as there were water, lizards, snakes, frogs, fish, insects, birds etc. In another pro-gramme the U.S. Agricultural Research Service studied the organochlorine residue distribution in soils from areas of regular, limited and no pesti-cide use at 51 locations in 1965, 1966 and 1967. By a further collabora-tive study conducted in five West Alabama Countries, the distribution ofpesticides in randomly selected soil samples taken from diverse environ-ments has been evaluated in 1973. Here, the range of the contaminants to be analyzed has been extended to several phosphorus ester insecticides, atrazine and 2, 4, 5-T. An investigation into the direction of the time axis had been presented by S. Voerman and A.F.H. Besemer (197o). They estimated soils applied with dieldrin, lindane, DDT and parathion each a year over a period of 15 years.

3. RECOMMENDATIONS FOR MONITORING PROGRAMMES TO BE PLANNED

3.1. Requirements with regard to the contaminants to be analyzed

As outlined in section 1 above, analytical samples should be taken for analyzing compounds of the organochlorine insecticide type, such that of PCB- and dioxin-type, chlorophenols and chlorophenoxy-alcane carbonic acid class, all fluoro- and several bromo-substituted pesticides and some of their metabolic products, furthermore the triazine herbicides, amitrole and substances of similar persistence. A possibility should be provided for investigating the so called "terminal residues",as e.g. poor soluble conjugates of pesticides or some of their degradation products.

In the opinion of the author it is not necessary to establish a monitoring progamme for analyzing heavy metals in plants and soil. By very many workers sufficient data have been elaborated which enable us to estimate the concentration of the three most important metals Pb, Hg, Cd in each crop of interest (or in soil) depending on the distance of the emitting source and its emitting intensity. If anyone - in spite of this argument - wishes to establish a monitoring system for heavy metal residues it must be done under separate aspect because the election of the sampling locations will differ from that of the organic compounds. While the occurrence of the organic pollutants mostly are determined by the human utilizations of the various parts of the district areas, the concentrations of the anorganic pollutants are depending on the lacality of the emitters. In any case determinations of the metal concentrations in samples at locations selected need not to be repeated there in the course of time.

It seems that the importance of selenium is not comparable with this one of the above discussed metals. Worth mentioning amounts of Se exist merely in some areas not widespread in the world.

3.2. Proposed Sample Types

The most important matrix within the topic of this working paper is the soil. It is the central medium for transfer of contaminants from air via rain water to the plants, and also from ground water to the plants, from soil-living organisms to the plants and from one plant culture to the following ones.

It seems a sufficient international agreement that agricultural biocides residue situation should be observed in wheat plants. This is because wheat is considered to be the most important food plant of the world. Besides that sampling of several additional food plants commonly used, e.g. potatoes and rice, is also desirable.

For investigating areas not used in food plant production, such as meadows and pasture-land, sampling of a grass species, Lolium multiflorum, is recommended. In addition, other objects of interest, e.g. (parts of) trees, bushes, flowers, should be sampled.

3.3. Proposed Sampling Localities

Programmes for monitoring environmental samples and for a specimen bank system should not exceed national frameworks. But the methods and criteria of the realization should be as similar as possible.

Sampling localities have to be selected carefully. About the designating of the localities decision should be made with respect to the surrounding ecosystem. The area to be included in the monitoring programme may be divided into sections (in the form of a network) according to biogeographical viewpoints. Number and locus of the discrete sample depend on the type and usage of the area as well as the geological properties of the field must be considered. In the case of soil samples these objectives are essential, and also is the depth of boring: Sample two separate layers of soil: o - 5 cm and 5 - 1o cm. The number of the individual samples belonging to one representative mixed sample depends on the heterogenity in the district and on the geological uniformity of the soil layers. Experiences lead to the conclusion that, generally, the number of single samples demanded by the rules of statistic for a high degree of confidence, cannot be fullfilled in practice. So, a representative result from a mixed sample may be obtained, only from very careful selected and described single specimen.

It should be appropriate to monitor at least moderately enlarged specific ecosystems separately, because each type, e.g. farming or industrial or woodland ecosystem, demands different methods for laying down the sampling localities. So, for determination of individual sampling lactions and evaluation of the results expected it may be useful to consider the following subdivided terrestrial ecosystems separately: orcharding, tillage, pasture and meadow, woodland, wasteland, and industrial ones.

3.4. Handling and Describing Samples

Drawing individual samples in the field should be made using a special car which provide with instrumentation to mix, to subdivide, to weight, and to freeze (-18°C) the analytical samples. Soil samples should be drawn by means of a grooved drill.

Samples destined for residue analysis of trace compounds should not to be stored in containers which may secret analytical interfering substances. For analysis or organic contaminants, e.g. paper bags covered with a thin film of aluminium, are suitable.

For all samples drawn a circumstantial description must be given. It should include the soil profile and soil composition of the area, data about the faunal and floristic society (including organisms in the earth) in the surrounding area, data covering the course of climate and the history of treatments in the respective area. Remarks about the pathological findings of the sample are also desirable.

4. RECOMMENDATIONS FOR ENVIRONMENTAL SPECIMEN BANKING

4.1. General Aspects

Criterions for environmental specimen banking of soil and plants generally, are nearly the same as outlined in the discussion about the monitoring programmes. But in banking it should be kept in mind that all must be done to keep the expenditure as low as possible. Therefore, the author would like to propose sharper defined requirements with regard to the samples.

The mixed samples of a plant of a certain species to be stored should be

an average each of at least 1o individuals. The analytical result at time
of sampling should be representative of the state of this species in an
area within a radius of 3o km. Therefore, precise description of the
scenery within a radius of 1, 5 and 3o km, respectively, must be given to
each sample in the bank.

4.2. Organizational Aspects

Design of banking system depends on the type of samples to be stored as
well as the class of contaminants to be expected to analyze in the
future. These two points of view have decisive influence on the storage
technology to be selected. For this reason, environmental banking should
be disintegrated into several specialized banks. In addition, at such
special banks the best know how about developments both in analytical
methods and storage technology (within a narrow limited part from the whole
field of trace analysis, e.g. environmental analysis of plants and soil
for residues or organic contaminants) may be linked together with the
respected banking requirements.

Furthermore, the region, covered by one specimen bank, should be visible
at a glance without trouble. An international bank seems to be not realistic. In the opinion of the author, the existence of several discrete specialized banks instead of one general bank does not lead to expanded costs,
because the cost - yield - relationship will be better by far in each
specialized bank, and the degree of correct results and conclusions will
be enhanced.

From the experiences obtained so far in circles of research collaborators
who do preliminary work or who presently try to built up a model of an
environmental specimen bank system in the United States, Japan and the
Federal Republic of Germany, no concrete guidelines for organization
banking systems in the future can be deduced.

Only one organizational aspect may be pointed out: All analytical work
to be done in monitoring and banking systems must be conducted exclusively by personnel periodically trained between the laboratories (exchange
basis). This should be worth striving for an international field. Methods
applied should be similar but need not to be identical. Obligatory
standardization of analytical methods prevent progress in this field.

Attempts made so far, to standardize the form of report on the analytical
results and the comments about the sampling did not succeed very well. From
the viewpoint of the author it seems more successfull to demand information
as much as possible to questions formulated referring to the requirements
stated in the above mentioned sections.

4.3. Storage Technology

At present time, in the United States and - to a smaller extend - in the
Federal Republic of Germany some work about storage of samples with traces
of heavy metals is under investigation. An agreement within the experts
whether to prefer deep freezing, freeze drying, ashing or other methods
has not been achieved, so far.

With respect to organic trace compounds stability studies conducted until now yield information only for 6 matrix-incorporated compounds to be analyzed as recommended in section 3.1. Presently, experts recognize deep-freezing, probably till -8o°C, as the only principle for longterm storage. But this has to be confirmed by experimental work in future.

5. LEGAL CONSIDERATIONS

Because of the recommendation of the reporter to organize monitoring programmes and environmental specimen banks within national borders we do not recognize any existing regulatory limitations between the countries which could have been touched by the systems proposed. But in the case of interchanging plant material samples between the countries attention has to be paid to the prespective quarantine regulations. Within the borders, regulations should be created, which declare the permission for any sampling officer to take samples even on private plots. Banking systems should be built up as a government enterprise.

6. COST ESTIMATES

At present time, it is very difficult to estimate costs of specimen banking, as the techniques for solving this task are not clearly recognized. In the case of a specialized sub-specimen bank for plants and soil, assuming storage could be sufficiently made by freezing to -8o°C, investments of about 15o.ooo,-- DM for a storage room of a minimum number of samples covering approximately the area of the Federal Republic of Germany by sufficient data material are required.

The following rough estmation of the costs for an environmental monitoring programme as recommended above is based of a calculation made for a soil monitoring programme, which had been intended in Germany but had not been realized, unfortunately.

Design of the programme	5o.ooo,-- DM
Selection of the sample localities and working out data for description of the surrounding	9oo.ooo,-- DM
Analytical equipment required	6oo.ooo,-- DM
Collaborative studies in analytical methods	35o.ooo,-- DM per year
Collection and transport of sample	2oo.ooo,-- DM per year
Sample analysis (personnel and material)	1.ooo.ooo,-- DM per year
Data processing	1oo.ooo,-- DM per year
Organization and project accomodation	1oo.ooo,-- DM per year.

7. SUMMARY

Monitoring programmes for organic chemical contaminants in plants or soil with regard to the description of the surrounding of the sampling locality and observing trends following a time course had not been conducted so far. In future, such programmes should be organized within narrow limits. It is reasonable to establish a monitoring programme and a respective small specimen banking system for a few plants (especially wheat and the gras species Lolium multiflorum) and soil, and for the halogenated compounds (non-volatile chlorinated hydrocarbons, chlorophenols, chlorophenoxyalcane carbonic acids) and slowly degradionable compounds (triazine herbicides). For heavy metal traces, monitoring is unnecessary for soils and plants, because pollution of these contaminants on that matrices depends on the distance of sample locality to the emitters and their emitting intensity. Very many papers described this data with respect to plants growing on soils. So for the most cases, heavy metal trace concentrations may be estimated by those data without further experimental work. In order to obtain best results and best cost-yield-relation sampling, description of the environment of the localities, analyzing and storage should be handled in narrow connection. The number of mixed samples to be stored for analysis should be kept samll. Deep freezing to -8o°C is expected to be the most favourable storage technique for the sample types considered. To realize the small monitoring sub-system proposed the costs per year will not exceed 1,75 millions DM. For investigations, selection of sample localities etc. once 1,55 millions DM must be added. A respective banking system requires about 15o.ooo,-- DM in addition.

8. ANNEX

8.1. Some additional remarks to sample selection, collection and sampling procedures

Within terrestrial plants no species is known as a pronounced accumulator for a broad spectrum of contaminants, e.g. from the soil. It may be pointed out, generally, that fast growing plants trend to collect residues to a somewhat higher degree than such ones with a more extended vegetation period. So, it would be useful to take e.g. cress, whereever it has been cultivated.

On the other hand, plants to be sampled should be selected in the first place with regard to the human beings living on the various continents. Therefore, wheat has been generally accepted as the food plant mostly spread over the world.

Besides this species another plant sample type occuring on areas not in use for agricultural plant production should be taken into consideration. So, a commonly spread grass species, as e.g. Lolium, should be sampled.

In the case of soil, the samples must be taken from indisturbed soil strate, exclusively.

As outlined in 3.3 and 3.4, the environment of this region, for which the mixed sample is representative, has to be described very carefully. This must be done with regard to the surrounding members of the plant society, the climate course, the anthropogenic influences, and the geological soil type. With respect to the latter the soil constituants, the organic carbon and moisture contents, and the pH-value are the most important data for characterization.

Both for monitoring and banking purposes sampling should be done in the same manner as outlined in 3.4 and 4.1. Sample collection should be carried out by the analysts in very near cooperation with biogeographic

scientists, biologists and soil scientists. In several cases, specialists
of the forestry governments have to make partners.

8.2 Some additional remarks to organizational aspects

For an initial period of monitoring as well as banking the number of samples should be kept within reasonable limits. So, it seems to be adequate
to take one mixed sample (containing an average of 1o individuals) each
of soil, wheat, and grass, respectively. If the three types of the average
samples represent an area within a radius of about 3o km, so, from a country like the Federal Republic of Germany covering 248.ooo km^2 about
27o samples have to be taken for the three types together. Analysis of the
several classes of compounds, which should be measured as outlined in 3,1,
requires the application of about 3 to 5 methods each consisting in about
3 single estimations yielding one analytical result. So, about 12oo samples
are needed for one screening just within this sub-system "plant and soil".
Monitoring should be repeated at least three-times a year continuously
throughout the future. In banking the samples of at least 3 years should
be stored. This concept seems to be of sufficient dimensions which can
be carefully handled and evaluated within national monitoring and national banking sub-systems.

8.3. Some additional remarks to cost estimation

Supported by some data of programmes projected in the Federal Republic
of Germany the author estimated the costs proposed for a country covering
an area of about 25o.ooo km^2 in section 6.

Monitoring sub-system "plant and soil":
Once, at the beginning of the work, investments of about 1.55o.ooo,-- DM
are required. The studies costs are 1.75 Mio DM for each year.

Banking sub-system "plant and soil":
If - as recommended by the author - banking is organized and subjected
in the same manner, banking- and occasional analyzing - may participate
in the monitoring programme. Just for storage containers, additional
investments of 15o.ooo,-- DM are required. Maintainance and energy costs
are not expensive. In the opinion of the author, the over-all-budget
of this banking sub-system including supervising, analytical work, evaluation etc., will not exceed 1.75 Mio DM per year.

NON-HALOGENATED ORGANIC COMPOUNDS IN AQUATIC AND TERRESTRIAL ECOSYSTEMS

Dr. R. Eckard
Institute of Pharmacology and Toxicology
University of Muenster,
Federal Republic of Germany

1. Past and current programmes

Although approx. 5o.ooo different organic chemical compounds are produced and processed by industry, little experience is available about the behaviour of these materials in the different ecosystems. With regard to the organic pollutants most of our knowledge is related to the persistent organohalogenated compounds while relatively little is known about the other organic compounds.

The knowledge about behaviour and monitoring of other organic substances is confined generally to the field of occupational health. Most of the work on distribution and occurrence of anthropogenic and/or natural pollutants is restricted to local areas and is often not incorporated into regular monitoring programmes. Apart from this, the provided data from different sources is often not comparable, partly due to different origin of the samples, partly because of inadequate standardisation of the analytical methods.

Of all the environmental pollutant categories of interest with respect to monitoring and banking, the phthalates, nitrosamines, organophosphate pesticides, mycotoxins and antibiotics are dealt with in this paper. The programmes carried out until now concerning these substance classes have dealt with the monitoring of different parts in the respective ecosystems but experience in environmental banking is minimal.

The increasing significance of some substance classes for the environment is being taken into consideration by national and supranational authorities. Programmes which deal with the ecological behaviour of the phthalates were carried out by the National Institute of Environmental Health Sciences (NIEHS). The nitrosamines problem is being investigated by the International Agency for Research and Cancer (IARC) as well as by the Kommission zur Prüfung fremder Stoffe bei Lebensmitteln der Deutschen Forschungsgemeinschaft (DFG). In the Federal Republic of Germany, studies

are undertaken on a national level by the Kommission zur Prüfung von Rück-
ständen in Lebensmitteln der DFG to investigate the residues of antibiotics
and mycotoxins in food.

Nevertheless, despite these efforts there are still large gaps in the
knowledge regarding distribution and residues of pollutants in the environment and the resulting influence on the different ecosystems including
a possible danger to human health.

2. Reasons for Interest or Concern

2.1. Phthalates

2.1.1. Chemical, metabolic, toxicological and environmental characteristics

The commonly used phthalate esters are liquids of very high boiling points
and very low vapour pressures. Due to their lipophilic character, they are
almost insoluble in water and readily soluble in non-aqueous media. They
are relatively stable towards light and oxygen at normal temperatures and
towards hydrolysis by water. The relationship of these characteristics to
environmental migration is considered later.

Metabolism:

Investigations on the metabolism of phthalates are mainly restricted to
the metabolic fate of di(2-ethylhexyl) phthalate (DEHP) and di-n-butyl
phthalate (DBP). Metabolism is fairly rapid in fish and rapid in mammals,
involving hydrolytic cleavage to the monoester and subsequent side chain
oxidation with the production of highly water-soluble metabolites. Upon
oral administration, most of the phthalate is hydrolyzed enzymatically
within the gastro-intestinal tract.
The microbial metabolism and biodegradation of phthalates is well established by the SCAS and RDA-tests, revealing a non-persistent character
of the phthalates.

Toxicological characteristics:

The acute toxicity of phthalates is low: There seems to be a direct correlation between water solubility and toxicity as well as an inverse relationship between molecular weight and toxicity. It has been suggested
that the toxicity of these compounds depends to a large extent on the nature of the alcohol released by hydrolysis.
Chronic toxicity studies revealed no carcinogenic effect. However, the teratogenic and mutagenic effects of phthalates at high dosages are well confirmed. The significance of these effects to human health by environmental
pollution still remains to be assessed.

Environmental behaviours:

The environmental behaviours of phthalates and their movement in terrestrial and aquatic ecosystems is mainly determined by the physicochemical
and metabolic properties mentioned above. Furthermore, the large extent
of industrial production of phthalates plays a significant role in their
environmental distribution and possible ecological disturbances.

In 197o, the total amount of US-phthalate-production was about 9oo million pounds, suggesting an approximate world production of 3.ooo - 4.ooo million pounds. C_8-phthalates (DEHP and DOP) - normally used as PVC-plasticizers - accounted for about 5o % of the total production. The annual production of DEHP alone is ten times that of all PCB's based on the 197o figures (the last year of unrestricted use of the PCB's).

Besides DEHP, the dibutylated phthalate (DBP) seems to be an important environmental pollutant, althouth it accounts for only 2,5 % of the total phthalate production (197o). This is mainly because of its relatively high vapour pressure and widespread nonplasticizer uses (pesticide carrier, insect repellant etc.), whereby a direct route of entry into the environment is made possible. Thus, environmental monitoring of phthalates up to now is mainly restricted to DEHP and DBP, both being considered as the most important phthalates with respect to environmental occurence.

The amounts of anthropogenic phthalates entering the environment from various sources are difficult to estimate. The following main sources should be taken into consideration:

- Direct entry through their non-plasticizer use, where the phthalates are not encased in a polymer matrix.
- Losses during manufacture and processing
- Vaporization by incomplete incineration of plastics
- Leaches and vaporization from plasticized PVC-items in use
- Migration from plasticized PVC-items from dumps into soil, air and water.

Vaporization due to incomplete incineration of plastics is estimated to account for 75 % of the total phthalate entry into the environment, leading to a widespread and nearly homogeneous distribution.

As the major reservoir of phthalates is plastic dumps, the rate of loss of phthalates from this reservoir is important. However, the extent of loss is difficult to estimate because it is influenced by several factors including local conditions e.g. temperature, soil, rainfall, watershed etc. as well as the form and surface of the plastic items themselves. The distribution and movement of phthalates in ecosystems is suggested to be similar to that of DDT and PCB's, as they have similar lipophilic characters. Indeed, biomagnification in lower aquatic organisms was similar to that found under identical conditions for DDT. The occurrence of high accumulation factors for DEHP (2o.ooo - 11o.ooo) for snails, algae and mosquito larvae and low factors (13o) for fish as evaluated in aquatic model ecosystems indicates that the highest concentrations would be expected at intermediate points of the food chain rather than at the top as occurs with DDT. This is probably because the metabolism of phthalates is fairly rapid in fish and rapid in animals. Thus, monitoring phthalate residues at lower trophic levels seems to be more adequate for environmental pollution monitoring.

2.1.2. Levels of environmental exposure

An increasing number of reports concerning the environmental appearance of phthalate esters, especially in aquatic ecosystems, has been published.

The reported data are mainly to DEHP and DBP, revealing relatively constant DEHP-levels in aquatic systems but widely varying DBP-levels.

The degree of environmental burden by phthalates in terrestrial ecosystems is largely unknown due to the problems of the extremely nonhomogeneous distribution of phthalates in non-aquatic systems.

The occurrence of phthalates in higher plants (cranberries, grapes, tobacco) as well as in fungi and bacteria (mycobact.-tuberculosis, corynebact.-diphteriae) has been reported. The occurrence in some plants is suggested to be of endogenous origin.

Typical levels reported in different samples are listed below [+].

	DBP	DEHP
River water Lake water (the concentrations may reach ppm-levels)	n.d.-1o (35o) ppb o.o4	n.d.-3o ppb n.d.- 5 (3oo) ppb
egg yolk (Cormorant) (Herring gull)	14,1 ppm 1o,9-19,1 ppm	
juvenile atlantic salmon (lipid)		12,9-16,4 ppm
salmon (canned)	37 ppb	63-89 ppb
tuna (canned)	78 ppb	4o-16o ppb
eel		1o4 ppb
channel catfish	2oo ppb	4oo-32oo ppb
dragon jelly naiads	2oo ppb	2oo ppb
tadpoles	5oo ppb	3oo ppb

[+] Some of the reported results may be affected by contamination during collection and analysis.

		DBP		DEHP	
fish food and components:	total diet			2ooo-7ooo	ppb
	casein	2o	ppb	19o	"
	corn starch	2o	"	17o	"
	gelatin	2o	"	14o	"
	bone meal	3o	"	4oo	"
heart muscle:					
	bovine			135	ppm
	rat			1,29	"
	rabbit			1,18	"
	dog			o,36	"
human adipose tissue		o,1-o,3	ppm	o,3-1	ppm
	blood			n.d.-1 (1o) ppm	

samples on direct contact with plasticized PVC-items:

stored blood	up to	6oo-7oo ppm DEHP
milk	ca.	1oo ppm DEHP
cheese	up to	15o ppm DBP

2.3.1. Pathways for human exposure

Phthalates may enter the human body through various channels including inhalation, absorption through the skin and dietary ingestion. The most important sources are likely to be lipophilic foodstuffs (e.g. milk, cheese) stored in plasticized PVC-containers or foil, as well as plastic items on direct contact with the human body. The possible accumulation within the food chain seems to be unimportant compared to the large amounts incorporated by direct or indirect contact with plasticized PVC-products.

2.2. Nitrosamines (NA)

All nitrosamines which are amenable to environmental monitoring are moderate polar liquids of relative high volatility, moderate water solubility and are remarkably persistent in abiotic systems, but sensitive towards light. Microbial degradation of NA in sludge is normally extremely slow and thus, NA may be classified among the relative persistent environmental pollutants.

NA are rapidly metabolized in animals, involving probably on oxidative dealkylation process, with the production of intermediate alkylating

moities of high potential carcinogenic risk and high organotropic specifity. Despite the powerful carcinogenic properties, the acute toxicity is relatively moderate, mainly affecting liver parenchyma.

2.2.1. Environmental behaviour

Environmental occurrence of NA is not likely to be a result of direct
NA-pollution but a result of different chemical processes, involving
a large number of natural as well as anthropogenic compounds. Knowledge
of the conditions and mechanisms of NA-formation in environmental systems has increased in recent years. Complex interactions of nitrates,
nitrites and nitrosable substrates such as secondary and tertiary amines,
ureas and carbamates to form introso compounds have been reported. The
formation of NA is not restricted to in-vitro-systems. Thus, nitrosation
may occur in the gastrointestinal tract of animals following administration of precursor materials in the diet. Furthermore, various bacterial species can form NA.
Nitrosamines and/or reactants capable of forming them are widely distributed in the environment but little is known on the migration and possible accumulation of nitrosocompounds in ecosystems. NA added to soil,
readily taken up by plants but accumulation in plants obviously does
not occur.
The widespread accumulation of nitrosable environmental pollutants including many herbicides and pesticides, as well as the increasing environmental levels of nitrate/nitrite could lead to the increasing formation of nonvolatile nitrosocompounds of potential risk to health. Unfortunately, however, until now no adequate analytical methods for monitoring non-volatile nitroso compounds at low levels are available.

2.2.2. Environmental levels

Monitoring of NA at present is mainly restricted to the extremely volatile
dialkyl-nitrosamines in foodstuffs with high precursor concentrations.
Some typical levels of dimethylnitrosamine (DMN) and diethylnitrosamine
(DEN) above the detection limit are listed below:

Sample	DMN (ppb)	DEN (ppb)
Air	0,033-0,96	
canned fish	up to 25	0,1-30
fresh fish	up to 9	0,1-30
smoked fish	4-6	
cheese	0,1-6	0,1- 5
fish meal	up to 500	
bacon, fried	1-30	1-30
Frankfurters	up to 84	

Extremely high values are reported in animal feed (up to 100 ppm).

2.2.3. Pathway for human exposure

The main source for human exposure is the dietary content of nitrosamines
and possibly the formation of NA in the alimentary tract following the
simultaneous ingestion of nitrite/nitrate and nitrosable substrate-inclu-

ding durgs. As NA are suspected to be causally related to human cancer in industrialized society, careful and intensive environmental monitoring of not only volatile NA but of nonvolatile NA as well is deemed necessary.

2.3. Organophosphate pesticides

2.3.1. Environmental behaviour

Most organophosphates are highly lipophilic compounds and yet freely soluble in water. Degradation by hydrolytic or enzymatic reactions occurs to a high extent. For this reason, organophosphates are relatively less persistent than organochlorine compounds in soil and aquatic environments. Nevertheless, low levels of organophosphates may be detected in soil even 16 years after the last application. The reported persistence in soil varies considerably, e.g. for parathion it varies from a few weeks to several years. The accumulation of organophosphate pesticides in soil and plants (coniferous foliage) has also been reported by various authors. Generally, organophosphates are known to be rapidly metabolized in plant and animal tissues. Degradation of the organophophorous pesticides in soil is normally mediated largely by chemical and/or biological means and is affected by ph, soil type, soil moisture and organic matter. Because of their moderate solubility in water, terrestrial application of organophosphate pesticides raises the problem of pollution of aquatic ecosystems by residues from surface run-off water. However, concentrations of organophosphorous pesticides detected in water do not generally exceed the lower ppb-range. Due to the low persistence and to the application to restricted areas, environmental levels of organophosphates differ remarkably. With respect to plants, concentration of pesticide residue is dependent on the surface area of mass ratio.

2.3.2. Environmental levels

The reported levels of fenitrothion may be considered paradigmatically, revealing possible routes of environmental distribution and accumulation within several hours after spraying.

Fenitrothion (after spraying at 14o-28o g/ha)

forest soil	4o	ppb
water	1-6o	ppb
coniferous foliage	2ooo-4ooo	ppb
terrestrial insects	2o	ppb
birds (quail)	2o-12o	ppb
rainbow trout	4oo-6oo	ppb

organophosphorous pesticide residues in food

| fruit and vegetables | o,o1 to 1 ppm |
| grain and flour | o,o1 to 1 ppm |

in general, concentrations are below o,o1 ppm.

2.3.3. Toxicity and pathway to human exposure

The main route for human exposure is considered to be the ingestion of contaminated fruit and vegetables, as well as occupational exposure during manufacturing, handling and spraying.
Acute toxicity to man due to the inhibition of acetylcholinesterase is well known. The chronic ingestion of subacute amounts is suspected to cause subclinical changes in the nervous system. Thus, monitoring of organophosphorous pesticides seems to be of high importance despite their rapid biological degradation.

2.4. Mycotoxins

2.4.1. Environmental behaviour

The widespread occurrence of mycotoxins as naturally-produced metabolites of different fungi is well confirmed. Of the mycotoxins, the group of aflatoxins (mainly B_1, B_2, G_1 and G_2) derived from ubiquitous Aspergillus strains have been intensively studied. Aflatoxins are compounds of high melting point. Their stability may be affected by fluorescent light, UV-radiation, heat and (alkaline) hydrolysis. The acute toxicity of aflatoxins is exceedingly high, mainly affecting the liver and kidney. In fact, they are among the most potent liver carcinogens known.

Aflatoxins have been found to contaminate many cereals, nuts and seeds, including maize, cottonseed, rice, soya, beans, wheat and barley. As they are stable under normal conditions of handling and food processing, many agricultural commodities derived from plants are susceptible to aflatoxin contamination. Metabolism in animals is rather quick. Biliary and renal elimination is nearly complete within 24 hours. The M-aflatoxins are the main products of metabolism in animals and they are usually found in milk and urine.

After chronic ingestion of moderate amounts of aflatoxins, the highest concentrations are reached in the liver and kidney. However, the level in these tissues still remains only 1/1ooo that in the diet. Such levels are usually not detectable by the analytical methods available at present.

2.4.2. Environmental levels

The reported contamination levels in agricultural commodities from plants and in grains vary considerably according to type, origin and storage of the sample and normally are in the lower ppb-range.
The normal level of contamination for some of these products is listed below:

Peanut	n.d. - 9o	ppb
peanut meal	n.d. - 1oo	(1ooo) ppb
cotton seed	n.d. - 3o	
cotton seed meal	n.d. - 1oo	ppb
comestic grains (normally low incidence of contamination)		

corn	3 -	3o ppb
soya beans	1o -	11 ppb
wheat		9 ppb

The main route for human exposure is the ingestion of mycotoxin residues in food derived from plant sources. Residues in food derived from animal sources are of subordinate significance. On account of the extremely high carcinogenicity of the aflatoxins, it is desirable to include also the extremely low residues (sub ppb-range) into the monitoring programmes.

2.5. Antibiotics

Antibiotic compounds of different chemical structure e.g. tetracyclines, streptomycin and penicillin are generally relatively unstable and sensitive towards heat and are not lipophilic.

They occur in the environment related to man, mainly however not be diffuse or incidental contamination but intentionally or as a result of medical use, food preservation or animal feed addition.

The chronic feeding of antibiotics especially to poultry in order to increase the feed efficiency as well as their parenteral administration to cattle before slaughter, results in tissue levels which are highest in liver, kidney, muscle and bones. The antibiotics are usually eliminated within a few days. The residue levels after feeding or processing lie generally in the range of o,1 - 1o ppm or lower.

The natural occurrence of antimicrobial substances is described in even higher plants which serve as food e.g. onions, bananas and cabbage. The natural occurrence in food derived from plants appears to be however of minor importance for the human environment.

Residues in meat, eggs and milk products are regarded as main sources for chronic ingestion of low antibiotic amounts by human beings even though a part of the antibiotic activity is destroyed through boiling.

3. Sample selection

Phthalates, nitrosamines, organophosphorous pesticides, mycotoxins and antibiotics are recognized as relatively low persistent organic environmental pollutants in comparison to, for example, DDT and PCB's.
Sample selection for monitoring low persistent and moderate or non-volatile organic pollutants is affected by the following facts:

- The distribution of these pollutants is markedly non-homogeneous in aquatic and especially terrestrial ecosystems.
- Pollution levels are not constant, but may increase or decrease within a relatively short period.
- Knowledge of organism or parts of them, which are able to accumulate the pollutants and reflect chronic environmental burden at high steady-state-levels, is very limited.
- "Normal" steady-state-levels of specimens which are not exposed to intentional or accidental high concentrations, are extremely low and do not, in general, exceed the sub-ppb and ppb-range.

Nevertheless, selection of indicator specimens which may reflect acute and chronic exposure to low persistent pollutants is important for real time monitoring as well as environmental banking. For that reason, integrating rather than accumulating properties of the specimen have to be taken into account.

Sample selection covering all organic compounds entering the environment is a difficult problem, because their distribution patterns are very different. Monitoring should therefore be restricted to a few types of samples for financial, analytical and storage reasons.

For each of the compounds mentioned in Chapter 2, which may be representative for other compounds of similar environmental properties, there are a variety of specimens including some of higher priority which appropriate for monitoring.

Phthalate residues in aquatic systems may be monitored in sludge and accumulating organisms e.g. snail, mussel, algae or mosquito larvae. Terrestrial systems e.g. wheat, grass and soil may also be useful but residues in animal tissues are normally low and not well suited for monitoring.

Knowledge of specimens containing measurable amounts of nitrosamines is confined mainly to food samples closely related to the human environment e.g. processed fish, meat. Concentrations of NA in sludge may correlate well with the exposure to aquatic systems while the NA content of plants (wheat, grass) may reflect the terrestrial NA burden. However, for analytical reasons, their adequacy for monitoring has not yet been well established.

As accumulating specimens for organophosphorous pesticides are not yet available, monitoring is rather difficult unless the concentration of residues is sufficiently high as a result of local pesticide application. Animal tissues are not very useful for monitoring. On the other hand, monitoring can be well conducted in soil and plant samples (wheat, grass, coniferous foliage). Soil and coniferous foliage may contain pesticide residues for a long time after application.

Mycotoxins and antibiotics, although probably compounds of ubiquitous occurrence, have been monitored till now mainly in ingredients of the human diet. Depending on their source and application patterns, monitoring of antibiotics seems more appropriate in domestic animals (muscle, liver, bone, milk, egg) rather than in other specimens whereas monitoring of mycotoxins is rather limited to cereals and seeds, at least until more sensitive analytical methods become available to enable the investigation of other specimens.

The previous considerations on sample selection with respect to phthalates, nitrosamines, organophosphate pesticides, mycotoxins and antibiotics are summarized in the following table:

Table 1: Selected specimen from aquatic and terrestrial systems

specimen \ compounds	Phthalates	Nitrosamines	Organoph. Pest.	Mycotoxins	Antibiotics
aquatic					
snails	x		(x)		
mussels	x		(x)		
sludge	x	(x)	(x)		
processed fish	(x)	x			
terrestrial					
wheat	x	(x)	x	x	
grass	x	(x)	x		
soil	x	(x)	x	x	
domestic animal					
blood	(x)		(x)		(x)
liver					x
kidney					
muscle					x
bone					x
milk	(x)			(x)	x
egg	x				x
processed meat		x			

x   appropriate specimen for monitoring

(x) usefulness not yet confirmed

4. Sample collection, preservation and storage

Sampling of specimens containing known and unknown organic pollutants in
the ppb- and sub-ppb range requires certain strict precautions to avoid
contamination and loss of volatile pollutants. This is particularly true
for phthalates, when sampling should be carried out meticulously to
avoid contamination due to direct as well as indirect contact with plastics.

Special cleaning procedures for materials and instruments used for sampling
are necessary, as well as special sampling techniques to avoid contamination of the sample by pollutants from the environment during sampling. Loss
of volatile compounds during sampling is a less serious problem with respect to phthalates, organophosphates, mycotoxins, antibiotics and even
nitrosamines, but should be considered in monitoring other organic com-
ounds of higher volatility.

As it is assumed that there is no homogeneous distribution of the pollutants to be monitored in the sample, sample size has to be large enough
to be representative of environmental burden. In fact the sample size
should be at least 1ooo g in most cases for specimens where special experience with organic pollutants is lacking.

Chemical preservation (e.g. by formaldehyde) as well as sterilization by
radiation is detrimental to sample integrity, as most organic compounds
are affected by these procedures.

Homogenization is necessary prior to analysis and/or storage. Unlike dealing with trace metals, the problem or contamination during this procedure with regard to organic compounds is of minor importance.

It should be emphasized that the material used for containers for samples
or aliquots of samples for environmental banking should show no interaction with the sample or parts of it. With respect to organic compounds of
high moderate lipophilic properties, polyethylene or even perfluoropolyethylene and similar materials are not convenient. The use of quartz or
borosilicate glass seems to be the best for this purpose. Nevertheless,
adsorption of some compounds, e.g. phenols, to the glass surface may
occur. Gold, aluminium or other metals without catalytic properties may
be appropriate, but there is no experience in this field. At least the
long-term storage of halogenated compounds in aluminium seems to be
problematic. Long-term storage of samples without alteration, as needed
for environmental banking, is a difficult problem with regard to organic
compounds of low persistence.

Lyophilization is not suitable, because there is a remarkable loss of
volatile and even moderate volatile compounds.

The storage of extracts may be an advantage in the case of some groups
of chemical compounds. But the extraction procedure may entail the loss
of some polar compounds, which are not amenable to environmental monitoring at present and which are therefore of great importance for environmental banking.

Rapid and deep freezing seems to be the most acceptable method for maintaining sample integrity. Storage at -2o° is certainly not adequate in
some cases. Thus, the concentration of phthalates in blood samples stored
at this temperature has been reported to decrease up to fifty percent
within a few days.

Temperature of -8o° or even -196°C as well as exclusion of oxygen seem
to be necessary for long-term storage of biological specimens.

5. Analytical procedures

A great variety of analytical methods including clean-up procedures for the determination of trace amounts of organic compounds in environmental material have been described in the literature. The methods are widely varying because of the different chemical behaviour of the compounds and because of the variation in equipment from one laboratory to another.

The standardization of analyctical procedures in environmental monitoring of organic compounds that are recognized as important pollutants leaves a lot to be desired.

Analytical methods of high efficiency and specifity have been developed in recent years, including computerized gaschromatography-mass spectrometry (GC-MS), capillary column gaschromatography (CC-GC) and liquid chromatography (HPLC). These methods are able to solve most of the analytical problems involved to environmental monitoring, but in many cases complex clean-up and concentration steps before analysis are still necessary. For the groups of environmental pollutants described in chapter 2., most acceptable analytical methods are:

5.1. Phthalates

Phthalates can be conveniently determined by gaschromatographic methods using flame-ionization-detection (FID). Electron-capture-detection (ECD) has been used as an alternative detection procedure but it offers no significant advantage over the FID-method. Sensitivity and specifity may be increased considerably using GC-MS single-ion or multiple-ion detection mode (SID;MID), since most of the phthalates are well suited for SID monitoring m/e 149.

5.2. Nitrosamines

Reliable NA-determinations up to now were performed by GC-NFID. More sensitive and specific detection can be achieved by Thermal Energy Analysis (TEA), which has been developed recently.

GC-TEA as well as HPLC-TEA-coupling seem to be the most specific methods for the determination of even non volatile nitrosamines at the present time. High resolution GC-MS monitoring of the NO^+ ion of m/e 29.9980, which is common to all the NA, corresponds well to the GC-TEA technique.

5.3. Organophosphate compounds

Residues of organophosphate pesticides are determined by GC-FID involving a large variety of modified ionization detection systems. In some cases, GS-separation is affected by the thermal decomposition of the compound to be monitored. For that reason, detection may be more complicated than flame ionization detection.

5.4. Aflatoxins and antibiotics

As the determination of these compounds is restricted to non gaschromatographic methods, monitoring of aflatoxins and antibiotics is not yet satisfactory.

In the determination of aflatoxins thin layer- and column chromatography using fluorescence detection have been the most accepted methods, but newer separation techniques e.g. HPLC involving detection by fluorescence or laser fluorimetry are in progress in an attempt to increase the sensitivity and specifity.

Separation of antibiotics is performed by TLC, agar electrophoresis or similar methods, then microbiological tests (e.g. Bac. subtilis) are used for quantification. Besides this, complementary chemical methods are urgently necessary in environmental monitoring. HPLC-techniques may be appropriate.

With respect to environmental monitoring as well as environmental banking, development and use of analytical systems with very high separating efficiency are desirable to reduce the need for complex clean-up procedures prior to analysis.

An increase in the separating efficiency coupled with a simplification of clean-up procedures has several advantages:

- simultaneous determination of many pollutants is made possible
- representativity and reproducibility of profile analysis will increase
- contamination, chemical degradation and losses during extraction and clean-up procedures will be diminished
- reduction of the number of clean-up procedures will reduce the sample size necessary for monitoring and banking.

6. Programme design and organizational aspects

The monitoring of selected samples from terrestrial and aquatic ecosystems should not only represent the universal burden but also reflect the burden in the human environment on a large scale.
Furthermore, it should be possible to obtain through environmental monitoring trend data which could indicate changes of the burden.
As to the lesser persistent organic pollutants which are subject to a largely differentiated non-homogeneous distribution as described in chapter 2, a statistically representative selection poses a difficult problem. In order to fulfill the above mentioned requirements, without having to examine an immeasurable number of samples, the samples have to be taken from districts which are exposed to a steady burden over a longer period. Moreover, it would be necessary to specify in as much detail as possible all steps of sample taking, transport, storage and analysis and to make such specifications compulsory in general.
In addition, a comprehensive collection of all data concerning sample type and sample origin should be made available.
In order to safeguard the correctness and continuity of the analytical determinations, the latter should be carried out exclusively by qualified expert personnel using recognized procedures of high precision.
An important aim to achieve is centralization of the investigation laboratories to only a few. These should be established in accordance with the high quality demands of real time monitoring and environmental banking at least as far as apparatus and personnel are concerned. A continuous inter-laboratory quality control appears to be necessary.

To raise the efficacy in carrying out the programmes, there should be more intensive cooperation and exchange of ideas between the parties concerned. This can be achieved by holding regular workshops as well as international symposia in collaboration with other supranational authorities.

7. Cost estimation

The cost of monitoring and banking of samples depends largely on the following:

- quantitiy of samples to be analysed and/or stored

- number and kind of pollutants to be monitored

- nature of the analytical tool necessary for monitoring

- number of analytical techniques involved.

Accordingly, cost estimation is rather a difficult problem and only rough figures can be given.
With respect to monitoring, the cost may amount to DM 8oo,-- to DM 1ooo,-- per sample, including collection, transportation and analysis as well as personnel.

Summary

There are large gaps in our knowledge concerning the distribution patterns and residue levels of the less persistent organic compounds, viz. -phthalates, nitrosamines, organophosphate pesticides, mycotoxins and antibiotics in aquatic and terrestrial ecosystems. Data available at present is mostly confined to their occurrence in some components of the human diet. Thus, some of these organic compounds have not yet been recognized as general environmental contaminants.
Sample selection for monitoring and banking is generally limited by the markedly non-homogeneous distribution patterns of these compounds, variation in their levels of pollution and the lack of accumulating organisms for them. Nevertheless, some specimens e.g. snails, mussels and sludge as well as wheat, grass and soil may reflect acute and/or chronic exposure to some of these less persistent pollutants.
The storage of the samples necessitates the use of glass or quartz containers rather than polyethylene or teflon ones. Rapid and deep freezing is the most appropriate method for maintaining sample integrity. Long-term storage at -2o°C is not an adequate measure by itself. Temperatures of -8o°C or even -196°C as well as exclusion of oxygen seem to be necessary for long-term storage of biological specimens with regard to the less persistent pollutants. Because contamination levels of these compounds are extremely low and usually do not exceed the ppb range and because they differ widely in their physicochemical properties, several analytical systems of very high sensitivity have to be used for monitoring, e.g. GC-MS, HPLC-(MS) and CC-GC involving a large variety of detection systems.
The centralization of the research laboratories to only a few efficient ones would serve to achieve the high qualtity standards which are required for real time monitoring and environmental banking.

226

References

1. Archer, M.C. and J.S. Wishnok: Quantitative aspects of human exposure
   to nitrosamines. Fd. Cosmet. Toxicol. 15, 233 (1977).

2. Armbrecht, B.H.: Aflatoxin residues in food and feed derived from
   plant and animal sources. Res. Rev. 41, 13 (1972).

3. Belisle, A.A., W.L. Reichel and J.W. Spann: Analysis of tissues of
   mallard ducks fed two phthalate esters. Bull. Environ. Contam. Toxicol.
   13, 129 (1975).

4. v. Bergner, K.G. and H. Berg: Zur Migration einiger Zusatzstoffe aus
   Kunststoffen in Triglyceride in Vergleich zur Extrahierbarkeit durch
   organische Lösungsmittel. Dtsch. Lebensm.-Rdsch. 68, 282 (1972).

5. Bogovski, P., R. Preussmann and E.A. Walker (eds.): N-Nitroso compounds analysis and formation. Internat. Agency Res. on Cancer,
   Lyon (1972).

6. Bogovski, P. and E.A. Walker (eds.): N-Nitrosocompounds in the environment. Internat. Agency Res. on Cancer, Lyon (1975).

7. Bull, D.L.: Metabolism of organophophorus insecticides in animals and
   plants. Res. Rev. 43, 1 (1972).

8. Crosby, N.T.: Nitrosamines in foodstuffs. Res. Rev. 64, 78 (1976).

9. Daniel, J.W. and H. Bratt: The absorption, metabolism and tissue
   distribution of di(2-ethyl exyl)-phthalate in rats. Toxicology 2,
   51 (1974).

1o. Dezeeuw, R.A., J.A. Jonkman and F.J. v. Mansvelt: Plasticizers as
    contaminants in high-purity solvents: a potential source of inter-
    ference in biological analysis. Anal. Biochem. 67, 339 (1975).

11. Diebold, G.J. and R.N. Zare: Laser Fluorimetry: Subpicogram Detection
    on Aflatoxins Using High-Pressure Liquid Chromatography. Science 196,
    1439 (1977).

12. Downes, M.J., M.W. Edwards, T.S. Elsey and C.L. Walters: Determination
    of a Non-Volatile Nitrosamine by Using Denitrosation and a Chemilumini-
    scence Analyzer. Analyst 1o1, 742 (1976).

13. Elespurn, R., W. Lijinski and J.K. Setlow: Nitrosocarbaryl as a Potent
    Mutagen of Environmental Significance. Nature 247, 386 (1974).

14. Fiddler, W.: The occurrence and determination of N-Nitroso compounds.
    Tox. appl. Pharm. 31, 352 (1975).

15. Fine, D.H., D.P. Rounbehler, N.M. Belcher and S.S. Epstein: N-Nitroso
    compounds in air and water. Forth IARC-Meeting, Tallin, Estonia, USSR,
    October 1+2, 1975.

16. Fishbein, L. and P.W. Albro: Chromatographic and biological aspects of the phthalate estera. J. Chromatogr. $\underline{7o}$, 365 (1972).

17. Giam, C.S. and H.S. Chan: Control of blanks in the analysis of phthalates in air and ocean biota samples. NBS Publ. $\underline{422}$, 7o1 (1976).

18. Giam, C.S., H.S. Chan, T.F. Hammargren, G.S. Neff and D.L. Stallin: Confirmation of phthalate esters from environmental samples by derivatization. Anal. Chem. $\underline{48}$, 78 (1976).

19. Hayes, J.R., C.E. Polan and T.C. Camphell: Bovine liver metabolism and tissue distribution of aflatoxin B_1. J. Agr. Food Chem. $\underline{25}$, 1189 (1977).

2o. Hites, R.A.: Analysis of trace organic compounds in New England Rivers. J. Chromatographic Sci. $\underline{11}$, 57o (1973).

21. Krauskopf, L.G.: Phthalates in the environment. Plasticizer Panel Meeting,Society of Plastics Engineers, Palisades Section, Saddle Brook, New Jersey, February 2o, 1974.

22. Lake, B.G., J.C. Phillips, J.C. Linnell and S.D. Gangolli: The in vitro hydrolysis of some phthalate diesters by hepatic and intestinal preparations from various species. Tox. appl. Pharm. $\underline{39}$, 239 (1977).

23. Lijinski, W. and S.S. Epstein: Nitrosamines as Environmental Carcinogens. Nature $\underline{225}$, 21 (197o).

24. Luepke, N.P. and R. Eckard: N-Nitroso-Verbindungen, Nitrit and Nitrat - Vorkommen, Bildung, Wechselbeziehungen und umwelt- und humantoxikologische Relevanz. Denkschrift für Forschungsgruppe Ökosystemforschungsanalyse beim Umweltbundesamt Berlin (West), 1977.

25. Luepke, N.P.: Phthalate esters: occurrence and toxicology (in prep.).

26. Maienthal, E.J. and D.A. Becker: A Survey of Current Literature on Sampling, Sample Handling and Long Term Storage for Environmental Materials. NBS Technical Note 929, Washington (1976).

27. Marth, E.H.: Antibiotics in foods - naturally occuring, developed and added. Res. Rev. $\underline{12}$, 65 (1966).

28. Mathur, S.P.: Phthalate esters in the environment.Pollutants or natural products. J. Environ. Qual. $\underline{3}$, 189 (1974).

29. Mayer, F.L., D.L. Stalling and J.L. Johnson: Phthalate esters as environmental contaminants. Nature $\underline{238}$, 411 (1972).

3o. Melancon, M.J. and J.J. Lech: Distribution and biliary excretion products of di-2-ethylhexyl-phthalate in rainbow trout. Drug. Metab. Dispos. $\underline{4}$, 112 (1976).

31. Mes, J., D.E. Coffin and D.S. Camphell: Di-n-butyl- and di-2-ethylhexyl-phthalate in human adipose tissue. Bull. Environ. Cont. Toxicol. $\underline{12}$, 721 (1974).

32. Mestres, R.: Occurrence of non-persistent organic compounds in water, soil and foodstuffs: pesticides. Report of a working group of experts Commission of the European Communities. Document EUR 5432e (1976).

33. Metcalf, R.L., G.M. Booth, C.K. Schuth, D.J. Hansen and P.Y. Lu: Uptake and fate of di-2-ethylhexylphthalate in aquatic organisms and in a model ecosystem. Environ. Health Perspect. 4, 27 (1973).

34. Morris, R.J.: Phthalic acid in the deep sea jellyfish Atolla. Nature 225, 1264 (197o).

35. Myers, R.P.: Antibiotic residues in milk. Res. Rev. 7, 9 (1964).

36. Nazir, D.J., M. Beroza and P.P. Nair: Bis-(2ethylhexyl)phthalate in bovine heart muscle mitochondria. Its detection, characterization, and specific Localization. Environ. Health Perspect. 3, 141 (1973).

37. Peakall, D.B.: Phthalate esters: Occurrence and biological effects. Res. Rev. 54, 1 (1975).

38. Perspective on PAES.: Phthalic acid esters conference, National Institute of Environmental Health Sciences, Pinehurst, North Carolina, Sept. 6-7 (1972). Environ. Health Perspect. 3, 1-182 (1973).

39. Purchase, I.F.H. (ed.): Mycotoxins. Elsevier Publ., Amsterdam (1974).

4o. Rowland, I.R., R.C. Cottrell and J.C. Phillips: Hydrolysis of phthalate esters by the gastrointestinal contents of the rat. Fd. Cosmet. Toxicol. 15, 17 (1977).

41. Schuller, P.L., W. Horwitz and I. Stoloff: A review of sampling plans and collaboratively studied methods of analysis of aflatoxins. J. Assoc. Off. Anal. Chem. 59, 1515 (1976).

42. Sethunathan, N., R. Siddaramappa, K.P. Rajaram, S. Barik and R.A. Wahid: Parathion: Residues in soil and water. Res. Rev. 68, 91 (1977).

43. Shimomura, K.: Toxicological and environmental aspects of phthalic acid esters 2. Nikkakyo Geppo 3o, 4o (197o); C.A. 86, 115678v (1977).

44. Shotwell, D.L.: Aflatoxins in corn. J. Am. Oil Chem. Soc. 54, 216A (1977).

45. Stalling, D.L., J.W. Hogan and J.L. Johnson: Phthalate ester residues, their metabolism and analysis in fish. Environ. Health Perspect. 3, 159 (1973).

46. Stickel, W.H.: Some effects of pollutants in terrestrial ecosystems. Environ. Sci. Res. 7, 25 (1975).

47. Symons, P.E.K.: Dispersal and toxicology of the insecticide fenitrothion; predicting hazards of forest spraying. Res. Rev. 68, 1 (1977).

48. Wogan, G.N. and S.R. Tannenbaum: Environmental N-Nitroso Compounds: Implications for Public Health. Tox. appl. Pharm. $\underline{31}$, 375 (1975).

49. Williams, D.T. and B.J. Blanchfield: The retention, distribution, excretion and metabolism of dibutylphthalate -7-^{14}C in the rat. J. Agr. Food Chem. $\underline{23}$, 854 (1975).

5o. Williams, D.T.: Dibutyl- and di-(2-ethylhexyl)phthalate in fish. J. Agr. Food Chem. $\underline{21}$, 1128 (1973).

51. Williams, P.P.: Metabolism of synthetic organic pesticides by anaerobic microorganisms. Res. Rev. $\underline{66}$, 63 (1977).

52. Wyatt, P.J., D.T. Phillips and E.H. Allen: Laser light scattering bioassay for veterinary drug residues in food producing animals. 1. Dose-response results for milk, serum, urine and bile. J. Agric. Food. Chem. $\underline{24}$, 984 (1976).

53. Vettorazzi, G.: State of the art of the toxicological evaluation carried out by the Joint FAO/WHO Meeting on Pesticide Residues. II. Carbomate and organophosphorus pesticides used in agriculture and public health. Res. Rev. $\underline{63}$, 1 (1976).

54. Zitko, V.: Determination of phthalates in biological samples. Internat. J. Environ. Anal. Chem. $\underline{2}$, 241 (1973).

ORGANIC AND INORGANIC COMPOUNDS - ANALYTICAL ASPECTS

H. Egan
Laboratory of the Government Chemist
London SE 1 9 NQ,
United Kingdom

In reviewing analytical aspects of the assessment of exposure to environmental pollution of human populations there are a number of variables which
must be taken into account. One feature is general however: the interest is
virtually exclusively confined to trace analysis. To begin with it is necessary to distinguish between analyses for various pruposes such as routine
health screening, screening for regulatory control, screening in emergency
circumstances following accidental over-exposure and reference measurements
for research purposes, perhaps at sub-clinical levels.

Physiological responses to exposure to environmental pollutants vary widely
in character and this fact has a substantial influence on the type of sample which is of interest. Toxicity problems which are obviously acute in
character will first involve the examination of the normal range of physiological fluid and other biopsy samples; this may extend to environmental
media to which the populace may be exposed including the atmosphere and the
dietary intake. Chronic situations may be relatively well characterised by
analytical parameters, though there is still room for considerable discussion even in some areas which have been studies for many years, such as the
relative significance (and the levels concerned) of lead in blood and urine.
On the other hand for chronic exposure situations the analytical interest
may in practice be more meaningful in relation to the source of exposure
rather than to human tissue. This is notably the case for the carcinogens
or potential carcinogens such as mycotoxins, polynuclear aromatic hydrocarbons and N-nitrosamine compounds: the analytical methods now in use for
these are among the most sensitive in regular use today; but this is not to
say that there may not be an interest in developing yet more sensitive methods which could, for research purposes, be applied to human tissue including physiological fluids. In considering pollutants I will try for each
group to give a brief understanding of the analytical approach, the levels
of interest and the limits of detection involved; but it is important to
realise that in most cases there is relatively little point in following
day to day levels in human tissues.

The general range of sample substrates of environmental interest thus varies
with the pollutant. Blood and urine levels may be of interest for trace metal pollutants such as lead, cadmium or mercury and subcutaneous fat for organochlorine pesticide residues and certain other persistent compounds including the polychlorobiphenyls (PCB's). Whether these substrates are of
interest for carcinogens such as polynuclear aromatic hydrocarbons is not
yet known, the presumption being that if they are, then the levels concerned
are below - perhaps substantially below - the normal current limits of detection. For such pollutants (if that is the right word in this context) the
amount in the environmental media to which man is exposed -air, water, food-
is at present of greater interest. And whilst it would be wrong not to re-
cognise that current trace methods of analysis can be improved as regards

sensitivity, specificity and accuracy, any substantially lower levels of special significance might be associated with new and as yet undiscovered species. To preserve biological tissue in storage for long periods against the possibility of the discovery later of better methods of examination for factors significant in this way has the added difficulty that (by the nature of the exercise) the storage characteristics of the substances involved are unknown. It is perhaps appropriate in this context to consider what materials, appropriately preserved a century (or a millennium) ago, one would wish now to examine using present-day trace analytical methods. Whilst this does not provide a full answer to the possibility that something completely new, as yet undiscovered, might not emerge later, the essential difficulty of not being able in advance to ensure that the unknown factors remain unaffected in long storage now is still daunting.

In the present context, the pollutants of intereset tend to be chronic in their action rather than acute. This is to some extent reflected in their relation to biological, chemical or physical stability to degradation, which varies among the synthetic hormones, antibiotics, so-called persistent organochlorine pesticides, mycotoxins, nitrosamines, polynuclear aromatic hydrocarbons, trace metals and asbestos fibres. Whilst the short-term stability afforded biological samples by simple chemical preservation or anticoagulant treatment in general may have no significant effect on any of these pollutants which may also be present, such treatment are not appropriate to longer-term storage. The latter calls for the lyophilisation (deep-freezing) of tissue or fluid samples; and freeze storage. However many contaminants, including pesticides, mycotoxins and industrial chemicals, are not stable indefinitely. There is evidence of solid state reactions even when stored ad very low temperatures: thus unsaturated fats may oxidise in freeze-dried samples. Such measures therefore may not provide stability over periods longer than a few month for the less stable of the pollutants and further work on storage stability over longer terms than a year or so is needed. There is no short cut to this: and there are some complications, notably the question of the standardisation of analytical methods and the need in many areas for reliable biological standard reference materials for analysis.

The question of the standardisation of analytical methods has given rise to considerable discussion in recent years. The International Federation of Clinical Chemists among others, have given the matter particular attention, to the extent that there are currently proposals for international definitions for types of method, a distinction being drawn between a method which after exhaustive investigation is found to have no known source of inaccuracy or ambiguity (definitive method), one that can be accomplished with generally available equipment and which after exhaustive investigation has been shown to have acceptable, know inaccuracy in comparison with a difinitive methods (reference method) and other less demanding types of method (1). The development of even a reference method is a major exercise, that conducted by the American Association of Clinical Chemists als illustrating the reference material problem: in this, diaceton glucose (1,2:5,6-di-0-isopropylidene-D-glucofuranose) was selected as a standard for glucose because of ease o proparation and its simple, well characterised mass fragmentation behaviour (2).

Instability on long-term storage is a limitation in the interest in analysis of samples treated in this way, except insofar as analysis is itself a measure of the instability: at the same time, there is considerable interest in the standardisation (perhaps the term 'stabilisation' also would not be appropriate) of analytical methods themselves. Whilst long-term storage thus presents some difficulty, it is doubtful whether in view of the high sensitivity of the methods now available that it would be worthwhile holding such samples (even if this were feasible) for long periods of time against the later development of more sensitive methods. The methods at present available in general offer adequate sensitivity although there may be some scope, as indicated above for the improvement of reproducibility between laboratories. It seems likely that storage of tissue samples to await the recognition of new factors and the development of analytical methods for their determination will also be of limited value, since the question of the stability of the factors and the significance of results from the stored samples will also arise. It is difficult enough to ensure that the trace environmental factors at present recognised are stable during long-term storage and more work is necessary here if this is considered to be a desirable objective. But, as already indicated, it is impossible to design long-term conditions such that factors as yet undiscovered will remain unchanged during storage.

Biological specimens and individual pollutants

The type of human biological specimen of interest in context of exposure to environmental pollutants can differ for different pollutants. For some there is uncertainty as to the relevance of human specimens, the main substrate of interest being the medium for the ingestion of the pollutant (air, water, food for example). The main substrates of interest are blood, urine and other physiological fluids (trace metals and possibly nitrosamines, toxic gases, polynuclear aromatic hydrocarbons and other hydrocarbons) muscle tissue (antibiotics, synthetic hormones), various organs including kidney and liver (trace metals, some pesticides, asbestos) and subcutaneous or other fatty tissue (organchlorine compounds). The relevance of biological samples, particularly in the long-storage context, is unclear for mycotoxins, nitrosamines and a number of organic meterials including polynuclear aromatic hydrocarbons and vinyl chloride. There are other complications such as the relative stability of sample substrate and trace pollutant and the long-term relevance of subclinical levels of significance. For these reasons it is the most convenient to deal with individual pollutants. The analytical aspects of these are considered in the following paragraphs with indications for each of the limits of dedettion and stability on long-term storage (6, 7). The picture is far from complete and there is something of a need to define the long-term storage problem - what substrates, what levels of pollutants and for how long.

Nitrosamines

Trace nitrosamine analysis has been the subject of considerable attention in recent years, mainly in relation to foods in the preparation of which nitrates or nitrites may have been used. Like most other procedures for trace analysis this involves a preliminary extraction or separation stage, a detection and estimation stage (which is the basic analytical observation) and a stage in which the identity of the species is confirmed. The letter is of particular importance in trace nitrosamines work because of the wide variety of possible interferences; and usually calls for the use of a mass spectrometer coupled to a gas chromatograph. Nitrosamine work is thus expensive. It is also relatively alow since the sensitivity requirement is high and the gas chromatographic analytical stage may have to be used near to the limit of detection; the gas chromatographic method is normally successful only if selective detection systems are used. For these reasons it is usual also to insert a concentration stage into the analytical procedure, so that the trace nitrosamines extracted or otherwise separated from the food sample at the beginning of the analysis are concentrated into approximately 0.5 ml of an appropriate solvent before gas chromatographic examination. The initial extraction stage, normally steam distillation or solvent extraction is the most time-consuming usually taking 2 to 3 h per sample. The length of the gas chromatography and mass spectrometry stages depends on the number and molecular weight of the nitrosamines sought. If a range of C_1 to C_4 and heterocyclic nitrosamines are included, chromatography may take 1 - 2 h but this can be shortened by the use of pressure programming and programmed elution techniques.

Samples of greatest interest are cured meats and fish and some cheeses. In some cases, for example fried bacon, formation takes place during the cooking of bacon. Some of these foods may contain 1 - 10 microgram/kg of nitrosodimethylamine or certain other nitrosamines, the lower limit of detection being about 0.1 microgram/kg. Nitrosamines are are decomposed by ultraviolet irradiation, initially to nitramines. Sample extracts in the course of examination are therefore stored (where necessary) in the dark at 5 - 10° C, preferably in a sealed container: extracts held in this way are stable for several months.

Pesticide residues

The principal area of interest has for many years been the organochlorine compounds, mainly dieldrin, HCH, DDT and its immediate degradation products. The interest has also extended to a number of other more-or-less persistent organochlorine compounds, notably the polychlorobiphenyls (PCBs) which have a variety of industrial uses. Analytical methods based on gas-liquid, thin-layer and more recently high-pressure liquid chromatography, supported as necessary by other techniques including high-resolution mass spectrometry, are now in regular and routine service. When used in conjunction with suitable extraction and clean-up techniques (of which the chromatographic processes themselves may form part), limits of detection down to about 0.05 mg/kg are possible with thin-layer chromatography. With gas-liquid chromatography limits of detection vary slightly with the retention time but levels down to 0.001 mg/kg (1 µg per kg) are usually attainable though for most purposes levels as low as this are not always appropriate. Hexachlorobenzene residues may be significant in some countries and have on occasion been confused with isomers of hexachlorocyclohexane (HCH) an account of similar retention times on some stationary phases commonly used in gas chromatography.

Abbott et al have described a gas-chromatographic procedure for the estimation of organochlorine compound residues in human fat based on the use of diethyleneglycol succinate on silanised Chromosorb P and a cyanolilicone column (9, 10). Samples may be held in deep-freeze storage for several months pending examination. They are then first freed from non-fatty tissue and dried with cellulose tissue, extracted with hexane and the extract cleaned up by dimethylformamide solvent partition followed by alumina column chromatography. An electron capture detector is used in the subsequent gas chromatographic examination; the identity of the residues found may be confirmed by thin layer chromatography (11). These aspects were also discussed at an earlier European Colloquium in Luxembourg (12). Although this is usually regarded as a satisfactory means of preserving samples for residue analysis, it may not always be convenient or practicable. Moreover it may not fully inhibit the breakdown of some compounds; pp'-DDT has been reported as breaking down to pp'TDE in liver (4). 4 per cent formaldehyde solution has been suggested as a preservative for tissue samples; 10 per cent phenol is also effective (5).

The PCB compounds are of interest for their ability to interfere with trace organochlorine pesticide residue analyses but at the same time they may be a convenient index of pollution (or potential pollution) situations. The methods of estimating levels differs from that used for pesticides since it is necessary to refer to some convenient standard mixture of material rather than to a single standard reference material: one approach has been to measure the total chromatographic peak area on the chart record and interpret this in terms of the weight of pp-DDE (which is not a PCB compound) which gives the same response. The limit of analytical detection for PCBs in biological media is of the order of 0.01 mg/kg or 0.002 mg/l for milk.

Organophosphorus pesticide residues, for the most part much less persistent can also be estimated by similar methods but detection limits in routine work tend to be somewhat higher, of the order of 0,003 mg/kg, but it is seldom necessary to work down to such levels. It is not normally appropriate to consider long storage for samples. Increasing attention is being paid to residues of other pesticides including triazine and chlorophenoxy compounds and a wide range of analytical techniques is used to cope with these mainly in water and plant tissue. Determination limits depend on the particular combination of compound and method, but normally fall between 0,1 and 0,01 mg/kg.

As regards the stability of pesticide residues in biological tissue during storage, experience relates mainly to organochlorine residues in human and fats such as dieldrin, DDT and DDE isomers, HCH isomers in deep freeze storage: no significant changes are found on re-examination at intervals of up to a year. The general review of stability published by Kanar, de Batista and Gunther (17) deals with the cold storage of foods and extracts of both organochlorine and organophosphorus compounds: stability is influenced by temperature, substrate and duration.

Vinyl chloride monomer

Vinyl chloride (vinyl chloride monomer, VCM) is a gas at normal temperatures and pressures but traces may be occluded in polyvinyl plastics materials and subsequently leached from these. The monomer polymerizes on exposure to light or under the influence of certain catalysts; and whilst relatively stable at room temperature, traces, where they occur in biological tissue, cannot be considered as stable indefinitely even when the tissue is held in deep freeze. The analytical approach is gas chromatographic, using a solvent extract (for example butan-2-one) of the sample material followed by direct injection, or headspace gas analysis. Levels of interest are below 1 mg/kg, the detection limit in food being of the order of 0.05 mg/kg or 0.005 mg/l for liquids.

Antibiotic residues

Antibiotic residues may occur in meats, including poultry meats, following the veterinary use of these materials, usually as injections or as additives to feeds. Veterinary usage currently permitted within the Community is confined to a few selected antibiotics at low levels as growth promoting feed additives. The methods of analysis available have mainly been used to establish that residues in food, where these occur, are so low as to be of no practical significance. Residues in muscle tissue are detected by direct application of the sample to seeded agar plates; using a agar-gel diffusion technique, the limits of detection vary depending on the potency of the antibiotic relative to the test organism used but are of the order of 0.1 to 0.5 microgram/g. Antibiotic residues arising from the treatment of farm animals may also occur in milk, due in most instances to failure to observe the recommended withdrawal periods between treatment of the cow and resumption of marketing the milk. Samples should be examined as quickly as possible. If storage is necessary chemical preservatives may not be used. Low temperature or drying can be considered but antibiotic activity may diminish. Freeze-drying followed by cold storage is to be preferred but frozen tissue samples may if subsequently transmitted unfrozen give 'false positive' reactions after a day or two, owing to the formation by normal spoilage microflora of natural bacterial inhibitory substances, perhaps including a C18 unsaturated fatty acid. Deep-frozen milk retains penicillin activity for a few months; dried milk powder shows a variable loss, possibly depending on the moisture content.

Synthetic hormones

Synthetic hormones such as hexoestrol, diethylstilbestrol(DES) and methyl testerone may be used in beef cattle and poutry meat production either by implantation in vivo or by incorporation in feeds. Both chemical and biochemical methods are available for residue detection. In biochemical testing, the uterine method depends on the increase in weight of immature female rats or mice after the ingestion of oestrogens; this assay is sensitive but not specific. An alternative method depends on the change in the histological character of vaginal smears after oestrogen treatment. This test is specific but not sensitive but in combination with the uterine method it can detect 2 to 10 microgram/kg of oestrogen. Both gas-liquid and thin layer chromatographic chemical techniques are available with similar limits of detection.

Radio-immunological methods are both specific and sensitive, being capable of detecting down to 2 - 1o ng/kg. They use a specific radio-labelled antigen for each hormone to be detected but, on account of their high sensitivity, are also liable to interference by hormones naturally present.

Mycotoxins

Toxic mould metabolites may arise as a result of the growth of spoilage mouds on foods and feeding stuffs. The aflatoxins result from a limited number of strains of Aspergillus and Penicillium species, and eight compounds of related molecular configuration are now recognised, aflatoxins B_1, B_2, B_{2a}, G_1, G_{2a}, M_1 and M_2. Over 100 mycotoxins are known in all, including also zearalenone, patulin and ochratoxin; these are potent carcinogens to many animal, piscean and avian species.

Analytic methods employed are generally based on chromatographic procedure, principally TLC, for the purification and separation of the individual compounds. Mixtures of chloroform and methanol in various proportions, together and with acetic acid, have been used as development solvents with silica gel as a support. Detection and semi-quantitative estimation have generally been achieved by the use of visual fluorescence techniques under illumination by UV radiation, the limits of detection and the relative fluorescence intensities of the various aflatoxins depending on whether the fluorescence is observed on a solid support or in solution. In methanol for example the detection limits for aflatoxins B_1 and G_1 are respectively $2 \cdot 10^{-2}$ and $5 \cdot 10^{-4}$ µg/ml, but on solid TLC supports about 0.2 µg per spot of aflatoxin B_1 (blue fluorescence) and 0.1 µg per spot of aflatoxin G_1 (green fluorescence) may be detected. The presence of non-characteristic palewhite fluorescence may be used to reduce the detection limits of TLC plates by approximately one order of magnitude. For conformation of aflatoxin B_1, adduct reactions using formic acid-thionyl chloride, acetic acid-thionyl chloride and trifluoroacetic acid have been proposed, fluorescent spots with modified R_f values being obtained with the adducts formed. Irradiation degradation of the aflatoxins B_1 and G_1 on silica gel has also been used as a means of confirmation, three products with reduced R_f values being revealed by UV irradiation for each. Other methods used include paper and partition column chromatography, but the limits of detection of silica gel have been found to be superior to those obtained on other supports. Similar analytical methods are used for other mycotoxins but gas chromatographic methods have also been used for zearalenone as the tri-dimethylsilylether derivative with a limit of detection of about 0.5 µg.

Substrates usually examined are foods, notably cereals for which partition methods, both liquid/liquid and liquid/solid have been used as a means of preparing extracts. Column systems using Celite, Florisil and silica gel have been described following extraction with methynol-water or aqueous acetone-hexane. Pigments and other interfering materials can be removed with hexane, tetrahydrofuran or diethylesther. Solvents for desorption of aflatoxins include chloroform-hexane and chloroform-methanol. Aflatoxin M_1 has been detected in milk at a level of 0.3 mg/l and has been directly related to the ingestion of approx. 1 mg of aflatoxin B_1 by a 500 kg cow. Aflatoxin M_1 has been detected in human urine from subjects known to have ingested contaminated peanut butter.

Asbestos fibres

Asbestos is a micture of silicates of iron, magnesium, calcium, sodium and aluminium. It occurs naturally as a fibre in various forms, the three most important being chrysotile, crocidalite and amosite. These are normally characterised and counted by purely physical means. Physical or chemical methods may be used for the preliminary removal of extraneous matter from the sample. Tissue counting techniques have been described by Oldham (21) and Pooley (22); the letter concludes that no single method of preparation for electron microscopy examination is yet available. Optical microscopy is normally used for identification, supported where necessary by X-ray diffraction spectrometry or scanning electron microscopy. The examination involves the measurement of fibre size (lenght to breadth ratio) and count, the latter normally being restricted to fibres of length greater than a specified minimum (say 5 μm) and exceeding a specified length to breadth ratio (say 3), and a diameter less than 3 μm. The limit of detection (length) by visual optical means is about 0.5 μm. The stability of the fibres is characteristic and any question of long storage of samples is a matter of the preservation of the substrate.

Trace Metals

Many methods have been developed over the past 50 years for the detection and estimation of traces of arsenic and such metals of environmental interest as copper, mercury, lead and cadmium. These have been principally colorimetric or spectrophotometric in nature, often based on the use of selective (if not specific) organic reagents especially developed for the purpose; but the methods also extend to almost every other technique in analytical chemistry, including for example coulometry, polarography, gravimetry and chromatography. The tecnnique which has become the general method choice in most control laboratories is atomic absorption spectroscopy. The usual method for biological tissue involves preliminary oxidative destruction of organic matter, either by wet oxidative with nitric ans sulphuric acids or by dry ashing in a platinum dish, although some fluids, for example, can be examined with no preliminary treatment at all. Where the highest sensitivity is required, the trace element from the sample or sample digest can be concentrated into a small volume by extraction with a suitable organic complexing agent, ammonium pyrrolidine dithiocarbamate being widely used in conjunction with 4-methyl-pentan-2-one solvent extraction for cadmium, lead and nickel. In this way lead and cadmium levels down to about 0.05 mg/kg and 0.01 mg/kg respectively can be measured in most tissues (15) and 0.002 mg/l for cadmium and 0.01 mg/kg for lead in fluids. Special interest attaches to the analyses of blood and other biological fluids for lead and their delta-aminolevulinic acid dehydratase (ALAD) activity as an indicative or supplementary test for this, both of which (for blood) are the subject of a current draft directive. Heparinized blood may be stored at 4° if necessary before ALAD estimation, but not for longer than 24 h.

Trace mercury analyses are also most conveniently done by stomic absorption spectrophotometry, special attention being necessary at the initial oxidation or digestion stage to avoid losses of mercury by volatilisation. Following oxidation (which converts all of the mercury present into the mercurio form) excess of reducing agent is added to liberate elemental mercury, which by a stream of sir is then carried through the cell of a flameless atomic absorption spectrophotometer. Levels down to 0.005 mg/kg can be detected (16). Special attention attaches to certain food fish, notably tuna, for the ability to concentrate mercury in an organically bound form (methylmercury compounds) regarded as distinctly more toxic to man than inorganically bound mercury. Methylmercury compounds are extracted from the sample with benzene, then extracted into aqueous cysteine solution, acidified and back extracted into benzene for gas chromatographic examination. Levels down to about 0.02 mg/kg may be estimated in this way. Atomic absorption techniques have also been applied to the estimation of selenium, arsenic and antimony. This involves the evolution of the element as the hydride from an acid digest with sodium borohydride. The hydride is swept by a flow of argon into an argon-hydrogen entrained air flame, or decomposed in a heated silica tube followed by atomic absorption spectrophotometry. Useful working ranges are 0.2 - 30 ng/ml for selenium and 0.7 - 50 ng/ml for arsenic. Another application of atomic absorption spectroscopy involves the use of the heated graphite furnace flamelese technique which is of particular value for the estimation of trace elements where sample size is limited.

Selenium may also be detected and estimated at levels down to between 0.01 and 0.03 mg/kg. The sample to be examined is digested with nitric and perchloric acids under strongly oxidising conditions; following this a fluorescent selenium complex is formed with 2,3-diaminonaphthalene-(naphtho-(2,3-d)-2-selena-1,3-diazole), which is extracted into cyclohexane, back-extracted into 0.1M hydrochloric acid and compated spectrofluorimetrically with standard selenium solution under similar conditions. Multi element analysis methods such as neutron activation analysis, spark source mass spectrometry may also be used. With the development of very high temperature plasma emission sources, matrix effects can be largely eliminated and emission spectrometry offers considerable promise for a cheap and reliable multielement analysis.

Great importance attaches to the avoidance of contamination during sampling particularly for such metals as iron, chromium, cobalt and manganese. Anticoagulant measures for blood involving heparin may also introduce trace metals and Folg has discussed the special care needed to avoid contamination from the laboratory environment itself (20). Tissue samples for trace metal analysis can be stored by most normally accepted methods although some migration can occur between phases and, in the case of mercury in particular, the balance between organically bound and inorganically bound metal may change with time. Few systems have been studied systematically with stability in storage in mind, however, and there is scope for further work in this field.

A number of possible variable factors have to be taken into account if long-term storage is to be considered. These may include the oxidation state of the metal if in solution or the relationship between particle size and dissolution if in micron or submicron particulate form. The effect of microorganisms should be eliminated by heat sterilisation or lyophilisation. Contamination can occur due to absorption of trace metals from the surface of the container or leaching of metal-containing additives from the materials from which the containers are made. Zinc, or occasionally cadmium, calcium or tin, may be present in some plastics compositions. A study of borosilicate glass or polypropylene shows that these materials are suitable for samples frozen at pH 2 to reduce interaction between metal ions and the container surface. On the other hand, adsorption from the sample solution of trace pollutant onto the walls of the vessel containing the sample may be a hazard, even in short-term storage. Adsorption onto a borosilicate glass surface of some trace metals can be prevented by acidification to pH 2 but may not be possible to use polypropylene or other plastic materials (3). The long-term storage problem is illustrated by Hamilton in a review

of strategies and tactics in relation to trace elemental analysis in biological tissue (18). He points out that the significance of the levels of
most environmental contaminants is not clearly known and many contaminants
have not even been identified. Whilst these conclusions can be justified,
they must be interpreted with some caution since it is only too easy to
postulate a problem the solution of which is beyond the reach of methodology
without the means of either proving or disproving it (19). Tölg has made a
special study of the calibration problems involved in the determination of
trace metals and other elements in various substrates and has concluded that
these are simplified by the use of dissolution techniques (20). These could
obviously also simplify the problem of long-term storage, provided the species to be measured is known with certainty and steps are taken to ensure
that the solution process takes these into account.

Polynuclear aromatic hydrocarbons

Some of the polynuclear aromatic hydrocarbons have been shown to possess
carcinogenic activity and synergism between compounds may occur. One of the
major problems confronting the analyst in this field is that it is the exception rather than the rule to find contamination by a single compound and
since levels of the order of μg/kg are of interest it has been necessary to
develop multicomponent methods of analysis. Methods for the simultaneous
determination of 13 compounds are available and have been studied on a collaborative basis. General procedures for food, sensitive to about 2 μg/kg,
are based on solubilisation of the sample with methanolic potassium hydroxide solution followed by solvent extraction and partition between dimethyl
sulphoxide and an aliphatic solvent. Column chromatography on Florisil followed by paper chromatography and thin-layer chromatography is used for removing interfering substances and for semiquantitative analysis by fluorescence techniques, a general method being available for a number of hydrocarbons including benzo(a)pyrene, benzo(g,h,i)perylene, benzo(a)anthracene,
benzo(e)pyrene, pyrene, fluoranthene and benzo(k)fluoranthrene (13) and a
specific method for benzo(a)pyrene (14). If evidence of the present or otherwise of a single indicator compound (usually benzo(a)pyrene) is sought, a
shortened procedure may be used. Solution techniques, UV and fluorescence
spectrometry and mass spectroscopy have been used as confirmatory methods
and a method based on gas liquid chromatography with flame ionisation detection has also been used.

Other hydrocarbons

Minute traces of aliphatic and aromatic hydrocarbons, of the order of 1 μg/kg
or less, may occur in foods from the natural decomposition of lipids, proteins, steroids and other organic substances (8). The normal analytical approach is gas chromatographic, with a limit of detection varying down to
1 μg/kg or less. Although for the most part relatively stable substances,
particularly at deep-freeze storage temperatures, insufficient work has
been done on the stability of the very large range of straight and branched
chain aliphatic and benzenoid compound concerned to know whether significant
changes occur in periods of time of the order of 1-10 years or more.

References
1 Mitchell,F.L. Pure Appl. Chem. 1976, 45, 59-62
2 Schaffer,R. Pure Appl. Chem. 1976, 45, 75-79
3 Struempler, A.W. Anal. Chem. 1973, 45, 2251-2254
4 Jefferies,D.J. et al. Nature 1966, 212, 533-534
5 French,M.C. et al. Bull.Environ.Contam.Toxicol. 1971, 6, 460-463
6 Egan,H. Food Cosmet.Toxicol. 1971, 9, 81-90
7 Egan,H. et al. Toxicology 1975, 4, 245-252
8 Johnson, A.E. et al. Chem.Industry 1969, 10-11
9 Abbot, D.C. et al. Brit.Med.J. 1968, 3, 146-149
10 Abbot,D.C. et al. Brit.Med.J. 1972, 2, 553-556
11 Abbot,D.C. et al. J.Chromatogr. 1964, 16, 481
12 Weston, R.E. "Problems raised by the contamination of man by persistent Pesticides", pp 355-362, EEC, Luxembourg 1975
13 Howard, J.W. et al. J.Assoc.Offic.Anal.Chem. 1966, 49, 595
14 Howard, J.W. et al. J.Assoc.Offic.Anal.Chem. 1966, 49, 611
15 "Environmental pollutants: selected methods of analysis, pp 180-183 SCOPE, Paris 1975
16 "Environmental pollutants: selected methods of analysis, pp 174-176 SCOPE, Paris 1975
17 Kawar,N.S. et al. Residue Reviews 1973, 48, 45-77
18 Hamilton, E.I. Science of total Envir. 1976, 5, 1-62
19 Egan,H. Chem.&Ind. 1975, 814-820
20 Oldham,P.D. "Biological effects of asbestos", p45, IARC Scientific Publication No 8, Lyon 1973
21 Tölg,G. Talanta 1972, 19, 1489-1521
22 Pooley,F.D. "Biological effects of asbestos", p50, IARC Scientific Publication No 8, Lyon 1973

ANNEX

This note supplements the paper on Analytical Aspects. It is concerned with fingerprint and profile methods, automated analysis and newer methods of analysis. In addition, there is a tabular summary of limits of detection for various pollutant species for a number of substrates of environmental interest (see Appendices 1 and 2). By way of general interest Analytical Chemistry each year publishes a comprehensive review supplement which in alternate years is devoted to applied aspects (Application Reviews) and fundamental aspects (Fundamental Reviews) of analysis. The 1976 review volume (15) included electroanalytical techniques, ion selective electrodes, electrophoresis, chromatography and spectrometry in their various forms, chemical and electron microscopy and elemental and thermal analysis with an ordered presentation of many thousands of references to original papers. The 1977 volume (16) included air pollution, clinical chemistry, fertilisers, food, pesticide residues, pharmaceuticals and water analysis (and many other aspects) on a similar basis.

Fingerprint and profile methods

Fingerprint and profile methods of analysis may involve the matching of the pattern of responses in a chromatographic separatory method of detection and estimation of the conversion products from an unknown substance, for example the glc response after hydrolysis (for example of a glyceride) or pyrolysis or the aminoacid response pattern from a polypeptide.

Alternatively they may involve the pattern of a suite of determinands such as the organic acids from citrus products or cations such as Na, K, Mg, Ca in a physiological fluid. Pyrolysis followed by mass spectrometry has similarly been used. Pattern recognition is a much wider concept, based on general mathematical principles but can be applied to such multi-response analytical techniques. It has for example been proposed as a method for the identification of micro-organisms or antibiotics, by study of the radial diffusion zones as a function of known antibiotic or known micro-organisms colonies (1). Kowalski and Bender (2) have discussed the general approach to the problem of predicting an obscure property of a collection of substances from indirect measurements, for example the prediction of atomic composition from emission spectrometry; or the molecular structure from NMR spectrometry; or the reactivity of a mixed system. Linear and non-linear mapping techniques are used, both for single source and multi-source data, the former being well established for mass, infra-red, NMR and gamma spectrometry. Pattern recognition techniques have also been suggested for the identification of oil spills (9) and have an obvious potential for the "recognition" of unknown compounds. The fatty acids characteristics of the glycerides from natural oils have long been used as a basic for the identitiy and commercial quality of such oils. GLC has substantial improvements to be made in the characterisation of individual saturated and mono-, di- and tri-unsaturated acids and has considerably increased the value of pattern recognition possibilities in this field. Pattern recognition based on chemical constituents has also been widely used for the characterisation of distilled alcoholic beverages (3) and various fruit products (4) and Kowalski has attempted to classify wines according to their trace metal profiles.

"Patient profiling" in clinical chemistry and "multiphasic screening" for disease (5) have been the subject of considerable study. Typically, the blood and urine may be examined for as many as 50 (or more) parameters. This approach may pose as well as solve problems and doubts as to the value of the technique for diagnosis for whole populations have been expressed (6).

Automation and mechanization

Mechanization has been applied to a wide range of analytical techniques, particularly in the field of clinical chemistry where in fact the subject was first developed. True automation, in which there is a feed-back of the analytical result to (for example) a production line, is possible in some industrial processes; but in most analytical fields of environmental interest the mechanization extends to the direct display or ordered print-out of results, often on a multi-element basis. The subject has been reviewed by Foreman and Stockwell (7), who cover electrochemical, colorimetric, spectroscopic, thermal, radiometric, X-ray and gas-liquid, thin layer, paper and ion exchange chromatographic methods. The same authors also deal with the on-line and off-line use of computers in analysis. For biological samples, particular interest attaches to the mechanization of the sample preparation stage and the presentation of the prepared digest or other solution to the analytical train (8). Applications of analysis to problems of diagnosis, prognosis and therapy in clinical chemistry have recently been reviewed by Buettner (10).

Some newer techniques

Newer methods of environmental analytical interest include inductively coupled plasma spectrometry and heated graphite atomiser flameless atomic absorption spectrometry. The latter is more sensitive than normal FAA by some
two orders of magnitude: detection limits for lead and cadmium are 0.5 ng/ml
and 0.1ng/ml respectively. Interferences require attention but the technique
can be used for sample volumes down to 100 microlitres. The detection limits
for various metals and other trace elements are given in Appendix 2. Selenium and arsenic can be determined in water down to 0.1 ng/ml, antimony
down to 0.5 ng/ml. Reid (14) has reviewed the general approach to sample
preparation for the microdetermination of organic compounds, including metabolites, in plasma or urine. This does not specifically deal with unknown
constituents but a wide range of techniques is considered. High performance
liquid chromatography (HPLC) has been widely used for trace and compositional
analysis in recent years and has proved to be an exceptionally versatile
and powerful technique. The use of chemically bonded active stationary phases has extended the range of separations which are possible, including in
the biological field a large range of medicinal compounds and their breakdown products as well as natural products (11) and many substances of contaminant interest such as polynuclear aromatic hydrocarbons. The basic difference between classical column chromatography and HPLC is in the particle
size of the column packing material, which for the latter at present average
5 µm or less. A wide variety of detectors, based for example on ultraviolet
absorption, fluorescence, polarography or electron capture characteristics,
has been developed to match the versatility of the separations which can be
achieved. Wheals and Jane (12) have reviewed the use of HPLC for the analysis of drugs and their metabolites, covering steroids, antibiotics, vitamins, alkaloids, prostaglandins and general ranges of O-, S- and P- containing compounds. The application of the technique to the low levels which
occur (or might occur) in body fluids still presents problems but the area
is still regarded as of great practical potential. The use of gas chromatography for the determination of metal complexes has also been reviewed (13),
covering 37 metals and the rare earths: the use of HPLC has also been examined and the attributes of the two techniques as applied to metal chelates
are suggested to be complementary.

References

1 MacDonald,J.C. Intern.Labor. 3/4 1978, pp 78-87
2 Kowalski,B.R. et al. J.Amer.Chem.Soc. 1972, 94, 5632-5639
3 Lisle,D.B. et al. J.Inst.Brewing 1978, 84, 93-96
4 Mears, R.G. et al. J.Food Techn. 1973, 8, 357-389
5 N.N. Lancet 1974, pp 1434-1443
6 N.N. Lancet 1978, p 29
7 Foreman,J.K. et al., Automatic Chemical Analysis, Wiley, London 1974
8 Stockwell,P.B. Automatic methods of food analysis, in: Developments in
   food analysis techniques, pp 223-259, Appl.Sc.Publ., Barking 1975
9 Duewer,D.L. et al. Anal.Chem. 1975, 47, 1573-1583
10 Buettner, H. Z.Anal.Chem. 1977, 284, 119-124
11 Cox,G.B. J.Chromatogr. 1977, 15, 385-392
12 Wheals, B.B. et al. Analyst 1977, 102, 889-916
13 Uden,P.C. et al. Analyst 1977, 102, 625-644
14 Reid,E. Analyst 1976, 101, 1-18
15 Fundamental Reviews, Anal.Chem. 1976, 48, 1R-444R

16 Application Reviews, Anal.Chem 1977, 49, 1R-286R
17 Lokke,H. Bull.Environ.Contam.Toxicol. 1975, 13, 730
18 Khan,S.U. J.Assoc.Offic.Anal.Chem. 1975, 58, 1027
19 Dupuy,A.E. et al. J.Agric.Food Chem. 1975, 23, 827
20 Munro, H.E., Pesticide Sci. 1972, 3, 371
21 Stewart,D.K.R. et al. Bull.Environ.Contam.Toxicol. 1977, 18, 210
22 Agemian, H. et al. J.Assoc.Anal.Chem. 1977, 60, 1070
23 Sherma,J. et al. Anal.Chim.Acta , 1977, 91, 259
24 Buser, H.R. Anal.Chem. 1977, 49, 918
25 Shadoff, L.A. et al. Bull.Environ.Contam.Toxicol. 1977, 18, 478
26 Mahle, N.H. et al. Bull.Environ.Contam.Toxicol. 1977, 18, 123
27 Committee on Analytical Methods, Analyst 1974, 99, 570
28 Bureau International Technique des Solvants Chlore, Anal.Chim.Acta
                                              1976, 82, 1

Appendix 1 - LIMITS OF DETECTION micrograms per gram (or litre)

		SUBSTRATE	TECHNIQUE/S	
DDT and derivatives aldrin, dieldrin		Animal or vegetable tissue	GLC	0.01 µg/g (1g sample)
		Water	GLC	0.001 µg/g (10g sample)
				0.01 µg/litre (1 litre Sample)
	Pentachloro-phenol	Animal tissue	GLC (1)	0.005 µg/g (50g sample)
PCB etc	Direct (2)	Animal tissue	GLC	0.02 µg/g (1g sample)
		Water	GLC	0.02 µg/litre (1 litre sample)
	As decachloro-biphenyl		GLC	0.01 µg/g (1g sample)
aflatoxin B₁		Animal Feeds	TLC	10 ng/g
antibiotics				
Stilbestrol		Cattle tissues	GLC	0.001 µg/g
		Beef liver	Spectrofluori-metry	0.001 µg/g
OP insectides		Animal or vegetable tissue	GLC	0.01 mg/kg
vinyl chloride		Food		0.05 mg/kg
		Water		0.005 mg/kg
PAH		Food		2 ng/g

	Substrate	Technique	Detection Limit	ref.
2,4-D 2,4,5-T Dichlorprop	Grain	GLC-ECD (Me ester formed)	0.02 - 0.05 µg/g	(17 ,18)
Mecoprop	Grain	GLC-ECD	0.5 µg/g	(18)
2,4-D 2,4,5-T	Tomato plants	GLC micro-coulometric	0.01 µg/g	(20)
2,4-D 2,4,5-T MCPA	Soil	GLC-ECD (Me ester formed)	0.005 µg/g	(21)
2,4-D 2,4,5-T 2,4-DB Dichlorprop MCPA	Water " " " "	GLC-ECD (2-chloroethyl ester)	0.03 µg/l 0.02 µg/l 0.1 µg/l 0.02 µg/l 0.25 µg/l	(22)
2,4-D 2,4,5-T	Water "	TLC "	1 µg/l 1 µg/l	(23)
Tetrachloro dibenzo- dioxin (TCDD)	Soil, grass Fish Water Human milk Bovine milk	GC-MS	0.01 ng/g 0.005 ng/g 0.0001 ng/g 0.003 ng/g 0.001 ng/g	(24) (25) (25) (26) (26)
Chloroform	Grain Water	GLC-ECD	0.05 µg/g 0.08 µg/l	(27) (28)
Carbon tetrachloride	Grain Water	GLC-ECD	0.002 µg/g 0.025 µg/l	(27) (28)
Trichloroethylene	Grain Water	GLC-ECD	0.05 µg/g 0.05 µg/l	(27) (28)

DETECTION LIMITS FOR TRACE METALS AND OTHER ELEMENTS OF ENVIRONMENTAL
INTEREST

2σ values, mg/kg

Element	AAS*	ICP-OES[+]
As	0.05	0.07
Ba	0.008	0.001
Be	0.002	0.0001
Ca	0.0005	0.001
Cd	0.0002	0.002
Co	0.01	0.02
Cr	0.003	0.002
Cu	0.001	0.01
Fe	0.005	0.002
Hg	0.25	0.02
K	0.002	10.0
Mg	0.0001	0.0001
Mn	0.002	0.0003
Mo	0.02	0.04
Na	0.0002	1.7
Ni	0.002	0.006
Pb	0.01	0.02
Se	0.05	0.03
Si	0.02	0.02
Sn	0.01	0.02
Sr	0.002	0.0001
Ti	0.04	0.002
V	0.04	0.005
Zn	0.001	0.001

The 2σ values were obtained using demineralized water and should be
multiplied by a factor of from 5 to 10 to obtain working detection
limits

* atomic absorption spectrophotometry

[+] inductively coupled plasma optical emission spectrometry

USE OF MACROALGAE AS A REFERENCE MATERIAL FOR POLLUTANT MONITORING AND SPECIMEN BANKING

Scott W. Fowler
International Laboratory of Marine Radioactivity
Musee Oceanographique
Principality of Monaco

Summary

An assessment of the properties of macroalgae for serving as a reference material in marine pollution monitoring studies has led to the conclusion that these organisms should be given top priority for use in the tissue bank pilot program. Macroalgae are considered attractive candidates for pollutant monitoring and specimen banking in that they are ubiquitous, sedentary integrators of many pollutants and are already being used as pollutant indicators in many pollution monitoring programs. International interest in macroalgae is witnessed by the use of these organisms as reference materials for world-wide pollutant intercalibraton exercises.

Widely distributed near-shore species such as the brown algae, Fucus, are proposed as the best group of macroalgae for use in monitoring and specimen banking. The red algae would be an equally good choice for monitoring deeper, off-shore waters. Recommendations are given on sample collection, tissue preparation and homogenization techniques which aim at reducing the possibility of contamination in the resultant homogenate. The prospects of long-term storage of dry homogenate appear good in light of previous tests made with macroalgae use for radionuclide intercalibration exercises.

Assuming a small initial monetary outlay, a pilot program for monitoring macroalgae is proposed which will result in the acquisition and processing of approximately 25 samples per year. An international coordination of the project is stressed, specifically within the framework of ongoing national and international pollution monitoring programs.

BACKGROUND

General

Increasing interest in the quality of our surrounding environment is witnessed by the growing number of national and international programs aimed at assessing marine pollution (IDOE, 1972; UNEP; Ambio, 1977). Integral to these programs is the acquisition of environmental samples on which to base changes in pollutant levels within a defined area. One of the difficulties in assessing pollution in a given component of the marine environment is the lack of "baseline" samples taken prior to the input of the pollutant.

Analysts continue to find new substances in the tissues of marine organisms. This leads to the question - are these substances due to man's activities and, if so, when did they enter the environment? For example, in the late sixties relatively high concentrations of mercury were found in large game fish such as tuna and swordfish.

Spreading alarm caused mercury standard to be set with the result that much of the fish was subsequently judged unfit for human consumption. However, when museum specimens of similar fish were examined and also found to contain high concentrations of mercury, it became evident that the "high"mercury content in these fish may have been natural and thus, was not a result of anthropogenic input (Miller et al., 1972; Barber et al., 1972). Although the quality of the museum-preserved specimens may be suspect, this example points up the need for baseline samples as a point of reference for assessing future trends of pollutants.

Macroalgae

For many reasons marine macroalgae appear to be an attractive candidate for use as a reference material in the proposed program of environmental monitoring and specimen banking. Macroalgae are ubiquitous in both estuarine and coastal waters throughout the world. Algae are key links in benthic food webs and are of direct economic importance to man as well. Their size and sedentary nature facilitates rapid collection of large amounts of material. Because they act as time-integrators of many pollutants, macroalgae have been considered in many marine pollution monitoring programs for use as biological "indicators".

Phillips (1977), reviewing the usefulness of biological indicator organisms in trace metal pollution studies, listed several criteria for an organism to qualify as a "bioindicator" for these substances. The criteria, which generally hold for most pollutants, can be briefly summarized as follows:

The organism should:

1) accumulate the pollutant without being killed by the levels encountered,

2) be sedentary in order to show levels of pollutant representative of the area under study,

3) be abundant in the region,

4) be sufficiently long-lived to allow sampling of more than one year class,

5) be of adequate size to furnish sufficient tissue for analysis,

6) be easy to sample and hardy enough to survive laboratory testing of pollutant uptake,

7) be able to tolerate brackish water,

8) exhibit high pollutant concentration factors allowing direct analysis without pre-concentration,

9) be able to show a simple correlation between the pollutant content in their tissues with that in the surrounding waters at all locations studied, under all conditions.

It is evident that in most cases, macroalgae could be classified as a biological indicator organism; however, as Phillips (1977) points out certain things must be known about them to correctly interpret the results from a monitoring study using these species. For example, macroalgae appear to concentrate only soluble metals; hence, for elements like lead and iron, which are mainly particulate in sea water, algae

will not accurately reflect changes in the environment. Furthermore,
recent studies have shown competition between metals for binding sites
in macroalgae (Foster, 1976). Excluding certain soluble metals from binding
can lead to spurious results concerning the relative abundance of
available trace elements at any one location. This could be one of the
greater problems to overcome in using macroalgae as a biological indicator
for monitoring trace metals.

Several other aspects, which pertain to variation in concentration of
metals and presumably other pollutants in macroalgae, should be considered.
Metal levels vary remarkably with species, therefore comparisons of tissue
concentrations are best made between the same species. The position of
the algae on the shoreline with respect to tide mark also can affect the
metal concentration (Nickless et al., 1972, Fuge and James, 1974; Bryan
and Hummerstone, 1973). This variability is thought to be controlled by
the amount of tidal exposure received by the plants found in the different intertidal zones. Several studies have shown that the distal (older)
parts of macroalgal lamina often contain higher metal concentrations than
the faster growing new tissue (Bryan and Hummerstone, 1973). In was suggested that the older, slower growing regions of the lamina with higher
dry weight have more metal binding sites. Furthermore, seasonal changes
in metal levels have been noted to occur in several species (Bryan and
Hummerstone, 1973; Fuge and James, 1974; Phillips, 1977). These fluctuations may be directly linked to the growth effects cited above since
macroalgal growth is seasonal.

All these examples which pertain to algae (and presumably other organisms)
point up one reservation about the monitoring and specimen bank concept;
real-time analyses can assess relatively large-scale trends in pollutant
levels; however, real, small-scale trends in pollutants may be confounded by natural fluctuations caused by numerous environmental factors.

Table 1 gives some values for heavy metals, PCB's and radionuclides
measured in a common brown algae, Fucus sp., from various areas along
the U.K. coast.

International importance

At present the only project dealing specifically with macroalgae was
a reference material appears to be the Radionuclide Intercalibration
Exercise which is supervised by the IAEA's International Laboratory of
Marine Radioactivity in Monaco. Brown algae, Fucus serratus, was collected in 1971, processed and distributed internationally to laboratories
for intercalibrating their methods for radioanalysis of naturally-conta-
minated, environmental samples. The program has proved to be highly successful and the technical aspects as well as the results of the intercalibration exercise have been published (Fukai and Ballestra, 1975; Fukai and Murray, 1975). Due to the increasing interest in the conventional
pollutants, the Monaco Laboratory has recently prepared a number of reference samples of marine origin for use as intercalibration material in
several on-going or planned pollution monitoring programs. Oyster, sea
plant, copepod and mullet homogenates have already been processed, tested for homogeneity and are currently being distributed to interested parties. Samples of this type will obviously play an integral role in both
nationally and internationally coordinated monitoring surveys. Experience
gained from the IAEA's intercalibration activities will be extremely useful in the future preparation of macroalgae samples for long-term storage
in the specimen bank.

Conclusion

In summary, the role of macroalgae as a primary producer, its current use as biological indicator for pollutants and its success as a reference sample for international intercalibration studies are strong points in favour of considering macroalgae as a top-priority organism for use in environmental monitoring and specimen banking.

SAMPLE PREPARATION

Macroalgae selection

Choice of algae depends to some degree on the region being considered for monitoring. In the near-shore environment, in general, representatives of the Phaeophyceae, or brown algae, would appear to be the most suitable. This most familiar class of algae contains members throughout the world. The largest forms of macroalgae belong to this group and, as a whole, most species are readily obtainable because they grow primarily in the intertidal zone. Of this group, members of the genus Fucus should be considered as a first choice principally because several of these species have already been widely used in pollution surveys and monitoring programs (see Phillips, 1977; Mitchell, 1977; Melhuus et al., 1978). Two other genera, Laminaria and Ascophyllum, have also been the subject of pollution surveys and could be considered as alternative species.

In the event that deeper coastal waters are intended for survey, members of the class Rhodophyceae should be used. The red algae typically live below the tidal zone to depths up to 2oo meters. As deep water forms, they live in a more constant environment and are normally not exposed to tidal cycles; hence, their pollutant levels probably do not vary as greatly as those in near-shore brown algae. The difficulties involved with collecting large quantities of the deeper-living species will more than likely limit their usefulness as a tissue bank specimen. Nevertheless, in areas where they are eaten or where brown algae are not readily obtainable, red algae should be considered for the reference material. Two widely distributed edible forms, Porphyra and Chondrus, which are cultured commercially would be suitable for this purpose.

Collection

The safest way to collect uncontaminated seaweed samples is by hand. This is easily done with species such as Fucus when the algae are exposed at low tide. Care should be taken to sample only the outer fronds (lamina) since the lower stipe and holdfast often contain sand and grit. During collection the lamina should be rinsed in clean seawater to remove as much of the adhering silt as possible. Samples are best shipped to the laboratory in large, pre-cleaned glass (or glass-lined) containers. In this way, inadvertant contamination by metals or organic substances will be minimized. Addition of filtered-seawater (taken at the site of collection) to the containers will serve as a final wash during transport and hopefully remove any remaining silt particles which will eventually settle to the bottom of the container. The algae can then be removed from the seawater bath, rinsed in de-ionized double-distilled water to remove much of the adventitious salts, and drip-dried on clean clothes line. As an alternative method, the algae could be washed and spin-dried in a domestic washing machine (Fukai and Ballestra, 1975); however, this isonly possible if procedural contamination is not a problem.

Tissue preparation

At this point it is necessary to consider whether to freeze or dry the tissues. Both methods of preservation have their advantages for long-term storage. Low temperature freezing (< -100°C) is best in that the samples retain their integrity for subsequent microscopic examination. However, adequate freezer space may become limiting in a long-term, expanded program; in this case storing dried samples would be the most logical solution. Whatever the case, algae samples will most often be dried prior to pollutant analysis.

The following points should be considered during the preparation of macro-algae for analysis and storage. Wet algae with excess water removed with paper towels are weighed prior to drying so that dry weight/wet weight ratios can be determined for future reference. The possibility exists that certain trace elements and organic compounds can be volatilized at temperatures normally used for oven drying (see Pillay et al., 1971); therefore, to guard against pollutant losses through volatilization it is preferable to lophilize the tissues (LaFleur, 1973). If preliminary tests indicate difficulty in powdering lophilized whole algae, the samples should be homogenized in a blender (Waring type) prior to lophilization (freeze-drying). This pretreatment usually results in obtaining a more homogeneous powder during the grinding process.

Commercial lophilizers are best suited for freeze-drying the relatively large amounts of sample required for a macroalgae reference sample. The algae homogenate is loaded into polyethylene or foil-lined trays and quick-frozen at -40°C. The frozen samples are placed under vaccum and lophilized for 24 hours. At the end of the end of the cycle the dried samples are thawed at a constant 30°C to avoid fusion of the lipids.

The dried product is broken by hand into small pieces (= 5 cm x 5 cm) and then ground to a fine powder in a comminuting machine or porcelain ball mill. The resulting powder should be carefully sieved through stain-less steel or nylon screens to remove both large refractory particles and ultra-fine sediment grains. This has been done successfully with several marine tissues at the Monaco Laboratory by collecting the fraction that passes a No. 20 mesh (500 μm aperature) and is retained on a No. 200 mesh size (63 μm aperature) sieve. Approximately 50 % of the total sample is recovered in this process.

Homogenization is best carried out in some type of commercial feed mixer which automatically divides the sample, mixes and recombines the mixed product. If these systems are not available the total sample should be quartered, homogenized, recombined and homogenized, quartered again and homogenized, etc., until good homogeneity is assured. At this stage homo-geneity can be tested for the pollutants of choice with random aliquots taken from bulk tissue samples. If homogenization is inadequate, the en-tire sample can be re-sieved and treated again in the manner outlined above; nevertheless, it should be kept in mind that each additional handling enhances the possibility of introducing contamination.

Homogeneity Testing

One of the criteria for a reference material is homogeneity for the pollutants under study. Controlling homogeneity from sample to sample is the first critical test. This involves analyzing several similar-si-zed aliquots from the bulk product. When inter-sample homogeneity has been assured the next step is to test homogeneity among different-sized aliquots of a single sample (intra-sample). This is necessary because relatively rare, refractory particles (sediment grains, etc.) are often missed in small aliquots whereas they will have a greater chance for inclusion in the analysis of larger amounts or the entire sample. Inclusion or omission of these particles can cause wide variation in observed pollutant concentrations in the same sample. This problem is more important for heavy metals and radionuclides which are often present in particulate form in many biological tissues. In spite of these difficulties, if care is taken during the preparation, homogeneity in marine samples ranging from loo to 5oo mg can be achieved to better than $\pm$ 5 % for many trace elements and radionuclides as well as with PCB and DDT compounds (Fukai, personal communication).

It is also recommended to verify sample homogeneity by more than one analytical method. Neutron activation, atomic absorption spectroscopy and X-ray fluorescence are three independent methods commonly used to measure trace elements. Alpha and beta-emitting radionuclides can be analyzed by various chemical extraction procedures and gamma emitters can be measured by Scintillation gamma-spectrometric techniques that require no pretreatment of the sample. Within limitations, cross-checks between radionuclide and trace element homogeneity tests can often serve as controls for one another. Furthermore, if tissue preparations are homogeneous for metals and radionuclides, they are also likely to be homogeneous for organohalogens and hydrocarbons which are not normally "particulate" in tissues.

Storage

Preserving the integrity of the stored samples is one of the more difficult obstacles to overcome. As mentioned above, low temperature freezing is preferred if adequate facilities are available. However, if space becomes a critical factor as may happen in a pilot project, then only dried samples should be considered. If dried algae are used, in order to reduce bacterial activity, the homogenate should be sealed under vacuum or inert gas in pre-cleaned glass vials (opaque to light) or polyethylene-lined foil containers. Fifty to loo gms of dried homogenate per bottle should furnish ample material for carrying out several sets of analyses.

Irradiation has been used to sterilize tissue samples. For example,in the preparation of the NBS Orchard Leaves; the samples were irradiated with 4.o Mrad from a cobalt-6o source (LaFleur, 1974). However, one disadvantage of this technique is that high level irradiation can alter the chemical structure of tissue and cause the breakdown of certain labile organic compounds, some of which may be the pollutants which are being analyzed in the monitoring program.

In the case of marine macroalgae, radiation sterilization may not be necessary if a storage life of only a few years is projected. The oven-dried Fucus serratus homogenate prepared by IAEA in early 1971 has been stored since then in glass bottles in the Musee Oceanographique, Monaco. During this time no special precautions were taken; the bottles were kept in a darkened room (partially de-humidified) in which the annual temperature varied from approximately 15 to 25°C. Random samples were periodically checked and to date, 7 years after its preparation, no significant changes in weight or radionuclide concentrations have been noted (Fukai, personal communication). These observations are encouraging and suggest that properly liphilized algae homgenates, stored under vacuum in de-humidified facilities might be expected to last at least lo years for certain categories of pollutants.

It is recommended that samples be stored centrally, i.e. in one central depot. This is advisable because any alterations resulting from slightly different storage techniques would lead to increased variability in mea-sured pollutant concentrations.

ANALYTICAL PROCEDURES

A complete compilation and detailed discussion of standard analytical techniques used in pollutant analysis of environmental materials is beyond the scope of this working paper. For a given class of pollutants, the analysts should be encouraged to use the "state-of-the-art" method and perhaps one alternative technique for confirmation.

Pretreatment

The sample size will be dictated by the analytical method employed, how-ever, in the case of macroalgae probably a maximum of a few hundred milligrams would be necessary for most analyses. Prior to weighing, the dried sample should be dessicated over silica gel for 24 hours to alleviate any weight change caused by humidity.

Trace elements

The two most commonly used techniques for measuring trace elements are atomic absorption spectrophotometry and neutron activation analysis. Both methods have been used with marine macroalgae and are excellent for measuring a wide spectrum of trace elements in relatively small ali-quots of sample (Robertson et al., 197 ;Phillips, 1977). Most authors make no mention of any difficulties encountered with either digestion or measurement of trace elements in macroalgae; however, Knauer and Mar-tin (1972) state that the kelp, Macrocystis pyrifera, can accumulate as much as looo ng Hg/g dry weight which is not released following standard wet digestion procedures that have been described in the lite-rature. The problems involved with incomplete digestion indicate that neu-tron activation may be the preferred method since, for many trace elements, the analysis is non-destructive.
A third method, equally reliable but not so often used, is X-ray fluores-cence spectroscopy.

Radionuclides

The radiative nature of the radionuclide will dictate which measurement method must be used. Gamma ray spectrometry is ideal for many gamma-emit ting isotopes since the entire sample can be counted non-destructively in a well-type scintillation crystal. Most beta and alpha counting tech-niques require decomposition and separation of the radioisotope from the matrix. Some species of macroalgae have high levels of calcium and phosphorus which may interfere in the separation of transuranium nuclides from these tissues (Fukai, personal communication). Similarly, caution should be observed in separating certain radionuclides form coralline algae which contain large amounts of calcium and magnesium. Standard ra-dioanalytical methods and their applicability to the measurement of a

variety of radionuclides in marine biota (including macroalgae) are
discussed in detail in two recent technical reports (IAEA, 197o; 1975).

Petroleum and chlorinated hydrocarbons

These classes of compounds are best analyzed by gas chromatography in
conjunction with mass spectrometry. Several recent publications outline
in detail methods for analyzing specific hydrocarbon compounds (Pesticide Analytical Manual;Goldberg, 1976). Although the methods for analyzing various hydrocarbons are straightforward, the degradable nature
of these compounds will pose the biggest problem to the specimen bank
concept of retrospective analyses. At present the storage life for hydrocarbon compounds in tissues such as macroalgae is not known. However,
stability tests on two IAEA reference samples prepared nearly 4 years
ago, sea plant SP-M-I (Posidonia oceanica) and oyster tissues MA-M-I
(Crassostrea sp.), have shown no changes in PCB and DDT concentration
during this period of time (Elder, personal communication). These samples were stored in a manner similar to that of the macroalgae homogenate
(AG-I-1) described above.

Analytical protocol

It is highly recommended that the activities involving real-time and retrospective analyses be as centralized as is feasible. It is well known
that values of reference materials obtained by different laboratories
vary widely. The results from a recent radionuclide intercalibration
exercise using the IAEA seaweed sample AG-I-1 illustrate this point
(Table 2). Values for 5 out of 1o radionuclides exceeded + 4o %, a degree
of scatter that would clearly not be acceptable in a specimen bank program designed to identify temporal or spatial trends in pollutant levels.
The obvious way to reduce variation of this type is to limit the analysts
to a small, welltrained group of people working under the same conditions
with the same instruments. Minimization of interanalyst variation coupled
with proper control of instrument calibration procedures and frequent checks
against known standards should assure the high degree of quality control required for a specimen bank program.

GENERAL ASPECTS

Program design

Only the feasibility of using macroalgae for monitoring and specimen
banking has been addressed in this paper. No attempt has been made to
design a detailed monitoring program since the acquisition of algae samples will depend entirely on the specific needs of the "monitoring environmental materials" project. In general, the magnitude of the program
will depend upon the funding and personnel available. As this is, at present, undecided, we will proceed under the assumption that a minimum
level of funding and personnel will be available for the preparation of
macroalgae specimens; hence, only some general guidelines for a global
project are outlined below.

Macroalgae will be only one of many aquatic and terrestrial specimens
comprising the 4oo samples envisaged for the first year. Because macroalgae are ubiquitous, an ideal sampling scheme should include a specimen
from high, temperate and low latitudes from each side of the major ocean
basins. If these specimens are sampled once per year they would number
roughly 25 considering that the principal marginal seas are also included.

In the event this number is too high, sampling should be restricted to temperate (highly industrialized) and tropical (non-industrialized) latitudes. This would effectively reduce the sample number to about lo, perhaps a realistic proportion of the total number when one considers the global importance of macroalgae. If further increases in total samples are projected, acquisition of macroalgae could then be extended to cover all major areas where seaweeds are found.

Since the specimen bank program will eventually be international in scope, some form of international co-ordination would be desirable. This could best be effected by enlisting the expertise of national and international bodies which have had experience in the preparation of aquatic materials for pollutant analyses. In the framework of several national and international pollution monitoring programs, a vast amount of information exists on such subjects as sampling protocol, descriptive data required, procedures to standardize data, interpretation of data and data storage and retrieval. Tapping the knowledge available from pollution studies in the Mediterranean (UNEP, 1977), the North Sea (ICES, 1974) and the coastal United States (IDOE, 1972, Mussel Watch Program, in progress) will enhance the prospects of success for the environmental specimen bank.

Costs

Without knowing the exact scope of the "monitoring environmental materials" program, it is not possible to accurately predict the costs involved in procuring and preparing macroalgae for the specimen bank. Working on the assumption that a minimum worthwhile effort can be achieved with lo separate samples during the first year, a rough estimate of the costs envisaged is presented in Table 3.

Certain points need clarification to properly interpret Table 3. First, the collection costs have been minimized by assuming that local personnel at each site will collect, wash and freight the wet algae to a central location which, in turn, will prepare the sample. If project personnel have to be sent to the sites for collection and handling, the costs will increase considerably due to the travel involved. Second, at first glance the prices for sample analyses might appear high. These are estimates for the initiation of an analytical program during the first year; and, thus, cover the expenses for the initial analytical outlay. In most cases the cost per sample or element will drop considerably after routine analyses have become established; nevertheless, the cost for transuranium nuclides will remain relatively high due to the analytical difficulties involved. Finally, it should be noted that further savings could be achieved through consolidation of some of the work (e.g. carrying out preparation and analyses) by a single organization that is collaborating on the program. Furthermore, if the expertise exists within the body co-ordinating the program, the major costs involved in designing the program (e.g. consultants' meeting) could be substantially reduced.

In the interest of economy, when planning and budgeting a program of this nature, the organizing body should profit from knowledge of the successes and failures of other large scale monitoring programs such as the North Sea pollution survey (ICES, 1974) and the U.S. EPA Mussel Watch.

References

Ambio: Ambio 6 (6): entire issue (1977).

Barber, R.T., Vijayakumar and Cross, F.A.:Mercury concentrations in recent and ninety-year-old benthopelagic fish. Science 178: 636-639 (1972).

Bryan, G.W. and Hummerstone, L.G.:Brown seaweed as an indicator of heavy metals in estuaries in South-West England. J.Mar.Biol.Ass. U.K. 53: 7o5-72o (1973).

Elder, D.L.:International Laboratory of Marine Radioactivity, IAEA, Monaco. (personal communication).

Foster, P. Concentrations and concentration factors of heavy metals in brown algae. Environ. Pollut. 1o: 45-53 (1976).

Fuge, R. and James,K.H.:Trace metal concentration in Fucus from the British Channel. Mar. Pollut. Bull. 5: 9-12 (1974).

Fukai, R.:International Laboratory of Marine Radioactivity. IAEA, Monaco (personal communication).

Fukai, R. and Ballestra, S.:Intercalibration of methods for radionuclide measurements on a seaweed sample. In: Reference Methods for Marine Radioactivity Studies II. Techn. Reps. Ser. No. 169, pp. 213-233, IAEA, Vienna (1975).

Fukai, R. and Murray, C.N.:Results of plutonium intercalibration in seawater and seaweed samples. In: Reference Methods for Marine Radioactivity Studies II. Techn. Reps. Ser. No. 169, pp. 1o7-12o, IAEA, Vienna (1975).

Goldberg, E.D. (ed.): Strategies for Marine Pollution Monitoring (Ed. by Goldberg, E.D.), 31o p., John Wiley & Sons, New York (1976).

IAEA: Reference Methods for Marine Radioactivity Studies. Techn. Reps. Ser. No. 118, 284 p., IAEA, Vienna (197o).

IAEA: Reference Methods for Marine Radioactivity Studies. Tech. Reps. Ser. No. 169, 239 p., IAEA, Vienna (1975).

ICES: Report of working group for the international study of the pollution of the North Sea and its effects on living resources and their exploitation. Cooperative Research Report No. 39, ICES, Denmark, 191 p., (1974).

IDOE: Baseline studies of pollutants in the marine environment. Background papers for a workshop sponsored by the National Science Foundation's IDOE Brookhaven National Laboratory, 24-26 May 1972, 799 p. (1972).

Knauer, G.A. and Martin, J.H.:Mercury in a marine pelagic food chain.

LaFleur, P.D.: Retention of mercury when freeze-drying biological materials. Anal. Chem. 45: 1534-1536 (1973).

LaFleur, P.D.: Standard reference materials for the determination of trace elements in environmental samples. In: Comparative Studies of Food and Environmental Contamination, pp. 489-496, IAEA, Vienna (1974).

Melhuus, A., Seip, K.L. and Seip, H.M.: A preliminary study of the use of benthic algae as biological indicators of heavy metal pollution in Sorfjorden, Norway. Environ. Pollut. 15: lol-lo7 (1978).

Miller, G.E., Grant, P.M., Kishore, R., Steinkruger, F.J., Rowland, F.S. and Guinn, V.P.: Mercury concentrations in museum specimens of tuna and swordfish. Science 175: 1121-1122 (1972).

Mitchell, N.T.: Radioactivity in surface and coastal waters of the British Isles, 1976. Part 1: The Irish Sea and its environs. Tech. Rep.ifiish. Radiobiol. Lab., MAFF Direct. Fish. Res., (FRL 13). 15pp (1977).

Nickless, G., Stenner, R. and Terrile, N.: Distribution of cadmium, lead and zinc in the British Channel. Mar. Pollut. Bull. 3: 188-19o (1972).

Parker, J.G. and Wilson, F.: Incidence of polychlorinated biphenyls in Clyde seaweed. Mar. Pollut. Bull. 6: 46-47 (1975).

Pesticide Analytical Naual, Vol. 1. U.S. Dept. Health, Education and Welfare, Food and Drug Admin., Rockville, Md. (undated).

Phillips, D.J.H.: The use of biological indicator organisms to monitor trace metal pollution in marine and estuarine environments - a review. Environ. Pollut. 13: 281-317 (1977).

Pillay, K.K.S., Thomas, C.C., Sondel, J.A. and Hyche, C.M.: Determination of mercury in biological and environmental samples by neutron activation analysis. Anal. Che. 43: 1419-1425 (1971).

Preston, A., Jefferies, D.J., Dutton, J.W.R., Harey, B.R. and Steele, A.K.: British Isles coastal waters: The concentrations of selected heavy metals in seawater, suspended matter and biological indicators - a pilot survey. Environ. Pullut. 3: 69-82 (1972).

Robertson, D.E. Ranceitelli, L.A., Langford, J.C. and Perkins, R.W.: Battelle-Northwest contribution to the IDOE baseline study. In: Baseline studies of pollutants in the marine environment. Background papers for a workshop sponsored by the National Science Foundation's IDOE. Brookhaven National Laboratory, 24-26 May 1972, pp. 231-273 (1972).

UNEP: Administrative report on the implementation of the co-ordinated Mediterranean Pollution Monitoring and Research Programme (MED-POL) and related projects of the Mediterranean Action Plan. UNEP/IG.II/INF.3, UNEP, Geneva (1977).

Table 1. Levels of heavy metals, radionuclides and PCB's measured in brown algae, Fucus sp., collected around the British Isles. Values in parentheses are ranges.

Species	Trace metals	Zn	Cd	Pb	Cu	Fe	Mn	Ni
Fucus vesiculosus	(µg/g dry)	(32-962)	(0.05-25.6)	(0.5-11.3)	1.6-36.0	(35-1517)	(33-3o1)	(1.2-29.6)
	Radionuclides (pCi/g dry)	^{60}Co ^{65}Nz	^{90}Sr ^{95}Zr-Nb	^{106}Ru	^{110m}Ag ^{134}Cs	^{137}Cs	^{144}Ce ^{238}Pu	^{239}Pu
Fucus serratus		1.9 1.7	1o.o 2.9	135	1.5 1o.1	75	17.1 3.8	27.o
Fucus sp.	PCB's (µg/g wet)	o.o3-o.31						

Refs.

Fucus vesiculosus	Preston et al., (1973) Fuge & James (1974)
Fucus serratus	Fukai & Murray (1975) Fukai & Ballestra (1975)
Fucus sp.	Parker & Wilson (1975)

Table 2. Average and ranges of reported values for radionuclides in the IAEA seaweed samples AG-I-1 (Fukai and Ballestra, 1975)

Radionuclide	^{40}K	^{60}Co	^{65}Zn	^{90}Sr	$^{95}Zr\text{-}Nb$	^{106}Ru	$^{110}Ag\,m$	^{134}Cs	^{137}Cs	^{144}Ce
No. of reported results	22	2o	9	24	23	36	12	31	41	29
Max. value (pCi/g)	79.2	11	25	15.6	5o	48oo	13.1	715	5o47	2o6
Min. value (pCi/g)	11.3	o.4	o.1	2.4	o.347	28	1.1	6	31.6[a]	7.9
Average (pCi/g)	42.2	3.1	4.3	9.6	6.o	287	2.6	34	213	3o
σ (Mean)	$\pm$ 3.4 (8 %)	$\pm$ o.6 (19 %)	$\pm$ 2.6 (6o %)	$\pm$ o.5 (5 %)	$\pm$ 2.5 (42 %)	$\pm$ 131 (46 %)	$\pm$ 1.o (38 %)	$\pm$ 24 (71 %)	$\pm$ 136 (64 %)	$\pm$ 8 (27 %)

[a] The value represents $^{134}Cs + {}^{137}Cs$

Table 3. Approximate projected costs for a 1 year program
of preparing macroalgae for specimen banking.
Budget based on 1o samples per year.

Category	* Average unit cost	Sample No.		U.S. Dollars
Program design (+ 2 day consultants meeting for 3 people)				5,000
Collection of 1o-2o kg wet algae from 1o locals	$1oo	x 1o	=	1,000
Transport (air freight)	$2oo	x 1o	=	2,000
Bulk lophilization, grinding, sieving				2,5oo
Analysis (including personnel & overhead)				
PCB, DDT	$ 2o	x 1o	=	2oo
Petroleum	$ 2o	x 1o	=	2oo
Trace elments ($2o/element x 5 elements)	$1oo	x 1o	=	1,000
Transuranium nuclide (Pu and Am)	$5oo	x 1o	=	5,000
Other radionuclides	$ 5o	x 1o	=	5oo
Data processing	$ 3o	x 1o		3oo
Storage (1 year + overhead)				5oo
		TOTAL	=	18,2oo

* Costs reflect 1978 prices

A COMPARATIVE ANALYSIS AMONG RESPONSES TO ACUTE TOXICITY IN STANDARD LABORATORY BIOASSAYS AND IN NATURAL STREAMS

P.F.Ghetti
Laboratorio di Ecologia, Universita di Parma
Parma (Italy)

Introduction

There is a permanent lack of studies concerning the comparison among responses to pollutants in the laboratory tests and in natural conditions.
We have initiated a research programme with the aim of testing the effects of parathion inducued toxicity upon a natural stream and some standard species used in laboratory tests.

Materials and methods

The environment used for our experiments is represented by a tract of a small stream, having a length of 1,300 meters, completely contained within a natural woodland preserve in the plains. During the course of three years experiments were carried out in order to establish the yearly dynamics of environmental factors, such as hydrological, chemical, physical, and biological parameters. The characteristics of the stream are those typical of a natural environment; the slope (21%) is constant and the average (adjustable) flow (1 l/sec).
The first section of the water body has always been maintained unaltered up to the first hydrographer, which serves to convey the water flow and permits at the same time the collection of drift organisms by means of special interchangeable nets having different mesh dimensions.
Immediately downstream of the first hydrographer the stream was artificially polluted by parathion.
A second hydrographer, similar to the first hydrographer, and fiited with a drift net with an equal efficiency of capture, was established at approximately 400 m downstream, in order to test the fluctuations of drift organisms both in natural and stream conditions.
The waters of the stream are collected, at a certain distance from the end of the experimental tract, by several canals, artificially constructed for irrigation purposes, where there is a high polluting load of agricultural, zootechnical and urban origin.
The controlled pollution experiments permit a comparison, in any given time, between the biological characteristics of the "blank" section (the upper section) and the lower section.
In particular we have tested the relation dose-response in the macro-invertebrate communities, by analyzing the structure of bottom communities and the structure of sampled drift organisms. Further investigation was conducted by sampling with a mud-sucker sampler the microbenthonic communities : Ciliata, Nematoda, and Rotatoria. Attention has been given to the changes in photosynthetic and heterotrophic activity on artificial substrata.

Present state and perspectives

At first controlled pollution tests on the natural stream have concerned uniquely the effects produced by acute stress conditions in a short period of time.
Concentrations and duration of exposure to toxic chemicals were defined on the basis of laboratory tests on three species : Lebistes, Biomphalaria, and Daphnia magna.

The future program is to carry out tests on chronic toxicity, both in the laboratory and in natural environments. This approach, even if possibly more complex at a methodological and organizational level, would seem more adherent to the nature of polluted environments.

SPECIMEN BANK RESEARCH AT THE NATIONAL BUREAU OF STANDARDS TO INSURE PROPER SCIENTIFIC PROTOCOLS FOR THE SAMPLING, STORAGE AND ANALYSIS OF ENVIRONMENTAL MATERIALS

T.E. Gills and H.L. Rook
U.S. Department of Commerce, NBS
Gaithersburg, MD
U.S.A.

In 1973, the U.S. Environmental Protection Agency conducted a review of analytical methodology used for sampling, storage and analysis of environmental samples. The major conclusion derived from that review was that the accepted procedures were completely inadequate. Deficiencies in trace analysis methodology were further documented by analytical data obtained from a number of EPA contractor laboratories on samples of SRMs 1632, Coal and 1633, Fly Ash. Many data on these materials were in error by more than an order of magnitude. Factors such as these point to the real need for critical evaluation of sampling, storage and analysis methodology for the National Environmental Sample Bank (NESB) program. For the successful implantation of an effective banking system, rigid quality control procedures ensuring comparability and traceability of results between methods and laboratories are required. Several occasions have arisen where environmental samples of known and documented history would have been valuable in assessing changes in trace constituents for the determination of their impact on human health; however, undefined or improper sampling and storage procedures were utilized. The National Bureau of Standards (NBS) in a cooperative effort with the Environmental Protection Agency (EPA) has directed several research efforts toward developing "state-of-the-art" protocols for proper sampling, storage and analysis of biological and environmental samples. This research, when completed, will provide creditable scientific protocols for the collection and storage of NESB type samples as well as improved analytical techniques for the determination of trace constituents. This coupling of proper sampling and storage to these improved analytical techniques will allow the accurate determination of trace constituents of importance to human health in addition to maintaining samples for retrospective analysis.

Since its existence, NBS has made accurate measurements of trace components in a variety of materials. However, in the early seventies, NBS embarked upon a trace element characterization and standards program that has yielded numerous Standard Reference Materials that over a broad spectrum of environmental material. With such a venture NBS has gained considerable expertise in storage and analytical methodligies for a variety of biological and environmental samples. This paper summarizes important areas of research in which NBS has participated that contribute toward the development of storage ans analysis protocols.

Definitions and Goals

The concept of the NESB is that of a well defined system of collection, analysis and long term storage of selected environmental samples. This concept and its implementation was recently evaluated at two workshops: one sponsored by NBS and EPA, the other by the Worls Health Organization, the European Communities and EPA. The conclusion of both workshop was that the NESB is viable from the standpoint of need and the availability of presents scientific knowledge. However, the workshop participants suggested that before the concept is fully implemented, evaluation of storage and analysis methodology utilizing a pilot bank program is needed. During the pilot program problems encountered in collection, transportation, analysis and storage will be carefully monitored and documented. Several tasks were formulated around the pilot bank program to insure creditable scientific protocols. These tasks include:

1. A Five Year Program of sample collection starting at a rate of (400) samples per year and increasing to a maximum rate of (2000) samples per year in year four of the program.

2. Real time analysis of a split set of collected samples.

3. Implementation of long term storage for all samples with a minimum projected storage life of five years.

4. Continued research in analytical methodology and sample preservation and storage.

5. Retrospective analysis of storage samples and comparison with split, real time analyzed samples for quality assurance comparison.

Research at NBS has evolved around these five tasks over the past three years and is at the point now where it is possible to scale up developed protocols from the "lab bench" operation to a modified banking program.

Research on Sample Storage

Research on sample storage had been directed toward the experimental evaluation of contamination or the loss mechanism of trace constitutents (namly trace elements) during storage. The initial research was that of Moody et al. (1) wherein twelve polymeric container materials were evaluated for their trace element content and for the possibility of renoving these trace elements when contacted by liquid samples. This study was made using three complementary trace analytical techniques; neutron activation analysis, atomic absorption, and spark source mass spectrometry. The results of this study indicate that many materials were grossly contaminated by trace elements from plasticizers, formulators and other process materials. However, conventional polyethylene and Teflon were found to be reasonably clean and it was generally found that less than percent of the bulk trace element content could be leached out.

A second and equally important part of the current research program has been a study and evaluation of long term storage techniques which would be adequate for tissue and other biologically active samples. The effects of microbiological action on trace constituents' concentrations and distributions are well doccumented. However, the mechanism for complete long term elimination of that microbiological activity has not been well documented.

Freezing has long been applied as a technique for storage; however, no study has previously been made to document the reliability of this method of storage for more than a short period of time. Recently, the analysis and subsequent reanalysis of a selected animal tissue (bovine liver) that had been stored frozen at -80° C for a period of one year gave us the first indication that our preliminary protocols for the storage of fresh tissue are valid, i.e. polyethylene sealed samples stored at -20° C. The original organ had been subset sampled and the remainder homogenized with a commercial food blender and portioned into six polyethylene ice cube trays containing 14 samples each. The trays were individually sealed in 1 mm thick polyethylene film and stored in a chest type -80° C freezer. Analyses were performed on the subjects of the liver tissue before freezing to provide initial trace elemental concentrations and to verify contamination free homogenization of the sample.

For the one year reanalysis, one tissue cube was removed each of the six trays and the trays resealed for future studies. The selected tissue cubes were freeze-dried and analyzed using the same analytical procedures utilized in the initial analyses. A comparison of the results of reanalysis to those originally obtaines is given in table 1. Several things should be noted in these analyses. First, no detectable losses occured during homogenization and freeze-drying of the liver tissue. These findings support recent studies (2, 3) that in freeze-drying minimal losses and/or contamination of trace elements occur. Furthermore, NBS experience with NBS Bovine Liver (SRM 1577) had been shown to be unchanged for more than five years. This material was analyzed and certified for trace elements in 1972. To the present time no documented evidence of trace element loss or alteration has occurred.

The technique of low temperature ashing (LTA) has been evaluated for long-term storage and found to have many advantages. A recent study at NBS (4) investigated the loss of trace elements during plasma before and after ashing. The results obtained indicate that over thirty (30)trace elements are retained quantitatively during LTA. Five elements, mercury, osmium and the halogens (chlorine, bromine and iodine) are quantitatively retained. It was also determined from the studies that contamination of the sample was not a measurable problem during ashing. An added advantage to the LTA is that resultant samples are easily composited and homogenized.

Research on Analytical Methodology

The complexity of the chemical composition of many environmental and biological materials and the extreme low levels of toxic elements pose a problem in selecting a method or procedure that would ensure precise and accurate analysis. Methods must be sensitive, specific and capable of measuring an analyte within required uncertainty levels. The Center for Analytical Chemistry has available more than 18 analytical techniques capable of measuring trace constituents at the part per million and lower (Table 2). While most of these techniques have been used in support of the Standard Reference Material program, many of these techniques have been used to analyze and/or characterize biological and environmental materials that have direct impact upon research affecting human health.

Recently new or improved analytical methodologies have been developed to analyze typical NESB type samples. The most promising methods include a new multi-element separation procedure coupled with neutron activation which enables the simultaneous determination of Cd, As, Sb, Se, Cu and Cr. As a test of the accuracy of results, previously certified NBS Standard Reference Materials were analyzed. The results are shown in tables 3 and 4. A second procedure currently under investigation will allow for the simultaneous determination of Hg, Pt, Pd, Au and Os. These multi-element techniques will greatly reduce the analytical cost when large numbers of samples are processed during the operation of the specimen bank.

A new research effort has begun on the quantitative determination of selected "classes" of trace organic materials. Due to the large number of individual organic compounds and their metabolic residues of interest in environmental samples, it was decided to devote initial efforts to developing a limited set of quantitative analytical procedures for selected classes of organic compounds. These will include chlorinated aliphatic and chlorinated aromatic compounds, phosphorus containing compounds, organo mercurial compounds and possible phthalates. These methods will then be used test for contamination or loss of organic compounds falling into the above "Classes" during extended sample storage.

Significant new challenges still exist in improving the measurement capability of trace constituents in samples of biological and environmental origin. This research at NBS will, in my opinion, result in improving upon the state-of-the-art methodology of the analysis of trace elements in biological and environmental samples.

References

1. Moody, J.R. and R. Lindstrom: Selection and Cleaning of Plastic Containers for Storage of Trace Element Samples.
   Anal. Chem. 49, 2264 (1977).

2. S.H. Harrison and P.D. Lafleur: Evaluation of Lyophilization for the Preconcentration of Natural Water Samples Prior to Neutron Activation.
   Anal. Chem. 45, 1534 (1973).

3. P.D. Lafleur: Retention of Mercury when Freeze-Drying Biological Materials.
   Anal. Chem. 45, 1534 (1973).

4. G.J. Lutz, J.S. Stemple, H.L. Rook: Evaluation by Activation Analysis of Elemental Retention in Biological Samples after Low Temperature Ashing.
   J. Radiological 39, 277 (1977).

Table I: Analyses of a Stored Bovine Liver - Storage and Analysis Protocol Tests
(Concentrations Reported on Dry Wt. Basis) μg/g

Sample Type	No. of Samples	Fe	Cu	Zn	Mo	Se	Co	As	Analysis Proced. Used
I. Subset Samples (+)	18	76 ± 7	68 ± 10	39 ± 3	.89 ± .12	.29 ± .05	.077 ± 0.006	4 ± 1	RNAA
II. Homogenate (*)	7	79 ± 4	69 ± 5	40 ± 2	.76 ± .04	.30 ± .05	.077 ± 0.005	6 ± 2	RNAA
III. Homogenate (+)	5	74 ± 6	69 ± 3	39 ± 3	.80 ± .05	.30 ± .03	.073 ± 0.003	6 ± 2	RNAA
IV. Subset Set	6	75 ± 4	--	39 ± 1	--	.29 ± .02	.075 ± 0.002	--	INAA
Average	36	76 ± 2	69 ± 1	39 ± 1	.82 ± .07	.29 ± .01	.075 ± .002	5 ± 1	
Error: Standard Deviations of Means									
III. Reanalysis after 1 yr (+,*)	6	69 ± 7	70 ± 2	38 ± 1	.82 ± .08	.27 ± .05	.076 ± 0.003	4 ± 1	RNAA

+ Fresh or Frozen Tissue
* Freeze-dried

Table 2: Techniques Available to SRM Program for Measurement of Traces

Conductimetry	Coulometry
Polarography	Potentiometry
Stripping Voltometry	Gas Mass Spectrometry
Isotopic Dilution Mass Spectometry	Spark Source Mass Spectrometry
Ultra micro chemistry	Electron Microscopy
Activation Analysis - fast neutron	Activation Analysis - LINAC
Activation Analysis - thermal neutron	Fission Track Techniques
Atomic Absorption & Fluorescence	Flame Emission Spectrometry
Optical Emission Spectrometry	Fluorimetry

Table 3: Determination of As, Sb, Se, Cr, Cd, and Cu in NBS Orchard Leaves and Bovine Liver. concentration in µg/g

Matrice   NBS SRM Orchard Leaves 1571   NBS SRM Bovine Liver 1577

Element	Certified Values	This Work	Certified Values	This Work
As	10 ± 2	9.7 ± 0.4	(0.055)	0.054 ± 0.004
Sb	2.9 ± 0.3	2.8 ± 0.1	(——)	0.010 ± 0.002
Se	0.08 ± 0.01	0.09 ± 0.01	1.1 ± 0.1	1.06 ± 0.06
Cr	2.60 ± 0.3	2.67 ± 0.15	0.090 ± 0.015	0.085 ± 0.009
Cd	0.11 ± 0.01	0.116 ± 0.008	0.27 ± 0.04	0.30 ± 0.02
Cu	12 ± 1	11.6 ± 0.4	193 ± 10	185 ± 7

Values in parenthesis are NBS information values.

M. Gallorini, R. Greenberg, T. Gills (1978). Procedure to be publish in Anal. Chem.

Table 4: Determination of As, Sb, Se, Cr, Cd, and Cu in NBS Subbituminous
          Coal SRM 1635

          concentration in µg/g

Matrice	NBS SRM Subbituminous Coal 1635	
Element	Certified Values	This Work
As	0.42 ± 0.15	0.44 ± 0.05
Sb	(0.14)	0.12 ± 0.01
Se	0.9 ± 0.3	0.82 ± 0.04
Cr	2.5 ± 0.3	2.48 ± 0.08
Cd	0.03 ± 0.01	0.029 ± 0.007
Cu	3.6 ± 0.3	3.56 ± 0.36

Values in parentheses are NBS information values.

M. Gallorini, R. Greenberg, T. Gills (1978). Procedure to be published in
Anal. Chem.

MONITORING ENVIRONMENTAL MATERIALS AND SPECIMEN BANKING
- STATE-OF-THE-ART OF JAPANESE EXPERIENCE AND KNOWLEDGE -

Miki Goto
Department of Chemistry
Gakushuin University
Tokyo, 171
Japan

ABSTRACT

The list of toxic chemicals is being made in the Environment Agency, which
will include about 5.ooo-6.ooo chemical substances. About 2.ooo of them
are to be selected from the standpoints of production amount, use pattern
and toxicity and submitted to screening tests for environmental survey
to examine degradability in the air, water and soil. Environmental survey
will then be performed on highly residual compounds at fixed survey points
in the country. Starting from 1974 Environment Agency is carrying out the
survey on the residues of selected chemicals in water, sediments and fishes
at about 5o monitoring places. The results of the survey in 1974FY, 1975FY
and 1976FY will be described in this paper.

The movement and transformation of chemicals in the environment is, however,
extremely complicated and it is therefore very difficult to predict the
kinds and levels of chemicals to be detected in the environment from the
statistics of consumption of chemcials and the data of ecological profile
analyses. Theréfore, a great effort should also be made on characterization
of hazardous compounds in environmental specimens. For this and for studying the trend of environmental contamination, the system to preserve specimens taken at fixed monitoring points for several decades should be established as soon as possible.

Survey on the residues of environmental chemicals has been performed since
1974 FY mainly be the Environment Agency. Survey was conducted on 33 chemicals at the estimated cost of 6o,21o thousand yen (approx. US$ 3oo,ooo,-)
in 1974 FY, and 78 chemicals at 95,4oo thousand yen (approx. US$ 48o,ooo,-)
in 1976 FY, that is, 153 chemicals were investigated in total for 3 years
by 26 Prefectural Laboratories for Pollution Studies (for monitoring
points, see Fig.1). The chemicals selected were mainly (1) those already
regulated by laws because of their toxicity, (2) those of low degradability and (3) those similar in chemical structure to substances such as
PCB which had previously caused environmental pollution or their substitutes. Survey was conducted chiefly on the water and sediment, but organisms
were also investigated when fishes and shellfishes were living at survey
points.

Sampling Methods

Since the purpose of environmental survey is to quantitatively grasp the distribution of residual chemicals in the environment, sampling points were placed at city rivers in densely populated areas and regions not directly polluted in manufacturing areas. The number of samples taken at survey points was as follows:

	Survey Points	the Number of Samples	the Total Number of Samples
Water	4	5	2o
Sediment	2	5	1o
Organisms	2	5	1o

In sampling of water and sediment, sampling points should be scattered as uniformly as possible within a 5o m radius. In sampling of organisms, those of the same species are collected within a 25o m radius.

1. <u>Sampling of water:</u> Samples are taken from rivers, lakes and marshes when the quality of water is stable after a long spell of fine weather. Sampling point is placed on the center of flow at a survey point and the surface water (o-5o cm below the surface) is collected. After the removel of rabbish, etc., samples are allowed to stand for about a day at dark place and supernatant solutions are used for analysis. Treatments using filter paper and centrifuge are not performed.

2. <u>Sampling of sediment:</u> Sediment is collected by Ekman-Birge bottom sampler or its equivalents, placed in a clean tray and sieved through No. 9 sieve (2 mm), if necessary, after the removal of foreign matters such as pebbles, shells and fragments of animals and plants. A part of the sample is weighed after drying (1o5-11o°, 2 h.). When sediment contains much water, it is allowed to stand on 3 pieces of superposed filter paper or gauze for 24 hours to eliminate suspended moisture and used for analysis (as a rule, air-drying or heat-drying is not applied).

3. <u>Sampling of fishes and shellfishes:</u> Fishes, crustaceans and shellfishes undergoing reproduction at survey points are collected as samples, regardless of species. Small organisms are washed fully and used for analysis. In fishes, edible portions (muscles) are taken as samples. About 1oo g or more of edible portion is sliced off from any part of a fish and homogenized. In fishes weighing 1oo g or less, sample is prepared by collecting edible portions of several fishes and homogenizing them. In still smaller fishes, sample is prepared by weighing 1oo g or more of complete fishes and submitted to analysis after homogenization. In shellfishes, edible portions corresponding to a desired weight are gathered and homogenized when the mud contained in shellfishes should be removed as much as possible.

<u>Survey Results:</u>

The chemicals investigated were phthalic acid esters, organochlorines, such as DDT and BHC and heavy metals in 1974 FY, organo-chloric solvents such as hexachlorobenzene, trichloromethane, and trichloroethylene, chlorinated benzenes, organo-phosphoric compounds, substitutes of PCB and heavy metals in 1975 FY.

The survey results are shown in Table 1 (1974 FY) and in Table 2 (1975 FY). Analytical results are expressed in μg/ml. The weights expressed are those after drying for sediment and those containing moisture for organisms. Those below the lower limit of detection are expressed in such a way, for example, < o.oo1 ppm.

In 1976 FY, 78 substances were investigated using 4937 water samples, 4o57 sediment samples, 544 fishes and shellfishes samples and 23o air samples, resulting in 4o substances detected and 38 substances undetectable from all the samples. It is to be noted that 6 of 13 PCB substitutes investigated were detected from the environment though these are used as raw materials in the chemical industry and are scarcely used directly as products in the environment. In addition, 1o of 12 aromatic nitro-compounds examined were detected from the environment and especially nitrobenzene and nitrotoluene were identified at high rates. Environmental pollution due to aniline compounds in and around large cities, suggesting that this pollution was not caused directly, but caused secondarily through the consumption of fine chemicals such as pharmaceuticals and dyestuffs or degradation of natural products including foods. Dibutylhydroxytoluene (BHT)* was always detected from the sediment of the aquatic environment in large cities in the range of o.87-1.69 ppm). Fron 11 and Fron 12** were detected at high rates from the air over cities. The survey results are summarized in Table 3.

Discussion

The environmental survey described above has a character of semi-quantitative analyses as the methodology in different laboratories was not always unified. The results show, however, the complexity of the behavior of chemicals in the environment. It is very difficult to predict the kinds and levels of chemicals to be detected in the environment (in air, water, sediment and organisms) from the statistics of consumption of chemicals and the data of simple biodegradation and bioaccumulation tests. The development of more sophisticated ecotoxicological profile analyses is very important; some useful procedures can be seen in the literature.

The above mentioned survey is based on the samples collected at present point of time and the number of measured compounds is only about 2oo. The survey should be performed on highly residual compounds including conversion products. For this purpose the studies on identification and determination of unknown pollutants in water, sediments and fishes are now being carried out. By a preliminary experiment using GC-MS it was shown that the fishes in Tokyo Bay and Sagami Bay (wellfish, croaker, gray mullet, young sea bass, etc.) are proved to be contaminated with at least 6o chemicals.
The study on environmental survey should be folbwed up with the passage of time and the system to preserve organisms taken at fixed survey points should be established.

REFERENCES

Chemicals in the Environment, The Report of Environmental Survey of Chemicals in 1976 F.Y., Japan, Ed. by M. Fujii, published by Environment Agency, Office of Health Studies. Report Series No. 3/1977, October 1977 (in Japanese).

---

* In Japan, 8ooo t of this compound is produced in a year and used as antioxidant for foods, oils, systhetic rubbers and plastics.

** This compounds are used as refrigerant for refrigerator and freezer, spraying agent for cosmetic hair spray and blowing agent for urethane foam.

Table 1 Environmental Survey of Chemicals in 1974 FY.

Name of Substance	Sample	A/B	Scope	Detection Limit
Di-ethylhexyl-phthalate (DEHP)	Water	176/375	$\sim$ 15	< o.1
	Sediment	224/37o	$\sim$ 17	< o.o5$\sim$ o.1
	Fish	92/332	$\sim$ 19	< o.1
	Rainwater	61/111	$\sim$ 13	< o.1
	Plankton	1/4	$\sim$ 6.3	
Di-*n*-butyl-phthalate (DNBP)	Water	2o8/375	$\sim$ 36	
	Sediment	154/37o	$\sim$ 2.3	
	Fish	114/332	$\sim$ 2.o	
	Rainwater	68/111	$\sim$ 52	
	Plankton	o/4		
Di-*iso*-heptyl-phthalate (DIHP)	Water	23/375	$\sim$ o.8	
	Sediment	3o/35o	$\sim$ 6.5	
	Fish	13/312	$\sim$ o.4	
	Rainwater	22/111	$\sim$ 8.5	
	Plankton	o/4		
Di-*n*-octyl-phthalate (DNOP)	Water	4/355	$\sim$ 41	
	Sediment	3/331	$\sim$ 4.4	
	Fish	o/292	–	
	Rainwater	1/1o5	$\sim$ 12	
	Plankton	o/4		
Di-*iso*-decyl-phthalate (DIDP)	Water	o/25o		
	Sediment	o/227		
	Fish	o/2oo		
	Rainwater	o/73		
	Plankton	o/2		
Di-*iso*-btyl-phthalate (DIBP)	Water	38/375	$\sim$ 12	
	Sediment	57/35o	$\sim$ 3.7	
	Fish	22/312	$\sim$ o.5	
	Rainwater	11/111	$\sim$ 34	
	Plankton	o/4		

A: No. of detection B: No. of samples

Table 1   (continued)

Name of Substance	Sample	A/B	Scope	Direction Limit
p,p'-DĐT	Water	o/55		< o.1
	Sediment	2o/5o	∿ o.oo73	< o.o1
	Fish	7/49	∿ o.oo13	< o.oo5
p,p'-DDE	Water	o/55	–	
	Sediment	22/5o	∿ o.oo79	
	Fish	43/49	∿ o.131	
p,p'-DDD	Water	o/55	–	
	Sediment	2o/5o	∿ o.o15	
	Fish	25/49	∿ o.o15	
o,p'-DDT	Water	o/55	–	
	Sediment	o/5o	–	
	Fish	6/49	∿ o.oo21	
α–HCH	Water	3/6o	∿ o.1	< o.1
	Sediment	5/6o	∿ o.o1	< o.o1
	Fish	16/6o	∿ o.o15	< o.oo5
β–HCH	Water	o/6o	–	
	Sediment	9/6o	∿ o.o5	
	Fish	2/6o	∿ o.oo7	
γ–HCH	Water	o/6o	–	
	Sediment	9/6o		
	Fish	2/6o	∿ o.o13	
δ–HCH	Water	o/6o	–	
	Sediment	4/6o	∿ o.o1	
	Fish	o/6o	–	
Dieldrin and aldrin etc.,	Water	o/6o	–	< o.1
	Sediment	o/6o	–	< o.o1
	Fish	o/6o		< o.oo5
HCB	Water	o/6o		< o.1
	Sediment	o/6o		< o.o1
	Fish	4/6o	o.oo7	< o.oo5

A: No. of detection   B: No. of samples

276

Table 1 (continued)

Name of Substance	Sample	A/B	Scope	Detection Limit
PCP	Water	2/55	∿ o.2o	< o.1
	Sediment	1o/5o	∿ o.36	< o.o5
PCT	Water	o/6o		< o.1
	Sediment	o/6o		< o.o5
	Bird	3/11	∿ o.12	< o.1
Mn	Water	45/6o	∿ o.o8	< o.oo5
	Sediment	6o/6o	55∿ 1.3oo	< 5o
	Fish	4o/4o	o.23∿ 63	< o.1
Se	Water	12/6o	∿ o.ooo2	< o.ooo2
	Sediment	36/6o	∿ o.19	< o.o1
	Fish	4o/4o	o.o4∿ o.87	< o.o1
V	Water	1/6o	∿ o.o2	< o.o2
	Sediment	6o/6o	6.o∿ 275	< 1
	Fish	o/4o		< 1
Ni	Water	17/6o	∿ o.o11	< o.oo1
	Sediment	59/59	1.6 ∿35	< 1
	Fish	51/6o	∿ 3.1	< o.o1
Sn	Water	o/6o		< o.o5
	Sediment	39/59	∿ 21o	< 1
	Fish	2o/6o	∿ 6.7	< 1
Fluorine	Water	3o/6o	∿ o.7	< o.1.
	Sediment	59/59	28∿ 188	
	Fish	47/59	∿ 113	< 1
Surface active agent	water	26/6o	o.16	o.o5
CHCI$_3$	Water	21/6o	∿ 7o	< 1
	Rainwater	6/18	∿ 118	
C$_2$HCI$_3$	Water	o/6o		< 1
	Rainwater	o/18		
C$_2$CI$_4$	Water	5/6o	∿ 3	< 1
	Rainwater	o/18		
C$_2$H$_3$CI$_3$	Water	o/6o		< 1
	Rainwater	o/18		
CCI$_4$	Water	o/6o		< o.1
	Rainwater	o/18		

A: No. of detection   B: No. of Samples

Table 1-1

Phthalic Acid Esters in Rivers of Various Type Cities
in 1974 FY.

Test Material	Location of River	Di-ethylhexylphthalte			Di-n-butylphthalate		
		A/B	Scope	Average	A/B	Scope	Average
Water (μg/1)	Large City	40/60	∿ 2.4	o.54	49/60	∿36	3.o6
	Medium City	28/75	∿ o.5	o.1o	42/75	∿ o.6	o.16
	Small City	24/8o	∿ o.8	o.12	53/8o	∿ 9	o.88
	Industr.City	53/8o	∿15	2.19	32/8o	∿ 4.4	o.59
	Others	31/8o	∿ 8	o.39	33/8o	∿ 2.1	o.31
Sediment (μg/g)	Large City	48/58	∿ 3.o	o.68	32/58	∿ o.4	o.o7
	Medium City	3o/73	∿ 3.2	o.17	21/73	∿ o.6	o.o3
	Small City	29/79	∿ 1.4	o.o8	24/79	∿ o.3	o.o2
	Industr.City	73/8o	∿17	1.36	56/8o	∿ 2.3	o.26
	Others	44/8o	∿ 2.o	o.11	27/8o	∿ o.3	o.o4
Fish (μg/g)	Large City	8/42	∿ o.4	o.o5	9/42	∿ 1.2	o.14
	Medium City	24/7o	∿ 1.1	o.11	3o/7o	∿ 1.o	o.1o
	Small City	16/8o	∿ 1.4	o.11	25/8o	∿ o.9	o.13
	Industr.City	28/6o	∿ 2.9	o.34	23/6o	∿ o.7	o.o4
	Others	16/8o	∿ 1.9	o.72	27/8o	∿ 2.o	o.23
Rainwater (μg/1)	Large City	16/18	∿ 6.8	1.51	9/18	∿ 9.2	2.47
	Medium City	11/2o	∿ 3.4	o.77	2o/2o	∿1o	1.55
	Small City	6/24	∿ 7.1	o.76	9/24	∿ o.6	o.12
	Industr.City	2o/25	∿ 8.7	3.16	18/25	∿52	8.58
	Others	18/24	∿ 1.3	o.65	12/26	∿25	4.68

A: No. of detection   B: No. of samples

Table 2   Environmental Survey of Chemicals in 1975 FY.

Water (μg/1)

Name of Substance	A/B	Scope	Detection limit
HCB	o/39o		<o.oo1∿<o.o1
Trichloromethane	86/395	∿ 17	<o.o8∿ <1
Trichloroethylene	75/395	∿ 12	<o.2∿ <1
Tetrachloroethylene	73/395	∿ 9.5	<o.o6∿ <o.2
1,1,1-trichloroethane	43/395	∿ 5.4	<o.o5∿ <o.4
Carbon tetrachloride	lo.5/355	∿ 1.o	<o.o1∿ <o.3
o-Dichlorobenzene	o/95		<o.3∿ <3
m-Dichlorobenzene	o/95		<o.1∿ <2
p-Dichlorobenzene	2/95	∿ 1.o	<o.3∿ <3
1,2,3-Trichlorobenzene	o/95		<o.o8∿ <o.3
1,3,4-Trichlorobenzene	o/95		<o.o3∿ <o.4
1,3,5-Trichlorobenzene	o/95		<o.o2∿ <o.2
1,2,3,4-Tetrachlorobenzene	o/loo		<o.o5
1,2,3,5-Tetrachlorobenzene	o/loo		<o.o5
1,2,4,5-Tetrachlorobenzene	o/loo		<o.o5
Pentachlorobenzene	o/loo		<o.o1
Tributylphosphate	16/loo	∿ o.71	<o.o1∿ <o.1
Tris(dichloropropyl)phosphate	o/loo		<o.o2∿ <o.25
Triphenyl phosphate	o/loo		<o.o2∿ <o.25
Tributoxyethyl phosphate	o/loo		<o.o2∿ <o.5o
Trioctylphosphate	o/loo		<o.o4∿ <o.5o
Tricredylphosphate	o/loo		<o.o5∿ <1.5
Tris(dibromopropyl)phosphate	o/2o		<lo
Trichloroethyl phosphate	8/4o	∿ o.34	<o.o15∿<o.lo
Diisopropylnaphthalene	o/loo		<o.17∿ <5
1-Phenyl-1-(3,4-dimethylphenyl)-ethane	o/loo		<o.13∿ <5
Acrylamide	o/95		<1
Formaldehyde	o/loo		<loo∿ <5oo
Terephthalic acid	6/loo	∿ o.7	<o.o2∿ <5
Dimethyl terephthalate	1/loo	∿ o.16	<o,oo2∿<o.5
o-Chloronitrobenzene	o/95		<o.1∿
m-Chloronitrobenzene	o/95		<o.1∿
Organic tin compounds	o/8o		<lo ∿ <25
Vinyl chloride	5/loo	∿ o.1	<o.o5∿ <4o
Total phthalates	54/115	∿ 77	<o.o1∿ <lo
Di-n-butyl phthalate	75/115	∿ 21	<o.o1∿ <3
Diethylhexyl phthalate	58/115	∿ 1.1	<o.1∿ <3
Total cobalt	o/loo		<lo∿
Total Sb	o/loo		<lo∿ <loo
Total Ti	69/loo	∿7oo	<2 ∿ <5
Total Te	2o/8o	∿ 7o	<2 ∿ <lo
Total TI	26/95	∿ 1	<o.o1∿ <2

A: No. of detection   B: No. of samples

Table 2   (continued)

Sediment (μg/g)

Name of Substance	A/B	Scope	Detection Limit
HCB	37/399	$\sim$ 0.12	<0.0001 $\sim$ <0.005
o-Dichlorobenzene	0/95		<0.02 $\sim$ <0.5
m-Dichlorobenzene	3/95	$\sim$ 0.05	<0.01 $\sim$ <0.5
p-Dichlorobenzene	1/95	$\sim$ 0.03	<0.02 $\sim$ <0.5
1,2,3-Trichlorobenzene	0/95		<0.002 $\sim$ <0.1
1,2,4-Trichlorobenzene	3/95	$\sim$ 0.022	<0.002 $\sim$ <0.1
1,3,5-Trichlorobenzene	0/95		<0.001 $\sim$ <0.1
1,2,3,4-Tetrachlorobenzene	0/100		<0.05
1,2,3,5-Tetrachlorobenzene	0/100		<0.05
1,2,4,5-Tetrachlorobenzene	0/100		<0.05
Pentachlorobenzene	0/100		<0.01
Tributyl phosphate	34/100	$\sim$ 0.350	<0.001 $\sim$ <0.025
Tris(dichloropropyl)phosphate	0/100		<0.002 $\sim$ <0.05
Triphenylphosphate	0/100		<0.002 $\sim$ <0.05
Tributoxyethyl phosphate	7/80	$\sim$ 0.54	<0.002 $\sim$ <0.10
Trioctylphosphate	3/100	$\sim$ 0.100	<0.05 $\sim$ <0.10
Tricredyl phosphate	1/100	$\sim$ 0.15	<0.01 $\sim$ <0.25
Tris(dibromopropyl)phosphate	0/20		<0.4
Trichloroethyl phosphate	1/20	$\sim$ 0.070	<0.025
Diisopropylnaphthalene	9/100	$\sim$ 0.19	<0.03 $\sim$ <0.25
1-Phenyl-1-(3,4-dimethylphenyl-ethane)	13/100	$\sim$ 0.089	<0.025 $\sim$ <0.25
Total Co	76/80	$\sim$15.9	<1.0
Total Sb	0/95		<1.0
Total Ti	100/100	120$\sim$6800	
Total Te	20/80	$\sim$ 4.78	<0.8 $\sim$ <3
Total TI	46/100	$\sim$ 3.6	<0.016 $\sim$ <0.6

A: No. of detection   B: No. of samples

280

Table 2   (continued)

Fish and shellfish (µg/g)

Name of the Substance	A/B	Scope	Detection Limit	
HCB	11o/369	∿ o.o28	<o.ooo1	∿ <o.oo5
o-Dichlorobenzene	o/75		<o.o5	∿ <o.5
m-Dichlorobenzene	o/75		<o.o2	∿ <o.5
p-Dichlorobenzene	o/75		<o.o5	∿ <o.5
1,2,3-Trichlorobenzene	o/75		<o.oo5	∿ <o.1
1,2,4-Trichlorobenzene	2/75	∿ o.2	<o.oo5	∿ <o.1
1,3,5-Trichlorobenzene	o/75		<o.oo3	∿ <o.1
1,2,3,4-Tetrachlorobenzene	o/95		<o.o5	
1,2,3,5-Tetrachlorobenzene	o/95		<o.o5	
1,2,4,5-Tetrachlorobenzene	o/95		<o.o5	
Pentachlorobenzene	3/95	∿ o.o38	<o.o1	
Tributyl phosphate	31/94	∿ o.o26	<o.oo2	∿ <o.oo25
Tris(dichloropropyl)phosphate	7/94	∿ o.o25	<o.oo5	∿ <o.o5
Triphenyl phosphate	o/1oo		<o.oo5	∿ <o.o5
Tributoxyethyl phosphate	o/74		<o.oo5	∿ <o.1o
Trioctyl phosphate	o/94		<o.o1	∿ <o.1o
Tricredyl phosphate	o/96		<o.o2	∿ <o.25
Tris(dibromopropyl)phosphate	o/2o		<1	
Trichlorethyl phosphate	o/2o		<o.o25	
Diisopropylnaphthalene	2/94	∿ o.o48	<o.o25	∿ <o.25
1-phenyl-1-(3,4-dimethylphenyl)ethane	o/94		<o.o2	∿ <o.25
Total Co	2/75	∿ o.2	<o.1	∿ <1
Total Sb	8/75	∿ o.48	<o.1	∿ <1
Total Ti	5o/1oo	∿ 3.15	<o.o5	∿ <o.1
Total Te	2o/75	∿ 4.o4	<o.o5	∿ <o.4
Total Tl	37/1oo	∿ o.93	<o.oo1	∿ <o.2

A: No. of detection   B: No. of samples

Table 2-1

Chemicals in River Water in Cities, 1975 FY

	Test Material	Location of River	A/B	Scope	Detection Limit
Hexachlorobenzene	Water (µg/l)	Large City	o/75		<o.oo5
		Medium City	o/8o		<o.oo2 ~ <o.oo5
		Small City	o/8o		<o.ool ~ <o.oo5
		Industr.City	o/8o		<o.oo5 ~ <o.ol
		Others	o/75		<o.oo5
	Sediment (µg/g)	Large City	5/8o	~ o.ol6	<o.oo5
		Medium City	17/8o	~ o.oo9	<o.ooo19 ~<o.oo5
		Small City	8/8o	~ o.oo3	<o.ooo1 ~ <o.oo5
		Industr. City	7/8o	~ o.12	<o.oo5
		Others	o/79		<o.oo5
	Biological quality (µg/g)	Large City	15/75	~ o.ol4	<o.oo5
		Medium City	39/8o	~ o.o28	<o.ool ~ <o.oo5
		Small City	25/8o	~ o.olo5	<o.ooo1 ~ <o.oo5
		Industr. City	2o/6o	~ o.oo4	<o.ool ~ <o.oo5
		Others	1/74		<o.oo5
Trichloromethane	Water (µg/l)	Large City	35/75	~17	<o.2 ~ <1
		Medium City	18/8o	~ 8.9	< o.2
		Small City	11/8o	~ 1.o	<o.2 ~ <o.4
		Industr. City	2o/8o	~ 1.5	<o.1 ~ <o.2
		Others	2/8o	~ o.3	<o.o8 ~ <o.2
	Rainwater (µg/l)	Large City	8/24	~43	<o.2 ~ <1
		Medium City	8/24	~11.2	<o.2
		Small City	1/24	~ o.5	<o.2 ~ <o.5
		Industr. City	7/18	~ 7.1	<o.1 ~ <o.2
		Others	1/24	~ o.1 -	<o.o8 ~ <o.2

A: No. of detection   B: No. of samples

282

Table 2-1 (continued)

	Test Material	Location of River	A/B	Scope	Detection Limit
Tetrachloroethylene	Water (μg/1)	Large City	35/75	∿ 12	<o.2 ∿ <1
		Medium City	5/8o	∿ 2.5	<o.2 ∿ <o.3
		Small City	o/8o		<o.2 ∿ <1
		Industr.City	35/8o	∿ 12	<o.2
		Others City	o/8o		<o.2
	Rainwater (μg/1)	Large City	1/24	∿ 1	<o.2 ∿ <1
		Medium City	o/24		<o.2 ∿ <o.3
		Small City	o/24		<o.2 ∿ <1
		Industr.City	o/18		<o.1 ∿ <o.2
		Others City	1/24	∿ o.2	<o.2
Tetrachloroethylene	Water (μg/1)	Large City	3o/75	∿ 9.5	<o.2
		Medium City	5/8o	∿ 5.4	<o.1 ∿ <o.2
		Small City	o/8o		<o.2
		Industr.City	31/8o	∿ 6.9	<o.2
		Others City	7/8o	∿ o.2	<o.o6 ∿ <o.2
	Rainwater (μg/1)	Large City	3/24	∿ o.3	<o.2
		Medium City	o/24		<o.1 ∿ <o.2
		Small City	o/24		<o.2
		Industr.City	o/18		<o.2
		Others City	o/24		<o.o6 ∿ <o.2
1,1,1-trichloroethane	Water (μg/1)	Large City	19/75	∿ 2.5	<o.1 ∿ <o.4
		Medium City	7/8o	∿ o.81	<o.1
		Small City	o/8o		<o.1 ∿ <o.2
		Industr.City	1o/8o	∿ 5.1	<o.1
		Others City	7/8o	∿ o.1	<o.o5 ∿ <o.1
1,1,1-trichloroethane	Rainwater (μg/1)	Large	o/24		<o.1 ∿ <o.4
		Medium	o/24		<o.1
		Small	o/24		<o.1 ∿ <o.2
		Industr.	o/18		<o.1
		Others	o/24		<o.o5 ∿ <o.1

A: No. of detection   B: No. of samples

Table 2-1　(continued)

	Test Material	Location of River	A/B	Scope	Detection Limit
Carbon tetrachloride	Water (µg/1)	Large City	32/75	∿ o.9	<o.o2 ∿ o.3
		Medium City	31/8o	∿ o.44	<o.o2
		Small City	o/8o		<o.o2
		Industr. City	4o/8o	∿ o.21	<o.o1 ∿ o.o2
		Others	2/6o	∿ o.o2	<o.o2
	Rainwater (µg/1)	Large City	2/24	∿ 3.6	<o.o2 ∿ o.3
		Medium City	8/24	∿ 3.o	<o.o2
		Small City	1/24	∿ o.o4	<o.o2
		Industr. City	6/18	∿ o.6	<o.o2
		Others	o/18		<o.o2

A: No. of detection　　B: No. of samples

Table 3 Environmental Survey of Chemicals in 1976 FY.

Name of Substance	Water (μg/m)			Sediment (μg/m)			Fish and Shellfish (μg/g)		
	A/B	Scope	Detection limit	A/B	Scope	Detection limit	A/B	Scope	Detection limit
1 Biphenyl	0/68		<0.0002 ~ <0.01	0/50		<0.05 ~ <1.0	0/20		<0.04 ~ <0.25
2 Ethylbiphenyl	0/68		<0.0006 ~ <0.02	0/50		<0.16 ~ <2.0	0/20		<0.12 ~ <0.50
3 Diethylbiphenyl	0/68		<0.0008 ~ <0.02	0/50		<0.2 ~ <2.0	0/20		<0.10 ~ <0.50
4 Triethylbiphenyl	0/68		<0.0035 ~ <0.05	0/50		<0.5 ~ <5.0	0/20		<0.70 ~ <20
5 Biphenyl ether	0/88		<0.0006 ~ <0.005	0/28		<0.1 ~ <0.74	0/20		<0.15 ~ <0.25
6 o-Terphenyl	0/68		<0.000004 ~ <0.025	15/63	0.00075 ~ 0.39	<0.00019 ~ <0.025	0/1		<0.05
7 m-Terphenyl	0/68		<0.000013 ~ <0.125	31/63	0.001 ~ 0.21	<0.001 ~ <1.25	0/1		<0.25
8 p-Terphenyl	0/68		<0.000025 ~ <0.125	21/63	0.001 ~ 0.18	<0.0015 ~ <1.25	0/1		<0.25
9 Polychloro-terphenyl(PCT)	0/156		<0.00001 ~ <0.0025	21/150	0.001 ~ 0.33	<0.001 ~ <0.2	0/39		<0.001 ~ <0.2
10 α-Methylnaphthalene	0/28		<0.0002 ~ <0.001	0/28		<0.02 ~ <0.1			
11 β-Methylnaphthalene	0/28		<0.0002 ~ <0.001	0/28		<0.02 ~ <0.1			
12 Polychloro-naphthalene (PCN)	4/143	0.00010 ~ 0.00045	<0.00002 ~ <0.002	23/138	0.005 ~ 0.47	<0.004 ~ <0.2	1/39	0.35	<0.0005 ~ <0.005
13 Dodecachlorododeca-hydrodimetano-dibenzocyclooctene	4/60	0.0004 ~ 0.0006	<0.0003 ~ <0.0005	0/53		<0.010 ~ <0.03	0/2		<0.015
14 α-Naphthylamin	0/60		<0.0001 ~ <0.0007	7/60	0.007 ~ 0.046	<0.003 ~ <0.01			
15 1,2-Dichloroethane	0/60		<0.04 ~ <0.2	0/40		<1.0 ~ <13	0/10		<8.7
16 1,1,2-Trichloro-ethane	0/60		<0.004 ~ <0.05	0/39		<0.3 ~ <1.0	0/10		<0.4
17 1,1,2,2-Tetrachloro-ethane	0/60		<0.001 ~ <0.05	0/39		<0.05 ~ <1.0	0/10		<0.2
18 Hexachloroethane	0/60		<0.0001 ~ <0.005	0/39		<0.01 ~ <0.3	0/10		<0.3

A: No. of detection   B: No. of samples

Table 3 (continued)

Name of Substance	Water (µg/m)			Sediment (µg/m)			Fish and Shellfish (µg/g)		
	A/B	Scope	Detection limit	A/B	Scope	Detection limit	A/B	Scope	Detection limit
19 1,2-Dichloropropane	0/60		<0.04 ~ <0.3	0/39		<1.0 ~ <20	0/10		<8.7
20 1,2,3-Trichloro-propane	0/60		<0.01 ~ <0.02	0/39		<0.2 ~ <2	0/10		<2.4
21 2-Metoxyethanol	0/60		<0.09 ~ <0.1	0/20		<0.4			
22 2-Ethoxyethanol	0/60		<0.09 ~ <0.1	0/20		<0.4			
23 2-Butoxyethanol	0/60		<0.09 ~ <0.1	0/20		<0.4			
24 Dioxane	0/60		<0.1	0/20		<0.4			
25 Aniline	40/68	0.00002 ~ 0.028	<0.00004 ~ <0.0002	48/68	0.0007 ~ 0.50	<0.0008			
26 N-Methylaniline	0/68		<0.00008 ~ <0.0006	11/68	0.003 ~ 0.012	<0.002 ~ <0.008			
27 N,N-Dimethylaniline	2/68	0.0011 ~ 0.0017	<0.0003 ~ <0.0024	6/68	0.011 ~ 0.21	<0.006 ~ <0.05			
28 N-Ethylaniline	2/68	0.00043 ~ 0.0017	<0.0001 ~ <0.0006	20/68	0.002 ~ 0.038	<0.002 ~ <0.008			
29 o-Chloroaniline	12/120	0.000028 ~ 0.00035	<0.00002 ~ <0.1	29/113	0.0007 ~ 0.098	<0.0003 ~ <1.0	0/2		<1.0
30 m-Chloroaniline	10/128	0.000013 ~ 0.00034	<0.00001 ~ <0.1	34/121	0.0003 ~ 0.038	<0.0001 ~ <1.0	0/2		<1.0
31 p-Chloroaniline	9/128	0.000024 ~ 0.00039	<0.00002 ~ <0.1	39/121	0.001 ~ 0.27	<0.0005 ~ <1.0	0/2		<1.0
32 2,4-Dichloroaniline	7/68	0.000032 ~ 0.00053	<0.00002 ~ <0.0003	12/68	0.0050 ~ 0.034	<0.0005 ~ <0.001			
33 3,4-Dichloroaniline	4/68	0.00024 ~ 0.00042	<0.00004 ~ <0.0003	31/68	0.0045 ~ 0.11	<0.0008 ~ <0.003			
34 o-Toluidine	8/68	0.00014 ~ 0.020	<0.0001 ~ <0.0006	27/68	0.002 ~ 0.072	<0.002 ~ <0.012			
35 m-Toluidine	4/68	0.000096 ~ 0.00026	<0.00008 ~ <0.0002	32/68	0.002 ~ 0.056	<0.001 ~ <0.004			
36 p-Toluidine	11/68	0.00004 ~ 0.00018	<0.00002 ~ <0.0002	35/68	0.0007 ~ 0.090	<0.0004 ~ <0.0008			
37 o-Anisidine	6/68	0.00020 ~ 0.0013	<0.0002 ~ <0.0008	27/68	0.0083 ~ 0.55	<0.003 ~ <0.004			

A: No. of detection   B: No. of samples

Table 3 (continued)

Name of Substance	Water (μg/m)			Sediment (μg/m)			Fish and Shellfish (μg/g)		
	A/B	Scope	Detection limit	A/B	Scope	Detection limit	A/B	Scope	Detection limit
38 m-Anisidine	3/68	0.000016 ~ 0.000028	<0.00001 ~ <0.0002	6/68	0.0004 ~ 0.018	<0.0002 ~ <0.0016			
39 p-Anisidine	4/68	0.00006 ~ 0.00072	<0.00006 ~ <0.0002	12/68	0.001 ~ 0.006	<0.0007 ~ <0.004			
40 2,3-Xylidin	0/68		<0.0001 ~ <0.001	6/68	0.006 ~ 0.090	<0.001 ~ <0.006			
41 2,5-Xylidin	0/68		<0.0002 ~ <0.0005	2/68	0.006 ~ 0.027	<0.001 ~ <0.004			
42 3,4-Xylidin	0/68		<0.00006 ~ <0.0007	8/68	0.001 ~ 0.043	<0.001 ~ <0.004			
43 3,5-Xylidin	1/68	0.00004	<0.00002 ~ <0.0002	5/68	0.002 ~ 0.01	<0.005 ~ <0.0016			
44 Nitrobenzene	27/70	0.0001 ~ 0.0014	<0.00003 ~ <0.0004	15/47	0.005 ~ 1.9	<0.002 ~ <0.0035	10/10	0.003 ~ 0.58	
45 o-Nitrotoluene	3/70	0.00015 ~ 0.00079	<0.00003 ~ <0.0002	16/50	0.02 ~ 0.14	<0.0002 ~ <0.002	0/10		<0.002
46 m-Nitrotoluene	3/70	0.00035 ~ 0.00086	<0.00005 ~ <0.0002	2/50	0.014 ~ 0.019	<0.004 ~ <0.01	0/10		<0.004
47 p-Nitrotoluene	1/70	0.0001	<0.00003 ~ <0.0004	3/59	0.011 ~ 0.038	<0.002 ~ <0.01	0/10		<0.002
48 o-Nitroanisol	3/70	0.000035 ~ 0.00069	<0.000025 ~ <0.0004	1/58	0.010	<0.001 ~ <0.01	0/10		<0.002
49 m-Nitroanisol	5/62	0.0001 ~ 0.0016	<0.00005 ~ <0.0001	1/50	0.015	<0.003 ~ <0.004	0/10		<0.004
50 p-Nitroanisol	0/70		<0.00008 ~ <0.0002	0/59		<0.006 ~ <0.02	1/10	0.013	<0.006
51 o-Dinitrobenzene	0/70		<0.00005	1/54	0.0008	<0.0002 ~ <0.01	0/10		<0.004
52 m-Dinitrobenzene	0/70		<0.0001 ~ <0.00025	1/51	0.03	<0.007 ~ <0.02	0/10		<0.01
53 2,4-Dinitrotoluene	0/70		<0.00008 ~ <0.0001	0/50		<0.003 ~ <0.01	0/10		<0.006
54 2,6-Dinitrotoluene	1/70	0.000054	<0.000025 ~ <0.00003	3/55	0.003 ~ 0.050	<0.0007 ~ <0.002	0/10		<0.002

A: No. of detection   B: No. of samples

Table 3 (continued)

Name of Substance	Water (µg/m) A/B	Scope	Detection limit	Sediment (µg/m) A/B	Scope	Detection limit	Fish and Shellfish (µg/g) A/B	Scope	Detection limit
55 3,4-Dinitrotoluene	0/70		<0.00005 ~ <0.000075	0/59		<0.002 ~ <0.004	0/10		<0.004
56 1,2,3-Trimethylbenzene	0/20		<0.0001	0/20		<0.01			
57 1,2,4-Trimethylbenzene	0/20		<0.0001	0/20		<0.01			
58 1,3,5-Trimethylbenzene	0/20		<0.0001	0/20		<0.01			
59 Dibutylhydroxy toluene (BHT)	0/68		<0.0004 ~ <0.005	10/68	0.066 ~ 1.69	<0.01 ~ <0.04			
60 p-ter-Butylphenol	0/68		<0.0002 ~ <0.005	0/68		<0.01 ~ <0.25			
61 2,2-Bis(4-hydroxy-phenyl)propane	0/60		<0.00005 ~ <0.0001	0/50		<0.0002 ~ <0.005	0/10		<0.005
62 Chlorobenzene	0/68		<0.04 ~ <0.2	0/61		<0.5 ~ <4	0/2		
63 Benzyl chloride	0/60		<0.03 ~ <0.1	0/53		<0.4 ~ <1.0	0/2		
64 Carbazol	0/20		<0.0002	0/20		<0.02			
65 Diphenylamine	0/80		<0.0006 ~ <0.005	0/20		<0.20 ~ <0.74	0/20		<0.15 ~ <0.25
66 N-Phenyl-2-naphthyl-amine	0/50		<0.003 ~ <0.04	0/40		<0.13 ~ <0.8	0/20		<0.3 ~ <1.0
67 Naphthalene	0/20		<0.0001	0/20		<0.01			
68 Anthracene	0/20		<0.0001	4/20	0.01 ~ 0.23	<0.01			
69 Methylbromide	0/60		<0.0018 ~ <0.019	0/40		<0.024 ~ <0.95	0/20		<0.012 ~ <0.05
70 Bromochloromethane	0/60		<0.0002 ~ <0.001	0/40		<0.005 ~ <0.065	0/20		<0.005 ~ <0.010
71 Tribromomethane	0/60		<0.0002 ~ <0.026	0/40		<0.005 ~ <0.39	0/20		<0.005 ~ <0.006
72 Ethyl bromide	0/60		<0.2 ~ <0.45	0/40		<1.54 ~ <23	0/20		<0.77 ~ <210
73 1,2-Dibromoethane	0/60		<0.0002 ~ <0.075	0/40		<0.005 ~ <0.17	0/20		<0.005
74 1,1,2,2-Tetrabromo-ethane	0/60		<0.0002 ~ <0.0005	0/40		<0.005 ~ <0.013	0/20		<0.005 ~ <0.0065
75 Tetrahydrothiophene-1,1-dioxide	0/60		<0.00016 ~ <0.001	0/55		<0.007 ~ <0.260	0/1		<0.02
76 Nonylphenol	0/8		<0.005	0/8		<0.25			
77 Trichlorfluoromethane	90/115	0.0005 ~ 0.45		air (ppb)					
78 Dichloro-difluoromethane	45/115	0.31 ~ 3.3	<1						

A: No. of detection   B: No. of samples

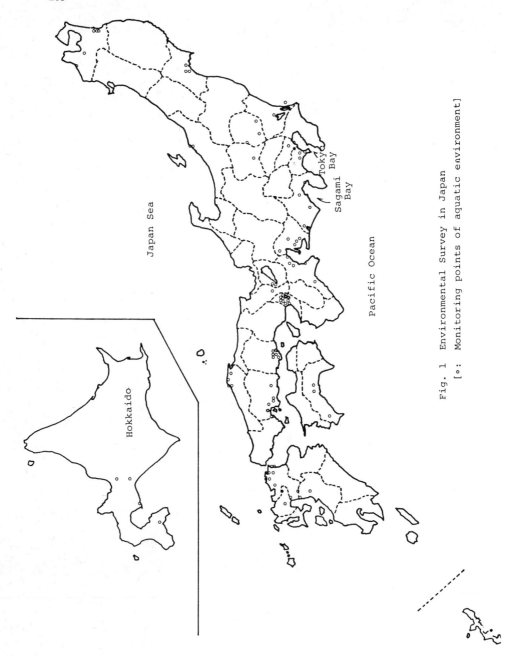

Fig. 1 Environmental Survey in Japan
[○: Monitoring points of aquatic environment]

ORGANO-HALOGENATED COMPOUNDS IN AQUATIC ECOSYSTEMS

P.A. Greve
Unit for Residue Analysis
National Institute of Public Health
P.O. Box 1
Bilthoven
Netherlands

Summary

Data from past and current monitoring programmes covering aquatic ecosystems, as well as from incidental investigations indicates that from the organo-halogenated compounds much emphasis has been laid upon the organochlorine pesticides and PCB's, which compounds have been investigated in water, sediments and a great variety of aquatic organisms. From the other organo-halogenated compounds the volatile organochlorine solvents and the chlorophenols have been studied most extensively.

Although many organo-chlorine compounds have been identified in aquatic ecosystems, still a large gap exists between the total amount of organochlorine found and the amount of organochlorine calculated from the compounds which have been identified thusfar. This fact forms an argument in favour of specimen banking, an other argument being the need for samples describing the status-quo-ante when calamities occur.

In any monitoring programme concerning aquatic ecosystems water samples, and sometimes also sediment samples, must be incorporated, as the water shed forms the vehicle which transports the pollutant from the source into the food chain. The monitoring programme must be supplemented with carefully chosen biota samples, concentrating on a few species of curcial interest, rather than on a broad spectrum of species. Local circumstances and the goal of the programme dictate the ultimate choice and number of samples to be investigated.

1. Review of past and current programmes

1.1. Sources of information

Monitoring programmes in aquatic ecosystems with regard to organohalogenated compounds have been or are being carried out in many industrialised countries. The fact that regular monitoring programmes are mainly confined to those countries is not surprising, as contamination of the aquatic ecosystem by organo-halogenated compounds, which by their nature are almost all man-made or derived from man-made materials, can be expected to be greatest near to the spots of production or handling.

It is to be expected that the current monitoring programmes will rather be extended in scope and frequency than cut down, as legislation is more and more demanding data on discharges by industries and users in general, and with regard to organo-halogenated compounds in particular due to the often persistent, toxic and bio-accumulating nature of these compounds.

They therefore invariably and in high priority appear on the different
"black lists" issued by official bodies supervising the quality of aquatic ecosystems. Many data on the occurrence of organo-halogenated compounds in aquatic ecosystems however do not originate from regular monitoring programmes but from more occasional sources, such as calamities,
incidental investigations or chance discoveries. These sources of information are naturally unpredictable and often not typical for a situation as a whole, but they can be of great significance as an incentive
for further investigations and, possibly, lead to incorporation of the
compound(s) involved into a regular monitoring programme.

In the following paragraphs use will be made of recent results from monitoring programmes as well as from other, irregular investigations.
The investigations cited can be illustrative only, as an exhaustive
review of the data available would far surpass the scope of this working paper (for literature older than 1972 see e.g. Edwards (1973)).

1.2. Type of information

1.2.1. Organochlorine pesticides and PCB's

An abundancy of data is available on the occurrence of organochlorine
pesticides and PCB's. Analysis of these compounds is, due to their low
polarity, low volatility and high stability, relatively easy and, due
to their electroncaptive properties, highly sensitive. To this fact,
the toxicological importance of these compounds must be added.

Thus, organochlorine pesticides (predominantly the HCH-isomers, dieldrin
and the DDT-complex) have been analysed in:

- water (Bevenue et al., 1972; Brodtmann, 1976; Eichner, 1973 and 1976;
  Engst, 1973; Environmental Protection Agency, 1972; Fay, 1972; Giam,
  1972 and 1973; Greve, 1972; Herzel, 1972; Lauderdale, 1969; Lenon,
  1972; Shea, 1969; Suzuki, 1972; Uhnāk, 1974; Wegman and Greve, 1978),

- fish (Addison, 1972; Bevenue, 1972; Bjerk, 1972 and 1973; Carr, 1972;
  Deichmann, 1972; Greichus, 1973; Huschenbeth, 1973; Jonczyk, 1972;
  Lunde, 1976; Minagawa, 1972; Muson, 1972; Neuhaus, 1973; Reinke, 1972;
  Shaw, 1972; Stalling, 1971; Stenersen, 1972),

- various intermediate organisms of the food chain (Bevenue, 1972; Bowes,
  1973; Fay, 1972; Giam, 1972 and 1973; Rice, 1973; Rowe, 197o; Ten
  Berge, 1974; Williams, 1973) and

- sediments (Bevenue, 1972; Fay, 1972; Lenon, 1972; Pfister, 197o;
  Routh, 1972; Shea, 1969; Weil, 1972),
  (cf also the monographs by Edwards (1973 and 1975)).

PCB's were analyzed in:

- water (Bauer, 1972; Dube, 1974; Eichner, 1973 and 1976; Giam, 1972
  and 1973; Harvey, 1973; Koch, 1974; Selenka, 1972; Tucker, 1975;
  Wiesner, 1973),

- fish (Addison, 1972; Bjerk, 1972 and 1973; Carr, 1972; Food and Drug
  Administration, 1972; Greichus, 1973; Huschenbeth, 1973; Lunde, 1976;
  Reinke, 1972; Stalling, 1971; Wiesner, 1973; Zitko, 1972),

- various intermediate organisms of the food chain (Bowes, 1973; Giam,
  1972 and 1973; McCloskey, 1973; Williams, 1973; Wiesner, 1973)and

- sediment (Wiesner, 1973),
  (cf also the monograph by Hutinger et al. (1974).

The data on the organochlorine pesticides and PCB's (the above-mentioned investigations represent a fraction of the whole body of data only) covers a great part of the world and, although not systematically planned and not always strictly comparable among each other (international.intercomparison studies often reveal drastic discrepancies), they give a fairly good overallpicture of the situation in the aquatic ecosystem with regard to this group of compounds.
More incidental investigations have been reported on i.a. endosulfan (Greve and Wit, 1971; Sievers, 1972) in connection with a massive fish-kill in the river Rhine and (Gorbach, 1971) in connection with field trials under tropical conditions, PCT's (Freudenthal and Greve, 1973; Zitko, 1972), mirex (Borthwick, 1973; Collins, 1973; Hawthorne, 1974; Kaiser, 1974; Markin, 1972; Ten Noever de Brauw, 1973), toxaphene (Durant and Reimold, 1972), TCDD (Baughman, 1973), hexachlorobutadiene (Laska, 1976; Yurawecz, 1976), polychlorostyrene (Kuehl, 1976; Lunde, 1976), kepone (Moseman, 1977) and pentabromotoluene (Mattson, 1975).

1.2.2. Volatile organo-halogenated compounds

Data becomes more scarce for organo-haloganated compounds of higher volatility, probably due to the more sophisticated analytical techniques which must be applied in order to avoid losses.
Examples covering this group of compounds include vinylchloride-monomer (Alberty, 1975), chlorinated solvents (Dietz and Traud, 1973; Nicholson, 1975) and chlorobenzenes (Lunde, 1976). Interestingly, volatile organochlorine compounds can be formed during the chlorination of surface waters at drinking water works or of effluents at sewage treatment plants (Glaze, 1973). Also volatile brominated products can be formed on these occasions when inorganic bromide is present in the treated water stream (Rook, 1975). The volatile organo-halogenated compounds are found mainly in the water itself, rather than in the sediments or in aquatic organisms, as generally they are less easily adsorbed, respectively more easily excreted or metabolised.

1.2.3. Polar organo-halogenated compounds

Organo-halogenated compounds of high polarity give still more problems in the analysis: even if they can be isolated by classical extraction techniques (as the phenoxy-acid herbicides and chlorophenols for example are), they must preferably be derivatised prior to gaschromatrographical analysis as otherwise sensitivity and reproducibility is generally poor. Available data suggests that contamination of the aquatic ecosystem is relatively low as far as the phenoxy-acid herbicides are concerned (Deleu, 1977; Soderquist, 1975), but that chlorophenols are often present in several parts of the aquatic food chain (Bevenue, 1972; Lindström, 1976; Tokunaga, 1971; Greve and Wegman, 1978). If the organo-halogenated compounds to be investigated become polar to a degree in which they can not be extracted anymore by conventional extraction means, adsorption techniques must be devised. Although much work has been done on this subject, treatment of this matter, being chiefly an analytical problem, lies beyond the scope of this working paper.

1.3. Usefulness of specimen banking

Despite of the vast amount of data published, a remarkable skewness of interest can be noted towards the organochlorine pesticides and PCB's. However, understandable this situation is, it should be borne in mind that only a fraction of the organo-halogenated compounds occurring in the aquatic ecosystem is known by name and concentration (Donkin, 1977; Greve and Haring, 1972; Kölle, 1972; Koppe, 197o), let alone by ecological significance.
A partly qualitative inventory of compounds identified in water has been issued by the European Communities (1976) and in e.g. the river Rhine and its tributaries regularly new organo-halogenated compounds are being identified and the results published (Internationale Arbeitsgemeinschaft der Wasserwerke im Rheineinzugsgebiet, Jahresberichte).
In view of the large gap between organo-halogen present and organo-halogen identified, banking of specimens for future reference seems attractive, but to the knowledge of the author this is not being done systematically on a large scale.
Specimen banking can also be of use in case of calamities, when background levels or the status-quo-ante need to be known in order to give a sound evaluation of the findings. In the next paragraph suggestions for specimen banking will be given.

2. Programme design

2.1. Monitoring programmes

Giving general rules for the design of monitoring programmes is almost impossible as circumstances vary widely; this is the more true if calamities and other unpredictable incidents are to be covered. Attempts can be made however to formulate a few minimum requirements which, according to the needs in the individual cases, must be supplemented with additional requirements.
At the outset, it must be clear that a monitoring programme never should be an analytical exercise on its own, but always a start to ecological evaluation, if needed followed by measures to improve the situation.
The effect of these measures then can again be followed by a new monitoring programme, a new evaluation and, possibly, new measures, and so on until the ecosystem is considered "clean".

2.1.1. Water

It will always be highly advisable to include water samples in any monitoring programme covering an aquatic ecosystem, even if, due to the often low concentrations in the water phase, water is not the easiest part of the ecosystem from an analytical point of view. Monitoring water samples is however often the only way to unambiguously locate a source of pollution and hence to improve a given unwanted situation. Sample size and isolation techniques must be adequate for the purpose envisaged and in many cases this will entail special development work. As this aspect is mainly analytical however, a discussion here would be out of place.

2.1.2. Aquatic organisms

Many organo-halogenated pollutants have not been identified for the first time in water samples, but in aquatic organisms or in fish-eating birds or mammalians. These organisms, owing to their higher place in the food chain, often contain higher concentrations of the compounds involved, which can facilitate the analytical work.

Fish and shell-fish are therefore often used as a monitor for aquatic pollution, also, in case of edible species, for economical and food-hygienic reasons. The species to be chosen in a monitoring programme depends in the first place on the ecosystem to be studied (streaming or standing, salt or fresh, climatological conditions, depth ect.), and advice from biologists familiar with the ecosystem involved should be sought before the ultimate choice is made.

For fresh water systems containing a large amount of fine sediment for example, eel often will be a good choice as an indicator organism for apolar organo-halogenated compounds; mussles have the advantage over eel of being sessile, but they are low in fat content, which can make analysis more complicated. For the same reason, mackrel is in many instances preferred over lean fish species if a salt water indicator organism is sought; livers or liver oils (e.g. from cod) on the other hand often contain too many contaminants on the fat phase (also metabolites and artefacts) for being of much value in a monitoring programme.

Organisms on intermediate stages of the food chain (algae, plankton, crustaceans etc.) can be incorporated in a monitoring programme, but costs can then quickly turn out to be prohibitively high. It can be argued that, given an amount of money available, it will in many cases be a good policy to concentrate on water and on one or two fish species, rather than on a large variety of aquatic organisms, which then necessarily will be investigated less frequently or more superficially.

2.1.3. Sediments

Special case of the aquatic ecosystem is the sediment. Many organohalogenated compounds which are sparingly soluble in water tend to get adsorbed on the sediment of the system (especially on the clay and humus fraction of the sediment) and bio-accumulation can find for organisms dwelling in the mud by preference its start there.

Incorporation of sediment samples in a monitoring programme is advisable when the sediment is abundant, small in size and liable to settle down (as i.a. in estuaries). This even can be mandatory, when the sediment is dredged up at regular intervals and used for other purposes. (e.g. on agricultural land), as in that case the adsorbed pollutants might migrate into crops, or into other aquatic systems by leaching or run-off. In general, still little is known about the migrating tendency of adsorbed contaminants (apart from common or recent pesticides) when the sediment is brought into a different environment).

2.2. Specimen banking

Much of what has been stated above on the choice of samples typical for the ecosystem is applicalbe to monitoring programmes as well as to specimen banking. However, in connection to specimen banking storage of the samples must be taken into account. Clearly, if samples for future reference are to be stored, the chemical composition of the samples must be kept unchanged as far as long as possible. Storage of extracts best fulfills this requirement, but has to disadvantage of limiting the range of pollutants which can be studied later to those which happened to have been extracted by the solvent used, and the same applies to storage of adsorbates or of freeze-dried materials. Storage of water samples as such seems unpractical due to the large volumes involved, so that, taking all arguments into account, the best advice is storage (at e.g. -180°C)

294

of a careful selection of biota samples, preferably high up in the food chain.

3. Organisational, legal and economical aspects

Implementation of specimen banking in existing monitoring programmes seems, if agreement is reached on the modalities discussed in 2., rather easily feasible for the programmes the author is familiar with, i.e. those concerned with Dutch surface waters. Difficulties may arise in transporting samples across national borderlines, as these samples might give information on industrial discharges which countries might not be willing to divulge. Obtaining samples generally will not give serious problems, although a number of analytical precautions must be taken which do not need to be discussed here.
As to the accessibility of the data obtained, publication of all results in an easily understandable form should be the general rule. Interpretation of the data from an ecological and/or toxicological point of view should always be tried, or otherwise investigations leading to such an evaluation should be started. In the meantime, measures can be envisaged to reduce the output of the pollutants into the ecosystem as far as feasible.
Costs of monitoring programmes and specimen banking will greatly vary from case to case, depending on the scope of pollutants to be covered; the following rough figures can give an impression of the amount of money involved (price level March 1978, in Hfl per sample):

analysis of:	organochlorine pesticides	PCB's	chlorophenols
in: water	24o	16o	16o
aquatic organisms	24o	16o	16o
sediment	24o	16o	16o

(these costs cover sample collection, transport, analysis and data processing, inclusive personnel, equipment, overheads etc.)

For specimen banking costs will be considerably less, specially if deep-freezing is chosen as the storage technique. Costs of analysis in the stored materials will be roughly the same as in the original samples.

References

Addison, R.F. et al., J.Fish.Res.Board Canada, 29, 349-355 (1972).

Alberti, J., Z. Wasser u. Abwasser-Forsch., 8, 14o-142 (1975).

Bauer, U., Gas- u. Wasser Fach, 113, 58-63 (1972)

Baughman, R. and M. Meselson, Environ.Health Perspect., 5, 27-35 (1973)

Bevenue, A. et al., Pest. Mon. J., 6, 56-64 (1972).

Bevenue, A. et al., Bull. Envir. Cont. Tox. 8, 238-241 (1972).

Bjerk, J.E., Nordisk Veterinaermedicin, 24, 451-457 (1972).

Bjerk, J.E., Bull. Envir. Cont. Tox., 9,89-96 (1973).

Borthwick, P.W. et al., Pest. Monit. J., 7, 6-26 (1973).

Bowes, G.W. et al., Envir. Health Perspect., 5, 191-198 (1973).

Brodtmann, N.V., Jr., Bull. Envir. Cont. Tox., 15, 33-39 (1976).

Carr, R.L. et al., Pest. Mont. J., 6 23-26 (1972).

Collins, H.L. et al., Bull. Envir. Cont. Tox., 1o, 73-79 (1973).

Deichmann, Wm. B. et al., Arch. Toxikol., 29, 287-3o9 (1972).

Deleu, R. et al., J. Chromatogr., 134, 483-488 (1977).

Dietz, F. and J. Traud, Vom Wasser, 41, 137-155 (1973).

Donkin, P. et al., Anal. Chim. Acta, 88, 289-3o1 (1977).

Dube, D.J. et al., J. Water Poll. Contr. Fed., 966 (1974).

Durant, C.J. and R.J. Reimold, Pest. Monit. J., 6, 94-96 (1972).

Edwards, C.A. (edit.), Environmental Pollution by Pesticides, Plenum Press, London-New York (1973).

Edwards, C.A., Persistent Pesticides in the Environment, 2nd edit., CRC Press, Cleveland, Ohio (1975).

Eichner, M., Z. Lebensmitt.-Untersuch. u. Forsch., 151, 376-383 (1973).

Eichner, M., Z. Lebensmitt.-Untersuch. u. Forsch., 161, 327-336 (1976).

Engst, R. and R. Knoll, Die Nahrung, 17, 837-851 (1973).

Environmental Protection Agency, Ecol. Res. Ser. EPA-R3-72-oo3, U.S. Gov. Printing Office, Washington D.C. (1972).

European Communities, Analysis of organic micropollutants in water, 2nd edit., EUROCOP-COST (1976).

Fay, R.R. and L.W. Newland, Pest. Monit. J., 6, 97-1o2 (1972).

Food and Drug Administration, Fed. Register, 37, 57o5-57o7 (18 March 1972).

Freudenthal, J. and P.A. Greve, Bull. Envir. Cont. Tox., 1o, 1o8-111 (1973).

Giam, C.S. and M.K. Wong, J. Chromatogr., 72, 283-292 (1972).

Giam, C.S. et al., Bull. Envir. Cont. Tox., 9, 376-382 (1973).

Glaze, W.H. et al., J. Chromat. Science, 11, 58o (1973).

Greichus, Y.A. et al., Bull. Envir. Cont. Tox., 9, 321 (1973).

Greve, P.A., Sci. Tot. Environ., 1, 173-18o (1972).

Greve, P.A. and B.J.A. Haring, Schriftenr. Ver. Wasser-, Boden u. Lufthyg., Berlin-Dahlem, 37, 59-64 (1972).

Greve, P.A. and S.L. Wit, J. Water Poll. Contr. Fed., 43, 2338-2348 (1971).

Greve, P.A. and R.C.C. Wegman, to be published (1978).

Gorbach, S. et al., Bull. Envir. Cont. Tox., 6, 4o-47 (1971).

Harvey, G.R. et al., Science, 18o, 643-644 (1973).

Hawthorne, J.C. et al., Bull. Envir. Cont. Tox., 11, 258 (1974).

Herzel, F., Pest. Monit. J., 6, 179-187 (1972).

Huschenbeth, E., Arch. Fischereiwiss., 24, 1o5-116 (1973).

Hutzinger, O. et al., The Chemistry of PCB's CRC Press, Cleveland, Ohio (1974).

296

Jonczyk, H. et al., Bull. Acad. Pol. Sci., Ser.Sci.Biol., 2o, 297-3o3 (1972).

Kaiser, K.L.E., Science, 185, 523-525 (1974).

Koch, R., Acta Hydrochim. Hydrobiol., 5, 447-448 (1974).

Kölle, W. et al., Naturwiss., 59, 299-3o5 (1972).

Koppe, P. and L. Rautenberg, Korresp. Abwass., 17, 53-54 (197o).

Kuehl, D.W. et al., Bull. Envir. Cont. Tox., 16, 127 (1976).

Laska, A.L. et al., Bull. Envir. Cont. Tox., 15, 535-542 (1976).

Lauderdale, R.A., U.S. Dept. Commerce Nat. Tech. Inform. Serv., PB 194,o56 (1969).

Lenon, H. et al., Pest. Monit. J., 6, 188-193 (1972).

Lindström, K. and J. Nordin, J. Chromatogr., 128, 13-26 (1976).

Lunde, G. and E. Baumann Ofstad, Z. Anal. Chem., 282, 395-399 (1976).

Markin, G.P.et al., Bull. Envir. Cont. Tox., 8, 369 (1972).

Mattson, P.E. et al., J. Chromatogr., 111, 2o9-213 (1975).

McCloskey, L.R. and K.H. Deubert, Bull. Envir. Cont. Tox., 1o, 261 (1973).

Minagawa, O. et al., Eiseigaku Zasshi, 13, 317-325 (1972).

Moseman, R.R. et al., Arch. Envir. Cont. Tox., 6, 221-231 (1977).

Munson, T.O., Bull. Envir. Cont. Tox., 7, 223-228 (1972).

Neuhaus, J.W.G. et al., Med. J. Austral., 1, 1o7-11o (1973).

Nicholson, A.A. and O. Meresz, Bull. Envir. Cont. Tox., 14, 453 (1975).

Pfister, R.M. et al., Proc. Conf. Great Lakes Res., 1, 82-92 (197o).

Reinke, J. et al., Pest. Monit. J., 6, 43-49 (1972).

Rice, C.P. and H.C. Sikka, J. Agr. Food Chem., 21, 148-153 (1973).

Rice, C.P. and H.C. Sikka, Bull. Envir. Cont. Tox., 7, 168-176 (1972).

Rowe, D.R. et al., J. Amer. Soc. Civ. Eng., 96, 1221-1234 (197o).

Selenka, F., Schriftenr. Ver. Wasser-, Boden- u. Lufthyg., Berlin-Dahlem, 37, 113-12o (1972).

Shaw, S.B., Calif. Fish Game, 58, 22-26 (1972).

Shea, T.G. and W.E. Gates, Prod. 24th Industr. Waste Conf., Purdue Univ., 1448-1463 (1969).

Sievers, J.F. et al., Environmental Quality and Safety, Vol.I, Georg Thieme, Stuttgart-New York, 239-243 (1972).

Soderquist, C.J. and D.G. Crosby, Pestic. Science, 6, 17-33 (1975).

Stalling, D.L., U.S. Dept. Int., Bureau Sport Fish. Wildlife, ISBN o 677 1216o 1, 413-438 (1971).

Stenersen, J. and J. Kvalvåg, Bull. Envir. Cont. Tox., 8, 12o-121 (1972).

Suzuki, M. et al., Kogyo Yosui, 166, 22-27 (1972).

Ten Berge, W. and M. Hillebrand, Netherlands J. Sea Res., 8, 361-368 (1974).

Ten Noever de Brauw, M.C. et al., Sci. Total Envir., $\underline{2}$, 196-198 (1973).

Tokunaga, S., Kagaku Keisatsu Kenkyusho Hokoku, $\underline{24}$, 136-138 (1971).

Tucker, E.S. et al., Bull. Envir. Cont. Tox., $\underline{13}$, 86 (1975).

Uhnàk, J. et al., J. Chromatogr., $\underline{91}$, 545-547 (1974).

Wegman, R.C.C. and P.A. Greve, paper to be presented at the International Symposium on the Analysis of Hydrocarbons and Chlorinated Hydrocarbons, Hamilton, Canada (1978).

Weil, L. et al., Schriftenr. Ver. Wasser-, Boden- u. Lufthyg., $\underline{37}$, 77-84 (1972).

Williams, R. and A.V. Holden, Mar. Poll. Bull., $\underline{4}$, 1o9-111 (1973).

Wiesner, H.J.C. et al., J. Res. U.S. Geol. Surv., $\underline{1}$, 6o3-6o7 (1973).

Yurawecz, M.P. et al., J.A.O.A.C., $\underline{59}$, 552 (1976).

Zitko, V. and O. Hutzinger, Schriftenr. Ver. Wasser-, Boden- u. Lufthyg., $\underline{37}$, 121-128 (1972).

STATEMENT OF POLYCYCLIC AROMATIC HYDROCARBONS

Prof. Dr. G. Grimmer
Biochemisches Institut
für Umweltcarcinogene
Sieker Landstraße   19
2o7o Ahrensburg
Federal Republic of Germany

General remarks:

There are good reasons to assume that many of the human carcinoma are
initiated by environmental carcinogens as e.g. polycyclic aromatic
hydrocarbons (= PAH), N-containing polycyclic aromatic compounds
(carbazoles, acridines), nitrosamines, aromatic amines, mycotoxines
and some anorganic compounds. From this the general question arises:
What is the sense of doing analytical chemistry of pollutants? The
answer is, to control harmful substances in the environment and first
of all to control acute and chronic toxic substances for man.
Epidemiological studies indicate that the environment significant influences the incidence of human cancer although many of the specific
causal agent have yet to be identified. Two major factors are known from
these epidemiological studies: inhalation of cigarette smoke and inhalation of air pollutants clearly increase the incidence of lung cancer in
men. By using animal tests, it is possible to identify and characterize
the carcinogens in cigarette smoke, automobile exhaust condensate or air
pollutants. In these cases, the fraction of PAH account for more then
the half of the carcinogenic activity of these environmental materials,
in automobile exhaust even for the total carcinogenic effect.
Since the PAH are common environmental pollutants, they are supposed
to contribute to cancer in other organs too. THERE ARE MANY SOCALLED
POLLUTANTS EXISTING IN ENVIRONMENTAL CONCENTRATION WITHOUT DETECTABLE
EFFECT IN MEN. BUT ONLY IN THE CASE OF CARCINOGENS AS POLYCYCLIC AROMA-
TIC HYDROCARBONS THERE ARE GOOD REASONS TO ASSUME THAT THESE ARE THE CAU-
SAL AGENTS FOR LUNG CANCER IN MAN. In 1975 more than 24 ooo men died in
the Federal Republic of Germany of lung cancer.

I think there is a need for definition of "environmental chemistry" and
for "pollutants".

Polycyclic Aromatic Hydrocarbons, widespread in the environment, are formed
in any incomplete combustion of all organic materials e.g. by burning
fossil fuels. Environmental samples may contain PAH preferentially from
hand-stoked residential furnances, open burnings e.g. from forest and
agricultural or coal refuse fires, and coke production. In contrast
to this uncontrolled combustion, power plants, gasoline- and Diesel-
fuel-powered cars contribute only few quantities of PAH. An assessment
of the contribution of PAH from all sources to air is not compiled. Only
an estimation of these emission of benzo(a)pyrene (BaP) is available,

shown in tab. 1.

Whereas the distribution of PAH and nitrosamines is fairly well investigated,there are few investigations of the distribution of aromatic amines
or nitrogen-containing aromatic compounds.One of the main reasons for this
is the difficult enrichment for the profile-analysis of N-containing
aromatic compounds. Recently gas-chromatographic profile analysis of
carcinogenic carbozoles, acridines and aromatic amines are published
(e.g. GRIMMER et al., z. Anal. Chem. 29o 147 1978).
As thereis large date material on the occurance of BaP in the environment, the question arise whether it can be used as a guide-substance,
representative for the carcinogenic activity of a product. Summarizing
the results of identifying the group of carcinogenic compounds in the
skin-dropping test model to proof the carcinogenicity in environmental
material as e.g. automobile exhaust condensate the situation hitherto
can be described as follows: the fraction of PAH which consists of
4 and more rings accounts for more than 9o % of the total carcinogenic
activity of automobile exhaust condensate. In contrast the benzo(a)-py-
rene of the condensate accounts for 8 to 1o % of the total carcinogenicity only. Using the same bioassay - dropping onto the skin of mice -
in case of cigarette smoke condensate, BaP accounts for about 1 %
of the total carcinogenicity only, whereas all PAH account for more
than 5o % of the total carcinogenic activity of this material. From
this it is obvious that BaP cannot be considered as a guide-substance,
representative for the carcinogenic activity of a product such as environmental material. More relevant information would be available if the
analysis involves all PAH and therefore a PAH-Profile-Analysis is necessary.

a. Review of Past and Current Programmes

Review of past and current programmes dealing with "monitoring environmental materials" and "specimen banking".
A huge number of investigations on the content of polycyclic aromatic
hydrocarbons (= PAH) in various environmental material is available.
Most of them are restricted to the determination of benzo(a)pyrene
(= BaP). During 1967 to 1977 several thousands of papers have been published dealing with the detection and metabolism of BaP (about 2ooo
titles in Chemical Abstract) or PAH (about 3ooo titles in C.A.), respectively. In the frame of this statement it is unpossible to discuss these
investigations critically. Determination of various PAH or PAH-profiles
have been performed with following environmental materials:

(a) Foods: fresh, broiled smoked and grilled meat, sausages, ham fish,
    poultry, single cell protein (e.g. yeast), baby food, coconut oil,
    oil of sunflower-seed, cottonseed, palm-kernel, palm, soyabean,
    olives, rapeseed and linseed; cocoa butter, margarine, beef tallow
    and butter; all kind of leaves as borecole, cabbage, salad; flour
    cereals, bread, seaweed etc.
(b) Aerosols: air pollutant, automobile exhaust from gasoline or Diesel-
    fuel engines, hand-stoked residential furnance, cigarette smoke, soot
    etc.
(c) Water, and soil: drinking water, water from river and lake, sediments

or drilling core of sediments, soil, sewage sludge etc.
(d) Petroleum and mineral oil products: gasoline, Diesel-fuel, heating
    oil EL and S, lubricating oil (fresh and used), cutting oil, paraffin,
    crude mineral oil ect.

"specimen banking"
A specimen banking is not available in Germany, but sediments of lakes
can be considered as a natural specimen bank. Well separated layers
of sediments resulting from the input of materials from rivers as well
from air dust can be observed in drilling cores from the ground of lakes
and calm areas of the sea, respectively. The age of these layers can
be determined by isotopes as Cs 137 and Pb 21o, or by pollen analysis.
Investigations on 2 lakes (lake Constance and Grosser Plöner See) show
that there is a moderate gradient from lower to recent layers, but a
dramatic increase since 19oo can be observed. From the end of the 6o'ies
the PAH-concentration in the layers seems to decrease again.

Comments on adequacy regarding utility and validity of these programmes

Most of the investigations on environmental material regards the content
of BaP only. This, however, is not sufficient for an estimation of the carcinogenic activity of this material. Only a few profile-analysis have
been performed by means of gas chromatography during the last years. This
technique gives the base to estimate the carcinogenic properties of a
material using chemical analysis data.

B. Rationale for Interest or Concern

Summarize briefly chemical, environmental, metabolic, and toxicological
characteristics of pollutants.

Chemical characteristics: PAH are widespread distributed in the environment
of men. The most frequent environmental PAH are naphthalene, biphenyle,
fluorene, phenanthrene, anthracene, fluoranthene, pyrene, benzo(a)anthra-
cene, chrysene, triphenylene, cyclopenteno(cd)pyrene, benzo(b)fluoran-
thene, benzo(k)fluoranthene, benzo(j)fluoranthene, benzo(e)pyrene
benzo(a)pyrene, perylene, indeno(1,2,3-cd)fluoranthene, indeno(1,2,
3-cd)pyrene, benzo(ghi)perylene, anthanthrene, coronene and methylderi-
vatives of these PAH, preferentially methylderivates from lower PAH
consisting of 2, 3 and 4 rings.
Chronic toxicological characteristics: Many of the PAH are carcinogenic
and mutagenic. To proof the carcinogenic effect of a PAH, a mixture of
PAH or an PAH-containing environmental material, are used the following
biotests on animals: Dropping onto the skin of mice, subcutaneous injection of a solution of PAH etc. in tricaprilin or a vegetable oil in mice
or rats, instillation into the trachea of rats or hamsters, implantation
into the lung of rats etc. All these different kinds of application produce local carcinoma or sarcoma in most cases. Only few of the before
mentioned PAH induce malignant tumors in all of these biotest. Intra-
veneous injection in rats induce malignant tumors in mammae, provided a
carcinogenic PAH as 7,12-dimethylbenz(a)anthracene etc. is applicated.
The carcinogenic potency seems to vary in different animal assays.
Metabolic characteristics: The metabolic pathway in microorganisms
and animal tissues leads to epoxids, diols, phenols, and quinones. The
oxidation of these aromatic compounds proceeds very rapid and therefore
no accumulation is observed in animal tissues. The metabolism of PAH is

effected by mixed-function oxygenases, enzymes widespread in all tissues of·men and animals. Mixed-function oxygenases are part of the endoplasmic reticulum and consist of a terminal cytochrom (P 45o) and electron transport chain. In case of BaP, the best investigated PAH, a specific diol-epoxide, the r-t, 7,8-dihydroxy, t-9,1o-oxy-7,8,9.1o-tetrahydro-benzo(a) pyrene is produced by the microsomes which has a very much higher mutagenic activity than any known BaP-metabolite, suggesting that this may be the "ultimate carcinogen" in the cell.

Environmental characteristics: PAH form a large group of chemicals, present in the atmosphere, soil, waterways and oceans and in most foods. Major source of PAH are heat and power generation with fossil combustibles, refuse burning, industrial processes, and oil contamination by crud mineral oil and mineral oil products.

Assess current and projected levels of environmental exposure

Epidemiological studies indicate that the environment significantly influences the incidence of human cancer. (see "general remarks" on p. 298). Especially in the case of lung cancer there are good reasons to assume that the PAH present in air are the causal agent for this cancer. From all these epidemiological studies, a correlation between the incidence of lung cancer in a definite area and the concentration of PAH in the air of this area for twenty years is not available. Therefore the "no-effect-level" is not known.

Discuss pathways for human exposure

Epidemiological studies show only in case of lung cancer a clear correlation between the incidence of cancer and the degree of air pollution or the number of cigarettes. The effect of PAH as the causal agent is to suppose but not proved. The effect of PAH on the incidence of other cancer diseases are e.g. stomach cancer has not been shown by epidemiological studies, but has repeatedly been discussed.

C. Considerations for sample selection, collection, containment, shipment and storage.

Idenfify and characterize specimens

A preselected number of environmental materials is supposed and accepted. From economical point of view, the number of kinds of specimens is limited to samples from "Aquatic Ecosystem" (1. fish, 2. mollusces, sediments and sludge, 3. seaweed, algae and plankton, 4. other aquatic wildlife) and from "Terrestrial Ecosystem" (1. plants, incl.moss and lichen, 2. soil, 3. wildlife as birds and insects, and other terrestrial animals, 4. farm and domestic animals).

In respect to the PAH, this choice is not efficient. The causal agent e.g. for pulmonary cancer or other chronic diseases of the lung is located in the "Air ecosystem". For storage a sample, it might be considered to adsorb the organic matter in air onto TENAX or other suitable materials.

Identify special precautions or techniques for obtaining specimens.

Special precaution for obtaining all the samples from the aquatic and terrestrial ecosystem, mentioned before, are not necessary.

Discuss special container (incl. material), preservative and/or processing requirements.

Container of glass, closed with glass-stopper, or of aluminium are suitable. Unfit for the storage would be container of plastic materials because of the immigration of the PAH from aquatic solutions into the wall of the plastic material.

Recommend storage procedures for short-term "monitoring environmental materials" and long-term "specimen banking".

It is not possible to suggest a "standard method" for storage of all kinds of specimens, mentioned before. Perishable material e.g. fish, food etc. must be protected against microbiological and oxidative decomposition by deep frozen e.g. at -20°C. In the case of long-term storage no experiences are available in respect to the stability of the PAH. A further possibility of storage would be the freeze drying. To control the possible evaporation of low boiling PAH from the sample during the freeze drying, it is necessary to investigate this method for this effect.

D. Analytical Procedures
Need for representative aliquot or sample.

In respect to the limited number of specimens of an environmental material only off-hand specimens are feasible.

AMOUNT, required to analysis

The amount of the specimen is determined (a) by the limit of detection of the method and (b) by the required limit of concentration in the material. The most sensitive methods for detection of the PAH are the glas-capillary-gas-chromatography, detection by flame ionisation-detector(=FID), the ultra-violett (=UV) and fluorescence spectrometry after separation the fraction of PAH, isolated from the material, by liquid-chromatography (e.g. high-pressure-liquid-chromatography, = HPLC). Only the FID is sensitive for all PAH in the same amount of a PAH. A full scaled signal of BaP require about 1o ng (o.o1 µg), other PAH are in the same range, depending on the retention time of the GC. Limit of detection for e.g. BaP is about o.2 ng. Therefore for a required limit of concentration of o.1 µg BaP/kg (= o.1 ppb), the required amount of the specimen must be about 1o g for one analysis.

Pretreatment requirements.

Provided that the sample solves without any residue, no complication arise for a complete extraction of the PAH. But few materials as e.g. oils and fats are complete soluble only. In other cases as e.g. high-protein materials, an initial digestion in methanolic potassium hydroxide is necessary to solve it homogeneously. Specimens of soil or soot are unsoluble in any organic solvent and therefore the exhaustive extraction must be precise controlled with regard to the adsorbtive properties of the unsoluble residue.

Interfering endogeneous or exogeneous substances

All known methods of the determination of PAH require a selective enrichment of the PAH from the material. The better the separation from other substances, the less interferences orginate by the quantification of the single PAH. Generally, the fraction of PAH comprise more than 1oo compounds. An exellent separation of this aromatic fraction is practicable by GC-capillary columns (usually more than 8o ooo HETP per 25 m), less effective are packed columns in gaschromatography (up to 25 ooo per 1o m) or high-pressure-liquid-chromatography (up to 1o ooo HETP).

Alternate analytical method that take into account specifity, precision, accuracy, reproducibility.

See section before. For determination of BaP in meat or for a PAH-Profile-Analysis in foods, recommended methods of the International Union of Pure and Applied Chemistry (= IUPAC) exist. In this cases e.g. collaborative studies has been performed and therefore data for repeatability (same operator, same apparatus, same laboratory and same time) and reproducibility (different operator, different apparatus, different laboratories) are known. A recommended method by IUPAC "Method for profile-analysis of polycycle aromatic hydrocarbons in (I) high-protein foods, (II) fats and vegetable oils, and (III) plants, soils and sewage sludge by gas chromatography is enclosed for information.

Availability or need for standards and quality control and interlaboratory check.

There is a need for some pure PAH for standards because many of them are not commercial (e.g. benzo(e)pyrene, benzo(b)fluoranthene, benzo(j)fluoranthene, benzo(k)-fluoranthene, anthanthrene, benzo(ghi)perylene, dibenz(a,j)-anthracene etc.).

E. Programe Design

Statistical considerations for programme design including: population groups and characteristics, choice of specimen, magnitude of programme.

I understand this means epidemiological studies for the occurance of PAH in environmental material and the correlation to chronic diseases. This is an important point, probably the most important point of the "monitoring environmental materials" to characterize the real harmful substances with chronic toxicity for men. See "General remarks" on page 298 The costs of an epidemiological study e.g. for a single chronic disease are extremely high, therefore that makes no sense to discuss more details.

F. Organizational Aspects

Assessment of extent to which existing and planned programmes may be utilized.

Nothing is known about Programmes on PAH.

Recommendation on centralized vs. decentralized approach (centralized: all samples to selected location(s) for analysis, storage and data control)

It is not necessary to storage all samples in a central place, but because of the high degree of difficulty of the PAH-Profile-Analysis a central laboratory for the analysis is recommended.

Desirability and feasibility of coordinated international programme (recommendations for implementation).

First of all it is necessary to collect experiences with national programmes.

Discuss need for quality control and reference standards

Because of the carcinogenicity of some PAH it is very important to monitor special environmental materials e.g. air pollutants, sewage sludge etc. for the content of PAH. Furthermore it is a need for some pure PAH for reference standards since many of them are not available. I suggest to establish a "Reference Standard Banking", which control the purity of commercial available PAH (better than 99 %) and synthesize non-commercial PAH's.

Needs for field and laboratory training and standardized form, nomenclature, etc.

In the case of a central laboratory for the analysis of all samples, a laboratory training and the standardization of the method is not necessary . The nomenclature of the PAH is recommended by the International Union of Pure and Applied Chemistry.

G. Ethical and Legal Considerations

This point of view is not relevant in the case of non-human-materials.

H. Cost Estimates

Nothing is known about the range of the "monitoring environmental materials" or the "specimen banking" in respect to the number of sampling per day. Therefore the estimation of the costs for the design of programme, collection and transport of samples, storage of samples and data processing is not possible.
The costs for the PAH-profile-analysis depends on the sort of material and the required limit of detection for PAH. The range would be between DM 5oo,-- and DM 1.ooo,--.

Encl.: (1) tab. 1 Source of benzo(a)pyrene in the USA
       (2) Method for profile-analysis of PAH in ....
       (3) Reprint "Simultaneous gas-chromatographic profile-analysis of carcinogenic ......"

tab. 1

SOURCES OF BENZO(A)PYRENE IN THE U.S.A.

tons/year

VEHICLES (1, 2)		
Gasolin-powered cars	lo	
trucks	12	
Diesel-fuel-powered trucks	o.4	
	22	= 1.7 %
HEAT AND POWER GENERATION (1, 3-9)		
Coal		
Hand-stoked residential	42o	
Intermediate units	lo	
Coal-fired steam power plants	1	
Oil		
Low-pressure air atomized etc.	2	
Gas		
Premix burners	2	
Wood	4o	
	475	= 38 %
REFUSE-BURNING		
Enclosed incineration		
Commercial and industrial (7)	23	
Open burning (4, 5, 7, 9)		
Commercial and industrial	lo	
Forest and agricultural	14o	
Vehicle disposal (3, 8)	5o	
Coal refuse fires (lo)	34o	
	563	= 45 %
INDUSTRIAL		
Petroleum (1, 11)	6	
Asphalt air-blowing	1	
Coke production (12) (1.8 g BaP per to)	2oo	
	2o7	= 16 %
total	1.267 to/year	

METHOD FOR PROFILE-ANALYSIS OF POLYCYCLIC AROMATIC HYDROCARBONS IN (I) HIGH-PROTEIN FOODS (II) FATS AND VEGETABLE OILS, AND (III) PLANTS, SOILS AND SEWAGE SLUDGE BY GAS CHROMATOGRAPHY

1. Scope

This method has been applied to a wide range of products such as (I) fresh, broiled, smoked and grilled meat, sausages, ham, fish, poultry, single cell protein (e.g. yeast), baby food (GRIMMER et al., 1975), (II) coconut oil, oil of sunflower-seed, cotton-seed, palm-kernel, palm, soyabean, olives, rapeseed and linseed; cocoa butter, margarine, beef tallow and butter, (III) all kind of leaves, cabbage, borecole, salad, flour cereals, bread, sewage sludge, sediment layers of drilling cores (GRIMMER et al., 1975b), and soil.
Collaborative studies of the International Union of Pure and Applied Chemistry, Applied Chemistry Division in 1975:
(a) Sunflower oil, fortified with 7 polycyclic aromatic hydrocarbons (= PAH) (range: μg/kg). The variation coefficients range from 9.4 % to 24.5 % (7 laboratories, 13 analysis)
(b) meat, fresh, fortified with 8 PAH (range: μg/kg). The variation coefficients range from 7.1 % to 26.9 % (6 laboratories, 12 analysis)
This method was accepted as a IUPAC recommended method in 1976.

2. Definition

In contrast to other methods, the gas chromatographic procedure allows the detection and determination of known and unknown PAH by the use of flame-ionisation-detector (= FID). For this way of simultaneous determination of all PAH in the sample, the term "PAH-Profile-Analysis" is suggested.

3. Principle of the method
Extraction:

To extract the PAH completely from the sample, it is necessary (I) in case of the high-protein foods: an initial digestion in methanolic potassium hydroxide and the extraction of this solution with cyclohexane, (II) in case of fats and vegetable oils: to solve in cyclohexane only, (III) in case of plants, soils and sewage sludge: after an initial extraction with acetone, to solve the acetone residue in cyclohexane.
Enrichment of the PAH:

From this cyclohexane solution, the PAH are concentrated by liquid extraction (N,N-dimethylformamide+water+cyclohexane), by filtration on silica gel and by column chromatography on Sephadex LH 2o/isopropanol.
Separation and determination of the PAH:

The PAH are separated by high-performance gas-liquid chromatography with columns containing 5 % OV 1o1 on Gas-Chrom and estimated by integration of the flame ionization detector signals in relation to an internal standard (benzo(b)chrysene or picene).
Identification of the PAH:

As the PAH profiles of different samples of the same product-group are very similar, it is normally not necessary to characterize the PAH by mass spectrometry, but it is sufficient to compare the retention

time.
Because the high selectivity of the enrichment procedure, only PAH are in this fraction for gas chromatography.

4. Reagents

All solvents are analytical grade and nevertheless distilled: methanol, water, cyclohexane, acetone, N,N-dimethylformamide, isopropanol; 2 N methanolic KOH.
Silica gel: WOELM for adsorption chromatography, 15 % of water was added 24 hrs before use. ICN Pharmaceuticals GmbH, 344o Eschwege.
Sephadex LH 2o: equilibrated with isopropanol > 4 hrs before used. PHARMACIA, Uppsala or Deutsche Pharmacia GmbH, Munzinger Str. 9, D-78oo Freiburg, Germany.
Internal standard: Benzo(b)chrysene (Biochemical Institute for environmental carcinogens, Sieker Landstraße 19, 2o7o Ahrensburg) or Picene (FLUKA GmbH, Lilienthalstr. 8, 791o Neu-Ulm).
Reference substances: Fluoranthene, pyrene, benzo(a)anthracene, chrysene, triphenylene, benzo(b)fluoranthene, benzo(j)-fluoranthene, benzo(k)-fluoranthene, benzo(e)pyrene, benzo(a)pyrene, perylene, dibenz(a,h)-anthracene, dibenz(a,j)anthracene, dibenz(a,c)anthracene, indeno(1,2,3-cd)pyrene, benzo(ghi)perylene, anthanthrene, coronene etc.
Reference solution: Solution of some of the reference substances in dimethylformamide (ca. o.5 µg/µl for injection)

5. Apparatus
Columns for chromatography: For silica gel (5 g) 1o mm id x 2oo mm (height of silica gel, 11o mm); for Sephadex LH 2o (1o g) 3o mm id x 1oo mm (height of gel bed, ca. 5o mm).
Gas chromatography: Bodenseewerk Perkin-Elmer & Co, Type F 2o FE or F 22 or Siemens AG, Type L 35o or 42o, or equivalent instrument, with flame ionisation detector and 2 mm id x 1o m coiled glass column packed with 5 % Silicone OV 1o1 on 125-15o um (= 1oo-12o mesh/inch^2) Gas Chrom Q or Supelcoport (Preparation of the column: GRIMMER et al., 1975a).
Mass spectrometer: (not necessary in most cases): Varian MAT 111 or 112 S, interfaced to Varian 144o GC (with capillary or packed columns)

6. Procedures
6.1. Extraction
6.11 Method for (I) (see scope): Digestion with 2 N methanolic KOH.
1. Grind 2oo g food sample e.g. in a meat grinder.
2. Transfer sample to 1 L round-bottom flask with 29/4o joint, add 3oo ml aqueous methanolic 2 N KOH (water-methanol, 1+9) and 5.o µg Benzo(b)chrysene, place in heating mantle, insert condenser, and reflux at a slow rate for 2-4 hours. Only complete hydrolysis leads to well separated phases in following partition.
3. Cool to room temperature and transfer material to 2 L separatory funnel with glass or Teflon stopcock. Rinse flask with total of 4oo ml methanol + water (4+1), transfer all washes to the separatory funnel, add 8oo ml cyclohexane, and shake the funnel 3 min.
4. Let layers separate, drain lower (methanol + water) layer, and discard.

5. To the cyclohexane in separatory funnel add 4oo ml methanol + water (1+1) for washing and shake 3 min.
6. Let layers separate, drain lower layer, and discard.
7. Repeat this washing of cyclohexane twice with 4oo ml total
   of water.
8. Evaporate cyclohexane on rotatory evaporator (bath temperature
   4o C, reduced pressure) until liquid volume is ca. 1oo ml
   (weight of the solid residue is ca. o.2-o.4 g for meat,
   sausages, fish, poultry)

6.12 Method for (II) (see scope):
1. Dissolve 2oo g oil in 1 L cyclohexane, add 5.o µg benzo(b)
   chrysene, and transfer to 4 L separatory funnel.

6.13 Method for (III) (see scope):
1. Homogenize plant material (e.g. fresh 4oo g) in a chopper
   or cut into small pieces.
2. Transfer sample to 1 L round-bottom flask with 29/4o joint,
   add 6oo ml acetone and 1o.o µg benzo(b)chrysene, place in
   heating mantle, insert condenser and reflux at slow rate for
   1 hour.
3. Cool to room temperature, transfer the extraction agent to
   a 1 L round-bottom flask and evaporate the acetone on rotatory evaporator to dryness.
4. Dissolve the residue of the flask in 1oo ml cyclohexane.

6.2. Enrichment

1. Extract the solution of cyclohexane (in case of 6.118 and
   6.134 : 1oo ml; in case of 6.121 : 1ooo ml) with 2oo ml
   (respectively 1ooo ml) of N,N-dimethylformamid + water (9+1)
   by shaking 3 min. Let layers separate and drain lower (DMF
   + water) layer into a second 1 L (4 L) separatory funnel.
2. Add 2oo ml (respectively 1ooo ml) water to DMF + water phases,
   add 2oo ml (respectively 1ooo ml) cyclohexane, shake the
   funnel 3 min. let layers separate, and discard lower (DMF +
   water) layer.
3. Wash upper (cyclohexane) layer twice with 1oo ml water and
   let layers separate.
4. Transfer the cyclohexane to round-bottom flask, and evaporate
   to o.5 ml (respectively 1 - 2 ml) under reduced pressure in
   rotatory evaporator. Weight of remaining residues in case
   of products of group (I) and (III) are 5 - 3o mg, in group (II)
   about o.5 g.
5. Place residue from 4., dissolved in 1 - 2 ml cyclohexane on to
   of the silica gel column, rinse the flask twice with cyclohexane and place it on the silica gel column too.
6. Allow extract and each rinse to flow into column, stopping when
   liquid is 1 mm above adsorbent.
7. Wash column with 1o ml cyclohexane and discard these first 1o ml.
8. Elute the PAH with 1oo ml cyclohexane, collect eluate in
   1oo ml round-bottom flask and evaporate to dryness under reduced
   pressure in rotatory evaporator.
9. Place 1o g Sephadex LH 2o in 5o ml isopropanol for 4 to 24 hours,
   rinse slurry into chromatographic column, and drain isopropanol
   until surface of Sephadex column is just covered with solvent.

1o. Place residues from (8.), dissolved in 1 ml isopropanol
     on top of column, rinse flask twice with 1 ml isopropanol
11. Allow extract and each rinse to flow into column, stopping
     when isopropanol is until surface of the Sephadex column.
12. Wash column with 48 ml isopropanol and discard the first
     48 ml.
13. Elute the PAH with 4 to 7 rings (fluoranthene to coronene)
     from 48 to 19o ml with isopropanol.
14. For gas chromatography, evaporate isopropanol in 1oo ml
     round-bottom flask to dryness under reduce pressure in ro-
     tatory evaporator.
15. Transfer the residue, solved in 1 ml acetone, into small
     flask with tapered neck (volume of the flask 1o - 2o ml).
16. Rinse the 1oo ml round-bottom flask again twice with 1 ml
     acetone and transfer the solutions into the small flask
     with tapered neck.
17. Evaporate the acetone to few drops with repeated washing
     of flask wall with acetone. Attention: avoid to splash
     the wall of the flask.
18. Add 5 µl N,N-dimethylformamide to solve the residue of the
     small flask.

6.3 Gas chromatography
Gas chromatography operating conditions are as follows: Iso-
thermal operation at 25o C°(or until 28o°C); nitrogen carrier
gas at ca. 3o ml/min (in cold condition) equivalent to 3 - 5 bar
= atm.) pressure. Benzo(a)pyrene elute after 3o to 4o min. If the
retention time of benzo(a)pyrene is too long, it is possible to
increase the temperature of the column or the pressure.
Temperature of the injection block and the flame ionisation detector : 25o°C - 28o°C.
1. Inject 2 µl of the N,N-dimethylformamide solution (of 6.2-18)
    into the gas chromatograph.

s. fig. 1

6.4 Check test
To check the accuracy of the response of the flame ionization detector it is recommended to inject a known standard mixture of
5 to 1o PAH (with known concentrations in the range of o.2 µg/µl
to 1 µg/. µl) before the analysis.

6.5 Blank test
To check the purity of the solvents, silica gel, and Sephadex
LH 2o a blank test should be carried out before the analysis itself, using the same procedure as in latter and same quantities
of all solvents and with added internal standard at the beginning
of the analysis, but omitting the product being tested.

7. Method of calculation
The PAH's are estimated by integration of the flame ionization
detector signals in relation to the internal standard (benzo(b)-
chrysene).
Beside an electronic integration of the FID-signals, other simple
methods are available e.g.

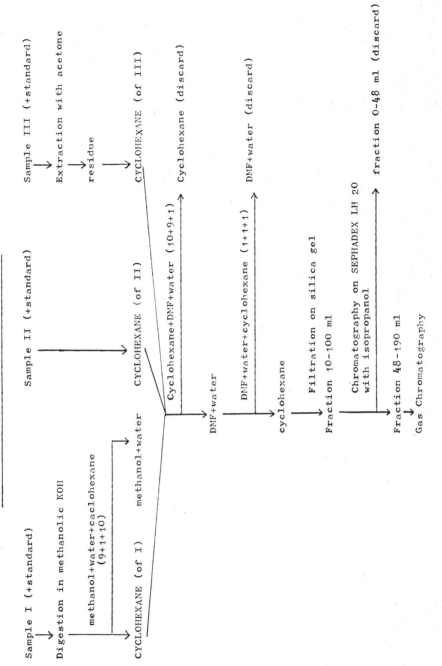

SCHEMATIC REPRESENTATION OF PROCEDURE

Sample I (+standard)   Sample II (+standard)   Sample III (+standard)

Digestion in methanolic KOH   Extraction with acetone

methanol+water+caclohexane (9+1+10)   residue

CYCLOHEXANE (of I)   methanol+water   CYCLOHEXANE (of II)   CYCLOHEXANE (of III)

Cyclohexane+DMF+water (10+9+1)   Cyclohexane (discard)

DMF+water

DMF+water+cyclohexane (1+1+1)   DMF+water (discard)

cyclohexane

Filtration on silica gel

Fraction 10-100 ml

Chromatography on SEPHADEX LH 20 with isopropanol   fraction 0-48 ml (discard)

Fraction 48-190 ml

Gas Chromatography

310

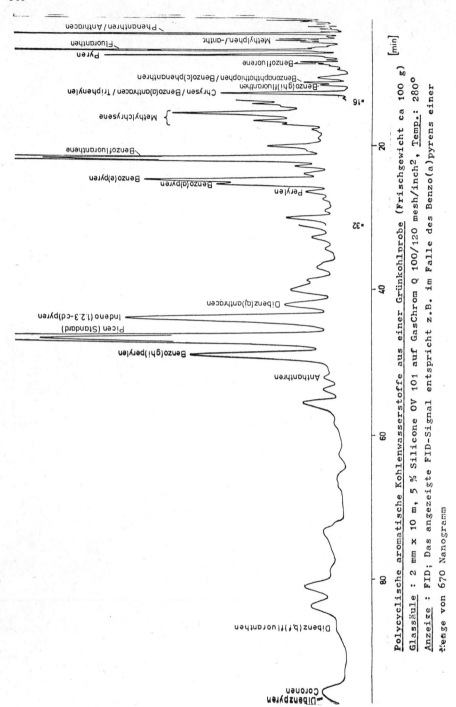

Polycyclische aromatische Kohlenwasserstoffe aus einer Grünkohlprobe (Frischgewicht ca 100 g)

__Glassäule__ : 2 mm x 10 m, 5 % Silicone OV 101 auf GasChrom Q 100/120 mesh/inch², __Temp.__: 280°

__Anzeige__ : FID; Das angezeigte FID-Signal entspricht z.B. im Falle des Benzo(a)pyrens einer Menge von 670 Nanogramm

$$\mu g(PAH)/kg = \frac{t(PAH) \times h(PAH) \times \mu g(IS)/kg}{t(IS) \times h(IS)}$$

t(PAH)	= Retention time of thePAH from the injection (in cm or min)
t(IS)	= Retention time of the Internal Standard
h(PAH)	= Height of the signal of the PAH to be calculated (in cm)
h(IS)	= Height of the Internal Standard
μg(PAH)/kg	= concentration of the PAH to be calculated
μg(IS)/kg	= known concentration of the Internal Standard

8.1 Repeatability

(same operator, same apparatus, same laboratory and same time).
Sample: Sewage sludge, ca. 5 g samples (freeze dried), 5 analysis;
determination of 19 PAH (range o.19 μg/g to 4.28 μg/g). The variation coefficients range from 2.4 % to 11.o % (GRIMMER et al., 1977).

8.2 Reproducibility (different operators, different apparatus, different laboratories) see: Collaborative Studies of the IUPAC with sunflower oil and meat (see Scope, page 1).

8.3 Limit of detection of PAH
In the range of the retention time of benzo(a)pyrene and by 1/8 of the highest sensitivity of the FID, the noise level correspond to 2 ng BaP, and therefore the minimum detectable amount would be about 6 ng (full scale: o.5 μg BaP in case of 1/8 of the highest sensitivity).

9. Bibliographical References

Titles for information about the content of polycyclic aromatic hydrocarbons in different foods, soils, and sediments.
A.-Enrichment as described, but determinated by UV-method:

1. KOHLENWASSERSTOFFE IN DER UMGEBUNG DES MENSCHEN.
   GRIMMER, G.& A. HILDEBRANDT 1965: Der Gehalt polycyclischer Kohlen wasserstoffe in Brotgetreide verschiedener Standorte.
   Z. Krebsforschg. 67,272-77.

2. GRIMMER, G. & A. HILDEBRANDT 1965: Der Gehalt polycyclischer Kohlen-wasserstoffe in verschiedenen Gemüsesorten und Salaten.
   Dtsch.Lebensm.Rundsch. 61, 237-39.

3. GRIMMER, G. & A. HILDEBRANDT 1966:Der Gehalt polycyclischer Kohlen-wasserstoffe in Kaffee und Tee. Dtsch.Lebensm.Rundsch., 62, 19-21.

4. GRIMMER, G. & A. HILDEBRANDT 1967: Der Gehalt polycyclischer Kohlen-wasserstoffe in Fleisch und Räucherwaren. Z.Krebsforschg., 69, 223-29.

312

5. GRIMMER, G. & A. HILDEBRANDT 1967: Content of polycyclic hydrocarbons in crude vegetable oils. Chem. & Industry 2ooo-o2.

6. GRIMMER, G. & A. HILDEBRANDT 1968: Der Gehalt polycyclischer Kohlenwasserstoffe in rohen Pflanzenölen. Arch.Hyg.Bakteriol. 152/3, 255-59.

7. GRIMMER, G. & G. WILHELM 1969: Der Gehalt polycyclischer Kohlenwasserstoffe in europäischen Hefen. Dtsch.Lebensm.Rundsch. 65, 229-31.

8. GRIMMER, G. & D. DÜVEL 197o: Untersuchungen zur endogenen! Bildung von polycyclischen Kohlenwasserstoffen in höheren Pflanzen. Z.Naturforschg. 25b, 1171-75.

9. GRIMMER, G., J. JACOB & A. HILDEBRANDT 1972: Der Gehalt polycyclischer Kohlenwasserstoffe in isländischen Bodenproben. Z.Krebsforschg. 78, 65-72.

B. - Enrichment and determination by gas chromatography:

1o. GRIMMER, G. & H. BÖHNKE 1975: Polycyclic Aromatic Hydrocarbons Profile Analysis of High-Protein Foods, Oils, and Fats by Gas Chromatography. J.Ass.Off.Anal.Chem. 58, 725-733.

11. GRIMMER, G. & H. BÖHNKE 1975: Profile Analysis of Polycyclic Aromatic Hydrocarbons and Metal Content in Sediment Layers of a Lake. Cancer Letter 1, 75-84.

12. MÜLLER, G., G. GRIMMER & H. BÖHNKE 1977: Sedimentary Record of Heavy Metals and Polycyclic Aromatic Hydrocarbons in Lake Constance. Naturwiss. 64, 427-431.

13. GRIMMER, G. & H. BÖHNKE 1977: Untersuchungen von Sedimentkernen des Bodensees. I.Profile der polycyclischen aromatischen Kohlenwasserstoffe. Z.Naturforschung 32c.

14. GRIMMER, G. & H. BÖHNKE 1977: Polycyclic Aromatic Hydrocarbons and Heterocyclics and their Relation to Maturity of Crude Oil from the Gifhorn Trough (Northwestern Germany).
Erdöl & Kohle, Erdgas 3o.

15. GRIMMER, G. , H. BÖHNKE & H. BORWITZKY 1977: Profile Analysis of Polycyclic Aromatic Hydrocarbons in Sewage Sludge by Gas Chromatography. Fresenius Z. Anal. Chem.

ORGANO-HALOGENATED COMPOUNDS IN FARM AND DOMESTIC ANIMALS

Prof. Dr. med.vet. H.-J. Hapke
Abteilung für Toxikologie
Institut für Pharmakologie der Tierärztlichen Hochschule
Bischofsholer Damm 15
3ooo Hannover

1. Past and current programmes

There are no programmes at all in the sense of an observing system. Systematic investigations with representative results are not performed till today.

But there is one exception: the food control. This control is prescribed by law. The datas of the residues in food are not published in general and are varying between different analysis laboratories. Today only those results are available, which are got without any system in the Public Food or Veterinary Analysis Boards. The purpose of these investigation is to control the residues in meat, organs, milk and eggs, whether they are without healthy effects upon the consumers. To control the maximal tolerated concentrations (tolerances) is the only purpose. But they give no information about the total environmental situation and don't allow any interpretion of the toxic condition, because the collection is not representative. Many datas are not acceptable without further confirmation by other investigators. The results often are not produced under controlled conditions and sometimes without relevant methods. The comparison between two laboratories or between two periods of time is very difficult or is impossible. In the very last years the laboratories of food control participate incircular control analyses systems.
Samples for further investigations and after-controls are not yet available. After residue analyses the probes will be destroyed. The election of the samples is without any system but accidentally distributed over a region. The results of investigations are collected in the reports to the government yearly (State Ministry of Food, Agriculture and Forest). Sometimes a connection exists between the investigating laboratory and the Central Collecting and Evaluating Board of the Federal Health Office. Many thousands datas are collected by this way in schedules. In some institutes like the Federal Research Institutions the results are stored in computers. It will be necessary to have a banking system in the field of residues in food from animals. That means not only a banking system of results, but also and mainly a system of specimens for later investigations. That system is necessary to compare different years and different areas. We may suppose that differences exist between residue concentrations in tissues from animals near industrial factories and those animals far away from an industrial area. We can suppose too, that a development take place in the values of the residues form year to year and that there is a qualitative change in the residue situation. But there is no proof.
Only by a banking system we may have an answer to these questions.
Today there are only datas resulting from very accidentally investigations, according to the technical arrangement of the institute or to the personnaly interest of the researcher. Concentrations of organochlorine compounds in farm animal tissues are determined since many years ago. Keeping in mind that the most persistent compounds of these group, DDT and related substan-

ces, accumulate in the food chain from feed to farm animals and than to men and at least to babies, this compound DDT was an object of intensive investigations. We can establish that the concentrations of DDT and of the more resistent metabolites DDD and DDE decrease in the very last years after banning the use of these pesticides in central Europe and in most industrialized countries.

It may be that instead of DDT other pesticides like HCH are used in the same indication as DDT before banning. In presence it will be more usefull therefore to determine HCH in the tissues instead of DDT.

The second of the most important compounds is HCB. It is not only important in regard to its toxicity, which is very low, but to its persistence and accumulating potency too. The isomeres of HCH, i.e. alpha, beta and delta, and other organochlorine pesticides are of less importance, because they are determined irregularly and not in all animals. Dieldrine, heptachlor-epoxide, endrine persist only in few animals. They are not fit and relevant for a specimen banking system. It will be usefull to reduce the sample examination to only some compounds, which can then be used as standard contaminants. The obove mentioned substances HCH and HCB are present always and everywhere, only in different concentrations. But firstly it should be sure that the concentrations of the standard contaminants indeed are related within narrow boarders to the concentrations of other organochlorine compounds and of pesticides in agricultural practice.

The storage of organochlorine pesticides in animal tissues, mainly in fat, underlies very small changes, due to the little metabolism of fatty tissues. The concentrations give therefore a correct picture of the general contamination of the last months.

2. Rational for interest

PCB's and PBB's are widely used in technique and industry, in household and in animal stables. Farm animals are contaminated by these persistent compounds only indirectly by eating residues in feed or by inhaling the compounds in gaseous forms. The toxicities of these substances are very low and are dependent on the degree of the chlorination of the molecule.

Other organochlorine compounds like TCDD or organic solvents are only of a local value and give no general information to describe the environmental condition. The concentrations in tissues are dependent on the contact of the animal with these compounds. The contact will be very seldom in farm animals and is only possible after an accident. It is not suitable to include these substances in a specimen banking system, though they are very toxic and dangerous and are therefore very important as environmental toxicants.

But in regard to the costs of the whole monitoring programm the determination should be restricted to those compounds which may be served as contamination standards or guide substances. The indicator compounds gamma-HCH and PCB's can be implemented for a monitoring system regarding farm animals by using adipose tissues, milk and eggs. The method of choice in the chemical analysis is the combination of gas chromatography with mass spectrometry.

The effects of environmental compounds on farm animals concern two different aspects: first the toxic action on the animal as a living being, second the accumulation and presence of the substance in eddible tissues of the farm animals including milk and eggs.

The investigation of food (meat control) is restricted today to determine only antimicrobial acting agents, estrogenes and thyreostatics. There is a proposal in the Federal Republic of Germany in connection with the EEC to

investigate meat for residues of some heavy metals like lead, mercury and
cadmium. But the changes of normal difficulties consist in the normal concentrations of ubiquitous substances in contaminated animals. Therefore
it is not yet possible to fix a maximal tolerated concentration for environmental chemicals today.
Many assays of the residues of environmental compounds in food were performed and today we know the amounts of the most important contaminants. In
summary these concentrations are:

	meat	liver	kidney	eggs	milk
DDT	o,1			o,o4	
DDD	o,o6			o,oo6	o,2
DDE	o,1			o,o5	
HCH	o,5			o,o5	o,o5
HCB	o,3	o,oo2	o,o15	o,o2	o,15
PCB's	o,2			o,3	o,3
Dieldrine	o,o2			o,o1	o,o2
Heptachlor-epoxide	o,o1			o,o1	o,o5

Dogs and cats as domestic animals are not representative for the whole contamination of animals, because they are exposed varying conditions in the
households. They do not indicate an ecological contamination, and should
not be included in the specimens banking system.
The category of organohalogenated compounds contains many different substances. They belong to different toxicological groups.
The classical substances related to DDT are Hexachlorcyclohexane, the
diene-group and the indene-group. These compounds produce similar reactions
in the animals, the domestic animals as well as in laboratory animals as
well as in men. Species-differences are not known in regard to the type of
actions. Differences may exist in the effective doses.
Many other pesticides are organohalogenated, even organophosphorous esters,
some nitrobenzenes (i.g. quintozene), coumarines, many herbicides like linuron and related compounds or chlorinated carbonic acids (phenoxy herbicides). The last mentioned pesticides show other reactions in the animals
than the classical organohalogenated pesticides mentioned above.
The toxic action of chlorine-containing organophosphorous esters is caused
by an inhibition of acetyl choline esterase. Coumarine interfere with the
blood coagulation system. Nitrobenzenes irritate the mucosa of the gastrointestinal tract. The toxicity is very low, but quintozene may be metabolized to hexachlorbenzene (HCB), which is a stable compound and accumulates
in the body. Urea-derivatives (e.g. diuron, linuron, monolinuron, monuron)
produce in animals unspecific ations after high doses only. Investigations
of tissues to determine these compounds are possible, but are not carried out
systematically in meat control up to this day. The presence of herbicides in
animal tissues is seldom, because herbicides are used to kill plants before
crop intake and before feeding the plants to animals. Residues may only
occure after application of persistent herbicides or their metabolites respectively, like HCB. Halogenated dioxines are not used in the agriculture
practice. Residues in animal tissues can only remain after contamination
with dioxinecontaining herbicides. Today the purity of phenoxyherbicides
is very high so that dioxine may occure only in very low concentrations of

neglecticable value.

3. Considerations for sample selection.

A monitoring system in the sense of systematical investigations is not performed till today. It can be established easily by an other organization of
the existing system of food control.
Additional informations are useful and necessary by reporting the following datas of the animals: Species, age, sex, geographical regions, type
of feed (corresponding to a banking system of plant contaminants), application of veterinary drugs, health conditions, date and time of sampling
(only before feeding). Only those farms should be included in the investigation programme, whose owners resign to use pesticides in the stables.

To standardize the storage programme and to reduce variations in results
it is necessary to choose only a small group of selected animals with uniform properties, e.g.(1) milk, kidney and perirenal adipose tissue from
female cows, more than two years old; (2) calfs not elder than 2o weeks:
kidneys and perirenal adipose tissue,(3) pigs of loo kg body weight($\pm$ 2o kg)
with the same tissues; (4) eggs of farm hens held in batteries and fed with
a standard feed.
Two alternative systems are possible: The first is, to build up a system
like a land-register including all regions by investigations of a representative quantity of animals distributed regular in the country. The other
system considers only populations at risk. With regard to the organochlorine
compounds it seems to be that all animals in a country are contaminated uni-
formely. Differences are not be recognized up to date. In case of heavy
metals (e.g. lead) or other industrial emissions the concentrations of
these compounds are very different depending on the station of the donor
animal.
Fat and kidneys should be taken as indicator tissues for analysis of organo-
halogenated compounds. Other tissues are abundant in the field of these
substances. To analyze heavy metals other tissues like hair or bones should
be taken. The present scientific knowledge about the presence of biocides
in animal tissues is based on available informations. To discuss other pollutants more informations are needed.
The analytical procedure is only successful by using gas chromatography
with capillary glas columns to separate the different types of organohalo-
genides, especially PCB's and DDT-compounds.
To minimize the experimental error it is necessary to compare the own
results of the laboratory with those of other labs, that means to participate in circular controls.
The collection and storage of specimens from farm animals is feasable by
the existing system of food control, prescribed by law.
After collection the samples are to be stored in uniform tubes with identification remarks.
A part of the sample will be analyzed immediately in the regional laboratory. This laboratory then will send the datas together with the rest of
the samples to a central laboratory for banking each data and specimen.
To provide statistically meaning full results and to have representative
results it will be necessary to gather 2o probes from a district out of
2ooo animals.
High costs are not to be expected by this proposal because already today
the investigations in meat control can be estimated. To perform the proposal about the collection of datas the actual costs will not increase significantly.

But new costs will arise by the storage of samples. The expansive cooling houses to store food supply perhaps may be able to take up the specimens. The programme of selecting donors and collecting specimens can not
be restricted to a single country but must consider several states of comparable technical situation.
It may be useful, to compare the concentrations,measured in the tissues,
with biological effects of the compound on the animal. But the low concentrations of organochlorines do not have any effect which could be determined
by simple methods. The first effect, the induction of enzyme activity, is
very expansive and difficult to determine in farm animals. Other possible
effects of some organohalogenated compounds, i.e. porphyria, are very seldom to be seen and can't be established.
The samples, fat and kidneys, are easy to get and to collect without danger
to come in quarrel with the owner of the slaughtered animal. It may be a
problem or may be impossible to have a piece of liver or meat. But the results will not be different from liver or kidney. Meat is not useful to analyze to determine residues, because this tissue shows only very low concentrations of the biocides.
The determination of lead and of PCB's should be chosen as standards to
which other compounds should be related. The determination of lead and of
PCB's are well established and standardized today and may be controlled
continuously by participating in a control system within the "good laboratory
practice".
To collect datas and specimens in a combined system it will be useful and
necessary to build up a monitoring system in the existing Offices for food
control, i.e. Chemical and Veterinary Analysis Boards of the towns or countries.
Today there are many samples and datas available in these laboratories. But
they are mostly won by different methods and they began to be collected in
the Federal Health Office in Berlin (Collecting and Evaluation Center).
These offices, the Center of the Federal Health Office and the Chemical
or Veterinary Analyses Boards of the states should prepare a data sheet in
a uniform type. With this data sheet it will be possible to guarantee a
data system representative for the whole country to observe.
The monitoring system as discussed here is primarily a collection of datas
and results (or specimens). But it is not only the purpose to have a huge
collection. The aim must be the interpretation of these datas and results.
The datas must have any rebound effect.
Afterwards we have to compare the datas of every year and to form the diffe-
rece. If this difference is negative in an arithmetic sense, that means
a reduction of the concentration of biocides. Is in contrast the difference
positive, the concentrations increase in the period under investigation.
This programme describes the situation in food for human consumption. It
does not describe an environmental condition. The organohalogene compounds
in fat tissues are not representative for the situation in the environment
because these substances are ingested by feed, which mostly is not gathered
in by the farmer. The modern way of feeding and holding practice in animal
production uses food produced by industry and partly imported from foreign
countries.
A second way of "false contamination" is the use of organohalogenated compounds as veterinary drugs, e.g. for parasite control.
These two ways of contamination make it impossible to take samples from farm
animals only for a monitoring system of environmental situation of the region observed.

In summary the equipment of a monitoring environmental materials and specimen banking may have the following form:

- Selection of farmers, who are representative for a region;

- collection of adipose tissue and kidney from slaughtered calfs, cows and pigs and of milk and eggs;

- first determination of HCH and PCB's in the above mentioned tissue in regional laboratories;

- storage of the results and the remaining specimen; supervised by the Collecting and Evaluation Center of the Federal Health Office, which is already established.
This system can be proposed (in the Federal Republic of Germany or in related Centres of other Countries).

- Current evaluation of the results (and their changes from time to time and from region to region) and redetermination of HCH and PCB's in the storaged tissues in the central laboratory.

- The determination of organohalogenated compounds in animal tissues does not give exact pictures of the environmental situation because foreign feed and veterinary drugs may introduce these compounds into the animals without taking the way through the environment.

Annex

to: H.-J. Hapke, Organo halogenated compounds in farm and domestic animals.

Programme Design

The country under survey is to be divided in different parts concerning to agricultural and technical situations (i.e. pure rural conditions without any industry on one side, a totally industrialized region on the other side and the different types between these extremes).
The results of analyses undertaken by the official investigation institutes of the states or of the cities are to be collected and stored in a centrally acting place, like the Federal Health Office in Germany. As these investigations are already in programme since many years, the only work in future is to introduce the above mentioned collecting system considering the representative way of specimens.

Statistics

As already mentioned (see above) one specimen should be taken out of an animal population of one hundred. The relation is already prescribed by law in the meat control act. For an exact description of an area or a country the results of the investigations of 2o specimens are representative for this area and they allow to see differences between two districts or between two investigation periods.

Organizational Aspects

The Federal Health Office (Bundesgesundheitsamt) may organize the banking and monitoring of materials in the Federal Republic of Germany. It will be no problem to establish a more effective system for collection, storing and recalling results. But it will be difficult at this time to collect and store specimens. I am unable to make a proposal for this item.

Cost estimation

The costs of the collection of results and the costs of the investigations are already present in this time. The total sum is unknown to me. New costs will arise concerning to the collection of specimens and to store them. It is impossible to make an estimation about the amount.

MONITORING ENVIRONMENTAL MATERIALS AND SPECIMEN BANKING FOR
ORGANOHALOGENATED COMPOUNDS IN AQUATIC ECOSYSTEMS

Dr. A. Holden
Freshwater Fisheries Laboratory
Pitlochry
Perthshire PH 16 5 LB
United Kingdom

Summary

Monitoring programmes must have specific objectives, and the sampling
and analytical procedures must be designed to provide data which will
enable the objectives to be attained with measurable precision. Both
physical and biological samples can be used, but the former will be difficult to interpret in respect of the effects of pollutant levels on aquatic life.
Biological samples must be clearly specified, and the species must be selected on the basis of abundance, easy accessibility and identification,
and where possible sexing and ageing, without risk to the population
sampled. Where trends in contamination level at a particular location
are to be monitored, a species appropriate to that site will be sufficient, but if comparisons are to be made between locations or areas,
species common to those locations or ecologically equivalent species
must be selected.
Samples will represent the site of sampling at the time, and not necessarily adjacent sites or other times. If pollution is localised, other sites at short distances must be sampled to determine the extent of the
polluted area, but for baseline contamination levels or low-level pollution sampling sites can be more widely spaced. In biological specimens
the pollutant level may vary with season and age, and also with the external pollutant concentration. Frequent sampling may be required if the
pollution level fluctuates, but even for annual sampling the specimens
taken must be in the same physiological condition.
Many organochlorine compounds are not very persistent in the environment
and some are not accumulated to a high degree. Others, particularly certain pesticides and high molecular weight industrial compounds such as
PCB's, are persistent and concentrated in lipids from the external aqueous
environment by several orders of magnitude. Only a few halogenated compounds are currently monitored, and new analytical techniques may be
necessary to extend monitoring to other compounds.
The factors influencing the selection of species and tissues for monitoring purposes are discussed, but in general shoaling fish and colonial invertebrates are preferred, taking advantage of their relative abundance,
accessibility and the possibilities of age and size selection to reduce
the variance among individuals. Experience with the OECD monitoring programme is described and costs assessed.

Organohalogen compounds

This large group of compounds includes both aliphatic and aromatic molecules containing one or more atoms of chlorine, bromine, iodine or fluorine, but the substances of greatest concern in the environment have been primarily synthetic chemicals containing chlorine (and in a few instances bromine or fluorine). Those which have had the most impact on living organisms in the aquatic environment are generally of a non-polar, lipophilic nature with relatively low solubility in water. The organochlorine pesticides DDT, aldrin, dieldrin, endrin, heptachlor (and its epoxide degradation product), hexachlorobenzene, hexachlorocyclohexane (mainly the α- and γ-isomers), toxaphene (chlorinated camphene), chlordane and mirex can be accumulated from water into organisms by factors of several orders of magnitude due to their high solubility in lipids. A second group of halogenated pesticides, the chlorinated phenoxy-acetic acids, are used in the form of amines and esters, but are less persistent and more easily degraded in the environment, although some degree of accumulation may occur in tissues for short periods. The same is true of the herbicids pentachlorophenol, used usually in the form of its sodium salt.

Another group of highly chlorinated non-polar compounds, the polychlorinated biphenyls (PCB), which have been manufactured for various industrial purposes since about 193o, have been discharged to the aquatic environment and have accumulated in biological tissue in the same manner as the chlorinated pesticides. The PCB group consists of a large number of isomers and homologues, the majority in environmental samples containing three to seven chlorine atoms, and sixty or seventy different compounds have been identified in commercial PCB mixtures. Other groups of compounds with similar properties are the polychlorinated terphenyls (PCT's), the polybrominated biphenyls (PBB's) and the polychlorinated naphthalenes (PCN's). These groups have been identified in only a few instances in environmental samples, but most analysts do not employ techniques which are certain to detect them. High molecular weight chlorinated paraffins are also manufactured on a large scale, and have been used as substitutes for PCB's.

Impurities in PCB mixtures are the chlorinated dibenzofurans (CDBF's), which are extremely toxic but so far have not been detected in significant concentrations in the aquatic environment. A second group of highly toxic impurities which may occur in the herbicide pentachlorophenol, the chlorinated dibenzodioxins (CDBD's), seem not to have been reported from aquatic samples. One extremely toxic tetrachlorodibenzo-p-dioxin has been found in technical 2, 4, 5-trichlorphenoxyacetic acid, a herbicide.

Other halogenated compounds manufactured in large quantities include the aliphatic chlorinated solvents and intermediates such as dichloromethane, chloroform, carbon tetrachloride, trichloroethylene, tetrachloroethylene, trichloroethane and hexachlorobutadiene. By-products of polyvinyl chloride manufacture have also been discharged to the marine environment, while more volatile halogenated compounds in large-scale production include the chlorobromomethane fire extinguisher fluids, and the fluorocarbon propellants. In general these lower halogenated aliphatic compounds show less tendency to accumulate to any degree in biological tissues, and are probably transported fairly readily to the atmosphere. The position of the lower chlorinated aromatic compounds ortho- and para-dichlorobenzene is obscure, and although they can be discharged to the aquatic environment they are likely to undergo degradation and are probably not persistent.

Existing monitoring programmes for organohalogenated compounds are capable of identifying and quantifying DDT (and its metabolites TDE and DDE); aldrin (rapidly oxidised to dieldrin), dieldrin, endrin; HCB and the HCH isomers; toxaphene, chlordane and mirex (these three with some difficulty); heptachlor and heptachlor epoxide; and the PCB group. Most of the other compounds referred to above are less persistent or used on a more restricted scale. Similarly, while knowledge of the accumulation, excretion, metabolism and degradation of the pesticides and PCB's is now fairly well understood, information on the occurrence and fate of the solvents, fire retardants, refrigerants, propellants and the other higher halogenated compounds in the aquatic environment is very limited.

PAST AND CURRENT PROGRAMMES OF QUATIC MONITORING AND SPECIMEN BANKING

a) Monitoring

Many programmes of sampling and analysis of aquatic samples, both freshwater and marine, have been undertaken for the study of organochlorine contamination, but very few have been designed to provide information over a period of years using a standardised procedure. Samples taken on one occasion, or at intervals unsystematically, are not considered here. Several countries have monitoring organisations with the specific function of examining samples of various food commodities for organochlorine and other residues, in fulfilment of programmes of human health protection, and in the course of such programmes freshwater and marine fish and shellfish (and possibly other aquatic products) are regularly examined. The samples, however, will be selected as representative of food supplies rather than of the marine or freshwater communities, and associated data relevant to the exact location from which the specimens were taken will not be available. In a few instances a monitoring programme has been designed to provide both information on fish as a human food resource and as a representative component of a defined area of the aquatic environment, but rarely have countries established monitoring programmes for the purpose of protecting aquatic ecosystems.

In the United States, a programme for monitoring pesticides in the freshwater environment was developed in the late 1960's, using a large number of species of fish, each being sampled where it is sufficiently abundant. A few of the species are present in most States, enabling a level of direct comparison to be made, but in general the information provided by the use of a wide variety of species would make interpretation of the analytical data difficult. Extension of monitoring in this form to other continentsemphasises the problem of selecting species which are sufficiently similar in their habitats and general behaviour to allow direct comparison of the analytical data obtained from them. Nevertheless, changes with time could be assessed at each individual sampling location.

In the U.S. National Pesticides Monitoring Prcgramme of which the above-mentioned sampling is a part, five whole fish of each available species at each site were taken as a sample, and wight, length and age recorded. The five individuals were then ground together to a homogeneous mixture for analysis. Such a procedure gives no information on residue levels in individual organs or tissues, or variation with size, sex or age. The groups of five fish cannot be regarded as of uniform composition and an element of variation due to this heterogeneity is almost inevitable. Age and size selection could be important in minimising the influence of these factors on residue levels.

In the United States, shellfish (oysters and mussels) have been used as
monitoring species in coastal waters since 1965. These species are known
to be able to lose organochlorine residues rapidly by flushing, but nevertheless their sedentary nature is a considerable advantage in monitoring
the local environment, and they are more easily sampled than mobile species such as fish. Samples were taken from selected sites on both the Atlantic and Pacific coasts at monthly or three-monthly intervals, and
good correlations between residue levels and the use of agricultural pesticides in adjacent drainage areas were found. The techniques of sampling,
preservation and preparation for analysis were standardised and a single
laboratory was initially responsible for the analyses. The large numbers
of sampled eventually taken necessitated the employment of other laboratories, but by the use of identical techniques and adequate training good
agreement was obtained between the analysts.

Other national monitoring programmes for organochlorine residues in the
aquatic environment have not been as extensive or as prolonged as that of
the United States. In the United Kingdom several marine fish species were
sampled from 1969 to 1972 from commercial landings at ports in England,
Wales and Scotland, and in Scotland these have been continued to the present time. Ten fish of each species were selected at random, muscle fillets
taken and from these a single homogenate was prepared for each species and
area of sampling, this being carried out twice yearly in winter and summer.
The samples were primarily for food surveillance but also provided an
assessment of the pollutant status of each area fished. No monitoring programme for freshwater species has yet been developed in the United Kingdom.

Analyses of freshwater and marine fish for organochlorine residues have
been made in Sweden for some years as part of a food monitoring programme,
these samples providing also in indication of the levels of DDT and PCB
in various parts of the Baltic Sea. No continuous sampling and analytical
programme specifically to follow trends in contamination levels of halogenated hydrocarbons in this area has yet been developed, although the possibility has been discussed by the Baltic Group of ICES (the International Council for the Exploration of the Sea).

Two baseline surveys of organochlorines in selected marine fish species in
the North Sea (the second also extended to the north-east Atlantic) have
been carried out by ICES, but although proposals have been made to extend
these in principle to a regular monitoring programme on an annual basis
with standardised sampling procedures, this has not yet begun. Similarly,
UNEP and FAO (GFCM) have planned a Co-ordinated Project on Pollution in
the Mediterranean, as part of a UNEP monitoring and research programme. Surveys of organochlorine residues in marine mussels in the northern part of
the Mediterranean Sea have been made by the International Atomic Energy
Agency laboratory of Monaco, sponsored by the United Nations Environment
Programme, but there is no indication that this type of survey will be extended to form the basis of a monitoring programme.

The Organisation for Economic Co-operation and Development (OECD) has since
1966 been developing collaborative programmes for the study of organochlorine (and mercury) contamination of the environment, involving up the 14
member countries primarily from Western Europe and North America.

The earlier programmes were designed to test the feasibility of international cóllaboration in this field, and intercalibration exercises tested the
extent of agreement among analysts reporting on the examination of organochlorine residues in prepared check samples. Comparison of contamination
levels between selected sites in various countries, using as far as possible the same fish (or bird) species,with standardisation of the individuals selected for each sample, have given valuable information on the practical difficulties involved in conducting such programmes, and also on the
extent of variation in residue contamination between individual fish or
birds in the samples.

The most recent OECD programme, which continued from 1972 to 1975 and has
in part been extended to 1977, involved a detailed and extensive sampling
and analytical programme for the determination of organochlorine (and mercury) residues in selected species of fish and birds at both uncontaminated
and contaminated sites in twelve countries. The data have been analysed by
computer with the aim of assessing the significance of trends with time in
levels of various contaminants, at each site sampled, in the freshwater,
marine and terrestrial environments. A considerable amount of valuable information was obtained from the initial four-year programme, both in respect of the trends of various organochlorine residues and also in the practicability of carrying out a programme in which the sizes, composition
and timing of the wildlife samples were clearly specified. Much of the information obtained is used in the present report, but a full report on the
OECD programmes has been prepared for publication, and all of the data
submitted for analysis together with the results of the computer analysis,
are available for further study. The programme was not designed to compare
levels of contamination in different countries, for which a more precise
selection of the sampling sites would be required.

b) Specimen Banking

Little information appears to be available on the existence of long-term
specimen banking operations at the present time. Survey and monitoring programmes usually involve the storage of samples under deep-freeze conditions
(generally -18°C to -2o°C) for such a period as is necessary before the
analyses are carried out, but surplus material is often subsequently discarded. The major difficulty is undoubtedly the lack of adequate storage
space, but there is also some doubt regarding the stability of samples
held at the temperature stated over periods greater than several months.
Possibly the use of commercial cold storage facilities with temperatures of
-3o°C or even lower would reduce the risk of deterioration to some extent,
but capacity is still a serious limitation. It is also necessary at the outset to decide whether specimens can be removed for sub-sampling and returned
to the storage facility without any deterioration. Multiple samples could
avoid the need to return any samples removed for analysis, but would require even greater storage facilities.

A scheme for storing specimens of various species of wildlife at low temperature, to provide representative samples over many years for purposes
such as the examination of trends in contaminant level, was in operation at
the Swedish Museum of Natural History in Stockholm in the 196o's, but it is
not known whether the scheme is still continuing. Preservation by freezing
is not always essential, and for some contaminants the use of formalin or
certain other preservatives could reduce the costs of storage considerably.

One major difficulty in designing a procedure for specimen banking, where one intended purpose is to provide material at a subsequent date for the analysis of pollutants not known or recognised at the time of sampling, is that organs or tissues most appropriate to the pollutant concerned must be selected for preservation. Organohalogen compounds known to be stored in fat can be examined in specimens of adipose tissue, or in organs or tissues with a high lipid content, and to a large extent concentrations in other organs will be related to the lipid content of those organs. However, degradation may take place by enzyme action in the liver (even during storage) but the presence of metabolites in fresh liver samples does not imply that these metabolites will be in similar proportions in other body tissues. Furthermore, it is known that concentrations in the brain are not directly related to lipid content, but as this could be a critical organ in respect of the toxic effects of pollutants it could be one which should be chosen for long-term storage.

For other contaminants such as heavy metals, liver or kidney may be the perferred organs, and in a programme designed to retain samples suitable for a wide variety of pollutants a number of organs and tissues may be selected.

It is essential, if samples are frozen, that they are individually sealed to avoid any possibility of desiccation. Significant weight changes will result in incorrect values of pollutant concentration on a fresh (wet) weight basis. If specimens are dried before preservation, it is essential that the wet/dry weight ratio is determined,and tests must be made to ensure that no residues are lost during the drying process (freeze-drying or grinding with a desiccant being preferable to ovendrying). Drying may only be suitable where the samples are required solely for chemical analysis, and it is preferable to sub-divide dried samples if in powdered form, to avoid the possibility of contamination or other deterioration .of the entire sample when the first examination is made.

PROGRAMME DESIGN

Non of the national sampling programmes appear to have been designed to allow for the statistical analysis of the data obtained from them. The OECD programme for 1972-75 was planned with the intention of processing the data by computer, and in consequence the types of sample taken and the method of reporting were specified at the outset. However, it was not always found possible to carry out the instructions as intended, and the statistical analysis proved to be more complex than was anticipated.

Purpose of Monitoring The design of a monitoring programme must take into account the purpose for which the monitoring is required. Essentially the samples taken are intended to be representative of a particular location at a specified time, and in the case of a species may also be chosen to represent that species as a commodity which is to be used for another purpose. Thus a sediment or water sample could be selected to represent the environmental conditions in respect of a pollutant level, but a fish or shellfish sample may be of value both as representative of contaminant levels in the environment and as a food resource for human consumption.

Monitoring itself implies the possibility that action in some form may be taken on the basis of the concentration of contaminant found, or that the information is required to assess the effectiveness of such action. Unacceptable levels of a contaminant in fish examined in a monitoring programme could lead to the rejection of commercial catches of that species, and to a consideration of measures to control the use or discharge of the pollutant in question, either because the chemical rendered the fish unacceptable as human food or because of its potentially harmful effect on the fish or other members of the aquatic community.

Types of Sample   The sample taken, whether of a biological nature or part of the physical environment (water or sediment), is assumed to be representative of the sampling location and of the time of sampling. Samples of water, while most appropriate in the freshwater environment if the primary purpose of monitoring is to assess the quality of water for human consumption or food processing, present difficulties in several respects if the aim is to determine the influence on other components of the ecosystem. The relationship between the concentration of an organohalogen compound in water and levels in living organisms is complex, and even the concentration/effect relationship is dependent on exposure time and the form in which the pollutant is present in the water (eg dissolved or particulate, whether ionised or not). Concentrations in water could vary more rapidly than those in organisms, and the determination of organohalogen concentrations in water at the levels which usually occur, particularly in the sea, is difficult and subject to qualification, eg whether or not the sample is filtered, and the imporatance to be attached to living or inert suspended matter.

Sediment samples are difficult to quantify in respect of contaminants which may be confined to the upper few millimetres of the deposit, although calculation on an areal basis rather than on a weight or volume basis may be more appropriate. Core sampling, and section cutting to define the depth within the core, is preferable to grab sampling, but care must be taken to avoid disturbing the sediment surface when operating the sampler. Sediment disturbance is perhaps a more serious problem where any form of demersal fishing takes place, as mixing of a deep layer of mud will be inevitable and pollutants could be dispersed through a considerable depth of sediment instead of being confined to the surface. Sediments which are of coarse sand, gravel or stones are unsuitable for sampling.

Samples of plankton, which may include suspended particulate matter and oil or tar droplets, can be very variable in composition, and depend greatly on the characteristics of the apparatus used (eg mesh size of net, efficiency of grab sampler). Of other invertebrates, small crustacea have been suggested as monitoring organisms in fresh waters, but they must be sufficiently abundant and easy to identify, so that an adequate quantity of the sample material can be obtained for analysis. Large pelagic invertebrates such as squid could also be considered.

While certain shellfish such as mussels or oysters are relatively sedentary, fish may migrate over considerable distances and their contaminant residues may thus have been assimilated in an area other than that in which the sample is taken. Moreover, the residues may reflect contamination at an earlier time, after an interval of weeks, months or even years, depending whether the chemical is one which is retained permanently in the tissues, is excreted slowly or rapidly, or is metabolised and subsequently stored or excreted.

The biological half-life in tissues depends on the nature of the chemical substance, the organ or tissue and the species in question. Thus PCP's may be retained in fish tissues for periods of months after the original exposure, and only slowly lost in clean water, whereas organochlorine pesticides can be excreted by fish in a few weeks. Oysters can accumulate concentrate DDT from water by a factor of 25.ooo in 96 hours, but can also lose 9o % of the residues by fushing in clean water in a week.

This ability to accumulate and discharge by flushing varies between species of molluscs. Accumulation in both aquatic invertebrates and vertebrates, in respect of halogenated organic compounds at least, may result from direct uptake from the water through respiratory surfaces or by ingestion in food particles or organisms. Thus the concentration of a substance found in an organ or tissue is not necessarily correlated with one particular concentration in the surrounding medium. Phytoplankton and algae, however, may contain residue levels more directly related to concentrations in the external medium, although the adherence of particulate matter to the external surfaces is likely to make accurate determination of concentrations in cell tissue difficult.

Few studies have been made of the short-term variations to be expected in fish or shellfish, although monthly samples or oysters taken in the United States were effective in revealing the seasonal use of DDT in the drainage area of river basins. Similarly, monthly samples of the freshwater roach in Sweden showed a marked increase in PCB levels in individual month, followed by equally marked decreases, although the reason for these fluctuations was not identified. These examples illustrate the difficulty of using yearly or even quarterly samples to represent the contamination of a particular aquatic location, if discharges of a pollutant or exposure to that pollutant are intermittent. The selection of a sampling site could be based on proximity to known discharge, but unless the discharge is at a sustained level it might be necessary to sample at frequent intervals, particularly if the half life of the pollutant in the species sampled is relatively short. On the other hand, sampling at sites distant from any discharge need only be made at long intervals.

Tissue concentrations are not only dependent on the external concentrations. Physiological changes in the species, whether due to sexual maturation or starvation, result in changes in lipid concentration and in metabolism of lipid reserves, in which organohalogen compounds are concentrated. It is possible for organochlorine compounds to be toxic at such times of stress, due to the transport of the compounds to target organs at concentrations which are high enough to take effect. However, the relationship between organochlorine concentrations in tissues and lipids is not clearly defined, despite the many studies made on fish and shellfish, but in any monitoring programme it is advisable to specify the physiological state of the samples required unless they are taken frequently. The proportion of extractable lipid on the tissue or organ analysed should always be determined, so that results can be expressed on both a tissue and lipid basis. In the OECD programme, lipid content was found to be a major factor in the overall variance between individuals.

Other factors which may influence the concentration of organochlorine residues in individuals include the size and age, although correlations between these parameters and concentration depend on the species and tissue examined. Age was found to have an important influence on the variance in almost half of the series of fish samples examined in the OECD programme when this parameter was measured, but some biologists were unable to determine age in their fish samples. Length and weight were usually less important, but could not be entirely dismissed.

Of aquatic species other than those referred to, only birds and certain mammals have been examined in detail for organohalogen compounds. Both groups, however, are difficult to sample and to select. No detailed sampling programme for birds seems to have been undertaken, although several programmes have used the eggs of birds which feed primarily in the aquatic environment (eg pelicans, terns, guillemots and cormorants). This type of sample can only be related indirectly to the contamination level of the appropriate area of the aquatic environment, and the feeding range of the adult birds may not be easy to define.

Of the marine mammals, seals have been examined in several areas of the world, but it is not normally possible to acquire sufficient specimens of a selected type to provide an adequate sample for regular monitoring purposes. Nevertheless, by virtue of their high fat content, such mammals often concentrate organochlorines to high levels over long periods and thus indicate a significant degree of pollution at some time in their lifespan, although it seems unlikely that they will respond very quickly to changes in their external environment. Their residues are, as with birds, derived entirely through the food chain and not from the water.

Choice of Species   The selection of a wildlife species suitable for use in a monitoring programme depends on several factors. As it may be necessary to obtain a large number of individuals of the same age, size or sex, the species must be widely-distributed and the individuals abundant, easily accessible and identifiable. Sampling itself must not have any detrimental influence on a population. High-density populations such as flocks of birds or shoals of fish, or of certain species of invertebrates, must be considered. Nestlings or eggs of birds nesting in colonies may sometimes be sampled without affecting the population size, and in such cases the age can be assessed fairly accurately. Commercial fisheries can sometimes provide specimens for monitoring purposes, although samples may not always be obtainable at the specified times and locations, and the sampling operation is not under the control of the monitoring authority.

For regional or global monitoring, few species if any are sufficiently widely distributed, although it should usually be possible to substitute alternative species filling similar ecological niches. Migration may create difficulties both in obtaining the species at the same site at different seasons (if sampling is required more than once a year), and in associating tissue residues with the local environment. Sedentary species, or those known to remain in one area throughout the year, clearly have an advantage in this respect.

If it is considered desirable to monitor several trophic levels at a site, to provide confirmatory evidence, the selection of a number of species each of which is abundant could be difficult. However, samples of water and substrate could be useful for this purpose.

In the freshwater environment many species of shoaling fish occur, especi-

ally among the cyprinids, although in selecting similar species for the
OECD programme only two closely related perch species seemed to be
appropriate for the European and North American continents. In other regions similar types of fish (carnivores feeding primarily on invertebrate
species) could be identified. Invertebrates such as amphipods and molluscs
are abundant in many waters, but may be naturally limited by water quality.
Planktonic species cannot usually be selected individually, and the differences in composition of plankton hauls could be a serious source of
variance both between sites and sampling occasions. Ageing of invertebrates is not normally possible.

The distribution of plant species in fresh waters depends among other factors on water chemistry, the type of substrate and water depth, and selection of a species for the comparison of sites may be difficult. Surface
contamination by particulate matter, which could be difficult to remove,
could be a significant cause of variability, and it might be necessary
to select particular parts of a plant (e.g. leaves) to eliminate the
difference in contaminant concentration between leaves and stems, for example. No monitoring schemes using freshwater plants seem to have been described.

For sampling the marine environment, mussels or other molluscs have already been referred to. They are usually abundant and easily obtained where
present, although in distribution they are limited to shallow coastal
waters. A technique for using mussels on artificial substrates (eg mooring
ropes) has been developed and could increase the usefulness of these species for monitoring. The individuals are difficult to age, and growth rates are partly dependent on the exposure of the colony to wave action and
probably other factors.Of pelagic invertebrates, squid are abundant in
many areas and are of potential significance both because they feed on
smaller invertebrates (thus sampling this trophic level) and are themselves food for larger carnivores. It may be difficult to select individual species as commercial collections are normally a mixture of species.
The same criticism applies to samples of smaller zooplankton.

Plant material is difficult to utilise for marine monitoring, only seaweeds being available in sufficient quantities. These have similar disadvantages to those described for freshwater vegetation, and in inshore
waters will be less suitable than molluscs.

Of marine fish species, shoaling fish such as the clupoids (eg herring,
pilchards, anchovy or sprats) are useful for monitoring organochlorines by
virtue of their high lipid content, but they are restricted to certain areas
of the oceans. Oceanic monitoring samples must represent large areas, and
the use of species taken commercially by extensive netting, such as various gadoids, could be suitable where available. The age of fish can usually be determined by well-developed techniques, and in many cases some
index of condition is also available. Several species of hake (genus
Merluccius) occur in the Atlantic, Pacific and Mediterranean and might
serve in a global programme.

It may also be necessary or desirable to sample bottom-feeding species.
Flounder, plaice and sole are commercially available in many areas, although some flounder species may enter freshwaters and thus be exposed for

a period to different and possibly greater levels of pollution.

Sample Collection It must be recognised that the samples taken can basically only represent to populations from which they are taken and the times
at which they are obtained. Extrapolation beyond this must be considered
with caution. It is likely that seasonal variations in physiological condition will influence metabolism and excretion processes and the lipid content if tissues, an important factor in organochlorine analysis. As pollution levels in the external environment, especially in coastal areas, will
vary with distance from the source of pollution, the concentrations in individuals of a species will also vary. Mussel samples taken at 15-2o km
intervals along the coast of Scotland showed considerable variation between consecutive sites, probably reflecting local discharges. Sampling at,
for example, loo km intervals along a long coastline would therefore be
incapable of detecting many small discharges, and a programme of this type
could identify only large-scale pollution. For open ocean sampling, the
sites can be at much larger intervals, perhaps looo km for the monitoring
of low-level pollution, or loo km where local areas of significant pollution
exist.

Estuaries could require a more complex distribution of sampling sites, depending on the sources of discharge and the movement of pollutants by tidal
action. For shallow areas mussels could again be considered, but in the
deeper areas fish species would be necessary, and the choice of species is
restricted to those commonly found in estuaries, many of which may not be
commercially exploited. Sediment sampling is of doubtful value here for
monitoring (as opposed. to survey) purposes, as the movement of sediments
by tidal action or river flow will create considerable variability in composition independently of contaminant level.

In fresh water lakes sampling sites must be chosen with the same considerations in mind. Samples taken close to river discharges may be influenced more by the river than by general conditions in the lake, and would
thus reflect only local contamination. Even in a small lake differences
may be detected over relatively short distances if a polluting discharge
exists at one point.

Sampling in rivers involves certain problems not relevant to lake or
ocean sampling. Dispersion from a point of discharge is normally only in
a downstream direction, and sampling sites will therefore be located accordingly. Suitable species for sampling are more difficult to suggest and
particularly in small rivers species of shoaling fish may be absent or
difficult to sample. Sporadic or intermittent pollutant discharges can result in fluctuations in contamination of biological material which are
difficult to detect by occasional sampling. In such cases samples of sediment, if undisturbed, or composite water samples collected over a period,
may be of greater value.

Selection of Individual Specimens In natural animal populations individuals differ in sex, age and size, and any or all of these factors may be related to the concentration of an organohalogen compound in an tissue or
organ. The mean concentration of an organochlorine residue in a sample of
a population comprising a number of individuals will therefore be dependent on the sex or age composition of the sample.

In an earlier OECD study, between 1o and 25 individuals (birds and fish) were required per sample, but no sex, age or size selection was made. Statistical analysis showed that to detect a significant difference of 25 % between the means of two samples, fifty individuals would be required in each, analysed separately. This is a considerable analytical burden, but in the hope that greater precision could be obtained a subsequent programme required 25 individual fish to be selected for age, condition and sex, to reduce the variance.

These requirements proved difficult to attain. To obtain 25 three-year-old male (or female) herring, for example, it may be necessary to examine 1oo-2oo individual fish. To select fish in a particular physiological state, it is essential that the population is sampled at intervals until that state has been reached, at which time the required number of individuals is selected. The fat content of fish tissue was shown to be of fundamental importance in organochlorine monitoring in the OECD programme, as this parameter was responsible for a large proportion of the variance among individuals of a population in respect of residue concentration. However, measurement of the fat content and expression of the residue concentration on a lipid basis may eliminate the need to select for a prescribed physiological condition.

Although sex may have little influence on organochlorine concentrations, age was found in the OECD studies to be an important parameter in influencing the variance among individuals. Several participants were unable to obtain 25 fish of the same age, but recorded the age of each individual to enable an adjustment to be made for this variable. Weight and length of fish are usually highly correlated, and one of these parameters should be measured (or specified) as residue levels are frequently correlated with size.

In some programmes whole fish have been analysed, but the influence of visceral residue concentrations and the variable contents of stomachs could be significant factors in the variance among individuals. For this reason an organ or tissue with a high lipid content should be sampled, and muscle or liver are those commonly chosen, depending on the fish species.

The need to analyse individuals rather than a homogenate results in considerable expenditure on analysis, but a high proportion of samples taken in the OECD programmes showed a skew distribution of residue concentrations. Transformation of the data may then be required before the statistical analysis. The use of homogenates gives no information on the variance between individuals, which is essential in making comparisons between populations, or between years at the same location. Using 2o-25 individuals per sample the OECD programme was able to identify trends in contamination to a 1 % level of significance. For locating areas of gross pollution or identifying large changes, however, smaller samples or homogenates may be sufficient.

Frequency of Sampling For regional or global monitoring, sampling once a year is probably adequate, although the precise time must be specified either from a temporal or biological standpoint. Samples of fish and shellfish taken before spawning may be preferred, as the specimens should then be in good physiological condition. For monitoring the influence of seasonal pollutant discharges more frequent sampling (eg monthly or quarterly may be advisable.

Data Reporting All reports should be made to a central authority which is responsible both for the organisation and administration of the sampling and analytical programme, and for the data storage and analysis procedure. Reports must be on a standard form designed for use by computer punch-operators, so that the data can be transferred to the storage facility without error. Reports must be typed and checked before submission, and the data-punching operation must be double-checked.

For water and sediment samples, the location, time, tide-state (if relevant), depth and method of sampling should be recorded, with a brief description of the position of known sources of contamination. For biological samples, weight, length, sex, age, location and time of sampling should be given, and the concentrations of each organohalogen residue measured must be recorded for each individual, together with the fat content. Duplicate analyses on every fifth individual (from the extraction stage onwards) can be requested, to give an estimate of the analytical variance as distinct from the overall variance between individuals. Several studies have, however, shown that the analytical variance in an experienced laboratory is much smaller than the overall biological variance.

ORGANISATIONAL ASPECTS

All current programmes are assumed to have been designed for a specific purpose. It may not be necessary in some cases for the data obtained to be suitable for statistical analysis, or for comparisons to be made between sites or sampling occasions with measurable confidence limits. However, if major decisions are to be made on the basis of analytical data obtained from monitoring, particularly decisions involving fundamental changes in agricultural, industrial or social practice, some degree of confidence in the data is essential and the design of the monitoring programme must facilitate this. The last OECD programme has indicated some of the factors which must be taken into account in designing and operating a monitoring system, but it would require some modification to improve trend analysis, and further changes if it was intended to provide a means of comparing different sites (for which it was not designed).

The precision and accuracy required to produce data from a number of analysts suitable for direct comparison can only be obtained if an appropriate inter-calibration system is operated within the monitoring programme. This system will require exchange samples which should be similar to the types of sample material examined in the programme, and some samples should be of known composition. The central authority must have confidence in the analytical data, and any change in technique or analyst must be reported with further testing using check samples. Adjustment of the analytical data from biological samples on the basis of errors found in intercalibration is questionable, and participating laboratories must first prove their efficiency before they are accepted in a monitoring programme. (It may not be possible to arrange for all samples to be analysed at one central laboratory).

The limit of detection for each residue on which information is required must be prescribed, and analysts must achieve the required level of sensitivity in order that a high proportion of the data is positively quantified. This is important for the success of the subsequent statistical analysis.

The forms containing all the data submitted to the central authority must
be scrutinised by a specialist group to ensure that the data are complete
and in the required form, and doubtful values should be questioned.

Apart from ensuring the appropriate degree of precision in the data, it
is also necessary to decide on both the frequency of sampling and the number of sites to be sampled. For a small programme with infrequent sampling
it is possible for one laboratory to analyse and store the samples, and
maintain the data analysis and storage facility. However, a large programme will involve several laboratories, and a central data storage and
data processing facility will be essential. (The subject of data reporting
was discussed in the previous section).

ETHICAL AND LEGAL CONSIDERATIONS

Experience with Western European and North American countries participating
in the OECD studies has indicated that, in respect of data obtained from
wildlife sampling and analysis, there are not problems of confidentiality.
The selection of species for analysis could be limited by laws protecting
wildlife, but difficulties arising from such laws are unlikely in view of
the need to choose species which are abundant. However, there may be restrictions (close seasons) on the capture of some bird or fish species.

Storage of specimens within the country of origin should not present difficulties, but any requirements to transport specimens across frontiers for
analysis or specimen banking may infringe laws of import and export, and
of disease control enforcement.

COST ESTIMATION

In the last OECD programme an attempt was made to estimate the costs of
sampling, analysis and administration in several of the participating
countries, and the cost of data analysis and of administration by the
central authority. It is not possible to estimate the cost of design,
and some costs of sampling were included with the analytical costs. A
breakdown of these costs will be made available at the Workshop, but the
following summary indicates the general levels.
The overall average cost per site, involving the analysis of twenty-five
individuals and five duplicates, was $2850 in 1975, the range over nine
countries being $650-4570. Current costs (1978) could be twice as large.
Collection costs averaged about 5 % of the total national cost, and administration another 2 %. The remaining 93 % was allocated to analytical
costs, primarily for organochlorine determinations. The secretarial costs
and those of the statistician, key-punching and verification, computer
time and of the co-ordinating group amounted to a further 11 % of the total of national expenditure.
These estimates should be regarded as conservative. The cost of organochlorine analysis per sample varied widely among the participating countries, from $45 to $150, and in some instances no allocation was made to
cover the capital costs of purchasing expensive equipment such as gas chro-
matographs.The full cost of collecting samples was also under-estimated in
some instances, but these vary widely between the terrestrial, freshwater
and marine environments. The specialist staff were only involved in the
operation for part of their time, but a permanent long-term monitoring system would require full-time operators, which could prove more expensive.

No estimate could be made of the cost of storing samples, but permanent storage at temperatures used in commercial cold storage (-30°C or lower) would require the construction of special purpose buildings and could be expensive to maintain.

Data processing could involve the purchase of a computer, but the alternative of purchasing computer time and data storage facilities should be less costly. A less ambitious data analysis programme that was used in the OECD study could also reduce costs significantly

ANNEX TO PAPER BY A.V. HOLDEN

Analytical Procedures

The basic analytical technique now used for all organo-halogenated compounds is that of electron-capture gas chromatography, the E.C. detector being particularly sensitive to halogenated substances. The chromatograph may be coupled to a mass spectrometer for identification and confirmation of specific residues, but rarely as a routine procedure. Although chromatographic columns can separate several halogenated compounds, and capillary is essential for most samples to remove interfering co-extracted materials prior to analysis. It is also usually an advantage to separate the halogenated residues into two or more groups prior to gas chromatography.

The various stages of the analysis are thus extraction, clean-up, pre-GLC separation, GLC analysis and sometimes residue confirmation. Extraction is normally carried out by partitioning into non-polar solvents in which both the halogenated compounds and lipids are very soluble. Steam-distillation has been used for particular groups of compounds, but normally extraction is effected by direct partition into the solvent at room temperature or by Soxhlet or similar extractors.

The co-extracted lipids and pigments are removed either by partition between the non-polar and a polar solvent (e.g. hexane and acetonitrile) or more commonly by passing the crude extract through an adsorbent column (alumina, Florisil, charcoal) and eluting the halogenated residues with an appropriate solvent while the lipids, etc., remain on the column. The pre-GLC separation is also performed on adsorbent columns (silica, Florisil alumina), various solvents being used in succession to elute particular groups of substances, especially in the analysis of organochlorines. For example, hexachlorobenzene, aldrin, DDE and PCB's can be separated from TDE, DDT, the hexachlorocyclohexanes, dieldrin and many other pesticides. The latter group can be further subdivided if necessary.

The extracts so obtained can then be injected directly into the gas chromatograph, the residues being identified by their elution times and their concentrations determined by comparison with reference standards.

Different stationary phases on the GLC columns can provide variations in retention times which assist in confirming the identity of residues. Chemical reaction of residues in the solvent (or after evaporation of the solvent), followed by further GLC analysis, can also be used for confirmation of some residues. More polar compounds (e.g. chlorinated herbicides and phenols) may require derivatisation to enable them to be chromatographed satisfactorily on non-polar GLC columns.

Alternative clean-up techniques have been used in some laboratories, primarily treatment with strong acids or alkalis to destroy the lipids. Such methods result in the destruction of a few halogenated compounds, but are adequate if these particular compounds are of no interest.

Automation is rarely used in environmental analysis, where both the nature and concentration of residues may vary very widely between samples, and in consequence the rate at which samples can be analysed is low, perhaps only 5 - lo samples daily per operator.

Where the concentrations to be determined are low, as in most environmental samples, precautions must be taken to ensure that no contamination of the samples or apparatus, causing interference in analysis, can arise from extraneous materials. For organochlorine analysis, for example, the solvent (normally hexane) must be specially purified, all adsorbents tested for freedom from electron-capturing contaminants, all glassware solvent-washed or otherwise pre-treated, and almost all plastic materials excluded from the entire procedure (plasticisers can interfere seriously in the analysis).

In the OECD programmes analysts have used a variety of GLC columns, but most extracted tissue samples by Soxhlet extraction, and adsorbent columns have almost invariably been used for both clean-up and pre-GLC separation (primarily to separate DDE + PCB residues from the majority of other residues). Confirmation has been limited to alkali treatment to confirm the presence of DDT, and occasionally acid treatment or demonstrate the presence of dieldrin, but most analysts have relied upon the use of two different GLC stationary phases if any confirmation was attempted.

The practice in both ICES and OECD programmes has been to allow analysts to use techniques of their choice, but to intercalibrate by the use of specially-prepared check samples. These have mainly consisted of vegetable or fish oils, both unspiked and spike samples being provided, the composition and concentration of the spike residues being known but not disclosed to the analyst until he has reported his results. The information has yielded both comparisons of the efficiency of extraction and of identification and quantification of the residues. In both organisations, laboratories with the longer experience of this form of analysis showed improved ability over those participating in intercalibration for the first time.

The procedures described are those used for pesticides, PCB's and related compounds. Aliphatic halogenated solvents, refrigerants, etc., require modifications to the basic technique to allow for their often greater volatility, and GLC analysis is usually conducted at a lower temperature. Apart from electron-capture detection, coulometric detection can be used for chlorinated substances, but is not widely employed.

(A reprint describing the results of OECD intercalibration exercises is attached).

Programme Design

Assuming that the function of monitoring is to identify levels of contamination which must be compared with accepted limits, and to measure changes in these levels over time or distinguish between levels at different locations, it is necessary to estimate the concentrations in individual samples or the mean concentration in a population of individuals, with measurable precision.

The variation in contamination level between individual samples may be due to differences in exposure to the pollutant, in rates of metabolism or degradation, or differences in tissue type or composition (including seasonal changes in physiology). One or more of these factors may be responsible in any individual sample. All determinations are made by some form of chemical analysis, and the technique itself will give rise to some degree of variance.

It is possible to distinguish the analytical variance from the inherent within-sample variance to a large extent, as replicate analyses of one appropriate sample (not too dissimilar in composition or contamination level from the field samples) can be used to determine the analytical variance. Experience in the OECD studies has shown that careful analysts can reduce the analytical variance to a small component of the combined analytical/field sample variance.

The variance between individual samples from a field population (whether from soil, water or a population of a species) can be reduced by careful selection of the individuals. Soil and water samples should be taken from one depth and in a pre-determined pattern by recognised procedures. Population samples should be selected for age, sex, and possibly size, as some pollutants may vary with one or more of these parameters. As organo-halogen compounds are lipid-soluble, specific organs or tissues must be selected if possible (but for small individuals wholebody samples may have to be used to provide sufficient material for analysis). For all samples the lipid content must be determined, and the residue concentrations expressed on both a lipid and tissue basis. The specimens must be stored under appropriate conditions until required for analysis, to ensure that no change in residue content can occur as the result of bacterial or enzymatic decomposition.

The number of individuals to be obtained for each sample depends on the precision required for the mean. To detect with confidence a 25 % difference between means, 5o individuals may be required in each sample, although with careful selection the number may be reduced to some extent. Numbers as large as this require that large populations are sampled, and species which occur in shoals or flocks are essential. They must also be easily accessible, easily obtained and identified.

The distribution of values in a sample may be Gaussian, but is more commonly skew. However, except for extreme cases (where logarithmic transformation may be used) normal statistical procedures are usually permissable.

It may be necessary to obtain samples more than once a year, but for biological samples the seasonal variation in lipid content (due to starvation or sexual maturation) must be recognised, and samples from different periods of the year may not necessarily be directly comparable.

In practice, a species representative of one location can be used to measure changes with time at that site, but different sites may require different species, especially when continents are to be monitored. It is suggested that comparisons between countries should not be attempted by using one species, as it is doubtful whether any species is sufficiently widely distributed and abundant to allow this. Related species can sometimes be substituted, but behaviour and feeding regimes may result in different residue accumulation patterns.

For some purposes sample selection as described may be inappropriate, e.g. when fish or birds are used for human consumption. Monitoring of food requires that the samples represent the food consumed, and a random selection of individuals is essential. However, food surveillance usually involves only comparison with a acceptable limit of contamination, and the extent to which values are above or below the limit may not be important.

Statistics

The basic statistical requirements have been referred to above. All chemical, physical and other relevant data must be reported on standard forms designed to enable computer punch-operators to transfer them to the computer easily and without error. The forms will require accompanying instructions to ensure that analysts or others can provide the data in a form understood by computer operators. As far as possible, measured concentrations (rather than "below the limit" values) should be reported, to assist in statistical analysis, although techniques are available to adjust for a small proportion (say 15 %) of "less than" values.. This requirement will demand a high degree of sensitivity in the analytical techeniques employed. Missing data can be represented by a appropriate code. The data print-out must be examined for errors, and a small expert group should be available to check whether abnormal data have been reported or other errors suspected. These should be checked with the reporting laboratory before further processing.

The preliminary data analysis should involve the determination of the mean, standard deviation and a measure of skewness for each variable. Outliers, which may be defined as observations greater or less than the estimated mean by three estimated standard deviations, can at this stage be rejected and the operation repeated as necessary. Where skewness is significant the process can be carried out with the logarithms of the observation. It may also be useful to combine residues of one group, e.g. DDE+ DDT, to give the total DDT concentration, and the statistical analysis performed with this parameter.

Correlation coefficients can be calculated to test the degree of association between variables, which may be two residues or a residue and a physical parameter. If it is not possible to select individuals for age, for example, the influence of age on residue levels can be tested.

If duplicate analyses are provided, an estimate of the analytical variance can be obtained and compared with the within-sample variance.

The procedure can be used for data from different years (or, if appropriate, from different locations), and t-tests are then run for significance between the residue levels of different years (or sites).

If, however, physical variables differ between the samples the significance is limited, and a multivariate analysis is necessary.

The multivariate model used in the OECD programme adjusts a measure of chemical concentration for those physical factors which may influence it. This procedure removes any bias due to a physical factor, and reduces the variance of the mean residue. The latter could allow of a smaller sample size than would be required without such adjustment. The programme used was an adaptation of the Biomed BMDO2R Stepwise Regression programme, which performs the stepwise regressions, transforms variables, lists residuals, plots residuals against input variables and allows the perturbation of the variance-covariance matrix.

Organisational Aspects

A permanent monitoring system must be designed in such a way that the sampling and analytical stages can provide data capable of adequate statistical analysis, and the purpose of the latter must be specified before the sampling programme is detailed. This mean that a statistician must be involved in the initial planning of any programme together with biologists and chemists.

It is considered essential, following the experience gained in this OECD programme, that any permanent monitoring operation should have an experienced executive group composed of biologists, chemists and statisticians who are responsible for the administration of the sampling data acquisition activities. This group should have authority to take action to ensure the necessary uniformity in sampling programmes, and to supervise the inter-calibration of analytical techniques. It must be capable of checking spurious data, calling for essential analytical or other information if not supplied, questioning data of doubtful validity, and ensuring that all data is provided according to a pre-arranged time schedule.

The executive group might consist of both permanent and temporarily-assigned staff, and must have adequate statistical, computer and data-recording staff and facilities. These facilities should be available during the entire period in which the programme is executed, and easily accessible to the executive group so that a check on the importance of the parameters and residues being considered could be made whenever necessary. The group would probably also be responsible for reporting periodically, but the reports would be produced by the parent organisation. All data should be submitted to the executive group on standard forms designed to be used directly by the statisticians and computer operators, but at the same time the forms should not be too complicated. Experience in the OECD programmes suggests that unnecessary complexity results in incorrect or misleading form-filling, and a risk that computer operators may enter incorrect data into the computer. Double-checking of data at all stages and particularly at computer entry, is imperative.

It should be possible to ensure that the homogeneity of individual samples is such that changes in contamination levels with time, or differences between sampling locations, can be identified with sufficient precision. Submission of inaccurate or inadequate data for subsequent statistical analysis will almost certainly result in an inability to distinguish changes or differences in contamination level, rendering the monitoring operation ineffective, and involving personnel in unnecessary effort and expense.

This part of the operation should ensure that the quality and completeness of the data provided by the monitoring programme are maintained at an adequate standard. Changes or extensions to the overall programme would be authorised by a superior body, to whom the executive group would report regularly, but such changes would be subject to recommendations from the experts of the executive group. Major extensions or amendments to the programme could be expected to result in an increased workload for the executive group and the computer staff.

The group should issue regular reports summarising (but not detailing) the data received, and detailing the results of statistical analyses performed by the computer. In particular, major trends or sudden changes in contamination level should be reported, and the effects of changes in pollutant lead, the control of a contaminant or the use-pattern of a pesticide in an area should be identified where possible. Failure to detect any anticipated change in contamination level should also be reported. Where maximum acceptable limits of contamination have been agreed or designated, the executive group should refer the results in excess of these limits to the superior body for action as appropriate. The executive group should not be required to take such action itself, beyond confirming with the source of the data that the information supplied was correct.

The procedure outlined assumes that many laboratories would be engaged in a large scale monitoring operation, and it must be recognised that different countries will give varying degrees of importance, authority and support to their sampling and analytical organisation. Nevertheless, OECD experience suggests that in the more advanced countries the difficulties in co-ordinating the work of such laboratories can be overcome provided that the staff can be encouraged to give full support. It must be emphasized, however, that routine analysis of samples which rarely contain unusual concentrations of contaminants is extremely tedious, and the quality of the analytical work can suffer as a result. All unnecessary work of this nature must be avoided, to ensure that the quality of the data will not deteriorate.

For a monitoring programme involving less advanced countries, it may be more difficult to obtain and maintain the necessary expertise. Rigorous training and supervision is essential, and intercalibration must be relied upon to ensure that the standards of operation are upheld. An alternative, but not always acceptable, procedure is for the analytical work to be contracted to special laboratories in other countries.

A further alternative would be the establishment of a central laboratory or several regional laboratories to carry out all the analytical work, these laboratories being responsible to an international monitoring organisation. At the present time, however, a more modest operation is required to justify the establishment of an international organisation by demonstrating that the results of monitoring are worthwhile, and can fulfil the intended purpose.

Cost Estimation

The costs of monitoring could be sub-divided under the following headings

a) location, identifiying and selecting samples

b) transport, storage and preservation

c) subsampling, sample preparation and analysis

d) calculating data and reporting on standard forms

e) computer punching and processing, including statisticians time

f) executive group operations

g) administrative group time

An attempt was made during the final OECD programme to obtain the costs of participation from the countries involved, subdivided into collection (a, b above), analyses (c, d above), and administration for one year (1975). To the returns made were added the costs of the statistician and the secretarial involvement. The national currencies were converted to U.S. dollars using relevant conversion rates.

Nine countries supplied information on costs in one form or another. Two could not separate collection or national administrative costs, these being included in the analytical costs or borne by the agencies responsible as part of their normal operating costs. Two other countries reported only one or the other type of costs. In all countries the costs of collection and administration were invariably the smallest portions of the programme, ranging from 6 to 17 % of the annual cost in the four countries reporting both costs. This portion included collection, ageing, sexing, measuring, weighting, freezing, labelling and shipment to the analytical laboratory, and occasionally the salary of the collector.

Administrative costs to a country included the salary of the national coordinator for the time spent on checking the accuracy of the data, attending national meetings connected with the operation, limited statistical analyses, and telephone, typing and photocopy expenses. These costs were probably underestimated.

Analytical costs were easier to assess, as some countries purchased service from commercial laboratories and others monitor such costs routinely. All nine countries provided estimates of this cost, and on average analytical costs were 89 % of the total cost of the programme, varying from 83 % to 94 % where collection, analysis and administration were subdivided. Analytical costs included staff salaries, chemicals and solvents, overheads for electricity, water etc., and a fraction of the purchase price of equipment appropriately amortised.

The OECD programme involved sampling each selected site once a year, twenty-five individual specimens being collected and thirty analyses being performed for organochlorine (and sometimes heavy metal) residues, every fifht specimen being analysed in duplicate. The average cost per site was $2850, ranging from $650 to $4570, in 1975. OECD bore the cost of the statistical analyses, distribution of reports and Working Group members, and other central administrative costs. The statistical costs covered checking data before key-punching, the key-punching, checking print-out accuracy, purchase of a computer programme, modifying the programme, computer time and the statistician's salary (6 man-months per year). The average cost of administration was $13716 per year, but this is an underestimate as typing, copying and communications costs were not included. Statistical costs would be expected to be double those included in this estimate if calculated in 1978.

If a permanent executive group were responsible for the monitoring programme, administrative costs would probably be greater, as attendance by the OECD Working Group members was supported by salary costs paid by their employers although subsistence in Paris and transport costs were borne by OECD. Salary costs were not always allocated to the cost of the Working Group meetings.

The cost of analysing one sample for a limited group of organochlorine residues in 1975 ranged from $45 to $15o, and combined organochlorine + mercury analyses from $6o to $22o, but generally the single metal analysis would cost about one quater of the organochlorine analyses. It is likely that a set of analyses of several metals would cost about the same as a set of organochlorine analyses, as the analytical techniques for different metals may vary, and the combined cost of organochlorine and metal analyses at 1975 rates would have averaged about $2oo per individual sample. At 1978 prices this would be nearer $3oo per sample.

Assuming that twenty-five samples are taken per site and sampling occasion, involving thirty analyses each for organochlorines and metals, and assuming national administrative costs to be about 1o % of the sampling and analytical costs, the overall national cost per site would be about $ 1o.ooo at 1978 prices.

EXPERIENCES IN MONITORING AND BANKING HUMAN BIOLOGICAL SPECIMEN

F.H. Kemper

Institute of Pharmacology and Toxicology
University of Muenster
Federal Republic of Germany

Summary
Amongst ecotoxicological influences on human beings halogenated organic compounds, e.g. chlorinated polycyclic hydrocarbons as well as inorganic substances, e.g. toxicological significant heavy metals are of importance.

Beside the features of hazards of exposure target organs of toxicity and depot compartments, the following aspects are mentioned:
a) Organochlorine pesticides: Results of analytical determination in human
   organs (blood, liver, fatty tissues) of several collectives and organs
   distribution of DDT and HCB are given (Real Time Monitoring and autopsy
   materials).
   Correlation to age and pathophysiological processes (arteriosclerotic
   disease, tumorchachexia) are discussed. Some analytical results are compared with regard to different reference systems ("extractable lipids"
   and "whole tissue").
b) Toxic heavy metals: Mechanism and symptoms of intoxication with lead,
   mercury and cadmium are described. Examples for epidemic environmental
   load with organomercurials and cadmium are reviewed. The extended halftime of cadmium in human organism leads to a rapid load of most tissues with
   cadmium. Some results of Cd-determinations in human liver and kidney specimens are discussed in relation to age.
   Interactions between toxic and essential trace elements may play an important role by toxification or detoxification the pollutants. Therefore
   the determination of a "metal fingerprint" containing the analytical results of essential and nonessential trace elements and bulk electrolytes
   is proposed.

1. Introduction

Numerous environmental pollutants must be classified as health hazards for
man. In fig. 1 sources of possible xenobiotic exposure are listed: e.g. domestic poisons (detergents, pigments, propellants), natural occuring substances (plant or animal toxins), food components (additives, bacterial
toxins, nitrosamines), stimulants (nicotin, ethanol, drugs). Human populations are increasing by exposed to substances that are potentially detrimental to health. Many of these substances are allready found in human tissues, fluids, secreta and excreta and some tend to concentrate in specific
parts of the human body. Biological Monitoring programmes can provide direct evidence of exposure and must therefore be implemented to supplement
physical and chemical monitoring programmes in areas where these are already
in existence. Specimen banking will be of great importance in analyzing
trends in exposure to previously unrecognized harmful pollutants or pollutants for which current measurement techniques are inadequate. Biological
monitoring and analysis of stored specimens can provide a warning for the
initiation of remedial measures before critical demage occures.

From the toxicologists and pharmacologists point of view it is of interest
in connection with xenobiotics to look for the target organs, the possibil-

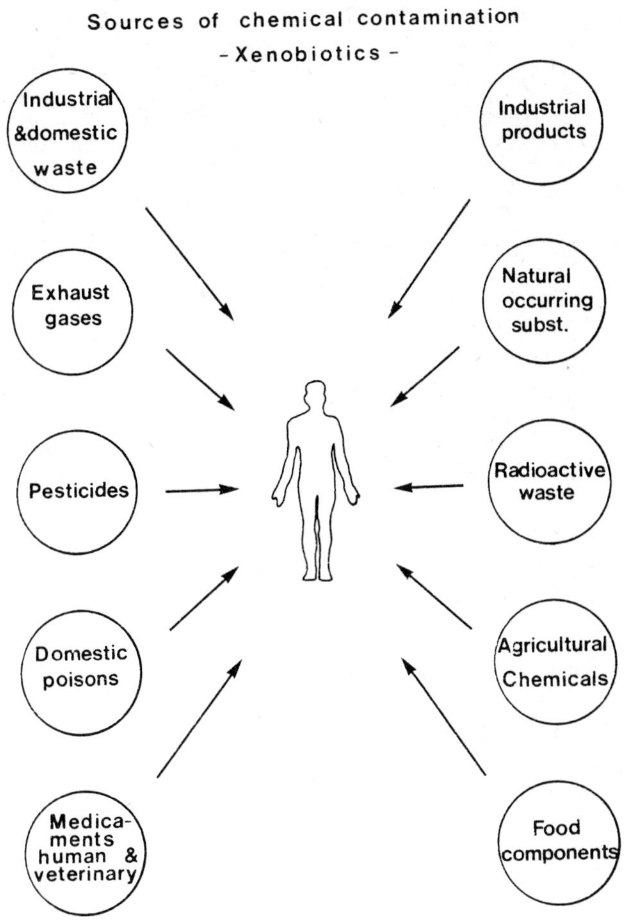

Fig. 1

ity of accumulation and moreover hazards of exposure. The results of analytical work in "Real Time Monitoring" as well as long-time-trend-analysis are the basis for medical estimation of the ecotoxicological risk concerning man's life.

Moreover possibilities of conversions of pollutants in different ecosystems must be taken in consideration. The conversions may result in substances with increased or lowered toxic qualities, as shown in fig. 2 for mercury and organohalogenated hydrocarbons.

In the following some points of interest concerning the toxicity of some non-essential trace metals and human exposure to organochlorine pesticides should be discussed.

344

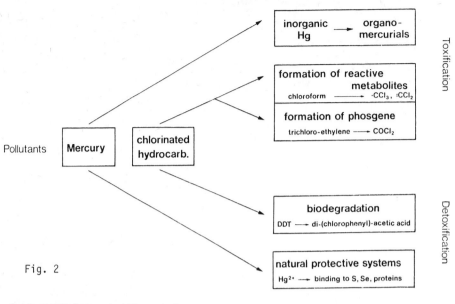

Fig. 2

2. Organohalogenated Compounds

Organohalogenated compounds are of important ecological and toxicological interest because of their presence in various parts of human environment. Fig. 3 shows the environmental and occupational pesticide exposure of man and newbon; fig. 4 shows the sources of man's exposure to pesticides.

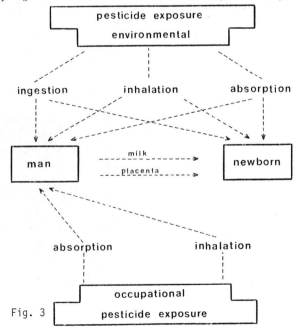

Fig. 3

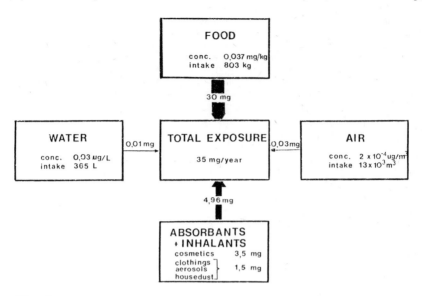

Fig. 4   Sources of man's exposure to pesticides

Among the possibilities of exposure, insecticides with prolonged halftime (DDT, hexachlorobenzene etc.) and substances with possible cancerogenic risk e.g. solvents (chloroform, dichloroethylene, vinylchloride) should have the highest priority in scientific evaluation. For that reason the observation of their ecotoxicological behaviour and not at last the respective environmental exposure of man is needed. Our institute is engaged in a programme testing the human exposure to organochlorine pesticides (OCP) as DDT, HCB, BHC etc. This program is divided in two parts, part 1, the "Real Time Monitoring" where the OCP-content in blood and subcutaneous fat of living people is measured, and part 2, the "Environmental Specimen Bank Program", where we measure the OCP-content in various organs of deceased people. The age of the persons analyzed was within 20 to 30 years. Most of them were students. The highest amount was found for HCB, the lowest for op-DDT. As usual the main part of total DDT is DDE. The maximum value measured is 13.5 µg/l for hexachlorobenzene.

In the "Environmental Specimen Bank Program" we analyzed human adipose tissue and human liver. The sequence is nearly the same as in whole blood, but the concentrations are about thousand fold higher.

An impressing example for the influence of some diseases on the distribution and concentration of pesticides in human organs is given in fig. 5. Shown is the HCB-concentration in human adipose tissue in tumorcachectic, in arteriosclerotic and in people, died by another disease. The reference is µg/g extractable lipids. The HCB content ranges of about 0 to 46 ppm. None of the cachectic patients has a HCB-concentration within the so-called normal range. The difference within the arteriosclerotic people are much larger but here none of the values is within the normal range, too. The explanation for the high content in cachectic people may be found in the shifted lipid content of the adipose tissue. The effect of starvation results in an increase of pesticid content in fatty tissue. The normal ratio adipose tissue lipids is about 1 : 0.6. In these patients however the ratio increased to 1 : 0.2. The conclusion of this condition may be: the pesticid level has diminished during the time of emaciation, but not with the same speed as the quote of lipids, so that the persisteng amount of OCPs, refered to a smaller portion of lipids, simulate higher values. Fig. 6 may be the proof for the former conclusion. It presents the HCB content in the fatty tissue of the same collective referd to tissue basis. The difference between cachectic and "normal people" is compensated although the content in arteriosclerotic persons is not effected by the changed reference basis. Probably the explanation for the latter group may be the restricted blood circulation in these people.

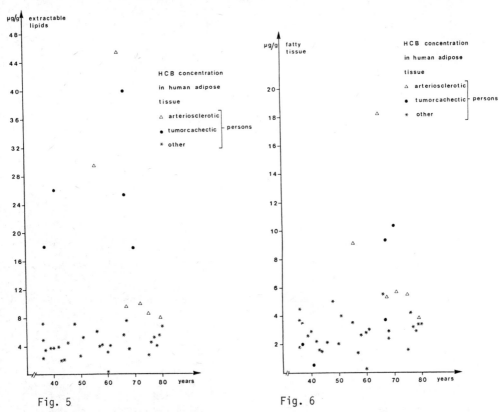

Fig. 5   Fig. 6

Analytical measurements of persisting pesticideš in the environmental and especially in human beings are important necessary for toxicological and legal evaluations. But it has to be considered, that the comparability of results gained by different labs, of the different collectives or different countries is difficult or even impossible because of the varying conditions and numerous other parameters influencing the results in a very high manner.

3. Inorganic Compounds

Unlike many man-made substances (mainly organic compounds), virtually all elements are normally present in most human tissues. Some elements (the so-called essential elements) are necessary for normal biological development and function, whereas others are not known to have anay useful function in the body. Since the human being is usually able to regulate the tissue levels

of the essential elements, non-essential elements are most likely to cause
environmental pollution problems. It is difficult to select which elements
should be considered of highest priority for study. With the present state
of knowledge the elements of greatest interest as environmental pollutants
are: arsenic, cadmium, chromium, lead and mercury. From the view of the toxicologists there are two forms of poisoning, in many cases differing in symptoms: the acute and the chronic intoxication. With regard to environmental
exposure the symptoms of chronic poisoning due to continuous or intermittent
incorporation of doses, are important and will be reviewed on the next pages
for lead, cadmium and mercury.

3.1. Lead

Target organs of toxicity of lead are: bone marrow, muscles of stomach and
gut and the central nervous system. The toxic mechanism of lead in these
organs is not yet clear in all points. In bone marrow lead involves a suppression of haem synthesis by interference with several enzymes. This results
in an increased urinary excretion of various precursors. Deposition of lead
takes place in bone (depot compartment). More than 90 % of the total body
lead is found here as relatively insoluble lead phosphates. It is particularly
found in the growing ends of long bones. For monitoring lead exposure, measurement of blood lead is the most obvious test, but must be combined with
other parameters. The resulting limits of exposure degrees are not defined
exactly in all countries. The upper limits of normal levels are considered
to be: blood lead 400 µg/l, urinary coproporphyrin 150 µg/l, δ-aminolevu-
linic acid 4 mg/l.

Values above these may be acceptable; the dangerous range of lead absorption
yields: blood lead >1000 µg/l, urinary coproporphyrin >1500 µg/l, urinary
δ-aminolevulinic acid >40 mg/l.

3.2. Mercury

All mercury compounds are poisonous, particularly the fat-soluble methyl
mercurials and the water-soluble mercury salts. From the toxicological and
environmental points of view this classification into fat- and water-soluble
compounds gives important characteristics for the difference in effects of
these two groups on human organism. Organocompounds of metals may pass more
easily the various membrans in the body, resulting especially in an increased toxicity to the central nervous system. The toxicity of organomercurials
must be mentioned separately because there is a complicated cycle of mercury
in nature. Micro-organisms are able to transform mercury salts to metallic
mercury, or methyl mercury compounds. The main target organ of toxicity of
mercury compounds is the central nervous system: the first symptoms often
false diagnosed as neurasthenic syndrome or hysteria are called micro-
mercurialism, because the clinical picture is based mainly on a minor intensity of classic symptoms of mercurial erethism. The massive form of central
nervous system symptoms is seen rarely and only in workers with excessive
exposure. One of the most characteristic features of mercurialism is the
presence of mercurial tremor in clinical symptomatology. The tremor develops
gradually in the form of fine trembling of the muscles beginning in the fingers.

3.3 Cadmium

Cadmium is surely the most dangerous heavy metal in the field of health aspects because of its extremly extended half time in human organism. For renal cortex a half time of about thirty years has been calculated. Investigations on the content of cadmium in different parts of all ecosystems are
therefore necessary with high priority to estimate the health risk and draw
up balances. A continuous load of most tissues with cadmium can be seen.
Fig. 7 shows some own results of autopsy material. Cadmium content of kidney
and liver from birth on to an age of 20 years or shown. A rapid load from the
first days or month of life is obvious. Maximum of kidney cadmium content is

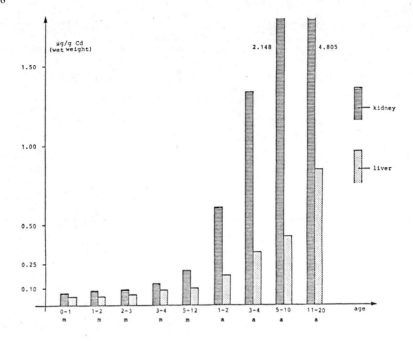

Fig. 7

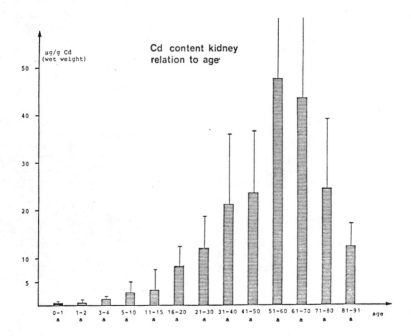

Fig. 8

reached in an age of 50 - 50 years (fig. 8), then a decreasing concentration of cadmium is observed. At present it is very difficult to explain
these changes. They might be connected with factors related to a low cadmium
intake a long time ago and with different food habits in older age groups.
Perhaps metabolic changes in kidneys in old age are of great importance.
The target organs of toxicity of cadmium are:
a) Main target organ is the kidney. Chronic cadmium exposure leads to a distinct increase in excretion of several proteins due to cell damage by
   cadmium. The excretion of the so-called "minialbumin" in chronic cadmium
   exposure was related to a defect in immunoglobulins, but this theory was
   not yet proved. The other target organs of chronic toxicity of cadmium
   are of lesser importance.
b) In the respiratory system cadmium oxide dust or fume may cause emphysema.
c) Chronic cadmium exposure as a cause for hypertension in humans is until
   now a controversial theory. There are only some animal experiments possibly indicating this effect.
d) Testicles are damaged mainly in acute poisoning.
e) Decalcification of bones may lead to serious clinical pictures, as seen
   in a severe environmental cadmium poisoning in Japan, called "Itai-itai-
   disease".
3.4. Metal Fingerprint
There are innumerous interrelations between trace elements, not only between essential metals, also in nonessential and in bulk elements. This
interactions may be kinetic or metabolic and are particularly powerful
among the environmental contaminants. An important aspect is for example
the detoxifying role of selenium for mercury and other heavy metals. Increasing cadmium content of kidneys is related to an increase of zinc in
the same tissue specimens, indicating the induction of certain detoxifying
proteins, which may bind cadmium, zinc and other metals in the same way.
To reveal possible interactions, we developed a "metal fingerprint", containing the results of analysis of several elements in one picture (fig. 9).
Interactions among the trace elements may be so powerful, that environmental studies involving single elements can lead to dangerously erreonous

350

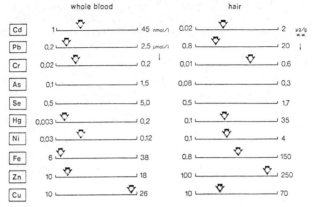

Fig. 9   ‹ metal fingerprint ›   RTM 2055

conclusions. Moreover the pattern of metals may give more detailed informations on possible pathogenetic processes and causal statements.

4. Technical and Organizational Considerations

In sampling, preparation, transportation and storage of environmental materials and specimens for monitoring and banking programmes certain precautions must be taken. Special cleaning procedures for materials and instruments used for sampling are necessary, as well as special sampling
techniques to avoid contamination of the sample and/or loss of pollutants.
All specimens should be transferred to permanent storage containers as soon
as possible and handled as few times as possible. Regarding the container
materials the following points should be observed:
- minimum interaction between specimen and container
- minimum interaction between specimen and external environment
- choice of container material is dictated by the sample to be stored and
  the substance to be determined
- conventional polyethylene, borosilicate glass, teflon and quartz should
  be considered
It is not possible to suggest a "standard method" for storage of all kinds
of specimens and related to all pollutants. Low-temperature ashing is not
advocated because of the possibility of volatile metal losses but may have
certain advantages for specimens such as bone. Chemical preservation, radiation sterilization and storage of extracts were not recommended as storage
methods. Freeze drying appears to be an excellent method for samples intended for inorganic analysis, but sample size may be limited to 25 - 50 g of
material. In recommending the rates of freezing, the rate of thawing should
also be considered and further investigation regarding these may be needed.
Nevertheless, temperatures of -80° C or even -196° C as well as exclusion
of oxygen seem to be the methods of choice for storing tissue specimens over
prolonged period. It is recommended that a centralized approach be taken to
problems of sample storage. Even smallscale sample alterations resulting
from slightly different storage techniques could lead to increased variability in measured pollutant concentrations.
One of the most basic and important of monitoring and banking problems is
how many specimens to collect to obtain useful results. The vast body of
data on important pollutants show that body burdens do not follow normal or
Gaussian distributions and have in general a more or less pronounced positive

positive skew. The importance of this finding must be taken into account in the design of future sampling programmes and in the interpretation of the results. Further more it must be considered that there is a minimum of sample weight regarding the development of "organic and/or metal finger-prints" (fig. 10).

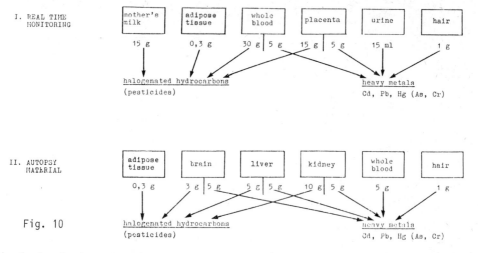

Fig. 10

5. Conclusions and Recommendations

Major activities are necessary of adequately ensure the protection of human health and the environment from the adverse effects of environmental pollu-tants. These activities include toxicological and ecological research, con-trol technology development, the promulgation of regulatory guidelines and

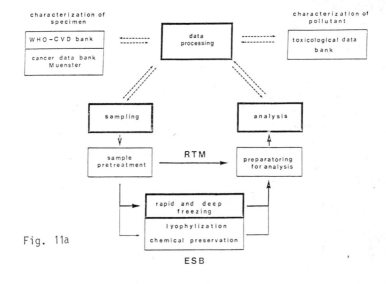

Fig. 11a

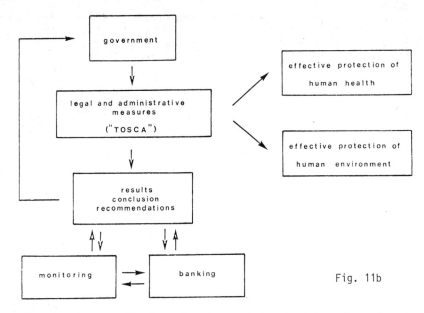

Fig. 11b

standards, and the monitoring of environmental materials and specimen banking. In the absence of effective monitoring environmental materials and specimen banking (as shown in figures 11a/b) the detection of serious environmental contamination from pollutants may occur only after critical damage has been done. The link between legal wants and scientific necessities must be found. Regulations must cover a maximum of safety and a minimum of scientific demands. Only in this way a practicable "environmental protection" man against environment versus environment against man can be established.

6. References

H.P. Bertram, F.H. Kemper, Ch. Zenzen: Man - a target of ecotoxicological influences, in print

N.P. Luepke: Monitoring Environmental Materials and Specimen Banking - Selection Criteria and Recommended Specimens, expert paper, UBA, Berlin

N.P. Luepke: Impact of Toxic Environmental Chemicals on Human Health, third meeting of the german-japanese panel on environment protection, Bonn 1978

F. Schmidt-Bleek, N.P. Luepke: Möglichkeiten und Grenzen von Langzeituntersuchungen von Fremdstoffen in Organen, Dtsch.Ges.Arbeitsmedizin 1978

A.S. Prasad, D. Oberleas (edts.): Trace Elements in Human Health and Disease, Vol. II, Ac. Press, New York, San Francisco, London, 1976

L. Friberg, M. Piscator, G. Nordberg, T. Kjellström: Cadmium in the Environment, 2nd. ed., CRC Press, Cleveland, Ohio, 1974

L. Friberg, J. Vostal: Mercury in the Environment, CRC Press, Cleveland, Ohio, 1972

L.J. Goldwater, W. Stopford: Mercury, in: J. Lenihan, W.W. Fletcher: The Chemical Environment, Blackie, Glasgow, London, 1977

M.R. Moore, B.C. Campbell, A. Goldberg: Lead in: J. Lenihan (s.a.)

H.L. Thron, N. Engbert, Ch. Krause, L.Laskus, M. Sonneborn: Bleibelastung von Bevölkerungsgruppen, Bericht des Instituts für Wasser-, Boden- und Lufthygiene des Bundesgesundheitsamtes, Berlin 1978

V.F. Guinee, B. Davidow, A. Tytun: Clinical and Environmental Correlations with Blood Lead Levels of Children in New York City, Proc. Internat. Symp. "Recent Advances in the Assessment of the Health Effects of Environmental Pollution", Vol.II, Luxembourg 1975

T. Tsubaki, K. Irukayama (edts.): Minamata Disease, Kodansha, Tokyo, Elsevier Sc.Publ.Comp., Amsterdam, Oxford, New York, 1977

M.Harada: Methyl Mercury Poisoning due to Environmental Contamination, in: F.W.Oehme (ed.): Toxicity of Heavy Metals in the Environment, Part 1, Marcel Dekker, New York, Basel, 1978

A.S. Curry, A.R. Knott: "Normal" levels of Cadmium in human liver and kidney in England, Clin.chim.Acta 30, 115 (1970)

J. Kobayashi: Pollution by Cadmium and the Itai-Itai-Disease in Japan, in: F.W. Oehme (s.a.)

E.F. Underwood: Interactions of Trace Elements, in: F.W. Oehme (s.a.)

ORGANOHALOGENATED COMPOUNDS IN PLANTS AND SOIL

W. Klein, GSF, Institut für Ökologische Chemie
D-8o42 Neuherberg

Summary

Within all organic chemicals, most extensive monitoring of organochlorine pesticides has been done for several years. An exhaustive review of this activity in several countries can not be given. Typical data for US are published in Pesticides Monitoring Journal. Results of monitoring these pesticides revealed e.g. a decline in DDT-exposure of the population. Assessment of monitoring data resulted in hazard lists: actual intake versus a.d.i. Similar data as for organochlorine pesticides are available for PCB's. For the larger number of solvents and other organohalogenated compounds, only random isolated data are available.

PCB's have been found in the flora of non-inhabited areas. Thus the occurrence of organohalogen chemicals must be expected generally in any plants and soil.

An appropriate specimen as long-term accumulator is soil from industrial, agricultural and non-inhabited areas. A seasonal accumulator, typical for human exposure, would be food grain, and a respective high-accumulator would be carrots. Suggested specimen for wild plants could be Cladonia or larch leaves or water hemlock (based on PCB). Proposed container for specimen is glass.

Freeze-drying reduces residues and changes analytical recovery. Therefore portional storage of original homogenized samples is proposed.

The large number of chemical individuals requires multimatrix-multiresidue methodology. Interference of non-halogenated chemicals can be overcome by glass-capillary GLC with internal standardisation. Convenient detection and determination is by GLC/ECD. So far no certified standards and reference materials are available.

For programme design it has to be decided large number of samples and good statistical representativity versus low number of specific local samples, enabling sophisticated analysis like GC/MS confirmation and no need for expensive development of routine analytical procedure.

The total national costs for a minimum programme would amount to about 5oo.ooo,-- DM annually.

a) Review of Past and Current Programmes

1. Monitoring

Apart from heavy metals, the so-called persistent organochlorine insecticides are the classical example of chemicals in the environment monitored for many years. Originally, this type of monitoring aimed in the assessment of human exposure to these chemicals. Consequently, human food of plant and animal origin as well as animal feed have been analyzed for their content of the respective chemicals in food quality and monitoring programs. With the sophisticated analytical methodology available today, it can be concluded that no additional activities are needed to be taken in respect to these chemicals. The U.S.National Pesticide Monitoring Program involves, for instance 3ooo soil samples annually which are carefully selected to pesticide usage, low- and non-use sites (Sand et al., 1967). Today, pesticide residues in food and feed are controlled in many countries. An exhaustive review of what has been achieved in this respect cannot be the topic of this paper; only a few typical examples are presented to emphasize the gap in knowledge between organochlorine pesticides and PCB versus other organohalogenated compounds.

Monitoring programmes for DDT to elucidate human average daily intakes have been started in the early fifties. Despite the difficulties in the interpretation of data, they have shown in the U.S.A. a decline in DDT exposure within ten years to about 3o % (DDT and analogues o.286 mg/man/day in 1953/54 to o.087 mg/man/day). By 197o, exposure had been reduced again to about half (DDT o.o15 mg/man/day; Review WHO, 1978, detailed data see Duggan et al., Pestic. Monit. J. 1967 ff.). Similar programmes have been carried out in Canada (Swackhamer, 1965) and in Great Britain (Egan, 1973, Abott et al., 1969, 197o). For cyclodiene insecticides, DDT, lindane, and inorganic bromide (which can be derived from methylbromide), the actual daily intakes have been compared with the respective a.d.i.'s, which is the final assessment of total diet monitoring programmes (van Thiel, 1972).

Realizing the need for international coordinated monitoring programmes and knowing the standardized tested analytical techniques are the basis to obtain reliable results, interlaboratory check sample analysis programmes have been carried out for organochlorine pesticides already more than 1o years ago. It should be mentioned that, within the first intercomparison programmes, not only the residue analytical methodology but also the sampling and evaluation procedure were recognized to need standardization. Under the aspect of soil monitoring for organochlorine pesticides in Canada, for instance, an intercomparison programme for aldrin, dieldrin, DDT, and DDE was carried out in 1967 with field-treated soils. It should be emphasized that already at this time fortification had been recognized as an inappropriate tool in the evaluation of analytical methods (Morley, 1968; review Hurtig, 1973). Results of the respective soil sampling and analysis programme started in 1966 and differentiating between soil types including relation to crop grown have been summarized by Hurtig (1969). Out of 36 laboratories analyzing for p,p'-DDT in three soil samples, for instance, more than 66 % of the results were out of the + 2o % range. Although the reliability of organochlorine pesticide analysis has been improved in the meantime and intercomparison of laboratories today would be better, it has to be realized that organochlorine pesticides including PCB's in plants and soil represent the least analytical difficulties as compared to other organohalogenated environmental chemicals.

1.1 Soil

Progress in organochlorine pesticides monitoring has been reviewed by Holden (1975). In this review it is stated that soil is an appropriate commodity for the monitoring of the terrestrial environment, that standardized sampling techniques for soil surveys are available. One problem remains for unintentionally contaminated soils - namely, that the depth of contamination is unknown, and it is therefore suggested that the soil burden is not expressed in concentration but in terms of unit area. There is no sediment monitoring programme in operation (Holden, 1975).

With the data available in the late sixties, especially for DDT, it was possible to develop a global model for the occurrence of DDT in the biosphere (Woodwell, 1971). Based on mean data of agricultural and non-agricultural soils and the respective amounts of biomasses and their DDT-concentrations, it is evident that by far the largest amount of DDT has been present on land, especially agricultural soil.This finding can be qualitatively extrapolated to other agricultural chemicals, but not to organohalogenated chemicals in general.

1.2 Plants

Apart from the specific pesticide sampling and monitoring programmes, national efforts in many countries to implement pesticide regulations and control residues in crops can be included in the inventory of knowledge. Obtained data are quite detailed and give, for instance, not only the food commodities analyzed but also their origin, the number of samples with nodetectable residues, the lowest, the highest, and the mean residues, etc. (for instance, Seibel, 1974; Ernährungsbericht, 1976). For organochlorine pesticides, monitoring data are included in the Joint FAO/WHO Expert Committee evaluations for the following substances: Chlordane, aldrin-dieldrin, endrin, heptachlor (FAO/WHO, 1971), technical BHC, lindane toxaphene, hexachlorobenzene, and quintozene (FAO/WHO, 1974). National programmes resulting from pressing problems with a chemical, for instance BHC in Japan, resulted in a complete map of the residues, differentiated for isomers, and including data on soil, air, rain, animal and plant products (Goto, 1972).

For the purpose of monitoring and specimen banking for organohalogenated compounds in general in plants and soil, data from pesticides monitoring are only of use where derived from non-treated cultures. Specimen selection, for instance, cannot be done on the basis of highest residues in those programmes, since they may result from high treatment or other agricultural factors which have no significance for the aims of this workshop. Therefore, data on PCB's which have never been significantly used in agriculture and residue data from vegetation are of greater importance. In the review on "Monitoring persistent organic pollutants" (Holden, 1975), it is stated that terrestrial vegetation is less suitable for monitoring pesticides and that concentrations found in plant material vary widely according to the exposure to dust, sprays, or effluent discharges. Being concerned with organohalogenated compounds in general, it is exactly this influence which should be assessed in the needed monitoring and specimen banking. Thus, influences infavourable for pesticide sampling do not affect the use of plants for organohalogen monitoring but need to be recognized upon sampling.

Taking PCB's as a model for non-agricultural organohalogenated compounds, selected food for human consumption (Sümmermann et al., 1978) and plant samples from two potentially exposed and from two remote biotopes have been analyzed in our Institute (Müller and Korte; Klein , 1973; Klein and Weisgerber, 1976). This work was not real monitoring but it is mentioned here since the data obtained can be used for specimen selection, etc. In table 1, the results of these investigations of samples taken and analyzed in 1971 are summarized.

Table 1: PCB in Flora

Sampling near Autobahn Pfaffenhofen or Irschenberg		Sampling Remote Area Alps, Tegelberg, or Hüttensee	
Plant	ppm dry weight	Plant	ppm dry weight
Moss	o.13	Moss	o.o6
Heathen	o.28	Heathen	o.o8
Raspberry leaves	o.15-o.27	Raspberry leaves	o.11
Larch leaves	o.95	Larch leaves	o.17
Rushes	o.12	Rushes	o.o7
Hay	o.13	Fern	o.o8-o.15
Grass	o.2o-o.46	Juniper	o.o7
Grass silage	o.4o-o.42	Dwarf fir	o.o9-o.1o
Clover	o.33	Alder leaves	o.o9
Mint	o.2o		
Strawberry leaves	o.16-o.46		
Blackberry leaves	o.49		
Fir apex	o.31		
Oak foliage	o.5o		
Pine leaves	o.11		
Water hemlock	o.23-o.57		

At this time, we had a laboratory background for PCB's of 5 ppb in the analytical methodology. This has been used for the correction of the results. The data show that PCB's have been present at this time in the vegetation of remote areas in concentrations of o.06-o.17 mg/kg plant dry weight, whereas near motor highways concentrations were in the range of o.11-o.95 mg/kg.

Since the samples were collected for immediate analysis, they were put in polyethylene bags. Non-used samples were stored in these bags at -18°C. Following the improvements of PCB analytical methodology, some doubt was put on the height of the found concentrations in remote areas, and part of the samples have been reanalyzed recently. The results of these analyses compared to the originally detected concentrations gave data which were somewhat below the values of Table 1. From this, it cannot be concluded whether the original values were somewhat too high or whether the recently found lower concentrations are due to PCB loss upon storage. In order to establish a trend of PCB burden, it is planned to sample the same plants in the remote biotopes again.

This experiment is mentioned here to emphasize the need for the use of a standardized trace analytical methodology in a specimen banking programme from itsvery beginning.

2.   Specimen Banking

2.1   Influence of Storage and Container Material on Organohalogen Material

Within the German/U.S. joint pilot programme on specimen banking, our

Institute has investigated the fate of organochlorine residues upon -18°C storage (Kilzer et al., 1977). For this purpose, samples containing grown residues of aldrin-^{14}C and its conversion products (dieldrin, photodieldrin, hydrophilic metabolites, unextractable residues) were available. Plant and soil samples containing residues of aldrin and conversion products were obtained from aldrin-^{14}C-studies under outdoor conditions in 1969, 197o, and 1971. Samples 1-1o (Tables 2 and 3) were packed fresh in polyethylene bags, sample 11 (Table 3) in aluminium foil; then, they were stored up to 1976. Samples 1-8 were analyzed before and after storage, samples 9-11 only after storage. After the storage period, the packing materials (polyethylene or aluminium foil) were also investigated. For analysis of the soils, the water content was determined by drying aliquots of 5o g in a vaccuum desiccator at room temperature until constant weight. The remaining soils (2oo-4oo g of each) were extracted wet in a soxhlet with methanol for 48 hours. The plants were cut into small pieces and homogenized in methanol with an Ultra-Turrax, then extracted in a soxhlet with methanol for 48 hours, using exactly the same extraction, clean-up, and determination procedure as in the original analysis. The polyethylene bags or the aluminium foil were cut into samll strips and extracted overnight in methanol, then rinsed several times with fresh methanol; the extracts were combined.

s.   Table 2
s.   Table 3

The differences between the data obtained before and after long-term storage are small for most of the soil and plant residues. The differences appear to be random analytical deviations probably due to factors like, e.g., uneven residue distribution within the plant parts, differences in fresh weight (water content), variations in extractability, etc., and do not justify the assumption of significant residue loss for these substances during the storage period investigated, when concentrations down to 1o ppb are considered.

For DDT, it had been demonstrated (Ecobichon and Saschenbrecker, 1967) that chemical changes are possible even at -2o°C. In our experiments, a significant decrease of aldrin and a parallel increase of hydrophilic metabolites was not observed within the range considered.

The residues of aldrin and conversion products detected in samples 1-8 after storage and, additionally, those of three other samples (9-11) were compared with the residues in the packing material which was polyethylene for samples 1-1o and aluminium foil for sample 11. Adsorption factors were calculated as % residue in the packing material, based on the sum of residues in sample and packing material (after storage). The results for aldrin and dieldrin are presented in Table 3.

The table shows, that, in the case of aluminium foil (sample 11), no adsorption of aldrin or dieldrin occured; traces of radioactive substances are probably due to minute soil particles fixed on the foil. Small amounts of aldrin and dieldrin were adsorbed onto polyethylene. In the case of two plant samples (6-7), the percentage of aldrin adsorbed is considerable, and for the plant sample 8, the adsorption is quantitative. However, the residues of unchanged aldrin in these samples were in the range of 1o ppb or less, as is the case for normal environmental plant samples, since aldrin is readily converted in plants.

Table 2: Residues of Aldrin-^{14}C and Conversion Products in Soil and Plants before and after 5-7 Years' Storage at -18°C (in mg/kg; mg equivalent to aldrin; based on dry weight for soils and on fresh weight for plants).

Sample Nr.	Material	Storage since (years)	aldrin before	aldrin after	dieldrin before	dieldrin after	photodieldrin before	photodieldrin after	hydrophilic metabolites before	hydrophilic metabolites after	unextract. residues before	unextract. residues after
1	Potato soil	5	0.04	0.04	0.39	0.33	<0.01	<0.01	0.07	0.06	0.13	0.13
2	Wheat soil	5	0.05	0.04	0.47	0.48	<0.01	0.01	0.08	0.09	0.11	0.20
3	Potato soil	5	0.23	0.17	0.80	0.74	0.01	0.02	0.12	0.11	0.21	0.29
4	Carrot soil	6	0.27	0.31	0.77	0.76	<0.01	0.02	0.16	0.11	0.17	0.16
5	Wheat soil	7	0.05	0.06	0.03	0.03	<0.01	<0.01	0.01	0.01	0.02	0.03
6	Wheat straw	6	<0.01	<0.01	0.16	0.17	0.04	0.03	0.22	0.16	0.07	0.05
7	Potato leaves	6	0.01	<0.01	0.08	0.07	0.02	0.02	0.03	0.02	0.02	0.01
8	Corn stalks	6	0.01	n.d.	0.04	0.05	<0.01	0.01	0.04	0.01	0.01	0.01

Table 3: Adsorption of Residues of Aldrin-^{14}C and Dieldrin-^{14}C by Packing Materials (in % of the sum of residues in the sample and in the packing material, both after storage).

Sample Nr.	Sample Material	Packing material	Storage time (years)	% Adsorption by the packing material aldrin	% Adsorption by the packing material dieldrin
1	Potato soil	Polyethylene	5	1.3	0.4
2	Wheat soil	"	5	0.7	0.3
3	Potato soil	"	5	2.2	0.6
4	Carrot soil	"	6	6.9	2.0
5	Wheat soil	"	7	5.1	1.6
6	Wheat straw	"	6	33.4	0.1
7	Potato leaves	"	6	67.0	7.6
8	Corn stalks	"	6	100.0	3.2
9	Wheat roots	"	7	10.1	2.3
10	Wheat roots	"	7	15.3	2.5
11	Maize soil	Aluminium foil	6	<0.1	<0.1

The amounts of photodieldrin and hydrophilic metabolites detected in polyethylene were even less than those of dieldrin; unextractable residues were
not detected. This may be explained by the assumption that the adsorption
occurs via the gaseous phase. For hexachlorobenzene, experiments had been
carried out which demonstrate that the substance is volatilized and adsorbed from the gaseous phase by polyethylene (Steinwandter, 1976). Systematic investigations on the loss of hexachlorobenzene upon freeze-drying of animal tissues have shown losses up to 75 % (Kraatz et al., unpublished).

It may be concluded from these experiments that no significant alteration
or losses of aldrin derived residues - that is at least 4 chemical of
different polarity - occur during five to seven years' storage of fresh
samples at -18ºC. However, this conclusion must not be transferred to
other contaminants.

2.2 Fingerprint Analyses with Emphasis on Polar Organochlorines

In the pilot programme, it was investigated whether a complete analytical
procedure can be developed to arrive at identical capillary GC fingerprints of plant and animal tissue samples (Vollner et al., unpublished).
Initially, spiked samples have been used for this purpose. Only the extractable portion was to be investigated under this topic (see below).

Lettuce was chosen as plant and pentachlorophenol-^{14}C as an indicator
chemical. In order to achieve a high recovery and reproducible chemicals' content of a fraction upon clean-up, counter-current partition
has been used in this experiment which is given schematically in Fig. 1.

The reproducibility for the indicator substance over the whole procedure
is good. But, what is even more promising, is the reproducibility of
the capillary chromatogram (fingerprint) over the whole procedure. This
is demonstrated in Fig. 2 which shows two chromatograms (a and b) obtained from a fraction of two extracts of the same lettuce sample after
5o-Step-Partition.

s. Figure 1
s. Figure 2

Further, similar experiments carried out with animal tissues hould be
mentioned for completeness. Stomach and liver of a Rhesus monkey which
had been treated with hexachlorobenzene-^{14}(were analyzed according to the
above described methodology using hexane /methanol/water as partition
phases. Since non-extractable residues in animal tissues are negligible,
recoveries were excellent (94-99 % upon extraction and above 9o % for the
whole procedure). The amount of sample material was only sufficient to
do the whole experiment with each sample twice. The capillary GC chromatogram of the HCB-fraction from each tissue has been exactly reproducible in qualitative and quantitative aspect. Quantitative deviations of
the non-identified fingerprint peaks were utmost in the range of about
5 %. For one of the fractions, the fingerprint peaks were additionally
characterized by their molecular weights from capillary GC/MS analysis.
This was just done for demonstration that it is feasible to characterize
the sample by fingerprint analysis.

2.3 Unextractable Contaminants

Despite great efforts devoted by several research groups to this problem,

Fig. 1: Scheme of Experimental Procedure for Fingerprint Analysis of
Polar Organochlorines Using PCP as an Indicator Substance

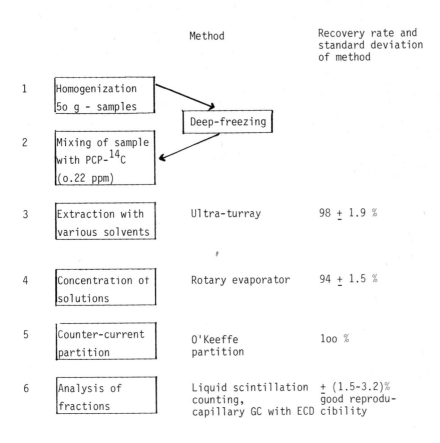

	Method	Recovery rate and standard deviation of method
1 Homogenization 5o g - samples		
Deep-freezing		
2 Mixing of sample with PCP-^{14}C (o.22 ppm)		
3 Extraction with various solvents	Ultra-turray	98 $\pm$ 1.9 %
4 Concentration of solutions	Rotary evaporator	94 $\pm$ 1.5 %
5 Counter-current partition	O'Keeffe partition	1oo %
6 Analysis of fractions	Liquid scintillation counting, capillary GC with ECD	$\pm$ (1.5-3.2)% good reproducibility

362

Fig. 2: Capillary GC Traces (ECD) of Fraction 43 Following 5o-Step-
Partition in Hexane/Acetic Acid 95:5 of two Ethylacetate
Ectracts of Lettuce

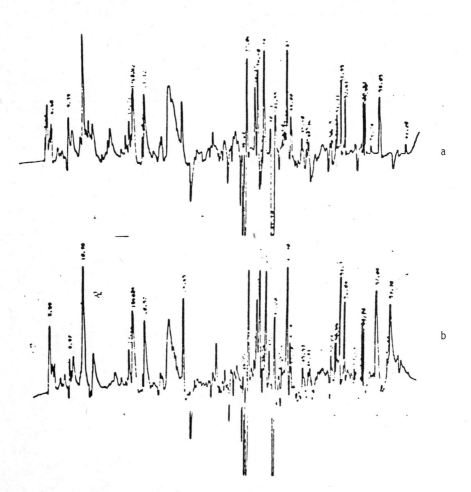

it has not been solved so far. For the purpose of specimen banking, according to our present knowledge, it would be appropriate for exclude "bound
residues" in the initial phase of banking for unknown contaminants from
the investigations. With the identification of a potentially hazardous
substance, the ratio of extractable to unextractable portion needs to
be experimentally established.

Table 4: Unextractable Residues* in Soil (o-lo cm depth) Following
Soil Treatment with ^{14}C-Chemicals (in % of radioactivity
present).

Chemical applied	Unextractable after 1 vegetation period	Unextractable after 2 vegetation periods
Dieldrin	< 1	3
Kepone	2	2
Kelevan	8	12
Aldrin	11	18
Imugan	32	68
2,2'-Dichlorobiphenyl	42	74
3,4-Dichloroaniline	84	89
Allylalcohol	91	not analyzed
p-CI-Aniline	95	92

* unextractable by 48 hours extraction with methanol, acetone or choro-
form in a Soxhlet

Table 4 shows some examples of our investigations and gives percentages
of non-extractable radioactivity one and two vegetation periods after
soil treatment with ^{14}C-chemicals. These percentages show that from a
balance point of view non-extractable portions have to be considered in
soil although their biological significance remains unclear.

b) Rational for Interest or Concern

There exists a great number of halogenated, especially chlorinated, organic commercial chemicals. In a compilation of chemicals identified in
surface-, sewage-, and other waters (Eurocop-Cost 64b, 1974), 112 organo-
halogenated individual chemicals have been listed. They include aromatic
and aliphatic substances, they include chemicals with low and high
halogen content, they include chemicals with low vapour pressure like
organochlorine pesticides and those with high vapour pressure like
chlorinated solvents. Their polarity varies in a wide range.

It can be generally stated that substitution of hydrogen by halogen increases persistence. Consequently, the rational for concern is different
from chemical to chemical and follows its likelyhood to occur from

- production and use pattern

- persistence

- dispersion

- bioaccumulation

- vapour pressure

- water solubility / lipophilic behaviour

- metabolic activation or detoxication

- toxicological significance of parent compounds.

It is likely that exposure levels increase with increased production. Significant exposure is known for organochlorine pesticides and punctually for others like PCB's via food. It is furthermore likely that a large number of chemicals occur in plants and soil, probably at least most of the compounds given in the Cost 64b or other respecitve lists.

Pathways for human exposure are food as the major source (fish > animal products > food crops) and drinking water (including compounds formed upon chlorination which have increased persistence). The exposure route via breathing is significant only for highly volatile solvents and propellents. Intake of pesticides, e.g. by air and water, is only about 5 % of total intake.

Since e.g. PCB's which have never been used significantly in soil or plants have been found in the flora of non-inhabited areas, "occurrence" of organohalogen chemicals must be expected generally in any plants and soil.

C) Considerations for Sample Selection, Collection, Containment, Shipment, and Storage

1. Sample Selection

1.1 Long-term Accumulator

Soil seems to be an appropriate specimen for the assessment of long-term accumulation. This is based on its property to sorb a number of chemicals and retain water-insoluble products. Since microbial degradation is low in poor soils, appropriate soil types would be those with lower humus content. A further advantage of soil as specimen is the fact that repeated samples can be taken any time in any requested amount from the same plot. Thus, there is no problem in relative representativity as regards time course. The selection of plots in industrial, agricultural and non-inhabited areas would give good typical samples for the exposure levels.

1.2 Seasonal Accumulator

A seasonal accumulator typical for human exposure as regards significance as food would be food grain. Since the "accumulation" of chemicals in food grain seems to be low, this specimen has no good predictive value. A respective seasonal high-accumulator would be carrots for lipophilic chemicals. However, they have no great significance in human food supply.

1.3 Wild plants

Based on the results reported above on PCB's, conifer leaves might be the best indicator besides Cladonia and water hemlock, which all seem to be high accumulators. Pines should be preferred due to their widespread occurrence and their feasibility of sampling.

2. Sample Collection

The general representativity of sampling is highly difficult and is not specific for the compounds discussed here. With the suggestions for specimen given above, however, the reproducibility of sampling and knowledge of sample history do not impose problems, except for food plants. Upon sample collection, shipment, and storage, there seem to be no severe contamination problems for this group of compounds if properly handled with glass and metal tools only.

3. Containment

Since organic chemicals migrate in the course of time into containers of organic material and since metal surfaces might catalyze unwanted chemical reactions in the sample, glass or other mineral containers only give the needed safety to avoid loss and minimize reactions.

4. Storage

Since freeze-drying reduces residues except for non-volatile compounds, and since it may change the extractability of chemicals (analytical recovery), fresh non-dried samples are preferred for storage. The storage temperature seems to be related with the persistence of the chemical of concern. Since the organohalogenated compounds considered here cover a wide range in this respect, low storage temperatures ought to be aimed at.

It is advisable to use portional stroage after homogenization which allows to draw samples for analysis at any time without disturbing the portions of the sample subject for continued storage. Furthermore, this procedure assures better homogenization and, in case of sorption of chemicals to the container walls, allows for their correct analysis in the sample portion.

d. Analytical Procedures

1. Since it is proposed to take aliquots of samples prior to storage, there is no problem to assure for the accuracy of the portion to be analyzed.

2. A large number of individual substances requires multimatrix-multiresidue methodology. Thus the used methods could possibly be reduced to 2-3 procedures, e.g. for volatile and non-volatile, or for polar and non-polar substances. This methodology, however, is not yet completely developed.

3. There exist only few chlorinated natural substances (e.g. in algae and fungi). Interference of non-halogenated chemicals can be overcome by glass-capillary GLC with internal standardisation or GLC-MS confirmation.

4. Convenient detection and determination of chlorinated and brominated substances is by GLC/ECD. For fluorinated chemicals sensitive detectors are being developed. Alternatives exist for clean-up: gel permeation, counter-current distribution, HPLC, etc.

5. So far no certified standards and reference materials are available. Interlaboratory check has been done for pesticides and PCB: variations by a factor of o.2 to 2 are typical.

e. Program Design

1. There exists one basic difficulty, namely, to bank and analyze a large number of samples and achieve good statistical representativity or to have a low number of specific local samples, enabling sophisticated analysis like GC/MS confirmation with no need for expensive development of routine analytical procedure. A small number of samples would be preferable at least for soil and wild plants.

2. For food plants, samples form different locations are to be combined to form one representative sample per area and allow for sophisticated analyses. This would be an alternative against many samples analyzed separately by routine methods.

3. Specimen suggested for banking are soil, food grain, and pine leaves or lichen.

4. The magnitude of samples must not be more than loo/year/area or country for complete analysis.

5. The sample description needs to include biological identification and exact local description with known data of chemical immission at the time of sampling.

f. Organizational Aspect

1. Pesticides are covered by existing programmes and actions. However, there exist no comprehensive programmes for other industrial chemicals, e.g. chlorinated phenols, hexachlorobutadiene.

2. The proposed small number of samples, randomly mixed samples, and the complexity of analytical procedure call forcentralized approach.

3. International coordination should include chemical species for monitoring, chemical species as regards storage, compatibility of analytical procedures. For the specimen discussed, full coordination might be too difficult.

4. Certified reference material is necessary for analytical work.

h. Cost Estimates

Annual national costs, provided the programme is limited to loo samples per year, including detection and determination of 2o chemicals, storage, and fingerprint analyses for major bulk chemicals:

1. Design including development of analytical procedures, where necessary, and data processing. This excludes basic instrumentation. (loo,ooo - 3oo,ooo DM).

2. Collection, transport:
   2.1 wild samples (3,ooo DM)
   2.2 food plants (8,ooo DM)

3. Storage:
   3.1 for monitoring (1,ooo DM)
   3.2 for banking   (8,ooo DM)

4. Analysis:
   4.1 monitoring   (8o,ooo DM)
   4.2 fingerprints (9o,ooo DM)

5. Data processing   (1o,ooo DM)

References

Abbot, D.C., Crisp, S., Tarrant, K.R. and Tatton J.O'G. (197o). Pestic. Sci. 1, 1o.

Abbot, D.C., Holmes, D.C. and Tatton, J.O'G. (1969). J. Sci. Fd. Agr. 2o, 245.

Ecobichon, D.J. and Saschenbrecker, P.W. (1967). Science 156, 663

Egan, H. (1973). Pesticide residues in food - the situation today. In: Environmental Quality and Safety, Vol. 2, Georg Thieme Verlag Stuttgart, Academic Press New York - London, 78 - 87.

Ernährungsbericht (1976). Deutsche Gesellschaft für Ernährung e.V., Frankfurt/Main.

Eurocop-Cost 64b (1974). Analysis of organic micropollutants in water. EUCO/MOU/4o/74; XII/825/74, Commission of the European Communities.

FAO/WHO (1971). 1971 Evaluations of some pesticide residues in food. The Monographs. Food and Agriculture Organization of the United Nations, World Health Organization, Rome.

FAO/WHO (1974). 1973 Evaluations of some pesticide residues in food. The Monographs. World Health Organization, Geneva, Food and Agriculture Organization of the United Nations, Rome.

Goto, M. (1972). In: Environmental Quality and Safety, Vol. 1,Georg Thieme Verlag Stuttgart, Academic Press New York - London, 211 - 216.

Holden, A.V. (1975). Monitoring persistent organic pollutants. In: Organochlorine Insecticides: Persistent Organic Pollutants, Academic Press, London-New York-San Francisco, 1 - 27.

Hurtig, H. (1969). Ecological chemistry implications of the use of pesticides. 1st International Symposium "Chemical and Toxicological Aspects of Environmental Quality", Munich, 1o - 11 July, 1969. Published by Georg Thieme Verlag, Stuttgart, 1969.

Hurtig, H. (1973). Chemicals in the environment - some aspects of agricultural chemicals. In: Environmental Quality and Safety, Vol. 2, Georg
Thieme Verlag, Stuttgart, Academic Press New York-London, 88 - 99.

Kilzer, L., Weisgerber, I., Klein, W., and Korte, F. (1977). Chemosphere
6, 93-98.

Klein, W. (1973). PCB's and environmental contamination. 3rd International
Symposium "Chemical and Toxicological Aspects of Environmental Quality",
Tokyo, 19 - 22 November 1973.

Klein, W. and Weisgerber, I. (1976). PCB's and environmental contamination.
In: Environmental Quality and Safety, Vol. 5, Georg Thieme Verlag Stuttgart, Academic Press New York-London, 237-25o.

Morley, H.V. (1968). The determination of organochlorine pesticide residues
in soil. Proc. 1st Seminar on Pesticide Residue Analysis, Eastern, Canada,
18 - 19 Nov. 1968. Published by Ontario Department of Agriculture and
Food, 1968.

Müller, W. and Korte, F. (1976). Chemosphere 5, 95-1oo.

Sand, P.F., Gentry, J.W., Bongberg, J. and Schechter, M.S. (1967). Pestic.
Monit. J. 1, 16-19.

Seibel, W. (1974). Getreide, Mehl und Brot 28, 257-259.

Steinwandter, H. (1976). Chemosphere 5, 241-244.

Sümmermann, W., Rohleder, H. and Korte, F. (1978). Z.Lebensm.Unters.-
Forsch. 166, 137-144.

Swackhamer, A.B. (1965). Pestic. Progr. 3, 1o8.

van Tiel, N. (1972). Pesticides in environment and food. In: Environmental
Quality and Safety, Vol. 1, Georg Thieme Verlag Stuttgart, Academic Press
New York-London, 18o-189.

WHO (1978). Environmental health criteria for DDT and its derivatives.
World Health Organization, EHE/EHC/78.9, VBC/TOX/78.21.

Woodwell, G.M., Craig, P.P. and Johnson, H.A. (1971). Science 1974.
11o1-11o7.

TERRESTRIAL VERTEBRATE ANIMALS AS BIOLOGICAL MONITORS OF POLLUTION

Drs. Robert A. and Carolyn W. Lewis
Office of the Assistant Secretary for Environment
U.S. Department of Energy
Route 8, Box 142, Frederick, Maryland

Summary

Properly collected and preserved, vertebrate specimens may serve in a number of ways as environmental monitors. The advantages, technical feasibility and special problems that attend such use are discussed, as are criteria for sampling, sample preparation and storage in a specimen bank.
Special emphasis is given to the problems of environmental dynamics, ecological sampling, and the retrospective evaluation of information.
Recommendations for the implementation of effective vertebrate specimen banking programs are made and the potential value of such systems is discussed.
Because the significance that can be attached to tissue, organ or whole organism concentrations of pollutants is confounded by many factors, we conclude that retrospective monitoring via chemical analyses of banked specimens will be of value in making environmental decisions only if it is used in conjunction with complementary methods of assessment, especially of biological effects.

Introduction

USE OF SPECIMEN BANKS HISTORICALLY AND PRESENTLY

The National Pesticide Monitoring Program

The Bureau of Sport Fisheries and Wildlife, U.S. Department of Interior, conducts the vertebrate animal component of the National Pesticide Monitoring Program (see Johnson et al., 1967). Numerous publications have resulted from this program (e.g., Dustman, 1966; Dustman et al., 1971; Kreitzer, 1974; Martin, 1969, 1972; White and Heath, 1976), which might serve as a partial point of departure for establishing goals and criteria for collecting and banking vertebrate specimens for analysis and evaluation of pollutants other than pesticides.
The primary objective of this program as it relates to fish and wildlife is to ascertain on a nationwide scale, independent of specific treatments, the levels and trends of certain pesticidal chemicals and other pollutants in the tissues of selected forms of vertebrate animals. Taxa employed in this continuing program include the European Starling (Sturnus vulgaris), the Bald Eagle (Haliaeetus leucicephalus), the Golden Eagle (Aquila chrysaetos), and the Mallard (Anas platyrhynchos); the closely related Black Duck (Anas rubripes) replaces the Mallard in regions where the latter is not sufficiently abundant to provide adequate samples.

The combined range of these ducks covers the continental United States.

The National Environmental Specimen Bank Survey

Oak Ridge National Laboratories, under the auspices of the U.S. Environmental Protection Agency, completed a survey in 1975. This survey identified 675 environmental specimen collections maintained by various institutions or investigators throughout the United States, including the following types of materials: atmospheric, geological, human tissue, animal tissue other than human, plant tissue, water. Taxonomic collections were not included in this survey. Results of the survey indicate that very few collections are suitable for retrospective chemical analyses because of the collection, preparation and storage techniques being utilized (Van Hook et al., 1976); many of these collections were not maintained for such purposes. However, the survey served a valuable function because it alerted the scientific community to a national interest in their collections; it caused some investigators to reexamine their practices; and, since the survey data base is being maintained, the NESB offers opportunity for information exchange among researchers who may find access to specimens or data from other locations useful.

The NESB was evaluated by Becker and Maienthal (1977). They concluded that few of the presently existing collections had adequate records to indicate that they were established and maintained under the exacting conditions necessary for retrospective chemical analysis.

The National Environmental Specimen Banking System

The U.S. Environmental Protection Agency and the National Bureau of Standards are working to establish a National Environmental Specimen Bank. This system is intended to provide "credible real time monitoring data for an environmental early warning system and well preserved and documented environmental samples for future retrospective analysis". The stated objectives are to: (1) conduct a survey and evaluation of existing specimen collections in the United States, (2) organize a planning committee to evaluate the feasibility of such a banking system, (3) develop a five-year plan for carrying out the work, and (4) develop a program to establish criteria for sample collection, preparation, storage, and analysis, (see Rood and Goldstein, 1977).

Needless to say, great difficulties attend the achievement of these goals. For example, more contrained and specific objectives must be defined and a limited number of specimen types must be selected. A pilot project would be a useful, and perhaps necessary, step. The design of field sampling rationales is a problem of particular importance.

Both the EPA and NBS bring needed experience to the design, development and implementation of a project of such scope.

Taxonomic Collections

Museum collections have been frequently employed in retrospective analysis of vertebrate materials. Laboratories assessing transport and effects of pesticides began using museum materials collected before the 1930's as "blanks" for purposes of chemical comparison. Vertebrate materials assayed in the past have included hair and other integumental structures such as skin, feathers, or nails; bone and even soft tissues. Products such as eggs have also been assayed. A number of special types of museum collections such as comparative serological collections, alcoholic tissues, and freeze-dried specimens which are now found in some museum practice, are also of potential importance.

Sampling strategies and methods of preservation and storage of general and research collections are not generally satisfactory for chemical analyses of pollutants that are widely distributed in nature. Nevertheless, used with care, museum collections may, on occasion, prove very valuable. Such collections are often more amenable to biological monitoring, and therefore, may play a supportive role in relation to specimen banks designed for retrospective chemical analyses. For example, the use of extensive ecological collections has proved invaluable in establishing those species of birds that are especially at risk from pesticides via egg shell thinning (and attendant disorders).

Integumental structures such as hair and feathers constitute a major excretory route for some chemicals such as methyl mercury, heavy metals and radionuclides. Various treatments and preservatives are employed for most museum skins to prevent infestations by pests (arsenic has frequently been employed); skins of fat birds such as waterfowl may be washed with organic solvents to remove lipid and thus delay decay. Other chemicals, notably boric acid and paradichlorobenzene, contaminate museum skins. Most integumental structures are, however, stable under normal museum management; some can be spared, washed, and together with appropriate controls, can provide valuable information on the extent of historical pollution by trace contaminants such as lead, arsenic, cadmium and mercury (e.g., Dorn et al., 1974; Gordus et al., 1973). Proper design of retrospective studies employing these materials makes it possible to evaluate the influence on pollutant concentrationsof a variety of variables such as age, sex, time of year, and diet. Hair has been accurately analyzed for various substances such as lead, arsenic, cadmium and mercury (e.g., Dorn et al., 1974; Gordus et al., 1973). Serial segments of hair have been especially useful in some cases. In birds that have a single complete annual molt, seasonal variations in flight feather concentrations should prove interesting.

Living Specimen Banks

Zoological Gardens. Relationships between disease, including carcinomas, pollutant burdens, other effects and air pollution have frequently been observed in zoo animals (e.g., Lombard and Witte, 1959; Snyder and Ratcliffe, 1969; Bazell, 1971; Tashiro et al., 1974). Zoos are generally situated in urban or suburban environments and the animals may be attended by full or part time veterinary staffs. Thus, specimen banks of tissues taken from healthy, ill, moribund, or recently dead animals would not be unusually difficult or costly to establish. Clinical records and vital statistics would be available on many of these animals and extensive life history information would also be available.

Because zoo animals are relatively long lived and often of known age (this includes indigenous as well as exotic species), they offer particularly good potential for the study of chronic pollution and accumulation of body burdens of environmental contaminants. Zoos are, of course, distributed throughout the world, and thus offer the possibility of global monitoring of vertebrate animals.

Surveys of Road Kills. Animals are frequently killed by automobiles. Because many mammals are nocturnal and shy, they are difficult to collect for study. Road kills represent fortutious samples of such animals. They must be regarded, of course, as non-random samples. Further uncertainties attend their use. For example, post-mortem changes in tissue concentrations of pollutants may occur. Surveys of road kills may nevertheless, provide provisional data on population variation, life cycles and other life functions of animals not otherwise easily accessible for study.

As part of a study of the distribution of selected toxic trace metals in vertebrate fauna of the State of Ohio, Curnow et al. (1975) collected and froze road-killed specimens of deer, rabbits, pheasants and squirrels. Tissue samples were later taken and subsequently analyzed. A variety of ecological or land-use relationships might account for the observed distribution of pollutant burdens among terrestrial habitats in Ohio.

Hunter's Bags. Hunter's bags have been extensively employed in wildlife management studies and surveys, including pesticide surveys. Wings of waterfowl (the Mallard and Black Duck) and of Mourning Doves (Zenaidura macroura) have been monitored nationwide for pesticide residues. In the Mallard/Black Duck survey, for example, wings that were collected nationwide during the 1965 and 1966 hunting seasons were assayed for organochlorine pesticides (Heath, 1969). DDE residues predominated; regional differences in residues were demonstrated, as were species and sex differences. This work was validated during 1969-7o (Heath and Hill, 1974). Residues of DDE, DDT, dieldrin, and PCB's in these species have declined in certain flyways since 1969 (White and Heath, 1976).

Tissue Banks. Tissue banks, maintained by medical institutions primarily for the purpose of maintaining viable tissues and organs for grafts, are of great importance to planning for the establishment of environmental specimen banks. Many of the methods of human tissue banking are suitable for use with vertebrates generally, to the extent indicated by the objectives of the environmental specimen bank system. Long-term (i.e., more than 25 years) preservation of various human and vertebrate laboratory animal tissue has already been achieved. Tissues such as skin have remained viable for such periods. One intriguing possible use of such methods of preservation is that of comparing (on a real-time basis) the long term trends in pollutant concentrations of particular sets of specimens, while at the same time via controlled in vitro experiments assessing altered sensitivity to pollutants of concern. Tests of tissue vigor and vitality might also be possible.

Use of Other Systems that Monitor Wild Animals. In the United States and many other nations, cooperative programs whereby large numbers of resident and migratory birds are banded and released on a continuing basis have been operating for many years. The possibility of conservative sampling (e.g., small drop of blood, toe clipping, feather sample, etc.) thus presents, together with the potential of repeat information on the same individuals. Such a monitoring system could be easily implemented in several countries at little cost if it were considered sufficiently important by the administering government agencies and the cooperators involved.

Tissues and Products of Domestic Animals. It is quite possible to collect and bank regulated animal products such as milk and eggs. The value of such a system is that it would involve sampling of materials consumed by man or non-destructive sampling of animals that are of high economic importance. Such a scheme might include blood samples, hair, urine, etc., of livestock on the way to slaughter. Both blood and milk represent tissues of potentially great usefulness. Milk is consumed in great quantities in some countries by both children and adults. A number of pollutants may be excreted in relatively large concentrations in milk. Lactation was inferred to be the major route of excretion of dieldrin in dairy cattle that were provided with contaminated diets (Braund et al., 1968).

CHARACTERISTICS OF TERRESTRIAL VERTEBRATES THAT MAKE THEM SUITABLE FOR BANKING

Terrestrial Vertebrates. Many environments, worldwide, are contaminated to the point that they present hazards to vertebrate animals including, in a few instances man. Environmental impacts of toxic materials are a matter of deep and urgent public concern. Terrestrial vertebrates are prominent among those biota that attract public attention. They are, furthermore, effective monitors of many pollutants as well as of pollution-induced ecosystem change (e.g., Bigler et al., 1975; Dieter, 1974; Dorn et al., 1974; Dustman and Stickel, 1969; Feriancova-Masarova and Kalivodova, 1965; Kreitzer, 1974; Martin 1969, 1972; McArn et al., 1974; Ohi et al., 1974; Selikoff and Hammond, 1968; Takemoto et al., 1974; Tansy and Roth, 197o; Tashiro et al., 1974). Vertebrates may prove to be especially valuable in registering and integrating transport, transformation and effects of chronic exposure of terrestrial environments to low levels of persistent pollutants. Use of fish-eating birds and mammals also offers an opportunity for assessing transfer of pollutants from the aquatic to terrestrial environments. And certain domestic and game species offer obvious opportunities to monitor potential transfer of environmental pollutants to man.
Vertebrate animals are exceedingly complex in their responses to environmental change. They rarely respond to a perturbation in a simple, linear fashion. Nevertheless, vertebrate responses are better understood physiologically and behaviorally than those of other comparable groups of animals. Life cycles and annual cycles are higly regulated and metabolic pathways, regulation and energetics are well known for many species. We are thus in a good position to interpret environmental pollutant dynamics as determined by vertebrate monitors, and to acquire needed experimental information to evaluate inferences or predictions drawn form monitoring data.
Terrestrial vertebrates have long been models in the study of the toxicity, pharmacology and physiology of drugs and other chemicals to which humans are exposed. The wealth of accumulated knowledge from such investigations will aid substantially in the interpretation of monitoring data and in the construction and validation of transport and effects models. We must caution, however, that much of this work has been done under environmentally unrealistic conditions and that the standard laboratory animals that are most frequently employed tend to be fairly pollution resistant and may not be representative of the responses of even closely-related taxa living in nature.
Residues of pesticides and related compounds such as polychlorinated biphenyls (PCB) have been demonstrated in vertebrate animals throughout the world. Adults and eggs or embryos as well as products such as milk may contain pesticide residues. Such residues sometimes persist much longer in vertebrates than in other portions of the environment (e.g., Keith and Flickinger, 1965).
Based on our interpretation of the literature of animal ecology, environmental physiology, toxicology, and to a lesser extent on health related studies of pollution effects, it is clear that we may anticipate effects at nearly all levels of animal organization (see Table 1). We do not know at this time, however, the "threshold" exposure rates that might be expected to produce the various kinds of effects, nor to what extent these effects may be indirect or due to secondary metabolites. This naivete speaks strongly to the need for an effective specimen banking system to take advantage not only of improved techniques for assay of low levels of tissue contaminants - but improved knowledge of pollutant effects and mechanisms of pollutant action.

Also of value is our knowledge of stress physiology of birds and mammals. Birds and mammals respond in similar ways to appropriate glucocorticoids and presumably, to chronic stress (see, for example, Buckley, 1972; Assenmacher, 1973). Thus, given appropriate allometry of tissues and organs of specimens collected for a specimen banking and monitoring system and especially if key tissues are spared for histological examination, it might be possible to establish the degree of non-specific stress. Such information can be at least as valuable as chemical assays themselves, and in some cases (e.g., non-persistent chemicals; inaccurate or insensitive analytic methods) can augment or replace chemical analysis. Depending upon the severity of stress, responses to environmental insults of a wide variety may include:

1) involution or degenerative changes in nearly any organ
2) altered liver lipid
3) increased protein catabolism
4) increased lipid mobilization
5) inhibition of growth and maturation
6) increased nitrogen excretion
7) a reduction in carcass protein of growing animals
8) decreased excretion of sodium and potassium with concommitantly reduced levels in urine and increased plasma levels
9) altered reproductive performance
1o) hyper- or hypoadrenocortical activity
11) adrenocortical enlargement
12) gastrointestinal ulcers
13) altered blood counts (e.g. lymphopenia).

Amphibians and Reptiles. These are probably least important among terrestrial vertebrates as potential monitors of chemical pollutants. Although they may be important components of ecological food chains, very little is known about the susceptibilities of these poikilothermous terrestrial vertebrates to sublethal effects of most environmental contaminants. They are sometimes killed by direct applications of insecticides, but are generally less sensitive than fish (see Fergusen, 1963; Herald, 1949; Smith and Glasgow, 1975; Wilson, 1972).

Declines of some amphibian populations have been attributed to treatment of breeding water or adult feeding grounds with pesticides. The findings of Cooke (197o, 1971, 1972, 1973a, 1973b) are consistent with this possibility.

Undoubtedly strong species differences occur with respect to pollution sensitivities and pharmacokinetics. Toads, for example, are far more sensitive than frogs (Cooke, op. cit.).

Healthy amphibians and reptiles may have extensive fat stores and might thus be especially sensitive to chronic exposure to lipophilic contaminants. They do indeed accumulate rather large residues of such pollutants (Fleet et al., 1972; Korschgen, 197o; Meeks, 1968; Rosene et al., 1961).

Birds. The most immediate dramatic point to be made here is simply to mention the well-known historic importance of the canary (Serinus) in sensing mine gases and anoxia (Neal and Olstrum, 1971). Unusual sensitivities and suspected sensitivities of birds to a wide spectrum of pollutants have been reported. Birds can, for example, absorb some toxicants through their feet. Indeed, roosts have been treated with fenthion and endrin to control birds.

Table 1

HYPOTHETICAL RESPONSES OR VERTEBRATES TO CHRONIC POLLUTION STRESS - EXTENSIVE

A. Direct Pathological Effects
1. Mortality
2. Morbidity

B. Physiological and Reproductive Effects
1. Fertility
2. Fecundity
3. Growth, metabolism and bioenergetics
4. Immunosuppression
5. Differential effects on life functions
6. Other factors affecting competitive ability

C. Biochemical Effects
1. Enzyme suppression or activation
2. Enzyme kinetics

D. Genetic Change

E. Behavioral or Physiological Effects
1. Dormancy
   a. Hibernation
   b. Estivation
2. Physical Movement
   a. Dispersal
   b. Migration
   c. Refuging
   d. Dispersion
3. Selective Behavior (e.g., feeding, habitat selection, etc.)

F. Adaptation and Resistance
1. Induced detoxication mechanisms
2. Altered rates of uptake and/or excretion
3. Sequestering
4. Behavioral adaptation

G. Indirect Effects Manifested Through Reduced Home Range Carrying Capacity, e.g., via:
1. Direct vegetation destruction
2. Factors affecting soil nutrients
3. Factors affecting nutrient quality of vegetation
4. Factors affecting climate
5. Other factors that interrupt energy flow or otherwise alter resource relationships

H. Other Effects
1. Dysfunctional phase-shifting (in time) of life functions
2. Preadaption
3. Non adaptive changes (e.g., ancillary or related to one of the above; pleiotropy).

Fowle (1972) demonstrated that birds that perch on phosphamidon-treated twigs can be killed. There have been alarming decreases in populations of certain waterfowl during the past two decades. Although causative agents remain largely unknown, anthropogenic chemicals and habitat alteration by man have undoubtedly contributed. Takemoto et al. (1974) reported that pigeons living in highly industrialized areas of Japan develop lung pathologies when aerial pollution levels are only one-tenth the value of those that produce analogous pathologies in human lungs.

Birds are aesthetically valued by many people and many of the larger birds (wildfowl, some doves and many gallinaceous birds) are valued as game birds. Many of the smaller birds in particular are very abundant and easily collected. Large numbers of bird species have become extinct over the past few centuries and many species are currently threatened or endangered. In a number of cases, pollutants have been linked with serious population declines.

Birds exhibit many characteristics that make them potentially good pollution monitors. They are conspicuous, generally day-active, typically live above ground and fly at levels where gaseous and other respirable pollutant levels may be highest. Indeed, birds provide a mechanism for separately assessing uptake and effects of aerial and dietary pollutants. The lungs and respiratory tract are particularly valuable for monitoring air pollution. In contrast, ingested pollutants probably affect the liver and perhaps the kidney selectively. Some species live in extreme environments; the class Aves has the widest distribution of any vertebrate class. Small birds, especially when in flight, have very high metabolic rates and the external respiratory system probably acts very much like a high volume sampler (discusses subsequently). Most birds are relatively long lived and life histories of most are well known. Of considerable importance, also, is the fact that the classification of birds is more completely worked out than for any other class of animal. Rarely do trained scientists fail to identify specimens to the species level. There is more information on the population biology and behavior of birds generally than for any other class of animals, and there is an excellent fund of knowledge on the physiology of birds. Many species are abundant and conspicuous with wide distributions. Some species or populations are migratory, some are partially migratory, and others are sedentary.

Birds typically are on a fat economy and some species deposit huge fat stores in winter or prior to migration. They are thus especially good accumulators of lipophilic pollutants and are often subject to delayed mortality, since the residue may be sequestered in the fat bodies until (e.g.,during molt, migration or incubation) they are mobilized.

The avian respiratory system differs greatly from that of other vertebrates. Because of a bellows-like air sac system, the air passes across the respiratory surfaces of the lungs twice during each respiratory cycle. Furthermore, the air is probably less well filtered than in mammals. Add to this the extremely high rate of air exchange during flight, and one should not be surprised at reports of death and illness of birds associated with urban air pollution (e.g., Takemoto et al., 1974; Tashiro et al., 1974).

Very little work has been done to date on the effects of air pollutants on wild birds, but available information suggests that they may be good monitors of both gaseous and particulate pollution (see Lewis et al., 1978; Takemoto et al., 1974; Tashiro et al., 1974, Takemoto, 1972; Neal and Olstrum, 1971).

A number of bird species have been repeatedly used or suggested as pollution monitors in North America. Among these are the Rock Dove (Columbia livia), the Mourning Dove (Zenaidura macroura), the European Starling (Sturnus vulgaris), the Canary (Serinus canarius), and various raptorial birds, notably the Golden Eagle (Aquila chrysaetos) and Bald Eagle (Haliaeetus leucocephalus).

Mammals. Mammals vary greatly with respect to behavioral and ecological characteristics, showing the greatest extremes in size, metabolic rate, and life span among terrestrial animals.

Small mammals, especially the more abundant rodents are extremely important links in terrestrial food chains. These animals can be collected easily in many parts of the world, although local distributions tend to be neurotic and populations may fluctuate widely from year to year. Many species of mid and high latitudes hibernate and are only seasonally available. Many are fossorial and thus may have limited exposure to many pollutants.

There is undoubtedly wide species variation among small mammals in susceptibility to pollutants. In the main, however, adults of the small rodent species that are most amenable to study (e.g. Peromyscus, Microtus, Rattus) appear to be highly resistant to direct acute and sub-acute challenge by most of the more common pollutants. The abundant and widely distributed White-footed deermouse, Peromyscus, appears to be practically unaffected by normal or even heavy applications of various pesticides (Robel et al., 1972). This species can tolerate ten times as much dietary DDT as the laboratory mouse (Cordes, 1971).

Snyder (1963) reported, however, a significant reduction in the number of litters produced by meadow voles (Microtus pennsylvanicus) two months following application of endrin to bluegrass meadows at the rate of o.6 to 2.o pounds per acre.

The potential use of small mammals as air pollution monitors has been given very little attention, although they are frequently the subject of baseline assessments. Elevated body concentrations of lead have been demonstrated in small mammals along major highways. Yamaoka et al. (1973) reported a number of increases in organ weights (e.g., lungs, kidneys, adrenal glands, and spleen) of experimental rats after 3o to 1oo days of exposure to urban air (relative to controls).

Medium-sized mammals, such as rabbits and hares, include recreationally valuable species as well as many fur bearers. These mammals are taxonomically and ecologically diverse. Many are nocturnal or secretive and difficult to collect in adequate numbers for quantitiative monitoring, though a few such as raccoons and hares because of special habits, unusual sensitivities and reasonable abundance might prove to be valuable monitors.

Most of the large mammals, those ranging in size from sheep to elephant, are economically, recreationally or aesthetically important to man. These animals may have large home ranges and move long distances daily, seasonally, or annually. Whereas large mammals do not lend themselves to local or narrowly delimited studies, some may prove to be effective monitoring of regional or subcontinental dispersion of environmental contaminants.

USE OF SPECIMEN BANKS FOR RETROSPECITVE MONITORING OF ENVIRONMENTAL POLLUTANTS

FEASIBILITY

Methods for collection, preservation and storage of vertebrate materials are well established and do not pose insurmountable problems. Thus, operationally specimen banking will be constrained solely by available resources, analytical methods, the choice of taxa and field sampling designs. Evaluations will be limited by the actual taxa selected, their relationships with other environmental components sampled, and environmental variables that tend to confound either analysis or the transport and fate of the pollutants of concern. Ultimately, feasibility will be tested by actual contributions of the system to environmental decision making.

Pollutants are widely dispersed through and by all environmental media - biotic as well as abiotic. We cannot catalogue all of these pathways and the transformations and effects that occur but must do so selectively both with respect to environmental components studied and the temporospatial scales employed. Specimen banking is an option that allows some choices in these regards that would not be otherwise possible. Its special value is in allowing us to compare the present and past, to predict the future and as importantly, to validate past methods and predictions and thereby to improve predictive ability.

In short, retrospective monitoring of terrestrial vertebrates via a specimen banking system is technically feasible. Benefits to man, however, will depend upon establishing appropriate operational goals and tailoring the system to these goals.

Environmental monitoring and assessment or prediction of trends and hazards requires a basic understanding of the systems that are monitored. This is especially true where the activity is one of monitoring only. Evaluation of the transport, fate and effects of pollutants based on monitoring alone invariably exhibits descontinuities and inconsistencies with established wisdom and with experimental results. It is essential to determine which of these are artifacts and which represent true environmental change.

A great deal is known about the biology of birds and mammals generally; this offers an opportunity to "measure" monitoring results against a wealth of physiological, biochemical, behavioral and ecological knowledge. Thus, our abilities to propose and then test plausible explanations or to make predictions may be greater than with many other ecosystem components.

Effective deployment and use of specimen banks required effective and credible field sampling rationales. This must rank equally with the accuracy of chemical analysis. Defensible sampling will be relatively costly and will require careful planning and execution. Otherwise there will be very little need for a specimen bank and the public's money and the time of talented scientists and decision-makers wasted.

If analytic precision is high (but no necessarily accurate) and a valid sampling design is employed, trend data will have credibility and will be useful. But if both analytic precision and accuracy are high, and sampling has not been carefully designed to meet system needs, the data will be essentially worthless and ultimately recognized as such! Sampling design is subsequently discussed.

Environmental systems are rarely stable and typically exhibit a high degree of random and non-random variability that will not only condition the design of any applied system of retrospective analysis, but will set limits on design, resolution and utility.

Numerous factors in addition to chemical species may influence the net uptake, tissue distribution and toxicity of chemical pollutants. Effects of such factors may be expected to vary seasonally, with life stage, geographically and often as a function of other conditions that will confound interpretation of chemical data alone. This may be further compounded by

adaptation and the development of resistance, including altered pollutant kinetics. Examples abound. Thus, selenium concentration in terrestrial vertebrates is site- and taxon-dependent and is also a function
of the available chemical form. For example, organically bound selenium is much more readily stored in sheep than is inorganic selenium.
Route of entry and size of individual doses also influence retention
as do a larger number of other environmental factors, including several
nutritional variables, most notably protein content of food (e.g.,
Cooper and Glover, 1974). Finley and Dieter (1978) and White and Dieter
(1978) provide further interesting examples.

DESIRABILITY COMPARED TO OTHER MONITORING OR DATA BANKING METHODS

There are desirable and interactive roles for all of the systems discussed in the first section of this paper. Moreover, retrospective monitoring via use of a specimen banking system will be of value in prediction and decision making only if it is used in conjunction with alternative
methods of assessment and prediction including appropriate assessment of
impact or biological effects, simulation modeling and appropriately designed field and laboratory experiments. Rarely do field surveys alone
have standing before the law, and never in science.

At the present time, most anthropogenic changes in the environment are
either intended changes as part of an environmental resource management
system or are the result of unintended and unanticipated byproducts or
effects of a technology. The latter changes often go unnoticed unless
or until the change becomes "significant". Needless to say, this latter
category generally requires some kind of retrospective analysis if the
sources, environmental distribution, fate, and effects are to be assessed.
An effective program of ecological monitoring coupled with a specimen
banking system offers the best possibility of screening for such pollutants and for retrospective monitoring, trend sensing, extrapolation
and evaluation.
A complete, continuing system of environmental monitoring must not only
register environmental changes, but must also register and accommodate
changes in our understanding of the environment. In other words, it is
important that specimen banking not be used to narrow the focus of scientists and decision makers, but rather to broaden our capabilities and thereby improve in some measure the effective information base upon which social, environmental, political and economic decisions are made.
Multiple Use of Samples. In line with the preceding statements, it is
clearly wasteful to collect, preserve and store specimens so that their
potential use is limited to chemical analysis. The potential value of
these tissues at little additional cost is greatly enhanced by use of
methods that will allow histological or pathological evaluation, bio-
chémical evaluation,etc.
Properly used, tissue banks will permit the detection of subtle biochemical or other indices that may reflect contaminants that would otherwise
remain unsuspected; or would indicate presence of transient, acute, non-
persistent contaminants; and in some cases the biological analyses might
prove to be more sensitive than direct chemical analyses. Most importantly, histological, biochemical or other biological measures would identify or confirm the significance of tissue concentrations. Where a well-
characterized, specific, quantitative relationship between the pollutant
exposure and a biological response is known, the biological response
may serve as a better sensor than direct assay for the pollutant.

COSTS INVOLVED

Can specimen banks save us from a glut of unnecessary data and publication? Or will it act as a driving force for repeated analyses of samples? Ideally, such a system will allow us to perform the most needed analyses when both the need and the technical capability exist; it can also provide information that may help to channel research into the most useful or potentially fruitful directions.

Frankly, in our view, a specimen banking system that is to contribute significantly to decision-making will be both costly and constrained with respect to goals. Such a system will therefore be complementary to other monitoring systems and will not be limited in use only to chemical analysis.

Depending, therefore, upon the ambitiousness of the system and its focus with respect to pollutants environmental components, and regions of interest costs could range from a few million dollars per year to several tens of millions.

Major determinants of cost are:

1. geographic boundaries
2. degree of resolution desired and consequent intensity of sampling
3. temporal boundaries to include both time horizons and the temporal scale of sampling
4. legal constraints
5. the nature of the environmental components sampled.

One must clearly then, establish precise operational goals for the banking system. Then the minimum boundaries, scales and scope of work that will satisfy the goals can be established.

The costs and benefits of any monitoring and specimen banking system must be weighed against the costs and benefits of alternate systems that might be employed and the net costs of decisions that are implemented on the basis of inferences derived from the results of the system in question.

Because we are in a period of stable or declining support for environmental research and assessment, the initiation of a specimen banking system probably would result in alterations in the environmental R&D budgets of the involved governments; what types of research, assessment and monitoring programs will suffer? Also, because of the potential gains for initiators and planners of the specimen banking systems at a probably high cost to environmental scientists generally, the cost-benefit analyses should be done by highly reputable private institutions with no vested interests (i.e., not by NBS, EPA, ORNL, as in the case of the NESB). In other words, the "Duchess Law" of K.E. Boulding should be applied: "the more there is of yours, the less there is of mine" (The Duchess in "Alice in Wonderland").

Finally, we would like to remark on a few budgetary considerations:

1. The available body of pollution monitoring and specimen banking practice should be examined. With respect to terrestrial vertebrates, this should include a review of the costs and constraints of:
   a) the National Pesticides Monitoring Program;
   b) large tissue banking systems such as that of the US Naval Medical Research Institute, Bethesda, MD, and others.

2. The potential future costs resulting from growth should be examined. This should include not only maintenance costs, but all costs relating to operations and access to systems.

3. What controls may be set to monitor the effectiveness of a combined
   monitoring and banking system so that its structure (including cost
   structure) may be made to evolve in directions that maximize cost
   effectiveness?

SHORTCOMINGS AND DISADVANTAGES

The ultimate driving force behind pollutant monitoring and research is
the undesirable effects of pollutants upon man - his health, his environment, his resources. Consequently, monitoring must directly or indirectly bear upon the question of these undesirable effects. Thus, the key
question posed is: What is the potential for transfer of environmental
pollutants or effects to man or to man's resources?
Components of ecological systems interact stochastically, yet specimen
banking and monitoring require a focus upon a relatively small number of
variables. Thus, a specimen bank comprised of lyophilized specimens of a few
selected taxa from a few locations over large areas of diverse climate and
habitat can be used reliably at best to assess the amounts of the selected
pollutants at the time of collection in the actual specimens of the taxa collected. Exposure rates and doses will remain unknown as will rates of
entry of the pollutant into the tissues and the biological effects. In
short, numerous factors as well as random variables may influence the registered net uptake, tissue distribution and toxicity of chemical pollutants. Furthermore, these functions may vary complexly with time and location to such an extent that they will confound interpretation of chemical data alone, regardless of the validity and intensity of field sampling methods. That this is widely recognized among real decision makers,
including the public, is evidenced by the fact that field data alone
generally have no standing under the law. Because environmental decisions
should be conservative, however, government agencies may set temporary
policies or issue warnings based upon such data (e.g., Fimreite et al.,
197o; Mussehl and Finley, 1967) and industries have occasionally participated in voluntary bans.
Assuming that we are both wise and fortunate in our selection of environmental components for banking, and the sampling is competent and suitable for assessing the pollutants of present concern, there remains the
possibility that the specimen banking techniques employed might not be
at all suitable for anthropogenic pollutants not now widely distributed
or otherwise not presently of concern.
We will thus always be forced to make decisions in an environment of risk
and uncertainty. It is crucial that we understand the nature of these
risks and make the best possible effort, consistent with available resources, to reduce uncertainty to acceptable or manageable levels with
respect to the practical problems that we face.
Wise use of specimen banks can help us to identify, localize and determine
the extent of environmental perturbation with respect to pollutant entry
and dispersion in the environment. Monitoring alone cannot, of course, relate these changes to actual exposure rates or dose nor to effects. Only
if specimen banks are structured and used wisely in conjunction with
appropriately designed research and assessments can they contribute to
our knowledge or understanding of impacts and our ability to establish
the sources of observed impacts or conversely the impacts, if any, of
observed pollutant burdens.

CHOICE OF TAXA AND METHODS

CRITERIA FOR SELECTION OF TAXA FOR SPECIMEN BANKING

The few taxa selected must have the highest possible potential for contribution to the goals of the monitoring system. This, of course, means that they must have a potential as sensitive, integrative monitors of environmental pollutants and be sufficiently common for the implementation of effective sampling design and for the desired scale of the program. They should have a high potential for use in prediction.

In the absence of precise program definition, it is not possible to set rigid exclusive criteria for selection of taxa. Compromises among a large set of criteria must be made.

Actual selection of taxa will depend upon the specific objectives of the banking system, what is possible, and the constraints that are acceptable or necessary in mounting such a system. We have elected at this time to discuss a rather large set of criteria. Some are not compatible with others. The terrestrial vertebrates ultimately selected will depend also upon the other taxa and environmental components that are selected for banking. We would further caution that there is a large array of existing species. The probability of selecting fairly representative, or even sufficiently sensitive species as environmental surrogates or indicators of transport and fate of diverse chemical species is low. Nevertheless, important decisions may be made on the basis of such choices. Clearly, in certain respects an effective monitoring program must be flexible, and new taxa may replace old as problems change. Even so, following careful design and a pilot period of perhaps one to three years, only changes that will clearly improve the effectiveness and credibility of the system should be permitted.

Bigler et al. (1975) summarized the minimum requirements for a wildlife monitoring system:

1. species selected for monitoring should be fairly common;
2. they should be sufficiently sensitive to be monitored;
3. baseline data on physiologic functions, reproduction, susceptibility to disease, parasite burdens, as well as pollutant concentrations of tissues should be available;
4. integration of this information with that of other monitoring systems should be possible;
5. analysis and evaluation of the combined material is desirable.

They are among requirements that we would recommend.

List of Criteria[1]

1. Moderate tolerance (i.e.,neither very high nor very low sensitivity) to one or more pollutant classes should be known or suspected.

2. There should be potential for pollutant exposure of a type that is especially enlightening regarding transport, fate or effects. For example, bioaccumulation and transport from the aquatic to the terrestrial sphere is frequently mediated by terrestrial animals that feed on fish or other aquatic organisms.
   Examples are many waterfowl and raccoons.

---

[1]These are not listed in order of importance. Weighting or criteria would depend upon program design.

3. The pharmacokinetics of one or more of the pollutant classes of concern should be well known.

   a. Taxa selected should not exhibit unusual pharmacokinetic behavior with respect to common pollutants.

4. Geographic distribution should be sufficiently broad to support effective study at the scale desired - regional, national or global.

   a. Suitable trophic, physiologic or ecologic equivalents should be available for use outside the area of common occurrence.

5. Specific habits or distributions should be considered. These may or may not be advantageous. Rock Doves and European Starlings, for example, are common in heavily industrialized settings and have thus been suggested as potential air pollution monitors. In Europe, House Martins might serve as especially sensitive pollution sentinals because of apparently low tolerance to urban air pollution (Anonymous, 1968).

   The advantages and disadvantages of resident versus migratory status should be considered on a case by case basis.

6. Food habits should be well known. While omnivory may be acceptable, widely varying habits in time or space are not usually desirable. Certain omnivorous species may actually be the best sensors of integrators of persistent, widely dispersed chemical pollutants.

7. Food web relationships and dynamics should be well understood. This is a key criterion for use as monitors of pollutants that are accumulated via food.

8. Selected taxa should be relatively long-lived. This is especially valuable in the case of accumulative poisons such as lead, cadmium and fluoride. Aside from improved potential for early warning, the possibility of "linking" body burdens to lesions or other biological effects, or to clinical signs is enhanced.

   a. Sex and age should be readily distinguishable in the field if possible.
   b. Sensitive annual cycle or life stages should be identifiable and easily collected.
      1. Early life stages are frequently sensitive to pollutants.
      2. Reproductive competence is often affected at ambient pollutant concentrations well below those that produce mortality among adults.

9. The taxa of choice should have an established information base, especially with regard to taxonomy, physiology, ecology and behavior. Knowledge of bioenergetics and metabolism is of special importance. Marked species differences in uptake, tissue distribution and toxicities will result from metabolic differences and/or receptor sites.

lo. It would be politic if some of the selected taxa were valuable to man. Thus species that are recreationally (e.g., game animals) or economically (e.g., domestic animals, fur bearers, etc.) valuable should be considered for banking.
    However, such species (other than pests) must be relatively abundant or life-sparing methods should be employed.

11. Use in other monitoring systems, such as the National Pesticides Monitoring Program.

STORAGE AND PRESERVATION

Methods of storage and preservation will depend upon the prospective analyses, and upon the mode of capture (e.g., live-trapping, shooting or snap-trapping) or of conservative sampling. Methods will also depend upon the tissues and organs of interest and upon the life stage of the specimen or the season of collection.

Nevertheless, excellent methods of preservation and long-term storage of vertebrate materials are available and well established. Principle problems relate to cost, to remoteness of sampling stations from processing facilities , the need for clean, rapid field processing and the possible end uses of the specimens.

The U.S. National Bureau of Standards, as part of the NESB, is surveying the recent literature on the problems and methods of sampling, transporting and storage of biological and environmental samples for purposes of chemical analyses. They are engaged in an ongoing program to study and evaluate methods of long-term storage that would be satisfactory for tissues and other biological materials (see Rood and Goldstein, 1977).

To get the greatest possible range of use from vertebrate materials, we recommend these options:

1. Collection of paired field samples, one to be processed in an conventional manner for future chemical analysis, the other preserved and stored for histological or other analysis.

2. Deep freeze all material for chemical analysis and prepare appropriate subsamples as needed.

ANALYTICAL METHODS

Sampling Design. The value of a monitoring system is no greater than the appropriateness and validity of the field sampling design. Only to the extent that the sample represents the set about which inferences are to be drawn are such inferences valid. And only to the extent that both statistical and biological significance can be confidently estimated, can we vouch for any chemical analytic results based upon use of a specimen banking system!

Furthermore, the problems of environmental sampling and analysis are extremely difficult in most instances and depend upon the taxa collected, the intended use of the data and numerous other factors.

The literature of vertebrate ecology is rife with information on field sampling design and analysis. Appropriate techniques are available and should be employed and the significance of constraints upon such designs should be fully understood and acknowledged. Furthermore, analytic precision that goes far beyond that which is necessary will not contribute to accuracy or credibility of results.

The high costs of intrumentation development for its own sake should not be countenanced.

Clearly, the full value of specimen banking will be realized only if statistically valid, quantitative data on body and tissue burdens and/or resultant transformation products or induced tissue or biochemical responses can be satisfactorily assayed in relation to pollution source locations and rates of introduction into the environment, and in relation to other measures of environmental quality and/or environmental pollution gradients.

Thus field sampling rationales and knowledge of life histories of the species of interest or structure of the ecological communities of interest must rank as equal in importance to chemical analytic capability.

Sampling design will depend initially upon the abundance, habits and distribution of the taxa selected, upon the geographic scale of the banking system and upon the desired degree of resolution.

As a minimum, the sampling design must take into account all of the factors that are likely to significantly affect tissue concentrations or burdens of pollutants. In most cases where reliable data are possible, features of the sampling design are likely to determine sample variance to a greater degree than will limits of analytical precision.

Sources of variance, even with a good sampling design, will be considerable. Ideally, the sample variance should be a measure of the true population variance.

As an example of problems relating to field sampling design consider the following: species-specific (indeed, population-specific) attributes will determine, quantitatively, not only the potential to accumulate specific pollutants, but will, for example, determine the precise temporal characteristics of such accumulation. Annual, seasonal and daily exposure potentials will vary with species as will accumulation potential under a given set of exposure conditions. Furthermore, some of the environmental parameters that modify uptake, transformation, and body distributions will affect different species differently. Additionally, both random and non-random variation will occur.

Design criteria must take into account such factors as the intended uses of the resultant data and the time of year and even the time of day that specimens are collected. Such factors will determine sampling time, location, frequencies and intensities.

Analytical Methods

Analytical precision and accuracy are of considerable importance, but the primary problems and limitations here lie not so much in the "state of the art", but rather in the use of available instrumentation by a diversity of analysts of varying skill. Thus a specimen bank that ultimately depends upon a variety of contractors and institutions for analysis will have a very real quality assurance and credibility problem. This is amply illustrated by Erdmann (1977) who found that of 28 laboratories no more than 5 were able to perform acceptable chemical analyses of a standard reference water.

Nevertheless (see preceding section), extreme accuracy of analysis is probably wasted for the most part because of problems of field sampling design and the stochastic behavior of natural systems and their component parts, both biotic and abiotic.

Quality Assurance

Inaccuracies and uncertainties in the system must be determined and specific in order to encourage improved technique, necessary research, and the development of complementary research and monitoring. We must also note that in most cases we will always live with substantial uncertainty. We won't be completely certain about the past and we can be assured of even less certainty with respect predicting to the future.

We must continually strive to monitor and improve the reliability and accuracy of the methods employed.

RESEARCH NEEDS

Following establishment of operating objectives of a specimen banking system and the approximate budgetary constraints, design and implementation of such a program is possible on the basis of present knowledge.

Further research should be directed primarily towared improved utility of the results of retrospective analyses and the improvement of methods of forecasting pollutant transport, transformation, effects and potential environmental irreversibilities.

For example, the significance that can be attached to tissue, organ or organism concentration or 'burdens is confounded by many factors. In each differently. Thus, extensive basic information is needed on the factors - both internal and environmental - that alter rates of uptake, retention and tranformation of chemical pollutants.

The screening and evaluation of new, potentially toxic chemicals should include studies of physiological and ecological persistence. Standard or reference measures of persistence are sorely needed, both at the level of the individual organism and at the ecosystem level. Model species and model ecosystems should be established in order to make early work on persistence manageable.

Knowledge of transport, fate and accumulation or biomagnification and the processes that control them are of great importance to the potential utility of a specimen banking and pollution monitoring system.

Also desirable are more information and improved understanding of terrestrial food web dynamics of persistent and accumulative pollutants. We are particularly in need of quantitative data on rates and routes of transfer and uptake, biological availability, food conversion efficiencies, retention times, trophic relationships, and factors that alter food web dynamics.

Greater knowledge of life histories and phenological stages of the component members of food webs are also needed, if the pollutant functions are to be understood. To make predictions based upon monitoring data, we need to identifiy the points of entry of pollutants into food webs, the chemical species and physical states upon entry, the specific pathways through the system of interest, transformations that occur, and assimilation and turnover rates at each point throughout the web (see also Reichle et al., 197o).

The pharmacokinetics of most anthropogenic pollutants remain unstudied in non-human vertebrates. Exceptions include certain of the more commonly employed organochlorine pesticides such as DDT and dieldrin (Kenaga, 1972). In order to make class predictions about the interaction of pollutants, pharmacokinetic studies should be conducted in both field and laboratory for several class compounds of interest in a wide variety of taxa. Both sensitive and resistant species should be included for comparative purposes.

Much better knowledge of metabolic pathways, including routes of uptake and excretion, is required.

Dose-response data are needed for key species and pollutants of concern. In particular, data are needed on differences due to route of entry or chemical or physical states of the pollutants. Data are especially needed on the relationships between exposure history and response.

Coupled with the above, is the need to develop more reliable and sensitive methods to discriminate early functional, subclinical, or prepathological changes.

Research is needed on pollutant traces, transformation products and subtle effects. Appropriate research can thereby enhance precision, accuracy and significance of monitoring in some instances and improve our ability to sense early trends. Thus, the development of methods to evaluate pollutant or products presence in single cells via microchemical, autoradiographic or other means should be explored in some cases.

Even small concentrations of toxic metals, for example, can displace essential metals from active sites on or within cells.

Research on the interactions of pollutant uptake, retention and natural stress (including disease and naturally occurring pollutants) are needed. Of importance, also, is the study of the adaptation and the development of resistance at both the individual and population levels. Self-regulating or compensating mechanisms are poorly understood. As part of such studies, it is important to establish the mechanisms and limits of resiliency. If predictive assessment is to be successful, it must as a minimum, identify irreversibilities that may result from long-term chronic pollution.
Modifiers of pollutant transport, uptake, transformations and effects that are importantly in need of study include nutritional influences (especially protein-calorie and mineral nutrition), climate, modes of exposure and routes of uptake, interactions among various pollutants, effects of physiological status, age, sex and stages of development.
The mechanisms and manner of ecosystem partitioning of anthropogenic chemicals are poorly understood. At the very least we need to develop a few model systems in which these processes are sufficiently well understood for purposes of prediction.

ACKNOWLEDGEMENTS

We are indebted to Dr. Burton E. Vaughan and colleagues at Battelle-Pacific Northwest Laboratories, Richland, Washington, for contributions to certain thoughts expressed here and to Ms. Sylvia Parket and Ms.Cynthia Barber, U.S. Department of Energy, for help in information processing.

REFERENCES

Anonymous. 1968: House Martins return to London. Sci. News, 95: 569.

Assenmacher, I. 1973: The peripheral endocrine glands. Pp. 183-286 in D.S. Farner and J.R. King (Eds.) "Avian Biology", Vol. 3. Academic Press, New York.

Bazell, R.J. 1971: Lead poisoning: zoo animals may be just victims. Science, 1973: 13o-31.

Becker, D.A., and E.J. Maienthal. 1977: "Evaluation of the National Environmental Specimen Bank Survey". U.S. Env. Prot. Agency Report EPA-6oo11-77-o15. Environmental Health Effects Research Series. vi + 291 pp.

Bigler, W.J., J.H. Jenkins, P.M. Cumbie, G.L. Hoff, and E.C. Prather. 1975: Wildlife and environmental health: raccoons as indicators of zoonoses and pollutants in southeastern United States. J. Am. Vet. Med. Assoc., 167: 592-597.

Braund, D.G., L.D. Brown, J.T. Huber, N.C. Leeling, and M.J. Zabik. 1968: Placental transfer of dieldrin in dairy heifers contaminated during three stages of gestation. J. Dairy Sci., 51: 116-118.

Buckley, J.P. 1972: Physiological effects of environmental stimuli. J. Pharm. Sci., 61: 1175-1187.

388

Cooke, A.S. 197o: The effect of pp'-DDT on tadpoles of the common frog (Rana temporaria). Environ. Poll. 1: 57-71.

Cooke, A.S. 1971: Selective predation by newts on frog tadpoles treated with DDT. Nature (Lond.), 229: 275-76.

Cooke, A.S. 1972: The effects of DDT, dieldrin and 2,4-D on amphibian spawn and tadpoles. Environ. Poll. 3: 41-68.

Cooke, A.S. 1973a: The effects of DDT, when used as a mosquito larvicide, on tadpoles of the frog Rana temporaria. Environ. Poll., 5: 259-273.

Cooke, A.S. 1973b: Response of Rana temporaria tadpoles to chronic doses of pp'-DDT. Copeia, 1973: 647-52.

Cooper, W.C., and J.R. Glover, Jr. 1974: The toxicology of selenium and its compounds. R.A. Zingaro and W.C. Cooper (Eds.), Van Nostrand Reinhold Co., New York. pp 654-674 in "Selenium".

Cordes, C.L. 1971: Comparative study of the uptake, storage and loss of DDT in small mammals. Ph. D. Thesis. North Carolina State University.

Curnow, R.D., W.A. Tolin, and D.W. Lynch. 1975: Ecological and land-use relationships of toxic metals in Ohio's terrestrial vertebrate fauna. Pp. 578-594. in "Biological Implications of Metals in the Environment". Conf.-75o929, Energy Research and Development Administration.

Dieter, M.P. 1974: Plasma enzyme activities in Coturnix quail fed graded doses of DDE, polychlorinated biphenyl, malathion and mercuric chloride. Toxicol. Appl. Pharmacol., 27: 86-98.

Dorn, R.C., P.F. Phillips, J.O. Pierce II, and G.R. Chase. 1974: Cadmium, copper, lead and zinc in bovine hair in the new lead belt of Missouri. Bull. Env. Contam. Toxicol., 12: 626-32.

Dustman, E.H. 1966: Monitoring wildlife for pesticide content. Pp. 343-351 in "Scientific Aspects of Pest Control". Publ. No. 14o2, Nat. Acad. Sci.-Nat. Res. Council, Washington, D.C.

Dustman, E.H., W.E. Martin, R.G. Heath, and W.L. Reichel. 1971: Monitoring pesticides in wildlife. Pestic. Monit. J., 5: 5o-52.

Dustman, E.H., and L.F. Stickel. 1969: The occurrence and significance of pesticide residues in wild animals. Ann. N. Y. Acad. Sci., 16o: 162-172.

Erdmann, D.E. 1977: Role of reference samples in the selection of a private laboratory to analyze water samples. WRD Bulletin, Oct-Dec 1976--Jan-Mar 1977: 21-23.

Ferguson, D.E. 1963: Notes concerning the effects of heptachlor on certain poikilotherms. Copeia, 1963: 441-43.

Feriancova'-Masarova, Z., and E. Kaivodová. 1965: The influence of fluoride emissions from an aluminium factory on the qualitative and quantitative state of birds (in Russian). Biologia, 2o: 397-4o3.

Fimreite, N., R.W. Fyfe, and J.A. Keith. 197o: Mercury contamination of
Canadian prairie seed-eaters and their avian predators. Can. Field Natur.,
84: 269-276.

Finley, M.T., and M.P. Dieter. 1978: Influence of laying on lead accumulation
in bone of mallard ducks. J. Toxicol. Env. Health, 4: 123-129.

Fleet, R.R., D.R. Clark, Jr., and F.W. Plapp, Jr. 1972: Residues of DDT
and dieldrin in snakes from two Texas agro-systems. Bio Science, 22: 664-
65.

Fowle, C.D. 1972: "Effects of Phosphamidon on Forest Birds in New Bruns-
wick". Can. Wildl. Rep. Ser., 16: 1-25.

Gordus, A.A., C.C. Maher III, and G.C. Bird. 1973: Human hair as an indicator of trace metal environment exposure. Pp. 463-487 in Proc. 1st Ann.
Natl. Sci. Found. Trace Contam. Conf., Oak Ridge, Tennessee, August 8-1o,
1973.

Heath, R.G. 1969: Nationwide residues of organochlorine pesticides in
wings of mallards and black ducks. Pestic. Monit. J., 3: 115-123.

Heath, R.G., and S.A. Hill. 1974: Nationwide organochlorine and mercury
residues in wings of adult mallards and black ducks during the 1969-7o
hunting season. Pestic. Monit. J., 7: 153-164.

Herald, E.S. 1949: Effects of DDT-oil solutions upon amphibians and reptiles. Herpetologica, 5: 117-2o.

Johnson, R.E., T.C. Carver, and E.H. Dustman. 1967: Residues in fish,
wildlife and estuaries. Pestic. Monit. J., 1: 7-13.

Keith, J.O., and E.L. Flickinger. 1965: Fate and persistence of DDT in
a forest environment. U.S. Fish and Wildl. Circ. No. 226: 44-46.

Kenaga, E.E. 1972: Guidelines for environmental study of pesticides: determination of bioconcentration potential. Residue Rev., 44: 73-111.

Korschgen, L.J. 197o: Soil-food-chain-pesticide wildlife relationships in
aldrin-treated fields. J. Wildl. Manage.,34: 186-99.

Kreitzer, J.F. 1974: Residues of organochlorine pesticides, mercury,
and PCB's in Mourning Doves from eastern United States -- 197o-71.
Pestic.Monit. J., 7: 195-199.

Lewis, R.A., M.L. Morton, M.D. Kern, J.D. Chilgren, and E.M. Preston, 1978:
The effects of coal-fired power plant emissions on vertebrate animals in
southeastern Montana (a report of progress). Pp. 213-279 in "The Bio-en-
vironmental Impact of a Coal-fired Power Plant. Third Interim Report (E.
M. Preston and R.A. Lewis, eds). EPA-6oo/3-78-o21.

Lombard, L.S., and E.J. Witte. 1959: Frequency and types of tumors in
mammals and birds of the Philadelphia Zoological Garden. Cancer Res.,
9: 127-141.

McArn, G.E., M.L. Boardman, R. Munn, and S.R. Wellings. 1974: Relationships of pulmonary particulates in English Sparrows to gross air pollution. J. Wildl. Dis., 1o: 335-34o.

Martin, W.E. 1969: Residues in fish, wildlife, and estuaries. Pestic. Monit. J., 3: 1o2-114.

Martin, W.E. 1972: Mercury and lead residues in starlings-197o. Pestic. Monit. J., 6: 27-32.

Meeks, R.L. 1968: The accumulation of ^{36}Cl ring-labeled DDT in a freshwater marsh. J. Wildl. Manage., 32: 376-98.

Mussehl, T.W., and R.B. Finley, Jr. 1967: Residues of DDT in forest grouse following spruce budworm spraying. J. Wildl. Manage., 31: 27o-287.

Neal, J.E., and E.G. Olstrum. 1971: "Birdlife-An Indicator of Environmental Quality". Ext. Bull. E-7o7, Natural Resources Series Cooperative Extension Service, Michigan State University. 4 pp.

Ohi, G., H. Seki, K. Akiyama, and H. Yagyu. 1974: The pigeon, a sensor of lead pollution. Bull. Env. Contam. Toxicol., 12: 92-98.

Reichle, D.E., P.B. Dunaway, and D.J. Nelson. 197o: Turnover and concentration of radionuclides in food chains. Nucl. Saf., 11:43-55.

Robel, R.J., C.D. Stalling, M.E. Westfahl, and A.M. Kadoum. 1972: Effects of insecticides on populations of rodents in Kansas -- 1965-69. Pestic. Monit. J., 6: 115-121.

Rood, H.L., and G.M. Goldstein. 1977: "Recommendations of the EPA/NBS Workshop on the National Environment Specimen Bank". U.S. Env. Prot. Agency Report EPA-6oo/1-77-o2o. Environmental Health Effects Research Series. vii + 54 pp.

Rosene, W. Jr., P. Stewart, and V. Adomaitis. 1961: Residues of heptachlor epoxide in wild animals. Pp. 1o7-113 in Proc. 15th Annual Conf. Southeast. Assoc. Game and Fish Comm.

Selikoff, I.J., and E.C. Hammond. 1968: Community effects of non-occupational environmental asbestos exposure. Am. J. Public Health, 58: 1658.

Smith, R.D., and L.L. Glasgow. 1965: Effects of heptachlor on wildlife in Louisiana. Pp. 14o-154 in Proc. 17th Annual Conf. Southeast. Assoc. Game and Fish Comm.

Snyder, D.B. 1963: The effects of Endrin on vole (Microtus pennsylvanicus) reproduction in bluegrass neadows. Ph.D. Thesis. Ohio State University, Columbus.

Synder, R.L.,and H.L. Ratsliffe. 1969: Primary lung cancer in birds and mammals of the Philadelphia zoo. Cancer Res., 26: 514-518.

Takemoto, K. 1972: Air pollution of the lungs of dogs and birds. Pp. 19-23 in "Histopathological Studies of the Human Lung Affected by Air Pollution".

Takemoto, K., H. Katayama, K. Namie, R. Endo, and K. Tashiro. 1974: Effects of air pollution on the ornithorespiratory system, part IV. Pathology of doves lung. (in Japanese). Nip. Eiseigaku Zasshi, 29: 1o6.

Tansey, M.F., and R.P. Roth. 197o: Pigeons. A new role in air pollution. J. Air Poll. Contr. Assoc., 2o: 3o7-3o9.

Tashiro, K., K. Namie, K. Takemoto, and E. Hisazumi. 1974: Effects of air pollution on the respiratory system of animals in a zoological garden. (in Japanese). Nip. Eiseigaku Zasshi, 29: 1o7.

Van Hook, R.I., and E.E. Huber. 1976: "National Environmental Specimen Bank Survey". U.S. Env. Prot. Agency Report EPA-6oo/1-76-oo6. Environmental Health Effects Research Series. iv + 281 pp.

White, D.H., and M.P. Dieter. 1978: Effects of dietary vanadium in mallard ducks. J. Toxicol. Env. Health, 4: 43-5o.

White, D.H., and R.G. Heath. 1976: Nationwide residues of organochlorines in wings of adult mallards and black ducks. Pestic. Monit. J., 9: 176-185.

Wilson, V.J. 1972: Observations on the effect of dieldrin on wildlife during tsetse fly Glossina morsitans control operations in eastern Zambia. Arnoldia (Rhodesia), 5: 1-12.

Yamaoka, S., M. Fukuda, and M. Oka (O. Fukase). 1973: Experiments of exposing animals to urban polluted air, part I. (in Japanese). Report Osaka Municipal Inst., Hygiene, 35: 134-135.

U.S. MUSSEL WATCH PROGRAM

THE MUSSEL WATCH BIOLOGICAL MONITORING RESEARCH PROGRAM

Frank G. Lowman
U.S. Environmental Protection Agency
Environmental Research Laboratory
South Ferry Road,
Narragansett, Rhode Island
U. S. A.

Introduction

Many pollutants which are introduced into the coastal waters of the United States are present a dilutions of lo to neg 12 to lo to neg 15 and are not easily analyzed at these levels without preconcentration and removal from the water. Although chemical and physical methods of preconcentration may be used, any one method is usually not applicable to several types of pollutants and the use of these methods may introduce errors into the analyses from contaminated regents or equipment. Many marine organisms are capable of concentrating dissolved or particulate material from seawater and the ability of marine animals to significantly concentrate nomerous pollutants has been demonstrated for several groups of pollutants and marine organisms. Marine animals have been successfully used in earlier monitoring programs (Butler, 1974 and Holden, 1973). Biological characteristics useful for monitoring all types of pollutants over a large geographical range are not found in single species and usually several species or genera of animals are required. For maximum utility the sentinel organism or organisms should:

(1) be capable of concentrating pollutants from seawater in a predictable manner to levels which can be analyzed by available methods,

(2) not regulate against the uptake of the pollutant throughout the range of water concentration to be measured,

(3) have turnover rates for the pollutants commensurate with the disired integration time-length of measurement,

(4) continuously monitor the pollutants throughout the year with a defined seasonal variation in turnover rates,

(5) not significantly alter ingested pollutants to forms not attributable to the original pollutant.

Additional samples were frozen and stored at the Scripps Institution of Oceanography, University of California, for future analysis. The program was managed by the Scripps Institution of Oceanography (E.D. Goldberg) under contract to the U.S. Environmental Protection Agency. Heavy metals were analyzed at the Scripps Institution of Oceanography (E.D. Goldberg) and the Moss Landing Marine Laboratory, California (J.H. Martin), radionuclides at the Scripps Institution of Oceanography (M. Koide) and the Woods Hole Oceanographic Institution, Massachusetts (V.T. Bowen), halogenated hydrocarbons at the Bodega Head Marine Laboratory, u. of California

(R.W. Risebrough) and at the Woods Hole Oceanographic Institution (J.W. Farrington) and petroleum hydrocarbons were analyzed at the Marine Station, u. of Texas (P.L. Parker) and the Woods Hole Oceanographic Institution (J.W. Farrington). The sampling, storage and analytical procedures were defined and standardised by a guidance committee whose members were the senior scientists in charge of the analytical work. Collection, preservation, transportation and storage annual collections were made on the three major coasts of the United States (Atlantic, Gulf and Pacific) by a single investigator using a mobile laboratory. Detailed descriptions and photographic records were made at each site so that subsequent sampling could be done at the same site. In addition to the annual collection, monthly samples of m. californianus were taken at Bodega Head, California, and six samples of m. odulis at Narragansett Bay, Rhode Island to assess seasonal changes in pollutant levels.

The monthly sampling at Narragansett Bay was interrupted during the winter by a covering of ice which killed the population of mussels at the collection site. When sampling was renewed, a near-by station in deeper water was used.

The annual collections from the three major coast lines provided a total of 1o7 samples with 29 from the Pacific, 34 from the Atlantic and 26 from the Gulf Coast. Samples were normally collected from single sites although composite collections from San Francisco Bay, California (2o stations), San Pedro Harbour (5 stations), Tillamook Bay, Oregon (5 stations) and Willpa Bay, Washington (2 stations) were made on the Pacific Coast. Samples were collected only at sites where there were large populations of molluscs and the collections removed only a small part of the total number of organisms. When possible, animals 5 to 8 centimeters (cm) in lenght were taken although some of the oysters were larger. Samples were collected from a variety of substances including rock ledges, large boulders, small stones, concrete structures, fine to coarse sand, old shells, subtidal reefs and mudflats. At a few sampling stations only creosoted pilings, metal pilings or metal buoys were available as substrates. These were avoided, when possible to reduce undue contamination of the samples.

About 25 kilograms (kg) of animals were collected at each station. Samples used for heavy-metal and transuranium measurement were placed in plastic bags and those petroleum and halogenated hydrocarbon analyses in hydrocarbon-free aluminium foil. Soon after collection the entire animals were placed in a freezer. The frozen samples from four successive stations were placed into styrofoam shipping containers with dry ice (solid CO_2) and shipped to the analytical laboratories. Approximately 5 kilograms of molluscs from each station were sent to the Scripps Institution of Oceanography to be placed in walk-in freezers as the reference collection. The reference collection now exceeds 1ooo kg and is maintained in a frozen condition.

Analytical Procedures

Frozen samples were placed in freezers at the analytical laboratories until they were thawed for analysis. The shells were removed, the liquid added to the soft tissues and wet weights determination for the two subsamples. Samples for analysis of heavy metals were freeze-dried in a drying oven and the dry weights determined. Aliquotes of the dried samples were wet washed in nitric acid and analyzed for heavy metals by flame atomic absorption spectrophotometry. Six metals (cadmium, copper, lead, nickel, silver and zinc) were measured by both laboratories, in addition, the Moss Landing Laboratory analyzed Pacific Coast samples for aluminium, iron, manganese and strontium. Interlaboratory comparison done on samples from the monthly samples and on those from point Fermin, California showed that the results from both laboratories were similar although the Scripps Laboratory dried the soft tissues at 11o degrees centigrade whereas the Moss Landing group freeze-dried the samples. Radionuclides analyzed in the mollusc samples included the transuranic nuclides pu-239 plus 24o, pu-238 and am-241. In addition, the Fission product cs-137 was measured, in some monthly samples the Woods' Hole Laboratory analyzed cm-242 and cm-244 and the Scripps Laboratory measured pb-21o in samples from the Pacific Coast. The samples were divided into two fractions, soft parts and shells, and dried at 11o degrees centigrade (Scripps) and 15o degrees centigrade (Woods Hole). The dried samples were dissolved in nitric acid, subjected to radiochemical separation and counted by alpha spectrometry or beta counting. Generally good agreement of results on interlaboratory comparisons were observed. Samples for petroleum hydrocarbons analysis were digested in a mixture of 1 1 n koh in 85 percent ethanol. The lipid extracts were purified by silica-gel chromatography in which the saturated hydrocarbons were extracted by a hexane eluate and the olefins, aromatic hydrocarbons and some sulfur-containing molecules by a benzene eluate. The two fractions were analyzed by gas chromatography and gas chromatography-mass spectrometry (Farrington et al., 1976). Tissues of pooled mussle samples for halogenated hydrocarbon analysis were weighed and dissolved for liquid extraction prior to gas chromatography. The compounds p, pl due and p, pl, ddd, two of the principal degradation products of biocide ddt and the polychlorinated biphenyls "1254" were measured. Systematic differences in the amounts of ddd and dde were observed in the analyses by the Bodega Marine Laboratory and the Wood Hole Oceanographic Institute but the labs were in close agreement on the pcb 1254 analyses. The Woods Hole analyses showed about twice as much ddd and appreciably lower amounts of dde compared with the analyses by the Bodega Head Laboratory.

Program Design

The "mussel watch"program is not a monitoring program but rather is a monitoring research program. Several parameters which limit the applicability of the method have yet to be defined including: the capability of the animals to concentrate the pollutants from the water in a predictable manner; the degree to which the molluscs regulate their uptake of pollutants; the biological half-lives of the different pollutants; the effects of biological age, sexual maturity, health condition, temperature, salinity, suspended sediments, dissolved organic matter and pollutant levels on the rates of uptake and loss and the effects of individual variability and population differences. Field and laboratory investigations are under way or are being started to define these variables. In the field program the effects of seasonal changes on the amounts of pollutants contained in the animals was assessed by monthly collections at two stations. These collections have been made during the second and third year of the project but the analyses of pollutants are not complete. Individual variation in uptake of pollutants has not been defined but pending further investigations, the investigators have assumed that composite sample of 25 individuals was adequate to reduce individual variance to a satisfactory level. In those samples analyzed from the second year's collection, the levels of

pollutants were, in most instances, the same as those of the first years'
samples, within the limits of analytical error. The effects of size and age
of the individuals on accumulation and loss rates are not known. Only
those individuals within a size range of 5 to 8 cm were used. Sampling
sites were selected along the open coasts and mouths of bays to include
areas of low expected contamination and other areas of high expected
contamination. In some cases, samples were collected inside bays for comparison with samples facing the open ocean. Four species of molluscs were
collected because no single bivalve occurred throughout the U.S. coastal
zones. Species differences in ability to accumulate the pollutants were
expected, so analyses were done on sets of two species that coexisted at
their geographical range boundaries to define these differences. The
degree to which moluscs regulate the uptake of pollutants, the effects
of differences in biological condition, age, reproductive stage and
biological half-lives on relative levels of pollutants in the water and
animals are being defined by laboratory experiments. Statistical analyses
of correlations between levels of different pollutants in the molluscs
as well as the interrelationships of the amounts of pollutants with the
levels of pb-21o, aluminium, iron, manganese and strontium are underway.

Costs

Collection costs, including packaging, freezing and shipment to the analytical laboratories averaged about looo dollars per sample, administrative costs, including the publication of a bibliography on pollution in
bivalves and maintaining the frozen "tissue bank" samples averaged about
2oo dollars per sample. The analytical costs per sample were as follows:

petroleum hydrocarbons and halogenated hydrocarbons	looo dollars
artificial radionuclides	5oo dollars
heavy metals	5o dollars

thus, the total costs average about 2,8oo dollars per sample.

Results

The analyses have been, in the main, completed for the collections made
during the first year and those for the second year are in progress.
Heavy metals analyses show that significant seasonal variations did not
occur in the heavy metal contents in the mussels from Narragansett and
Bodega Bay. In the samples from the three coasts of the United States,
no sited of significantly elevated metal contents were observed in the
animals, however, the analyses showed that oysters concentrate copper,
nickel, silver and zinc to much higher levels than do the mussels but
the reverse os true for lead. Extremely high levels of ddt residues were
measured in mussels collected in the San Pedro-Los Angeles area (17 ppm
for p,pl dde and 1,2 ppm for p,pl ddd) and elevated levels were observed
in the mussels collected between San Francisco and San Diego, California
(Fig. 1). The Pacific Northwest and the Atlantic coast molluscs contained "normal" amounts of pollutant (figure 1, figure 2). Relatively
large amounts of pcb's were measured in animals from San Francisco Bay
(o.59 ppm), Rincon Point, California (o.13 ppm), Point Fermin, California (o.25 ppm), San Pedro Harbour (o.44 to 8.7 ppm) and San Diego
Harborage nine (o.36 to 1.4 ppm). On the Atlantic coast elevated amounts
to pcb's in the molluscs were observed at Narragansett Bay, Rhode Island

(928 to o.63 ppm), Boston,Massachusetts (o.64 ppm), Plymouth, Massachu-
setts (o.23 ppm), Cape Cod Canal, Massachusetts (o.22 ppm). Millstone,
Connecticut (o.32 ppm), Manhasset Neck, New York (o.84 ppm), Rerod Point,
New York (o.32 ppm), Great Gull Island, New York (o.27 ppm), Fire Island,
New York (o.24 ppm), Roackaway, New Jersey (o.58 ppm) and Saint Augustin,
Florida (o.15 ppm). The Pacific Northwest and the Southeast Atlantic
coast molluscs contained relatively small amounts of pcb, ranging from
(o.oo7 to o.o9 ppm). Petroleum hydrocarbons were measured in four out of
eighty-three samples from the Pacific and Gulf coasts of the United
States, three in the Gulf coast area of Texas (Espirity Santo Bay, Mata-
gorda Bay and Galveston Bay and one at Boundary Bay, Washington).

References

BUTLER, P.A. 1973: Residues in fish, wildlife and estuaries, pest. Monit.
Bull. 6: 238-262.

FARRINGTON, J.W., J.M. TEAL and P.L. PARKER. 1976: Petroleum hydrocarbons.
pp. 3: 34 in "Strategies for marine pollution monitoring" (ed. E.D. Goldberg) John Wiley-Interscience, N.Y., N.Y. 31o pp.

GOLDBERG, E.D., V.T. BOWEN, J.W. FARRINGTON, G. HARVEY, J.H. MARTIN,
P.L. PARKER, R.W. RISEBOURGH, W. ROBERTSON, E. SCHNERDER and R. GAMBLE.
1978: The Mussel Watch. 22 pp. in press.

HOLDEN, A.V. 1973: International cooperative study of organochlorine and
mercury residues in wildlife, 1969-1971. Pest monit. bull., 7: 37-52.

COLLECTION, STORAGE, AND ANALYSIS OF FRESHWATER FISH FOR
MONITORING ENVIRONMENTAL CONTAMINANTS

J. Larry Ludke
Columbia National Fisheries Research Laboratory
U.S. Fish and Wildlife Service
Columbia, MO. 65201
U.S.A.

Introduction

The National Pesticide Monitoring Program came into being about 1964
as a cooperative effort of the federal departments making up the membership of the Federal Committee on Pest Control. This cooperative, multi-
administered program continued until the passage of the Federal Environmental Pesticide Control Act of 1972 (Public Law 92-516) at which time
the program received legislative status under the Environmental Protection Agency.

The U.S. Fish and Wildlife Service (FWS) is responsible for the fish and
wildlife subprograms of the National Pesticide Monitoring Program. The
primary objective is to ascertain on a nation-wide basis, and independent of specific treatments, the levels and trends of selected environmental contaminants in the bodies of freshwater fish, and certain bird
species over a period of time.

There are several ambiguous terms often used to describe monitoring, therefore, we include the following definitions as they pertain to this document:

(1) National Pesticide Monitoring Program (NPMP) - A national program to
undertake monitoring activities, including but not limited to monitoring
levels of chemicals in air, soil, water, man, plants, and animals. Agencies that participate in the subprograms of the NPMP are the Environmental Protection Agency, U.S. Geological Survey, Food and Drug Administration, U.S. Department of Agriculture, and the U.S. Fish and Wildlife
Service.

(2) Trend Monitoring - The process of repetitive observation of one or more
segments or indicators of the environment according to prearranged schedules in space and time, and using comparable methodologies for environmental sensing and data collection.

(3) Investigative Surveys - Studies of varying scope and duration usually
comprising only one period of sampling and intended to focus on local
or regional contaminant problems that require more intensive effort than
can be provided via trend or ambient monitoring.

History & Background

The U.S. Fish and Wildlife Service has participated in the National Pesticide Monitoring Program since 1967. The intent and overriding purpose of

the program is to reflect ambient trends of pollutants in the freshwater fishery. Monitoring of freshwater fish has undergone progressive
change and modification. Initially fish were collected from 5o sampling
stations located in the Great Lakes and major river basins throughout
the United States. Five adult fish of each of three species were collected in the spring and again in the fall of both 1967 and 1968. The samples
were divided among three private contracting laboratories without arrangement for cross- checking shared samples. Belatedly a separate collection
of samples was made with aliquots of each sent to five different laboratories including the three involved in the major analytical projects.
The residues reported on the shared fish samples sometimes varied by
several orders of magnitude (Henderson et al., 1969) (1).

In 1969 all residue analyses were made by a single contracting laboratory,
Wisconsin Alumni Research Foundation (WARF), with selected samples shared
with a government laboratory, (Columbia National Fisheries Research Laboratory), formerly the Fish-Pesticide Research Laboratory, Columbia,
Missouri) for a cross-check on accuracy. The results of the cross-check
analyses showed reasonable agreement, but differences related to specific pesticides continued to exist. The results of the 1969 program were
reported by Henderson, et al., 1971 (2).

In 197o the number of collection stations was increased to 1oo, with a
single collection comprising three species of fish (three pooled analytical samples) made in the fall of each year. Residue analysis was replicated on each of the 3oo samples for a total of 6oo samples. Residues of
organochlorine insecticides and polychlorinated biphenyls have been determined in fish collected from 197o through 1974 and the necessary cross-
checking completed. Manuscripts for the results from 197o-71 and 1972-73
are presently undergoing review and a manuscript for 1974 trend monitoring is in preparation. Collections were suspended in 1975 when freshwater fish monitoring was undergoing an internal review and reorganiza-
tion.

In 1969 the determination of mercury residues in fish was added to the
program. A total of 145 composite samples was collected from 5o sampling
stations, while in 197o there were 393 samples representing 55 species of
fish from 1oo stations. Samples from both years were analyzed for total
mercury by Wisconsin Alumni Research Fondation. In addition, 25 selected
samples from the 197o fish collection were analyzed for total mercury
content. For confirmation of results, 4o selected homogenated from the
197o collection were sent to a government laboratory for cross-checking.
The results of this study were published by Henderson et al., in 1972 (3).

Residues of five heavy metals (mercury, lead, arsenic, selenium, and cadmium) in fish samples collected from 1oo freshwater sites from 1971
through 1973 is completed (Walsh, et al., 1977).

For economic and administrative reasons the analytical work was shifted
to the Fish and Wildlife Service's laboratory at the Denver Wildlife
Research Center in 1972. Selected phthalates were temporarily added to
the previous list of contaminants monitored,which included eleven organochlorine insecticides, four metals, and PCB's.

Sample collections were suspended for the 1975 sampling year to allow for
a technical and administrative review of fish monitoring activities. The
freshwater fish monitoring program was reviewed internally and restructured.
In 1976 sampling was resumed with new stations added to give a more exten-

sive coverage of the Great Lakes. There are now 117 sampling stations; 55 stations were sampled in 1976 and the remaining active stations will be sampled in alternate years. Analysis of samples was transferred to the Columbia National Fisheries Research Laboratory (CNFRL), in Columbia, Mo.

Sample Selection and Storage

Choice of Species
Samples for trend monitoring should be collected at predesignated times of the year and at predesignated sampling stations located along major fresh water drainage systems. Fish collected for monitoring purposes should be chosen according to the following criteria:

(1) a highly ubiquitous species representative of the most widespread geographical distribution,
(2) different, but closely related species with similar in natural history and feeding habits,
(3) ecological equivalents, but not necessarily closest in phylogenetic relationship.

Other factors to be considered include ease and cost of collection, availability, size, and sex.

Sample size

Samples should be replicated, with a minimum of three samples per collection site.For interpretive purposes some distinction according to age and/or size should be made. Fish of different size, age, etc., should be distributed equally among the sample replicates and should remain constant from year to year with regard to random representation of the population.

Enough individuals should be collected to obtain a minimum of one or two kilograms. The number of fish per sample should be no fewer than 2o, but preferably 5o to loo individuals. Weight of individuals within samples should not exceed plus or minus 25 % of the sample average weight.

Sample Collection

No chemicals may be used to collect fish samples. Samples should be collected by shocking, seining, trawling, or trapping.
The fish should be wrapped in the field with clean aluminum foil or in polyethylene bags and then frozen. Composite samples are packed in dry ice, air shipped to the laboratory and stored in a freezer until they are removed for grinding and homogenization. Collection information enclosed with each sample should include the station number, date, collector's name, brief description of the collection site, and any other pertinent information noted by the collector. When the samples are received at the analytical lab or tissue bank, a log book entry is made for each composite sample containing the following information:
(1) date received, (2) date of shipment, (3) sample and station number, (4) collector's name and affiliation, (5) date of collection, (6) method of collection, and (7) any other meaningful information.

All fish selected for composite sample should be washed off and care taken to insure that fish do not contact contaminated surfaces (plastics, printed

papers,metal, mud)prior to wrapping. Each fish is individually weighed
and measured for total length and, where possible, the age of each fish
determined or estmated. Weights should be recorded to nearest gram and total length to nearest centimeter (o.1 inch).
The fish comprising a composite sample are then double-bagged in heavy
plastic bags and quick frozen as soon as possible. Each composite sample
also must be provided with proper identification tied on the outside of the
plastic bag. Information required includes sample code, date collected,
and collector's name and address. If these procedures are not adhered to,
the chain of custody is not established and the samples would then have no
legal validity.

Sample Shipment

The composite samples from each station may be shipped in the same container. Fish should be handled and processed for shipment in such a manner as
to avoid any contamination by pesticides, metals, or chemicals such as
oil or PCB's. The sample should be delivered directly to the analytical laboratory or shipped by air. If air shipment is made, the samples from each
station may be shipped in the same container. Fish should be handled and
processed for shipment in such a manner as to avoid any contamination by
pesticides, metals or chemicals such as oil or PCB's. The sample should be
delivered directly to the analytical laboratory or shipped by air. If air
shipment is made, the laboratory should be notified prior to the expected
time of arrival at the airport nearest the laboratory. No samples should be
shipped to arrive at the designated airport later in the week than noon
Thursday unless prior arrangements have been made for special pickup by
personnel of the laboratory. Samples should be packed in styrofoam containers
with adequate dry ice to maintain the sample in a frozen condition during
transit. The styrofoam container should be packed in cardboard cartons for
additional support. All shipping containers should be labeled as to their
frozen contents and presence of dry ice. As a safety precaution in packaging fish samples, make certain that containers holding the dry ice are
not sealed completely. This will prevent a build-up of CO_2 gas pressure
and prevent possible serious explosion in transit.
Each sample is inspected (discrepancies are noted in a log book), labeled
and immediately stored in the freezer. Samples should remain in the frozen
state at all times. For homogenation, frozen fish from each composite are
band-sawed into pieces which are passed twice through a meat grinder.
The pieces are forced into the grinder with a clean wood mallet. Between
samples the band saw and disassembled grinder components are washed with
hot water or steam and rinsed with deionized water and finally distilled
acetone. Homogenized tissues should be rapidly frozen and stored in conta-
minant-free, labeled containers which are air-tight and preferably purged
with nitrogen or another appropriate inert gas or mixture.
A written request should be required to withdraw and archived sample for
analysis. The sample is logged out, the amount required for analysis is
removed and the remainde of the archived sample is logged back into storage. The weight removed and purpose of the analysis is recorded for each
sample aliquot, to provide an up-to-date record of the quantity of archived sample on hand. A working log book is maintained at the storage facility. Each working log book is filed after checking and updating a separate central file which is maintained for all archived samples.

Sample Analysis

Sample analysis will necessarily vary according to the chemical, tissue matrix and quantity, and most certainly according to "the state of the art".Accepted procedures exist for many of the halogenated hydrocarbons and metals. However, the organometalics, natural and synthetic hydrocarbons, and volatiles present special problems with respect to handling, storage, extraction, separation(s), and analysis. Analytical procedures must be developed to reliably measure many compounds of present and future interest. This fact is the overriding justification for developing an extensive tissue bank, so that contaminants of the future can be placed into some historical perspective.

The sample should be maintained in as nearly a natural state as possible since the actual digestion extraction, and analytical methods cannot always be anticipated.As new techniques of analysis develop,new or different modes of extraction and sample preparation will undoubtedly be dictated. The following scheme outlines a typical preparatory and analytical procedure presently used for many halogenated hydrocarbons.

Extraction. Extraction procedures may vary slightly from laboratory to laboratory, but adequate recovery checks and quality control measures must be employed to insure consistent, reliable, and efficient recovery of the chemical(s) in question.

Gel permeation chromatography (GPC).

Lipid materials are removed from organic residues by a column of SX-3 Biobeads (2oo/4oo mesh) which fractionate compounds on the basis of molecular size. A commercial unit (GPC Autoprep 1oo1), designed to sequentially process 23 samples, is used for GPC fractionation. Before use, the GPC column must be characterized to establish the relative elution patterns of high molecular weight components (e.g. lipids) to be discarded (or saved as required) and the residues which are collected.

Portions of the mixed "lipid" extract are transferred to a sample loop (5 ml volume)of the GPC unit. The sample is indexed on the system and successive samples are added to the unit. The system is activated after the collection flasks are placed in position.

After a series of samples have been purified by GPC, the solvent is removed from each collection flask by rotoevaporation. N-nonane (1 ml) may be added as "keeper" to prevent loss of volatile pesticides and to keep the extract from going to dryness.

Lipid analysis. An aliquot (2 ml) of the "lipid" extract, remaining after GPC loading, is transferred to an accurately weighted vial. The solvent is slowly evaporated on a hot plate and the vial is reweighed for lipid determination.

Florisil fractionation. For analysis Florisil (Fisher, 6o-1oo mesh) is stored at 135°C until columns are prepared shortly before use. The concentrated GPC eluates (in n-nonane) are diluted to 5.0 ml in the calibrated collection flasks. After mixing, 4.0 ml are transferred to a column containing 5 g Florisil. Non-polar and moderately polar residues are eluted with ca. 35 ml of 8 % diethyl ether in petroleum ether. More polar compounds (e.g. dieldrin, endrin, phthalates) are eluted with ca. 45 ml of 2o % diethyl ether in petroleum ether. Both fractions are collected in 125 ml double reservoir flasks. The volume of the 2o % fraction is reduced in the collection flask, brought to volume (5.0 ml) with isooctane and transferred to a culture tube (teflon-lined cap) for gas chromatographic analysis. The 8 % fraction is reduced to 2-3 ml and brought to volume (5.o ml) with solvent (petroleum ether or iso-octane) for transfer to a silica gel column.

Silica gel fractionation. Silica gel (Silicar CC-7, Mallinckrodt) is placed on a 4 g silica gel column. The PCB fraction (including the Arochlors, aldrin, heptachlor, HCB and 5o to 9o % of the DDE), is eluted with o.5 % benzene in hexane. Remaining residues are eluted with 4 % ethyl acetate in benzene. Bot fractions are concentrated to 1-2 ml in double reservoir flask, diluted to 5 ml with iso-octane and transferred to culture tubes for gas chromatographic analysis.

Identification and quantification of contaminant residues are based on retention times and peak magnitude (area or height) or external standard compounds. Confirmation analyses with alternate liquid phases (e.g. 4 % SE 3o + 6 % QF-1 on Gas Chrom O, 8o-1oo mesh) may be done on some of the samples. Further confirmation and/or identifications of unknown compounds are done for some samples by gas chromatography-mass spectrometry or other appropriate method(s).

Organizational Aspects

Development and standardization of methods of an international tissue bank should be coordinated by a joint international committee. The determinations for site selection, analytical methodologies, collection and handling procedures, species selection, etc., require multidisciplinary input from biometricians, analytical chemists, biologists, and toxicologists. Lead roles for the various desciplines should be shared internationally. The tissue bank should be located in conjunction with a laboratory (or laboratories) which reflect the ultimate state of the art in analytical techniques. Separate banks might be established specializing in different types of tissue matrices. Strategies regarding the decision-making processes must first be developed - e.g. What species are selected? What analytical procedures should be employed? When is a portion of an archived sample to be removed for analysis and on what justification? How will information be shared? How often will samples be collected? etc.

STATE-OF-THE-ART OF BIOLOGICAL SPECIMEN BANKING IN THE FEDERAL REPUBLIC OF GERMANY

N.-P.Luepke
Institute of Pharmacology and Toxicology
University of Muenster

F.Schmidt-Bleek
Federal Environmental Agency
Berlin

Introduction

Ever since the industrial revolution, man has been subjecting the earth's biosphere to an increasing variety of chemical insults. Some, such as naturally occuring toxic elements and compounds, are reentering the environment via industrial processes at rates much greater than their natural rates of degradation or removal from the biosphere; other hazardous pollutants are being synthesized with molecular structures never before encountered by living organisms. However in the last decade, increasing attention, has been focused on the occurence and effects of pollutants and pollutant categories in the environment. Refinements in analytical techniques have resulted in the discovery that many substances are more widely distributed than previously reported. Serious accidents which have involved exposure to acutely toxic materials have resulted in a public demand for more effective governmental control and industrial mitigation.

A list of all presently suspected environmental hazardous substances would contain thousands of chemical compounds; and industry is adding to that list new compounds every year. Up to now we are in no position to analyze environmental samples for all 50000 or so man-made chemicals and their metabolites circulating in the environment today. In order to adequately ensure the protection of human health and the environment from the often subtle effects of these materials it is necessary to perform several major activities. These include toxicological research, control technology development, regulatory guidelines and standards promulgation, and monitoring environmental materials and specimen banking. There are at least three vital services which such a biological specimen bank could render:

1. Provide up to date information on the spread of man-made chemicals in the environment, including man;
2. Allow extrapolation of concentration trends with respect to chemicals considered to present threats to man and his environment;
3. "Preserve the presence" by "fossilizing" selected environmental specimens in a repository so as to be able to analyze them for specific chemicals and histological details of urgent interest in the future originating from chemicals scavenged in past years.

These major activities are extremely important because without an effective monitoring environmental materials and specimen banking the detection of serious environmental contamination from pollutants may occur only after critical damage has been done.

Activities toward establishing a biological specimen bank

At present the number and variety of environmental chemicals are such that a sytematic and all-encompassing determination of their ecotoxic behaviour and discernible effects is all but impossible. Neither is it feasible to account for their circulation and accumulation in the environment. It seems furhtermore self-evident that the same must hold for their decomposition products and metabolites.

In order to obtain more realistic information about the threats posed to man and his environment by environmental chemicals, however, it seems logical and highly desirable to consider the systematic and repetitive collection of such environmental specimens which are known to scavenge and accumulate hazardous man-made compounds from their respective environment. Systematic and repetitive analyses over time of comparable samples will yield three most important types of information with respect to environmental chemicals already recognized or believed to be harmful:

1. Real time information as to the distribution of man-made chemicals and perhaps some of their decomposition products in the environment;
2. Trends with respect to increasing threats posed by certain environmental chemicals believed to be deleterous to the environment, incl. man;
3. The long-term preservation of aliquots of such samples which were originally analyzed for mapping out the present-day distribution of known harmful chemicals and interpreted to determine any trends which may exist. The possibility to analyze well preserved samples ("fossils of the past") when need arises in the future for the clarification of specific problems will help greatly to develop action plans as they will then be required and also to improve public policies.

Having recognized the potential importance of environmental specimen banking, the Government of the Federal Republic of Germany began developing plans for exploratory research late in 1974. An important impetus was provided by several ongoing R & D activities in the US which has originated in 1971 and German research proposals based upon these. Under the US - German environmental Agreement of 1974 detailed plans began to take shape in 1975 for a joint R & D effort. The German decision for funding 9 selected projects was reached in January 1976. In its official Report on the Environment, dated 14 July 1976, the Government of the Federal Republic of Germany has specifically stated its intention to support the preparatory work toward establishing an environmental specimen bank. The German research programme concentrates at present on the intake and metabolism of selected groups of environmental chemicals recognized to be harmful (e.g., group-fingerprint analyses with multiple apparatus linkups) and on basic research regarding sampling techniques, container materials and storage techniques. The expansion of the German research efforts is currently being considered. The German environmental specimen bank pilotprogramme is coordinated, developed and evaluated by the Federal Environmental Agency. Funds are provided by the Federal Ministry for Research and Technology through an interagency agreement. Findings from a considerable number of R & D projects from the UFOPLAN (Environmental Research Plan), administered by the Federal Environmental Agency (some 500 current projects) as well as from many pertinent R & D activities sponsored by the Federal Ministry for Research and Technology are also utilized.

Function and operation of an environmental specimen bank programme are shown in the figures 1 and 2.

Selection of specimens

The scientific and technical problems associated with development of selection criteria, biological sampling and specimen banking programmes are generally recognized as being exceedingly profound and complex.

1. Human tissues

According to the above mentioned suggestions and in regard to the selection and characterization of a "best" human sample for monitoring and banking the following summarized factors, some more obvious than others, should be

considered in attempting to meet objectives :
- sex
- age
- ethnic origin
- social and economic level
- past and acute health status (incl. available informations on children's diseases, operations, clinical chemistry etc.)
- past and acute medication (kind and frequency)
- past and acute nutritional status
- smoking habits (kind and frequency, also formerly habits)
- drinking habits (kind and frequency)
- history of employment (incl. if possible the nature and concentrations of the pollutants to which the donor has been exposed)
- past and present residential environment (incl. if possible, the nature and concentrations of the pollutants to which the donor has been exposed)
- use of cosmetics
- hair colour and skin status
- available further data.

2. No-human species

Generally it must be indicated that considerable thought must be given to establishing criteria for selection of biological specimens for biological specimen banking in aquatic and terrestrial ecosystems. Major considerations in selecting or recommending sensitive species or tissue sampling for biological specimen banking revolve around a set of broad biological problems including but not limited to the following points:
- importance to man and environment
- position in the food chain
- availability and collection costs
- distribution and abundance
- mobility and action radius
- accumulation of environmental pollutants

These factors and perhaps some further similar ecological considerations must be addressed as criteria along with the physical-chemical factors of collection methods, transportation, analysis, storage, and cost considerations.

3. Selection of recommended specimens

According to the conclusions and recommendations made during international workshops and further bilateral (EPA - UBA) symposiums, which were held 1976 in Muenster, 1977 in Weihenstephan (Munich) and also 1977 in Gaithersburg, it was pointed out the species for a specimen banking pilot programme should be selected with regards to monitoring programmes. In regard to these suggestions and regarding the environmental specimen pilotbank the following bioindicators were discussed and taken in priority (1 - 3 = grade of priority; 1 = selected and recommended for environmental specimen pilotbank) :

a) human tissues
    1 : liver, blood, fatty tissue
    2 : kidney, brain, placenta
b) aquatic ecosytem
    marine: 1 : macroalgae
            2 : Mytilus spec., Ostrea edulis, Pleuronectes
    fresh : 1 : Dreissena polymorpha, Cyprinus carpio, sludge
c) terrestrial ecosystem
    1 : wheat/soil, cow milk, Carabids, earth worm, grass culture
    2 : cabbot, carrot, moss
    3 : meat, lichen

The following considerations influenced these decisions:
The liver has to be prefered to the kidney because of the size of organ and because of its homogenity as shown by trace element distribution studies. The fatty tissue and the brain are interesting for the lipophilic compounds. Because of ethical and legal considerations the fatty tissue should be prefered. For the "Real-Time-Monitoring-Programme, there are suggested milk, whole blood, hair, skin, urine, because they are more available.
An important fact for the choice of different kinds of mussels is their worldwide availability and the extensive experiences regarding bivalves as an indicator of water quality. The carp and the buttfish can be used as a predicator for the constitution of sediments and water. This is important as long as sediments are not tested directly also. The macroalgae are interesting because of their ability to accumulate heavy metals. The sludge was chosen because it is a very important indicator for industrial and urban pollution. It was found in a German basic research study that there are no great differences in the composition of different sludges taken from various areas.
In the area of food chain, the combination wheat/soil is of the same priority as cow milk. Here it should be seen that wheat is spread all over the world as important corn and that the concurrent investigation of the soil can yield important informations. Carabids and earthworm were selected as known indicators for the quality of soils and the front soil-atmosphere.
In the area of air quality, the grass cultivation should get the first priority. For many years extensive experiences have been gained in Nordrhein-Westfalen about grass cultures as indicators for air pollution.
Because of the importance and the heterogenity of samples of human origin it was recommended to take a number of samples above average from liver, blood and fatty tissue. On the other hand the number of samples taken from sludge can be limited because of the similar composition which is nearly independent from origin.
For the portioning of samples we should consider that depending on the analytical methode to be used different amounts of sample are needed. Therefore it seem reasonable to store the total amount of sample in portions of 100g, 25g, 10g and 1g.

Technical considerations

There have been numerous studies performed in recent years directed toward the identification of suitable container materials and optimum storage conditions, but much of this work is contradictory.
According to our experiences gained so far rapid and deep freezing and storage at temperatures of at least -80 degrees centigrade seems to be superior to other methods and also quite economical. Low-temperature ashing and freeze drying (lyophilization) lead to substantial losses of material in several cases, whereas chemical preservation (e.g. addition of CH_2O) or radiation sterilization caused chemical alterations. Beside this, ferment inactivation (e.g. by adding $HClO_4$) as well as conservation of ferment activity (e.g. by protective colloids or acetone/water exchange at low temperatures) are still to be discussed.
We do not expect a generally acceptable answer to the problem of container materials. Regarding the container materials the following characteristics should be considered:
- minimum interactions between biological sample and material
- minimum interactions between biological sample and external medium.
The choice of container material is dictated by the biological specimen to be stored and the compound to be determined.
It is quite clear that very rigorous sampling protocols have to be developed

and strictly adhered to. As a good number of epidemiological studies have furthermore shown, reliable sample collection as well as chemical analysis can very likely only be achieved by well trained and permanently employed personnel. This is particularly true for animal and human tissues. We therefore foresee also the use of mobile laboratories which are also equipped to do rudimentary analyses on the spot as well as sample preparation for storage and freezing.

Conclusions and recommendations

The establishment of systems for the monitoring of the actual environmental exposure to substances which have or may have adverse effects on the environment is recommended.

The establishment of environmental specimen banks which are important in analyzing trends in exposure to previously unrecognized pollutants or pollutants for which analytical techniques may at present be inadequate is recommended.

In order to ensure the efficient and economical operation of specimen banks sample collection, storage, analysis and quality control of data should be centrally located or at least coordinated for each programme and the number of storage sites and analytical laboratories kept to a minimum.

The above activities should be harmonized internationally as much as possible. They should utilize the resources and experiences of closely related programmes which already exist, e.g. the U.S. - German Environmental Tissue Bank Programme, the U.S. Pesticide Monitoring Programme and the Mussel Watch Programme. All highly industrialized countries and increasingly developing nations too, have yet to come to grips with the complex problems of providing facts and figures for establishing ecological criteria as base lines for environmental impact assessments. This is as much true for human installations and activities already impacting upon the ecosphere as it is true for the prejudgement of the future ecological consequences of plans as yet to be implemented.

International cooperation in this endeavour is most desirable. The Government of the Federal Republic of Germany is grateful for the excellent cooperation with the United States in the development of the basic knowledge necessary to implement an environmental specimen bank. The Government of the Federal Republic of Germany would welcome any additional constructive international cooperation.

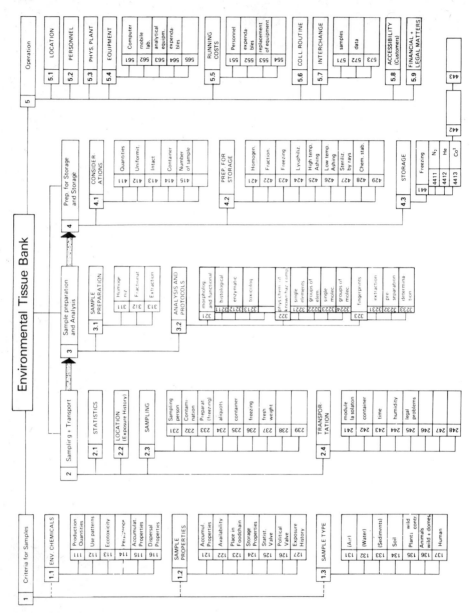

Fig. 1

Environmental Specimen Bank
Function and Operation

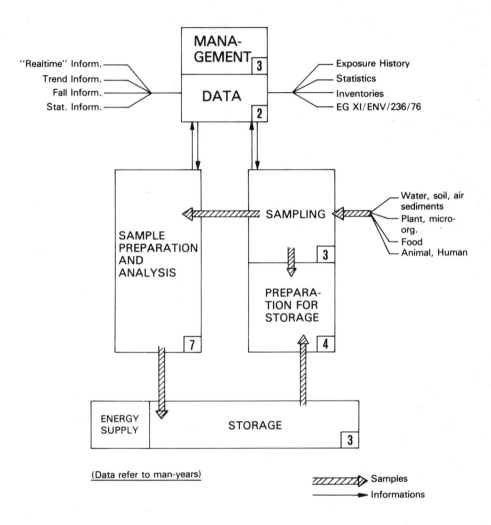

Fig. 2

ECOLOGICAL ACTION OF MERCURY BY-PRODUCTS ON DIFFERENT ANIMAL
TISSUES
KEYWORDS: MERCURY, LIVER, BLOOD, MEMBRANES

R. Marty and A. Boudou

Laboratory of Animal Ecology and Ecophysiology
Bordeaux I University
33405 - Bordeaux - Talence
France

Transfer ways from the sources of pollution to run are numerous and they
vary according to the environment and the pollutant. All living beings present, to various degrees, the property to accumulate in their tissues substances which are little or not at all biodegradable. Therefore in a contaminated ecosystem, there appears phenomena of pollution biological amplification as the different levels of trophic chain are gradually reached.

The increasing contamination of the environment by more and more unbiodegradable toxic products (heavy metals, organic components, pesticides,
additives P.C.B., biological components) requires the presence of ecotoxicological research in order to know better, in a both fundamental and practical purpose, the answer of natural ecosystems and their adaptative capacity to the different sources of pollution.

Our group of research has been working for more than 2 years for the building up of an ecotoxicological model in freshwater environment. The main
purposes we have are:
- creating a complete experimental trophic chain from the primary producers (autotroph) to the consumers of the third or fourth rank.

Clorella vulgaris → Daphnia magna → Gambusia affinis → Salmo gairdneri
                                          → Esox lucius

- using animal or vegetable species which are characteristic of the different trophic levels, frequent in natural environment, presenting a good
  genetic homogeneity and compatible with a breeding or stocking in laboratory.

- controlling as many abiotic factors as possible in order to reduce
  "parasitical variabilities" and to define with precision the experimental conditions (reproducible and comparative results).

- adding a toxic product for which the quantity determination techniques
  permit to detect,in the environment and in the organisms, very slight
  concentrations approaching those which can be found in natural systems.
  The pollutant we study: mercury by products ($HgCI_2$, CH_3HgCI) radioactives
  (Hg^{203}). One ppb in water.

- studying the sunergy effects, positive or negative, among the only or the different pollutants tested and the abiotic factors (for instance temperature: 1o⁰, 18⁰, and 26ºC.

- analysing, on the physiological and biochemical levels, the ecotoxicological incidences upon the terminal links.

- conceiving and designing, later, a complexification of these models.

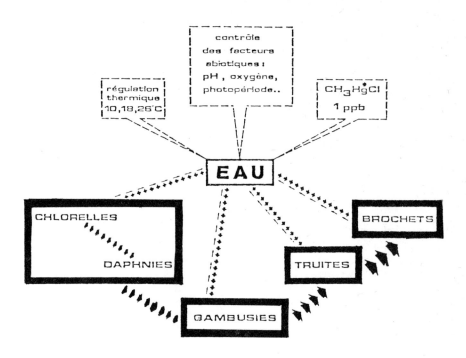

Experimental trophic chain in freshwater environment

These studies have two complementary orientations:

- one, <u>fundamental</u>, relying on the notion of "Biological model" as a means to know more about the phenomena of bioaccumulation and about their ecotoxicological incidences on ecosystems and on man.

- the other, <u>applied</u>, to improve biological tests of pollution and make them clear and reproductible enough to be used in the "industrial environment - natural systems" inter relations. Our experimental models comparatively complex and of long and costly use, could be located on the second level of the analysis, after a first detection by more simple tests of bioaccumulation (one or two species taken alone for example).

In a parallel direction to a precise quantification of concentration factors of the pollutant for each link and of the effects of positive or negative synergy of the environment temperature on the different transfers,
we study the ecotoxicological incidences of contamination on the superior
trophic levels (Salma gairdneri and Esox lucius):

- investigation on the tissue repartition of mercury and of the fixation
  capacity of the studied organs (gills, brain, liver, intestine, muscle,
  serum, figured elements), according to the time factor and the temperature of the water (1o,18 and 26°C).
  As an example:

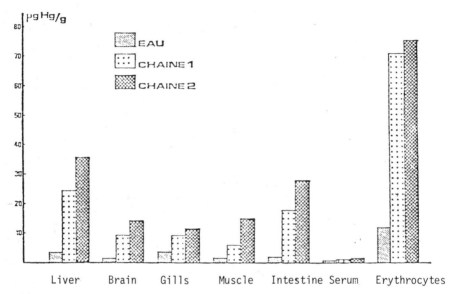

Repartition of mercury in the different organs of Salmo gairdneri

18°C - 3o days.

Chain 1: controlled food.

Chain 2: the eat as much as they want.

- analysis, from a structural and biochemical point of view, of the consequences of intoxication on trout liver and blood parametres.

1 - ACTION OF THE MERCURY BY-PRODUCTS ON TROUT LIVER: SALMO gairdneri
----

1.1 - Intoxication condition

The "third-rank consumer" link is intoxicated during 3o days thanks little combined action of the environment (1 ppb of CH_3HgCI in water) and
of the experimental trophic chain.

As an example, mercury elements found in liver are:

10,6 $\pm$ 2,1 µg Hg/g fresh weight ⟶ Chaine 10°C - 30 days

26,8 $\pm$ 5,6 µg Hg/g fresh weight ⟶ Chaine 18°C - 30 days

1.2 - Results

1.2.1 - Histopathology in optical microscopy

Liver fragments taken on prealably anaesthetized subjects (MS 222) are fixed during 24 hours in BOUIN. After including in paraffin, 5 µ sections are coloured either with hematocine-eosine or with PAS in order to identify vacuolar reserves. Comparation examination of the histologic sections of reference fish and intoxicated ones permits to set forth the structural modifications induced by the intratissular accumulation of mercury and by the more or less important increase of environment temperature (cellular homogeneity, state of cytoplasmic reserves vacuoles - glycogenes ...).
The general cellular architecture is preserved. The main fact of the methyl-mercury action is the appearance of intracellular vacuoles. Intoxication by methyl-mercury at 10°C histologically evokes the action of temperature at 26°C.
There is also a tendancy to make bile "thrombi" similar to what is observed in human retentional bile cirrhosis.
Intoxication by methyl-mercury frequently gives a turgescence of the hepatocytes evoking human hepatic steatose.

1.2.2 - Histopathology in electronic microscopy

Fixation of liver fragments taken "in vivo" on anaesthetized trout is made in buffer modified KARNOVSKY type fixer (glutaraldehyde + formaldehyde). The addition in the buffer of calcium salts permits to improve the quality of the fixer by avoiding a dilatation of cellular structures (Chondriome reticulum) and the "wash out" of glycogene.

Trout hepatocytes in relation with its major metabolic part in the organism presents a great interest as a "target organ" of mercury contamination at middle term.

1.2.3 - Enzymatic quantity determination

The quantitation study of tissular enzymes is a good indication of more or less important alterations in intracellular metabolic different ways. On each fish, a liver fragment is taken "in vivo" after anaesthesia and stocked in a buffer at +4°C. Then the fragment is ground and centrifugalized in order to isolate what is on top and which enzymatic quantity determination will be performed.

Studies enzymes:

- lactic dehydrogenase (LDH)
- malic dehydrogenase (MDH
- glutamic-oxaloacetic transaminase (GOT)
- glutamic-pyruvic transaminase (GPT).

These quantity determinations are based on a spectrophotometric method

which quantifies, at the end of the reaction, the oxydation of nicotinami-
de on hepatic functioning.
Moreover, the quantity of these enzymes is determined in blood in order
to detect a possible enzymatic "leak" (hepatic or renal level for instance).

2 - ACTION OF MERCURY BY-PRODUCTS ON BLOOD PARAMETERS

2.1 - Blood proteins

Qualitative and quantitative variations of circulating proteins present
a great interest in toxicology.
Their quantity determination is performed on blood samply (after centri-
fugation of blood taken on heparine by intracardiac puncture) by means
of a specific colorimetric reaction (GORNALD reagent). The average quantity
dose in trout blood (1o°C) is 35 $\pm$ 5,7 mg/liter
Among the different techniques of separating circulating proteins, electrophoresis in polyacrylamid gel is now the best one. We use the "disk
electrophoresis technique" of ORNSTEIN and DAVIES, adapted to the particularities of fish blood; it permits from blood microsamples (1o μl), to
obtain an electroproteinogramme presenting 23 fractions which are per-
fectly separated.

2.2 - Circulating enzymes

3 - ACTION OF MERCURY BY-PRODUCTS ON CELLULAR MEMBRANES

These studies, we just begin with, are carried on with the collaboration
of le Paul Pascal Research Center (C.N.R.S.) of Bordeaux.

3.1 - Blood globules

For 6 months, we have been studying thanks a new experimental protocol
we have achieved the impact of mercury by-products ($HgCI_2$ and CH_3HgCI)
on membrane fluidity and the transitions of phase observed in the course
of thermic variations.
In relation with the phospholipidic bi-layer of membranes, fluidity is
studied thanks to biophysical techniques such as electronic para-magnetic
resonance (RPE) with SPIN markers (stearic acids), nuclear magnetic
resonance (RMN), fluorescence, etc...
It must lead us to know better the molecular action of these toxics on the
cellular barrier.
Species we study: trout, pike, rat and man.

3.2 - Olfactive nerve of pike

Today, this biological "material" represents the best structure we have
to study axonal membranes from a biophysical and electrophysiological
point of view. This comparatively complex dissection permits to obtain
a 5 to 7 cm long nerve considering about a 2 kg heavy pike.
We study the impact of unorganic and organic forms of mercury ("in vitro"
and "in vivo") on three levels:

* ultrastructural modifications by electronic microscopy study and histo-
  autoradiography (location of 2o3 radioactive mercury). In one olfac-
  tory nerve of pike: $5.1o^6$ axons in each nerve - average diameter of

the axones : o.2 μ.

* incidences of the toxic on the electrophysiological properties of the nerve
* incidences on the membrane fluidity phenomena

Recent publications

BOUDOU,A., CAMBAR, J. et MARTY,R. (1975): - Symbioses 7(2), 111-125.

BOUDOU, A., CAMBAR, J., and coll. (1975): - Eur. J. of Toxicology 8(4), 2o1-2o4.

BOUDOU, A., DELARCHE, A., RIBEYRE, E. et MARTY, R. (1977): - Symbioses 9(1), 57-7o.

BOUDOU, A., DELARCHE, A., RIBEYRE, F., et MARTY, R. (1977): - Bull. d'Eco logie 4, 2o p.

DELARCHE, A., et RIBEYRE, F. (1978): - Chaine trophique expérimentale en milieu mimnique: recherches écotoxicologiques sur les dérivés mercuriels (bioaccumulation, synergie termpérature-toxité) - Thèse 3ème cycle (in press).

ECOLOGICAL ACTION OF MERCURY BY-PRODUCTS ON DIFFERENT ANIMAL TISSUES

(Complément)

1.- Mercury Elments in Aquatic Ecosystems

The ecosystem is a functioning unit which includes the communities of
living beings (biocenosis) and their environment (biotopy). The inter-
dependent organisms constitute a network of trophic and chorologic interactions.
In comparison with the terrestrial ecosystem, the aquatic ecosystem presents a greater homogeneity within the environment. The influence of the
terrestrial environment is more evident in the continental aquatic ecosystems than in the oceanic ecosystems. Certain particularities of the
coastal systems are strongly associated with the characteristics of the
river basins (topography, pedology, vegetation, antropic influence). The
lake represents one type of continental ecosystem which is relatively simple and well-defined, and, due to this fact, it is particularly vulnerable
to every change in the environment.
The introduction of a contaminant leads to a disorganisation, more or less
profound, of the system, but which can be compensated for by its capacity
for homeostasis. During the biogeochemical cycles the elements pass from
the abiotic environment into the organisms (absorption, retention), and
then back again (excretion, decomposition, sedimentation). The length of
the cycles depends on the number of levels participating in their transfer and on the amount of time of retention at each of these levels. In the
biosphere each element follows its own characteristic path during which
it is incorporated into the living organisms and there undergoes transformations.
Mercury, which is present in its natural state, can become dangerous for
the ecosystem when the biogeochemical cycle is modified. With the massive
use by industry and agriculture of this element and of its organometallic
combinations, the risk of pollution has been considerably increased during
the last decades.
The consequences of mercury contamination are linked to the numerous variables as concerns this pollutant, its mode of contamination and the ecosystem into which it is introduced. They are bound up with the physicochemical characteristics of the implicated element and controlled by its
atomic or molecular formation. S. Jensen and A. Jernelov (1969) have shown
the existence of a biological process of methylation. This is carried out
by the micro-organisms in the aquatic sediment starting from the mercury
ion (Hg++). The biomethylation appears as a fundamental stage in the biogeochemical cycle of mercury. In effect, starting from various organic
and inorganic forms, this biological transformation produces the form of
mercury which is the most toxic and which is the most easily accumulable
by a living thing: methylmercury.
Penetration into the organisms is affected by direct means and by indirect
or trophic means. The two means of contamination put into play the meca-
nisms of absorption and different physiological functions (respiratory,
cutaneous, digestive ...). In the course of the cycle in the organism
the pollutant may undergo metabolic transformations (biodegradation, excretion...). The biodegradability of a contaminant is closely associated
with its physico-chemical nature. Its remanence, or that of its metabolites, that is, its retentivity within the living things, is greater in

proportion to it.s capacity to contain it. The property of bioaccumulation is the result of the capacity of penetration of the pollutant into the organism and its ability to be excreted.

Samples from natural ecosystems contaminated by mercury elements have shown, in general, that the tissulary concentrations increased through-out the trophic network, from the primary producers to the final consumers. This appears to be the consequence of several processes intervening in the pyramid of biomasses: bioaccumulation at each trophic level, alimen-tary transfers, the expectation of higher forms of life in the higher species. In the literature on this subject this phenomenon is called "bio-amplification".

When mercury is introduced into the system, there is no direct ratio bet-ween the induced effects and the present concentrations in the environment. The ecotoxicological consequences of the pollutant under consideration result from the combination "dose-time of exposure". For the higher con-centrations in the environment the immediate effects of the pollutant are shown by critical toxicity at the level of the organism. On the other hand, chronic toxicity is seen in the case of prolonged exposure in the sublethal concentrations; the tissulary contents can then be very much higher than that encountered in the case of critical toxicity. The final consuming links undergo an important trophic contamination.This distinc-tion between critical and chronic toxicity assumes great importance in eco-toxicology; the effects due to the micro-doses manufested over a long pe-riod of time and which are most often the least understood.

The incidences of contamination can be shown in many ways and can be classified as

- primary effects on the species directly exposed
  (metabolic disturbances, mortality ...).

- secondary effects which are more insidious and
  difficult to discern, and which are manifested generally over a long period of time. They affect particularly the
  structure of the network of the interrelations within the
  ecosystem (Biocenotic distribution, chorologic relations ...).

The risk of contamination is not only at the level of dependence of intrin-sic characteristics of the contaminant, but also in relation to the "inte-grity" of the ecosystem. Notably, the modification of abiotic factors may have synergic or antagonistic reactions with the pollutant under conside-ration.

The bioaccumulation of the element appears as a fundamental aspect in the contamination of ecosystems. It is necessary to conceive of a methodology which allows the understanding of the process of contamination, the evalu-ation of risks, and, in the applied objective, the definition of threshold values above which the induced disturbances in the ecosystem may be con-sidered as "unacceptable".

2 - Natural and Artificial Chains

Among the different methods of approach possible in order to understand the process of contamination of ecosystems by the elements of weak bio-degradability, four are brought to light from the bibliography consulted:

- study "in site" in natural ecosystems
- use of toxicologic tests
- elaboration of microecosystems

- production of experimental trophic chains.

These methodologies are complementary since they each deal with a different level of perception.

Studies "in situ"

This widely-used method is based on the analysis of the global structure of the ecosystem, by observation and quantification of certain abiotic and biocenotic variables. The proportion produced in different organisms appropriated from the ecosystem allows us to define the state of contamination and to follow its chronological evolution. These studies also have allowed us to bring to light the process of bioaccumulation in the alimentary networks and the elevation of factors of concentration of mercury in relation to the trophic position of the species.
However, the difficulty with this approach resides in the "representativ-ness" of the system, notably by a judicious and restrained choice of stations, and in the analysis and interpretation of the data. The important number of variables and their reciprocal influences do not always allow us to define the cause and effect relationships.

Experimental models

The miniaturised ecosystems give us the advantage of diminishing the number of variables in order to more easily follow their evolution. Still they have their own dynamic which may be quite different from that seen in natural ecosystems. Also, because of the miniaturisation the state of biocenotic equilibrium is difficult to or may never be attained; the reproducibility of such models is affected. In addition, the difficulty in mastering the productivity makes it practically impossible to introduce carnivorous species of the second order.
The experimental trophic chains are based on the simplification of the trophic networks described in the natural ecosystems. They are made up of several successive trophic levels. They may designate short chains of two links as well as long chains comprised of a primary producer and consumers of various orders. The ties which unite the different links are uniquely trophic, the transfer of matter completed only in the direction from the primary producer to the final consumer.
Nonetheless the use of alimentary chains does not allow us to foresee the biocenotic changes induced by a contamination in the natural ecosystem, notably the secondary effects since they do not take into account the chorologic relations. These models should be envisaged as a preliminary approach to more complex experimental systems. On the other hand, they do permit us to quantify precisely the bioamplification in relation to the previously defined variables. Owing to their simplicity, the incidences of the abiotic factors and the participation of methods of direct and trophic contamination can be easily discerned.

3 - The "tuning" of an experimental chain in order to study the bioaccumulation and the bioamplification of methylmercury

---

The study of the bioaccumulation and the bioamplification of a pollutant in relation to the abiotic factors being the objective of our work, we will define the fundamental points which permit the use of an experimental model. The directives which we have retained concern the structure of the chain,

the nature of the pollutant, the modalities of the contamination and the
incidences of an abiotic factor on the ecotoxicologic mechanisms.

Definition of the Structure of the Chain

The ecotoxicologic role played by the plant life within the aquatic ecosystems is most often primordial. In effect, the phytoplanctonic biomasses
are important; the one-celled algae notably possess the capacity of high
fixation (adsorption or absorption) vis-a-vis the mercury present in the
environment. The use of an autotrophic organism at the base of the alimentary
chain allows us to obtain a trophic autonomy for the entire system.

The study "in situ"of the mechanisms responsible for the bioamplification
of a contaminant in the alimentary network generally shows that the
highest concentrations are encountered in organisms of an elevated trophic level. It is imperative to have a "long" alimentary chain up to the
carnivorous level of the second or third degree.

In addition, the different species chosen to characterize each trophic level should fulfill certain specifications:

- sufficient sensitivity in order to detect physiological or biochemical
  incidences of contamination, especially at the level of the last chain.
- the production of a culture either breeding or stock-piling at the laboratory stage. Taking into account the pyramid of biomasses, the productivity of the first links should represent a nutritional contribution sufficient to assure the complete nutrition of the last links.
- homogeneous populations at one's disposal, of one genetic strain, size,
  age, sex, in order to assure the reproducibility of the obtained results.

The trophic linear chain is composed of four chains. Among the species
which fulfill the criteria defined above, we have retained:

- primary producer: Chlorella vulgaris sp.
- 1st order consumer: Daphnia magna S.
- 2nd order consumer: Gambusia affinis.
- 3rd order consumer: Salmo gairdneri R.

Modalities of Contamination

In order to estimate the direct and indirect absorption of mercury by the
organism, each consuming link will be contaminated at the same time by water and by trophic means. Few researchers clearly define the respective
parts played by each of these. "However, this information should be essential to the comprehension of the mechanisms and especially the rate of
transfer of these pollutants into the various sectors of the ecosystem"
(J.M. Bouquegneau and F. Noel-Cambot, 1977).

The contamination by direct method, at the level of each species, is produced by the introduction of methylmercury into the environment.The indirect method is brought about by the transfer of contaminated food from
the primary producing link to the final consumer.

The concentration of methylmercury in the environment (1ppb) has been chosen according to the following criteria:

> The use of sublethal concentrations for the most sensitive organisms of the chain. This concentration will be defined by the results of the tests for acute toxicity produced in each species.

> Reference to the concentrations encountered in the samples of water taken from the natural aquatic ecosystems.

> Limits of sensitivity to the detection of the pollutant in the water and in the organic matter (use of a radioactive tracer--2o3 Hg).

If one wants to bring to light the process of bioaccumulation and "to explain" the factors of concentration, it seems fundamental to us to maintain the concentration of the contaminant at a constant level during the whole length of the experiment (1o days and 3o days).

* Influence of an Abiotic Factor

Among the different abiotic factors which define aquatic environments (pH, rate of oxygen dissolution, temperature, photoperiod, physicochemical composition) the temperature factor is a determining variable. Subjected to natural cyclic variations it influences the majority of biotic and abiotic factors. Each organism, when confronted with a change in temperature, reacts according to its capacity for adaptation, shown especially by the degree of specificubiquity. The thermal incidence on bioaccumulation of mercury will be analysed in each link at three temperatures: 1o°C, 18°C and 2o°C. This range of temperatures puts the species in hypo- or hyperthermal situations.

The preliminary experiments dealing with the toxicologic characterisation of each of the links have allowed us to establish a protocol of contamination for the whole of the trophic chain.

* Level of Observation and of Quantification of Bioaccumulation

The phenomenon of bioaccumulation in relation to the means of contamination to the duration and to the temperature of the environment will be analyzed from the following points of view:

1) concentration of mercury, by the determination of factors of accumulation for each link and by the tissulary distribution of mercury at the level of the final consumer. The quantification of the transfer of the pollutant along the chain, by the measure of "entries" and holders, at each trophic level should permit us to establish the balance of mercury in the system.

2) ecotoxicologic study of the last chain, begun by the observation of incidences of mercury contamination at the biochemical (enzymatic, plasmatic and hepatic proportions, molecular characterisation of plasmatic proteins) and structural (hepatic histology) levels.

4--Program

The results obtained from the previously defined model (A. Delarche and F. Ribeyre, 1978) show the complexity of the process of bioaccumulation and bioamplification of methylmercury.They demonstrate the predominant role of one contamination by trophic means and the importance of the effects of the temperature factor.

Some later studies should allow an increase in the repetitions of this model, on the one hand for a better understanding of bioaccumulation in a natural ecosystem, and on the other for a more complex modelisation of the system in an applied objective:

The following objectives will be studied on different levels:

- structural complication of the model
- new levels of analysis
- greater mastery of the abiotic factors
- increased control.

ORGANO-HALOGENATED COMPOUNDS IN TERRESTRIAL WILDLIFE

F. Moriarty, Monks Wood Experimental Station, I.T.E.
Natural Environment Research Council
Abbots Ripton
Huntingdon, England PE17 2LS

Introduction
Past and current programmes
Reasons for interest or concern
Samples
Selection
Precautions and techniques for obtaining specimens
Special requirements for containers, preservatives and processing
Storage procedures
Analytical procedures
Programme design
Cost Estimates
Design of programme
Collection and transport of sample
Storage of samples
Analysis of samples
Data processing
Summary
References

Introduction

This paper excludes material that relates only to birds: my collea-
gue Dr.R.K. Murton will cover this aspect in his paper. He will also
discuss the organizational aspects and the ethical and legal considerations. This paper considers all of the other topics requested in the
information note of October 1977.
The feasibility and nature of any monitoring or banking programme depends on the precise nature of the questions being asked, and because
of this, combined with the very large range of compounds to be considered, and the limited number of pages, may review of the relevant factors for monitoring and specimen banking is expressed in general terms.

Past and current programmes

There are none that I am aware of. This reflects the preoccupation with
species that are important for food, sport, or that are of popular wildlife interest. The terrestrial animals that come into one of these categories have not in general been considered to be at risk.
This lack raises one immediate question: are we concerned about too
restricted a range of species? The interdependence of species is the
basis of much if not all ecology, and serious thought needs to be given
to the range of species to be studied. Herbicides for example are often
unlikely to have much direct impact on terrestrial animals, but indirectly, by altering the flora, their impact can be enormous.

Reasons for interest or concern

The organochlorine insecticides were the first group to arouse interest
as potential pollutants, and for many of them their key characteristic
is a high degree of persistence, as with some other halogenated compounds.
It is important however to distinguish between three types of persistence:
1) Persistence within an organism or in a specific part of the environment. This is conventionally measured by "half-life", which is useful but can be misleading. Both in the abiotic environment (Edwards,
   1975) and within animals (Moriarty, 1975a) residues do not decrease
   at an exponential rate- the rate of loss tends to decrease with
   time. This means that a small part is much more persistent than the
   conventional half-life indicates.
   Disappearance of a pollutant does not necessarily mean of course
   that it has been lost altogether. This brings us to the other two
   facets of persistence.
2) A molecule of pollutant may in due course be converted into other
   molecular forms. It is too simplistic to assume automatically that
   the new compounds or metabolites will necessarily be less persistent
   and less toxic than the original. Thus p,p'-DDT is commonly converted to p,p'-DDE, which is much more persistent than the parent compound.
   Studies on DDT commonly combine all DDT-residues together, which can
   confuse the issue: it is important that studies on pollutants do
   not group related compounds together. PCB's provide another example
   where it is important that closely related forms be distinguished -
   their toxicity and persistence can differ appreciably.
3) Disappearance of pollutant from one part of the environment may
   merely indicate that it has been transported to another part. On a
   global scale, calculations for rates of transfer and break-down
   are very difficult to make. Even for p,p'-DDT there are major discrepancies in our current calculations, and it is difficult to make satisfactory estimates for rates of transfer between different components of the environment (Junge, 1975, Moriarty, 1975b). McClure &
   Lagrange (1977) have recently suggested a possible cause for the discrepancies: aerosol transport may only occur over relatively short
   distances.
Fluorocarbons, and their effects on stratospheric ozone concentrations
again illustrate the difficulties of making realistic global models,
of which terrestrial animals are one part.
It is important, if we are to predict amounts within terrestrial animals, that we know both the amounts of pollutant released into the
environment, and the sites of release. Organo-halogenated compounds have
three distinct patterns of release:

1) Pesticides are released deliberately into the environment.
2) Many compounds, such as fluorocarbons and chloroform, inevitably
   find their way into the environment.
3) For many applications of PCB's release occure by negligence.

Whatever the pattern of release, we need to know the quantities involved
but it is very difficult to get accurate figures. Manufacturers are often
reluctant, unless compelled, to give such data, and indirect estimates
can often be of uncertain accuracy. Thus estimates for agricultural
uses of pesticides in England and Wales are based on surveys of pesticide usage, and assume that pesticides are applied at the rate recommended by the manufacturer (Sly, 1977).

Samples

Selection

The essential purpose of any set of samples is to detect changes, or the
lack of change, with time. So we need to know the relationships between
exposure of an organism and the amount to be found within the body. Most
studies have been made with organochlorine insecticides and, to a lesser
extent, PCB's. Many of these results have been summarised (Moriarty, 1975a),
and some important considerations emerge.
Given a constant pattern of exposure, residues tend to reach a steady-state
concentration within the organism:

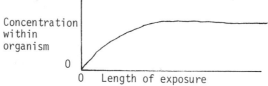

Concentration within organism — Length of exposure

It must be borne in mind that this is a gross simplification of any real
field situation. No animal is static - it is growing, maturing or senesc-
ing; its physiological condition will vary with time of day and with season; exposure may well be variable or intermittent over short periods of
time. Any or all of these inevitable changes can be expected to influence
residue levels. However, the concept of a study-state does suggest:

a) Before there has been time for a steady-state to be attained the ratio
   of pollutant within an animal to that in the abiotic environment is
   constantly increasing. In other words, the amount within the organism
   gives little indication of how much pollutant is present in its environment, although it may indicate a minimum amount that must be
   present. For species that traverse relatively large areas there is
   also the difficulty of deciding from where the residues were obtained.

b) The simple compartmental model tends to break-down when residues
   approach the toxic level. If amounts in the abiotic environment are
   sufficient to kill organisms, the main value of analysing such species for residues is to show whether they are at risk - results will
   indicate that, for that species, there is too much pollutant in the
   environment, but will not give an index of how much is present.

It follows that the time of year, and the age, sex, weight and physiological condition of a specimen can all affect the amount of residue found,
and consistency in all of those characteristics is highly desirable.
Where possible, it is also better for a single tissue or organ to be
analysed rather than a whole organism.

Precautions and techniques for obtaining specimens

Speed is of the essence if one wants to minimise the errors in estimates
of pollutants within organisms that are caught in the field.
Analytical results are commonly expressed as concentrations. Animals
that remain alive for any appreciable time after capture are likely
to mobilise much of their fat reserves, and thus may alter considerably
the distribution of many organohalogens between tissues.

It is also important to minimise post-mortem changes or loss of pollutant, which implies rapid preparation and storage in a suitable condition. Rizicka (1973) reviews the requirements for pesticides.

Special requirements for containers, preservatives and processing

Containers are commonly, and ideally, of glass with polypropylene tops. Containers should not be re-used, to avoid the risk of contamination. Solvents and reagents should also be tested for contamination.

Storage procedures

In general, the lower the temperature at which specimens are stored, the better. An alternative approach is to freeze-dry specimens, which can then be stored in air-tight dry containers at room temperatures. Freeze-drying is however, on a large scale, likely to involve a lot of time and effort. It may also sometimes have the risk that materials volatilise during the freeze-drying process.
It is highly desirable, before any monitoring programme starts, that the proposed storage procedure be tested in preliminary trials - samples of the proposed materials should be stored for different lengths of time before analysis to see whether any changes occur in the analytical result. If feasible, it is better to dissect out the appropriate tissues, grind up, and store in the extractant fluid, rather than to store the whole corpse and dissect out the appropriate tissues later. It is difficult to get accurate fresh weights for tissues from corpses that have been stored, there is always the risk of metabolism, and some organs such as the brain, do not store very well.

Analytical procedures

With such a range of compounds and organisms to consider, it is only practicable to make a few general comments.
We must accept that few techniques can be applied routinely without careful consideration, and checks should always be included in the analytical programme. These can include:
1) Addition of known amounts of the pollutant(s) to tissues - if the analysis does not detect the appropriate increase one may suspect interference from other compounds, or loss of pollutant during the extraction and clean-up process. Two main defects of this approach are:
    i)   Pollutant added to a tissue may not be in the same condition as pollutant already combined with tissue components, so added pollutant does not necessarily behave in the same way as that already present.
    ii) Consistent results from this test do not necessarily imply that analyses for lower concentrations are equally reliable. This can of course be overcome provided that specimens are available with residues below the minimum level that it is wished to detect.
2) Use of two or more independent analytical techniques, if available, to confirm the identification. The word independent should be stressed. Thus use of two different columns in gas-liquid chromatography does not necessarily check that two components are not being confused: relative retention characteristics for compounds on different columns tend to be

correlated. Truly independent techniques will test whether more
than one compound is being measured at the same time.
With organochlorine pesticides for example, interference from PCB's
has been a major problem.
A common technique, where funds are available, is to use gas-chroma-
tography linked to a mass spectrometer.

3) It cannot be stressed too much that the analyses are of pivotal
importance: any long-term monitoring programme stands or falls by
the consistency of the analytical results. This implies constant
built-in checks within the laboratory that the analytical procedures
are working properly. If more than one laboratory is involved, the occasional inter-laboratory checks are also highly desirable. The "double-
blind" technique, commonly used in medical research, should be applied,
so that the analysts do not know, until after the event, the "correct"
answers for control or test samples, nor should they know when such
checks are included.

Programme design

The types of statistical tests that may be made for a monitoring scheme
will depend on the questions being asked, but in essence as always one
will need to know the magnitude of the residual errors, their type of
distribution e.g. normal and log-normal, and their constancy or otherwise. These questions can only be answered by actually doing some monitoring, so a pilot scheme is necessary before any adequate design can
be implemented.
One aim will be to minimise the residual errors, so as to maximise the
sensitivity of the statistical tests. All the comments in the section
on selection of samples (pp. 4-6) are relevant here. In some instances
the use of "physiological time" may be more appropriate than "absolute
time". For example, the time of year at which the various phases of the
cycle of seasons occur differs from year to year. If, say, adult specimens of a species of grasshopper were to be sampled each year, it might
be better to collect specimens that have reached a certain degree of
sexual maturity rather than to collect them on the same day each year.

Some other general points should be made:

1) There should be sufficient individual animals for the sample not to
appreciably affect the population.
2) Where possible, it is likely to be advantageous for samples to be
taken from several trophic levels.
3) If samples are to be taken from a large area, it may be difficult
to find suitable species that occur throughout the area. Different
species, even if closely-related, may have quite different exposure-
residue relationships: it cannot even be assumed with complete confidence that populations of the same species from different areas
have identical responses to pollutant exposure.

In brief, all that can usefully be said at our present state of knowledge,
for terrestrial animals, is that a pilot scheme is essential before any
large-scale monitoring scheme is initiated.

Cost Estimates

It is difficult to give accurate estimates for the cost of a proposed
monitoring programme. Difficulties from inflation are conventionally
avoided by calculating current costs, and extrapolating to future costs
by use of an index of inflation. A rather more serious difficulty arises
from differences of economic philosophy. In the broadest terms, should
a proposed new additonal programme of work be considered as a marginal
cost, or bear its full share of all relevant costs? An example may make
the distinction clearer.
Let us suppose that samples from a monitoring programme are to be stored
in a deep freeze until analysed. The running costs are affected very
little by the degree of use to which it is put. If, without the monitoring programme, the deep freeze would be used at lo % of its storage
capacity for one year, whereas this monitoring programme would utilise
another 4o % of the storage capacity for one year. Then two alternative
costs for storage of samples from the proposed programme could be quoted.
If the deep freeze costs £loo per year for depreciation, interest on capital, running costs, maintenance and so forth, then storage of samples
for one year costs £loo x $\frac{4}{5}$ i.e. £8o, as a full economic cost, or virtually nothing as a marginal cost. Currently this difference of approach
is of great concern in the U.K. Universities tend to quote marginal costs
for contract research, wehreas government deparments quote full economic
costs.
It is not possible to estimate marginal costs - they are determined so
much by the particular individual circumstances. Full economic costs
will also vary -for example, the ages and seniority of staff employed
for a project will affect the salary costs - but the current costs
charged by the Institute of Terrestrial Ecology may serve as a guideline, at least for the UK.
Costs can be considered under five headings, and for each headings
costs are quoted in appropriate units of, for example, time or materials.
The total estimate of cost for any monitoring programme will of course
depend on the estimates of how many such units of time, materials, etc. will
be involved.

Design of programmes

On the assumption that sufficient preliminary information is available
to plan a monitoring programme, this will be a cost on people's time.
A senior biologist, statistician and chemist are likely to be involved,
Their cost, with overheads, is at present,
for a PSO £85/day
for an SPSO £11o/day
Allowance must be included for any money and time spent on travel to
meetings to discuss the programme.

Collection and transport of sample

This again can be costed in terms of

i)   People's time - likely to be more junior grades
ASO) £28
SO) £38   /day
HSO) £5o

SSO) £65

ii) Subsistence.

iii) Cost of transport. If private vehicles are used, the cost is
£12/1oo miles.

Storage of samples

Routinely samples are stored at about -2o°C, and the total cost will
depend principally on the amount of space occupied in cold rooms or
deep freezes, and is at present £2oo/cu metre/year.

Analysis of samples

The standard analytical method for most of these pollutants is gas-
liquid chromatography. Provided that a standard method has been developed that is suitable, with adequate sensitivity and freedom from
interference by other compounds, then the cost is £74/sample.

Data processing

The use of a small computer with terminals in £7o/day. To this should
be added the cost of the staff using the computer.

Summary

We lack detailed knowledge on which to design reliable monitoring or
specimen banking schemes for terrestrial animals (excluding perhaps
some species of birds - see paper by Dr. R.K. Murton). Any pilot
scheme will need to consider:

1) What range and types of species should be sampled.
2) What aspects of persistence we are interested in.
3) Whether pollutant levels in the environment are such that organisms
   will or will not be appreciably affected.
4) The timing and exact types of samples to be taken.
5) How to avoid artefacts from the method of capturing specimens, minimise contamination, prevent post-mortem changes, store samples, avoid
   interference from other compounds, and confirm analytical identification.
6) The nature and magnitude of sampling errors.

Some of these points pose difficult technical and research problems.
By comparison, estimates of cost appear to be relatively simple.

References

Edwards, C.A. (1975): Factors that affect the persistence of pesticides
in plants and soil. Pure & appl.Chem. 42, 39-56.

Junge, C. (1975): Transport mechanisms for pesticides in the atmosphere.
Pure & appl. Chem. 42, 95-1o4.

McClure, V.E. & Langrange, J. (1977): Deposition of heavy chlorinated hydrocarbons from the atmosphere. Bull. environ. Contam. Toxicol. 17, 219-224.

Moriarty, F. (1975a): Exposure and residues. In:'Organochlorine Insecticides: persistent organic pollutants', ed. F. Moriarty, Academic Press, Londoh, 29-72.

Moriarty, F. (1975b): The dispersal and persistence of p,p'-DDT. In: 'The ecology of resource degradation and renewal', 15th symposium Br. Ecol. Soc. 1o-12 July, 1973, 31-47, Blackwell Scientific Publication.

Ruzicka, J.H. (1973): Methods and problems in analysing for pesticide residues in the environment. In: 'Environmental pollution by pesticides', ed. C.A. Edwards, Plenum Press,11-56.

Sly, J.M.A. (1977): Changes in use of pesticides since 1945.In: 'Ecological effects of pesticides', ed. F.H. Perring & K. Mellanby. Academic Press, 1-6.

BASIC ECOLOGICAL CONCEPTS AND
URBAN ECOLOGICAL SYSTEMS

General paper, and definitions prepared for the International
Workshop on Monitoring Environmental Materials and Specimen
Banking.

Prof. Dr. rer.nat. Paul Müller
Chair for Biogeography
University of Saarbrücken, Federal Republic of Germany

Basic ecological concepts and urban ecologcial systems.

From the scientific and experimental point of view the program "Monitoring
Environmental Materials and Specimen Banking" as a whole - which means sampling, sample pretreatment, real time monitoring, analysis and banking - may
be regarded as a very difficult task. But methods for collection, preservation and storage of Environmental Materials are well established and do not
pose insurmountable problems. International and national biological monitoring programs were performed in the years 1966 to 1976. Difficulties in
selecting representative indicator organisms, regions and seasons for valid
interpretation, the necessity of including other biolgical information and
a deficit in basic ecological facts finished this projects. A representation of "Basic Ecological Concepts" implies a thorough study of autecological, synecological and ecosystemic findings and discussions with research
teams. Because of the specific problems in the workshop, however, I will
confine myself to those whose paradigmatic consideration and methodological
approach are of importance for the evaluation of landscape and urban systems.

1. Ecosystems, Burdening Capacity and Stability

A knowledge of the burdening capacity of ecosystems is a basic prerequisite
for any of planning which takes the environment into account. But the
"burdening capacity" as well as the "stability" of ecosystems can only be
defined reasonably with regard to certain relationships (Fränzle, 1978,
Müller 1977).

Just like other systems, ecosystems can be differentiated from their surroundings in that their elements are more closely related to each other
than to their environment (Abbott and Van Ness 1976). Therefore, three
parameters are of fundamental importance for the description of ecosystemic
structures:

a) linkage type of the organisms (takes into consideration the kind of
   functional relationships; ecological niche)

b) density of connections (as a measure for the webbing, takes into account the number of in- and outputs of the system's elements; food-web)

c) type of webbing (describes the ratio between the in- and outputs of an element, of a system and those outside the system).

These three parameters demonstrate at the same time that as an example bioindication using wildliving species is possible in three fields (Müller 1976, 1978):

a) chorological indication via surveys of occurrence (area system)

b) population-ecological indication by means of studying population fluctuations

c) biochemical-physiological indication through observation of the organisms' reaction, e.g. in relation to their intake of pollutants (accumulation indicators) and position within the food-web.

Since the elements of ecosystems are organisms with a history of evolution in some cases thousands of years old, it makes sense to speak of the genetic and ecological structure of an ecosystem. In hierarchical order according to their adaptation to exogenous factors, ecosystems are open systems, because they transfer matter as well as energy to their surroundings.

As with thermodynamics, the conceptual state of balance plays an important role with ecosystems. Ecosystems are characterized by internal and external states of balance. The stability of the relations between elements determines the elasticity of the system's structure (Margalef 1975). The range of stability of an ecosystem therefore can be described in terms of the number of stages in which disturbances caused by limited inputs can be compensated for without permanent structural changes. Webster, Waide and Patten (1975) therefore proposed replacing the term "stability" with "relative stability". "The argument that ecosystems are asymptotically stable focuses attention on the critical area of relative stability". Their "asymptotic stability" of an ecosystem is dependent upon the balance between all the structural elements of the system, its substance turnover and energy flow. This approach leads to an examination of the burdening capacity and elasticity of a system according to structural as well as energetic aspects. "Resistance is related to the formation and maintenance of persistent ecosystem structure. Resilience results from the tendencies inherent in ecosystems for the erosion of such structures" (cf. among others Hall and Day 1977, May 1972, 1973, 1977, Patten 1974). In ecosystems with an abundance of species, single elements generally have an greater density of connections than in ecosystems with species paucity. It follows from this that ecosystems abundant in species can have a greater internal stability. With respects to external influences, however, they can be more labile or instable than ecosystems with a dearth of species. Stable ecosystems are able to overcome transformations caused by limited inputs, while labile ones depart permanently from their original states. The quantitative expression of a load is the degree of disturbance (Fränzle 1978). This indicates the measurable amount of the disturbance. Burdening therefore is the state up to which ecosystems can still overcome transformations forced on them.

We do not consider it practical to limit the term "burdening" to anthropogenic effects, because many of the "loads" produced by man also occur
naturally. Through an ecosystemic approach, the subjective concept of
environment is replaced by a variable number of measureable parts and
factors. One special case can be observed in key-species ecosystems.
These are different in that their essential structural characteristics
are decisively impressed by one element (e.g. animal or plant species,
man). This means that the distribution of key-species ecosystems is
identical to the area systems. We understand an area system as an adaptive
subsystem of the biosphere defined by the ecological valence, genetic
variability and phylogeny of populations and the spatially and temporally
changing effect of abiotic and biotic factors, that has ecological as
well as phylogenetic functions and whose spatial dimension can be
characterized through a three-dimensional distribution area of variable
size and structure. Since all systems are closely related for example to
atmospheric happenings, the question as to how far man can change local
systems without changing global processes irreversibly (among others
Flohn 1977) is of increasing interest.

Systems whose ranges of stability are overstepped through the effects of
exogenous impacts, can no longer recover (Ellenberg 1973, Ellenberg,
Fränzle and Müller 1978). A system's ability to regenerate is decisively
dependent upon the spatial effect a certain disturbance factor (e.g. pollutant; cf. Blau and Neely 1976) has on the density of connections and
the type of webbing. During the last few years experimental biogeography
was able to prove the existence of a close relationship between the size
of an area and genetic structure (Calow 1977, Lack 1976, Macarthur 1972,
Macarthur and Wilson 1971, Simberloff 1976, Wilson and Bossert 1973,
among others). Numerous studies show that the rate of extinction in a system is contingent upon its size (Simberloff 1976). These findings led to
the establishment of a catalogue of demands with respect to sizes of protected areas (Diamond 1975). They allow the conclusion to be drawn that in
general only large areas can maintain their genetic structure rather constant over an extended period of time. The marked decrease in populations
of numerous animal and plant species in RFG can be attributed in a considerable number of cases to effects of area sizes.

2. Abiotic Factors Complexes and Ecosystem Behaviour

Ecosystemic behaviour is determined by endogenous element fluctuation and
exogenous factors. This means that I can limit myself to one section of a
system (e.g. element relations; factors behaviour) in order to describe
and control essential structural elements and energy flows. This is true.
But before I can talk about the "essential structural elements", I have
to know the system (among others Hall and Day 1977, Ellenberg, Fränzle
and Müller 1978).

Therefore, it is necessary to know more about city climate, especially
however, about radiation conditions and their interaction with living
systems and immission type (cf among others Jost 1974, Junge 1972, Lamb
1977, Lane and Katz 1977, Larson et al. 1975, Nguyen et al. 1974, Stern 1977,
Suffet 1977, Umplis 1978). Equally important is knowledge about cycles
of matter and the behaviour of chemical elements (cf. among others Meyer
1977; further references in Müller 1977). Gaseous and particulate emissions,

radioactive substances and/or noise affect humans, animals and plants living in the cities and things as well. Interacting with spatial and climatic factors, they form the immission type (Hartkamp 1975, Fortak 1977, Kellogg 1977 among others). Photochemical processes and a great number of organic carbon compounds (cf. 1972 emission register of Cologne show that in establishing limits for air pollutants according to "TA-Luft" and models of air pollution distribution (cf. among others Fortak 1977, Giebel 1977, 1978), obviously we are only working on the tip of the iceberg.

For every system, energy transfer and substance exchange are important parameters for describing and understanding its behaviour. It seems to me that a fair amount of research has been done on many special climatological problems relevant to planning (among others behaviour of resh air; local wind systems) and their relation to immission type (e.g. how long pollutants stay in the atmosphere, modification and chemical composition of precipitation). However, not enough work has been done on the relationship of these problems to the most important ecosystems via radiation belance and dose effect relations. But especially these relationships are of great importance to the stability of the system (Müller 1977).

This does not underestimate the importance of other climatological and aerological research. For it was this kind of research that proved, for example, that the pollution of systems with sulfur compounds (e.g. SO_2, SO_4) can show very different distributional patterns. Among other things such research explained the low percentage of survival in organisms exposed at places that evidenced (at least according to gas analysis) equally small concentrations of SO_2.

3. Urban Ecosystems, "Biotopes of Human Activity"

For pragmatic, methodological and historical reasons ecology as a science should only attempt to examine the interactions between living systems (organisms, man, populations, biocoenoses) and their environments, as far as they obey natural laws (for further information see Müller 1974, Müller and Mann 1978; cf. also Schmithüsen 1976). Such a statement naturally has effects on an ecological approach to work in a city. In principal there is no rational argument that would hinder an application of the term ecosystem to a city. One has to take into consideration, however that ecological work will only do justice to one particular level of information, namely the one that can be described with natural laws and not the comprehensive ecosystemic concept. Therefore, there are really at least five, in part very different approaches to ecological work:

a) a "city complex approach", which encompasses all the levels of human life and activity and attempts to describe the city as a complex system with man as the center point. The development of this conception of a system can be traced from Park (1916) to Berry and Kasarda (1977), Burkhardt and Ittelson (1978) or Chapman (1977) and can also be found in the evaluation matrix of many city simulation models (cf. e.g. Schönebeck 1975, Wilson, Rees and Leigh 1977).

b) ecopsychological approaches, which begin to see everyday life as the

434

"biotope of human activity" (Boesch 1976), in which many, but not all things can be described in terms of natural laws (Eckensberger 1977, Rapoport 1977)

c) epidemiological approaches, dealing with the health of humans in urban areas (cf. among others Ehrlich et al. 1973, Rees et al. 1977, Rosmanith et al. 1975, Schlipköter 1977), based on distributional structures for example of illnesses (cancer, chronic bronchitis, cardiovascular diseases). In spite of some positive beginnings (e.g. Heiselberg, Münster), so far these projects have failed because the analyzed groups were not sufficiently well known (for instance social and genetic structure; cf. also Cherrett and Sagar 1977, Howe 1977).

d) energy analyses of cities and sites, which attempt to make prognoses for urban systems about energy flow and burdening capacities by way of in- and output analyses, biomass distribution, productivity and examination of radiation conditions (among others Döllekes 1977, Duvigneaud 1974, König 1977, Niehaus 1977, Voss 1977)

e) evaluation of urban ecosystems through decoding the ecological information content of the organisms living in them (summarizing literature among others in Ellenberg, Fränzle and Müller 1978, Müller 1978, Steubing et al. 1974, Sukopp et al. 1974). Besides registering all living systems in a city, bioindication (e.g. monitoring) and the analysis of food chains as pollution integrators are emphasized in regard to man. Pollutant accumulation, conversion and breakdown are also given special attention (Allen and Miller 1978, Booth and Ferrell 1977, Dougherty 1978, Khan 1977, Khan, Korte and Payne 1977, Kutz, Murphy and Strassman 1978, Matsumura 1977, Metcalf 1977, Rao 1978, among others).

I personally think that all of these approaches are important and I would not reject any one of them unless claims of preeminence were made for it at present. This is also true for cybernetical models, which certainly are only at the beginning of their development. In this connection we must not forget that "there has to be a compromise between effort expended on a model study and the envisioned possibilities for results. Such a compromise does not allow for investigating all the interesting scientific details" (Voss 1977).

At the same time we are only at the beginning of our possibilities for ecological statements. Personally I believe that the analysis of epidemiological and energetic processes, the evaluation of city systems using bioindicators and the definition of the burdening of ecosystems through food chain analyses will help us progress most at the present, because right now it is necessary for us - more than ever before - to define the limitations for our decisions and actions and to recognize the fact that we ourselves and our systems are subject to biological laws.

4. Wildliving Populations and Area Evaluation

Seasonal and daily population dynamics and densities, in many cases perennial population cycles and/or species-specific population strategies determine the presence and therefore the verifiability of populations in their habitat. Without a knowledge of these population variables in space and time

we cannot use the informational content of living systems for the evaluation of areas and area surveys yield diametrical results (Berthold 1976,
Diamond and May 1977). To put it "sensitively", the "duck" (Vester 1976,
p. 38, "The Duck Model") is not decisive: we have to know what species
of duck or ducks live in a certain system in order to be able to estimate
what is endogenously or exogenously controlled.

As an example I would like to use the present distribution in the Saar
River of the hemerochorous water snail Physa acuta, which was unintentionally introduced. This species can live under beta to polysaprobic
conditions and obviously can also take high water temperatures. This
caused problems with its classification according to the saprobic system (cf. among others Mauch 1976),but it enabled the species to colonize
the Saar and its larger tributaries. In 1977 we found Physa acuta almost
everywhere in the Saar, but there were considerable differences in its presence and population density during the course of the year, which fact can
lead to misinterpretations of the water quality.

This example of Physa poses the question of the representativity of random samples, e.g. as proof of the water quality. A survey of the 221 invertebrates of the Saar - which we easily identified - and their classification according to substrate and saprobe groups provides us with an
exact picture of the quality of the river's water. Once these relationships are known and for example the position of Physa acuta in the food
web of the Saar has been clarified, Physa can be our "indicator duck".
This requires total mobilization of effort for the task, while at the same
time the methods of the causal analysis have to do justice to the complexity of the subject. "Without a solid biological foundation regional planning,
ecological expertises, suggestions for measures of environmental protection can only be quackery:
dangerous quackery, because simple and hasty solutions are so plausible"
(Remmert 1978).

Today we know that besides the genetic structure, the biological abilities
of populations are responsible for the synamics of area systems. Knowing
the biological abilities, however, means knowing the population growth that
varies according to species, knowing the very different population regulators and knowing the population structure (age and sex ratios). It means
a sure classification according to r- or k- strategies of their life style
(Pianka 1974), knowledge about their intra- and interspecific population
behaviour and about seasonal and daily rhythms as well as about their
distribution. Populations are usually not distributed by chance, yet normally is closely correlated with the pattern of the habitat islands. Every
organism and therefore every population chooses optimal habitats in a
landscape first. Food supply, population density, territorial behaviour,
mates and pressure of enemies, among others, often result in a coloniza-
tion of even suboptimal or pessimal habitats, something that my co-worker
Dr. Hermann Ellenberg (1978) painstakingly proved for the roe deer (Capreolus capreolus) in Central European cultural landscapes.

In this regard the selection of a "best species for monitoring and banking"
is seldom a simple matter, and at least the following factors, some more
obvious than others, should be considered in attempting to meet monitoring
objectives" (Ohlendorf 1978):

a) Availability - A species must be available in numbers sufficient to provide statistically adequate sample sizes and to insure no harm to their population as a result of the repeated sampling.

b) Distribution and Abundance - If the primary interest is in monitoring residue trends on a regional basis rather than in a particular species, it is highly preferable that a candidate species occur throughout that region. When an otherwise suitable species is not available throughout an entire part of the region, it may be possible to substitute an alternate species that is closely related or ecologically similar.

c) Mobility and Action radius - The mobility of a species is a necessary consideration in determining if the species will serve to meet the objectives of a survey. One must consider the extent of daily and seasonal movements and, if a migratory species, the timing and pattern of migration.

d) Position of the species in the food chain.

e) Diet - Food habits are a primary consideration in selection of a species, since the principal route of pollutant exposure in the wild is undoubtedly through the diet. Because many persistent pollutants tend to become progressively concentrated through successive levels of food chains, a species' food habits must be representative of the segment of the environment at which the monitoring is primarily directed. Beside of the Nutritional status it must be guarantied that the animals allows deposit - fat sampling in the collection season.

f) Habitat and Home range - The habitat preference of a species is an obvious factor, for if the intent of monitoring is to evaluate residues in a wetland ecosystem, the investigator does not select an upland species.

g) Physiology - The physiology of a species must be considered with regard to its propensity to acquire and retain residues of those pollutants to be monitored.

h) Population-genetic - The importance that the interaction of population-genetic and ecological factors has for the decoding of the informational content of living systems for the evaluation of areas was elucidated by a number of recent scientific projects, at least for some of the major indicator species (synoptical treatment in Müller 1978).

i) Environmental chemicals - The species to select must be sensible against the noxious agents. The time lag from exposure to accumulation should be characteristic. Special features of accumulation and metabolization of noxious chemicals are of interest.

j) Relations to mankind - regarded as food; in respect being food consument of similar pattern as humans; in respect to toxicological model studies.

k) Feasibility of laboratory tests and/or relations to experimental animal species; Valid interpretation of monitoring residue data require studies of the dose, accumulation, effect relationships in the assigned indicator species.

5. Genetic Structure and Spatial Distribution

The intense preoccupation with present environmental problems, pollution limits and/or tests for compatability with the environment made us overlook that evolutionary processes take place at present in our cultural landscapes (and especially in our urban conglomerates), whose explanation is of the greatest importance for the evaluation of noxious substances. Of course each change in allele number already means evolution in the final analysis (Jain 1975, Lees et al. 1973, Kettlewell 1973, Maruyama 1977), but the isolation barriers and selection gradients that we built up accelerate this process. While we are watching, the "ducks" ("The Duck Model"; Vester 1976) change. It proves wrong in many cases to talk about the ecological valence of a species, because this species may be composed of many populations with different ecological valences, which were only developed as a reaction to different burdening gradients. The subjects in question here go far beyond resistance problems with staphylococci or diptera strains, as well as coincident distributions of urban conglomerates and industry-melanistic lepidoptera or coleoptera (among others Biston betularia, Adalia bipunctata). They point to questions that are partially connected with the differing bioaccumulation properties of pollutants and thus with the representativity of biological samples, as well as the validity of mutagenic, cancerogenic and teratogenic tests.

Beginning with the question why certain Coleoptera species, e.g. in Saarbrücken, are able to penetrate far into the urban area and why just the inner-city populations of these beetles prove to be more resistant in fumigation experiments, my co-worker, Dr. H. Steiniger (1978) examined the genetic structure of 7 Carabid species in different sites. Using modern electrophoretic separation methods (disc electrophoresis with polyacrylamide gels), he was able to prove a correlation between allele-polymorphism and habitat diversities with 54 Carabid populations of urban and close-to-natural habitats (especially close with Carabus violaceus, C. Problematicus, Abax parallelepipedus and Abax parallelus as well as Carabus nemoralis). But so far it was not possible to establish a causal relationship between isozyme-polymorphism and its selective advantages. It is possible that the differing reactions of "bioindicators" in various areas of our country are mostly due to genetic differences in populations, even through varying immission types and the related additive and synergistic behaviour of pollutant combinations and climate types also play a role (among others Guderian 1977, Guderian, Krauss and Kaiser 1977, Müller 1978).

6. Monitoring Programs and Residue Analyses

Genetic variability of wild populations and their daily and seasonal
population fluctuations allow conclusions to be drawn about the quality of a particular area only if a high standard of information is
achieved. Therefore, establishing effects monitoring programs with
"standardized" organisms and substrates is necessary as an additional source of information (Arndt 1974, Guderian 1977, Müller 1975,
Prinz 1975, Schönbeck and Van Haut 1974, Sorauer 1977, Steubing et
al. 1974, 1976 and others).

In theory the necessity of effects monitoring programs was recognized
early, because this technique shows the interaction of the ecologically
important factors at one site especially well (among others climate type
and immission components). For a large number of pollutants and pollutant combinations a dose-effect relation could be established and close
correlations between specific pollutants, rates of accumulation in exposed organisms and their relative toxicity (e.g. as measured by the
death rate of the exponates) were described. Most recent research also
aims for correlations between emissions and reactions of exponates
(among others Steubing et al. 1974, 1976, Rgu 1974, Scholl 1978).

Independent of which parameters of reaction are finally chosen as a
guideline (among others CO_2 gas exchange; chlorophyll a; phenology)
we can already say that effects monitoring programs with e.g. Hypogymnia physodes or Lolium multiflorum are suited for practical tasks of
area evaluation.

For the surrounding communities of Saarbrücken (Stadtverband) my co-worker, W. Erhardt was able to establish significant correlations between
air pollution and death rates of lichen thalli by means of a specific
arrangement of exposed Hypogymnia physodes. The results of the 72 exposed
series of lichens also pointed out air hygienic dangers in places where
they were not recognized before. Similarly to other exposition series,
it also showed up here that the exact definition of the lichens at the beginning of the experiments, the duration of the exposition, treatment of
the lichens and effects of the exposure site may have a strong influence
on the reactions of the exponates. The question of representativity of an
exposition site for a larger area therefore has to be established individually.

If the results of the exposition of Hypogymnia physodes for 14o days are
compared with a map of the natural lichen vegetation that was constructed
using different methods and a map of forest growth damage, one can see
direct correlations. This is also true for the results of residue analyses (Pb and Cd)of Picea abies, Picea omorica and Picea pungens, which
were disclosed by my co-worker G. Wagner.

Effects monitoring programs for the Saar with limnic organisms were attempted (Müller and Schäfer 1976). After initial difficulties due to the
choice of organisms, boxes and exposition sites, we were able to develop methods which allow a differentiation of the increase in biomass and
the physiological condition of the exposed fishes, crawfish and molluscs

as well as a correlation with the river's burdening pattern, resembling a mosaic.

Naturally death rates and pollutant accumulation can only indicate relative toxicity in regard to human populations and thus can only reflect a relative risk in certain sites (Kates 1978). But this is just as true, for instance, for all of our toxicological laboratory tests. Of course monitoring programs with exponates can only provide information about one system factor complex (e.g. relative quality of the air or water), but I think this information is more important than the 12th annual series of SO_2 measurements in an area whose climatic type and emittent behaviour I have known for a long time. In my opinion it is essential to establish the comparability of the different effects monitoring programs on a transnational scale as rapidly as possible and to come up with guidelines for their use in planning.

7. Food Chain Analyses as Indicators for the Burdening of Areas

The populations and substrates linked in food-webs are integrators for the burden of areas and ecosystems. But area-related analyses of food-webs - at least in the RFG - have not progressed beyond their early stages. It is obvious that exclusive consideration of the benzpyrene content in the air (Hettche 1975) without an account of its derivatives in the human food chain (e.g. smoked herring; cf. Grimmer 1977) leads to area evaluation for which "air" is a factor with unjustified decisiveness. This thought can easily be extended at least to recognize that all the substances we can measure have already been used as "key substances" for burdening prognoses for air and water; the obvious question about transfer of substances within food chains, however, has not even been considered.

We know that the accumulation and breakdown of pollutants in individuals, populations and food chains can be accomplished in very different ways according, for example, to species, age and sex. While there are organisms whose pollutant accumulation is correlated with the concentration of the respective pollutant in their habitat, there are others that deposit selectively e.g. heavy metals and/or protect sensitive enzyme systems binding the pollutants to proteins and thus reducing their toxicity. Consequently, if the area-specific food chains are not analyzed, residue analyses with birds (among others Baum et al. 1975, Conrad 1977, Joiris and Martens 1973, Koeman et al. 1973, Moore 1969, Prestt and Ratcliffe 1972), game animals (Brüggemann 1974, Drescher-Kaden 1976, Drescher-Kaden et al. 1978, seals (Drescher Kaden et al. 1977) or invertebrates (among others Matsumura 1977) can only show how dangerous a pollutant is for a particular species but cannot indicate the burdening of an area. Coshawks (Accipiter gentilis), which mostly live on rabbits in one area, must necessarily have different PCB-contents than those of a different area where their main prey is wood pigeons (Columba palumbus).

For short food chains continuous analyses can be carried out; for food-webs, however, they can only be done sensibly via continuous ecosystem analysis and monitoring. Such a control can encompass essential environmental chemicals (among others Bevenue 1976, Gish and Christensen 1973, Martin and Coughtrey 1975, Metcalf 1977, Müller 1978, Po-Yung et al. 1975) and radionucleids. Thus Miettimen (1976) for example examined and surveyed

the whereabouts of the plutonium isotopes $^{239,240}Pu$ and ^{238}Pu over a period of ten years in a terrestrial food chain (lichens - reindeer - man)
and an aquatic food chain (sediments - benthic invertebrate fauna -
fishes). Similar analyses were carried out by Brisbin and Smith (1975)
with American Odocoileus virginianus populations and with a soil arthropods food chain by Crossley, Duke and Waide (1975), in which cases ^{137}Cs
was the main target (cf. among others also Dahlman, Francis and Tamura
1975). The influence of potassium on the whereabouts of cesium in Rangifer
tarandus was studied by Holleman and Luick (1975) under controlled food
intake conditions.

Transfer in food webs certainly has an influence on the chemical constitution and thus on the effectiveness of some pollutants. The methylation
of mercury belongs in this category, as does the activation or the temporary inactivation of organic compounds (Wegler 1977).

Food-webs are the basic structure for energy and matter transfer in ecosystems. This is why we think that the analysis of such food-webs is the
main task we will have to work on in order to give a realistic answer to
the question about the real pollution burden and endangerment for human
populations. Especially research done in the last few years shows that it
becomes more and more difficult to integrate all the multidimensional processes, that take place, for example, just within the immission type of
a city, into a matrix for evaluating the situation for man. Improvement
of already existing "environmental compatibility tests" are being demanded
more and more plainly. But these can only be used as relative reflections
of a real risk to city life if the metabolism of this substance is analyzed in food chains of the respective system (among others Beavington 1975,
Blau and Neely 1976, Jefferies and French 1976, Lagerwerff and Specht 1970,
Williams and David 1976). Parallel to this we have to evaluate areas by
means of monitoring programs with standardized organisms, the reactions
or pollution residues of which yield information made transferable to human
populations by epidemiological examinations (among others Guderian 1977,
Guderian et al. 1977, Scholl 1978, Steubing et al. 1976).

8. Specimen banking and Terrestrial Ecosystems

The environmental specimen bank concept has to be incorporated into an ecological monitoring program, for which only those specimens can be used that
have been collected within the framework of ecosystematic complex research
in representative regions of a country by one central post (if for no
other reason than for the analytics). An ecosystem specimen bank can only
be worthwhile as far as indication of a momentary state of the environment
concerned if the samples are chosen according to the following criteria:

8.1. Samples from a comprehensive effects inventory program with organisms
standardized as much as possible, which allow a transfer to the
human food chain,

8.2. Samples from food-webs in representative ecosystems of a country
(cf. Ellenberg, Fränzle and Müller 1978),

8.3. Development of safe methods for preserving specimens,

8.4. Certified reference material is necessary for analytical work.

"Effective deployment and use of specimen banks requires effective and credible field sampling rationales. This must rank equally with the accuracy of chemical analysis".

Literature cited

Abbott, M. and Van Ness, H. (1976): Thermodynamik, Theorie und Anwendung. Mac Graw-Hill, New York.

Allen, J.R. and Miller, J.P. van (1978): Health Implications of 2,3,7,8-Tetrachlorodibenzo-p-dioxin Exposure in Primates. In: RAO, Dentachlorophenol, 371-379, Plenum Press, New York.

Arndt, U. (1974): Langfristige Immissionswirkungen an ungeschütztem Nutzholz. Staub 34: 225-227.

Atkins, E.L., L.D. Anderson, D. Kellum and K.W. Neuman (1976): Protection Honey Bees from Pesticides. University of California, Division of Agricultural Sciences Leaflet 2283.

Baum, F., B. Conrad and U. Schneider (1975): Rückstandsuntersuchungen auf chlorierte Kohlenwasserstoffe in Eiern wildlebender Vögel. Transact. III. Wildlife Disease Conf. (Ed. L.A. Page), Plenum Press 841-848.

Beavington, F. (1975): Heavy Metal Contamination of Vegetables and Soil in Domestic Gardens Around a Smelting Complex. Environm. Pollut. 9: 221-227.

Beery, B. and Kasarda, J.D. (1977): Contemporary urban. Ecology. Macmillan Publ., New York.

Berthold, P. (1976): Methoden der Bestandserfassung in der Ornithologie: Übersicht und kristische Betrachtung. J. Ornithol. 117, (1): 1-69.

Bevenue, A. (1976): The "bioconcentration" aspects of DDT in the environment. Residue Rev. 61: 37-112, Springer, Heidelberg.

Blau, G. and Neely, W. (1976): Mathematical Model Building with an Application to determine the Distribution of Dursban Insecticide added to a Simulated Ecosystem. Adv. Ecol. Research 9: 133-163.

Boesch, E. (1976): Psychopathologie des Alltages. Zur Ökopsychologie des Handelns und seiner Störungen. Huber, Bern.

Booth, G.M. and Ferrell, D. (1977): Degradation of Dimilin ® by Aquatic Foodwebs. In: Khan, Pesticides ..., 221-243, Plenum Press, New York.

Brisbin, I.L. and M.H. Smith (1975): Radiocesium concentrations in Whole-Body Homogenates and several Body Compartments of naturally contaminated White-Tailed Deer. Mineral Cycling in Southeaster Ecosystems, Springfield, Virginia.

Brüggemann, J. (1974): Pestizid- und PCB-Rückstände in Organen von Wildtieren als Indikatoren für Umweltkontaminationen. Z.Jagdwiss. 2o: 7o-74

442

Buchwald, K. (1977): Landschaftsplanung als Beitrag zur Standortbeurtei-
lung und Standortfindung für Energieanlagen aus ökologischer und gestal-
terischer Sicht. In: Energie und Umwelt 58-61, Düsseldorf.

Burkhardt, D. and Itterlson, W. (1978): Environmental assessment of Socio-
economic systems. Plenum Press, New York.

Calow, P. (1977): Ecology, Evolution and Energetics: A Study in Metabolic
Adaptation. In: Ecological Research 1o: 1-62.

Chapman, G. (1977): Human and Environmental Systems. AGeographer's Appraisal. Acad. Press, New York.

Cherrett, J.M. and Sagar, G.R. (1977): Origins of Pest, Parasite, Disease
and Weed Problems. Blackwell Publ., Oxford.

Conrad, B. (1976): Die Giftbelastung der Vogelwelt Deutschlands.- Vogel-
kundliche Bibliothek, 5, Kilda-Verlag, Greven.

Crossley, D., Duke, K. and Waide, J. (1975): Fallout Cesium-137 and Mine-
ral-Element Distribution in Food chains of Granitic-Outcrop ecosystems. In:
Mineral Cycling in Southeastern Ecosystems, 58o-587, ERDA.

Cumberland, J.D. (1977): Boundary condition and influence on area planning
of the power generating industries. In: Energie- und Umwelt, 43-45,
Düsseldorf.

Dahlmann, R., Francis, C. and Tamura, T. (1975): Radiocesium cycling in vegetation and soil. In: Mineral Cycling in Southeastern Ecosystems, 462-
481, ERDA.

Diamond, J.M. (1975): The island dilemma: Lessons of modern biogeographic
studies for the design of natural reserves. Biol. Conserv. 7: 129-146,
Applied Science Publ., Great Britain.

Diamond, J.M. and May, R.M. (1977): Species turnover rates on islands: dependence on census interval. Science 197: 266-27o.

Döl_lekes, H. (1977): Ein multisektorales Energie- und Umweltplanungsmodell.
In: König, Ch. 1977, Energiemodelle..., Birkhäuser Verl., Basel.

Dougherty, R. (1978): Human Exposure to Pentachlorophenol. In: RAO, Pentachlorophenol, 351-361, Plenum Press, New York.

Drescher, H.E., Harms, U. and Huschenbeth, E. (1977):Organochlorines and
Heavy Metals in the Harbour Seal Phoca vitulina from the German North
Sea Coast. Marine Biology 41: 99-1o6.

Drescher-Kaden, U. (1976): Nationale und internationale Forschungsaktivi-
täten und Ergebnisse auf dem Gebiet der Nutzung freilebender Tierarten als
Indikatoren für die Belastung der Umwelt - insbesondere des Menschen - durch
Umweltchemikalien. Bundesministerium für Jugend, Familie und Gesundheit,
Bonn-Bad Godesberg.

Drescher-Kaden, U., R. Hutterer and E. von Lehmann (1978): Rückstände von Organohalogenverbindungen in Kleinsäugern verschiedener Lebensweise aus dem Rheinland. Decheniana 131: 266-273.

Duvigneaud, P. (1974): L'écosystème "URBS"! Mèm. Soc. roy. Bot. Belg. 6: 5-35.

Eckensberger, L. (1977): Die ökologische Perspektive in der Entwicklungs-psychologie: Herausforderung oder Bedrohung? Symp. Entwicklung in ökologischer Sicht, Konstanz.

Ehrlich, P., Ehrlich, A. and Holdren, J.P. (1973): Human Ecology. Problems and Solutions. Freeman, San Francisco.

Ellensberg, Heinz (1973): Die Ökosysteme der Erde, Versuch einer Klassifikation der Ökosysteme nach funktionalen Gesichtspunkten. In: Ökoystemforschung, Springer, Heidelberg.

Ellenberg, Heinz, Fränzle, O. and Müller, P. (1978): Ökosystemforschung im Hinblick auf Umweltpolitik und Entwicklungsplanung. Denkschrift erstellt im Auftrag des Bundesministers des Innern vertreten durch das Umweltbundesamt UBA, Berlin.

Ellensberg, Hermann (1978): Zur Populationsökologie des Rehes (Capreolus capreolus L., Cervidae) in Mitteleuropa. - Beiheft zur Zeitschrift für Zoologie "SPIXIANA", Zool. Staatssammlung, München (im Druck).

Flohn, H. (1977): Großräumige Beeinflussung des Klimas durch menschlichen Eingriff? Historischer Überblick und künftige Aussichten. In: Europa und Umwelt, 11o-113, Düsseldorf.

Fortak, H.G. (1977): Beeinflussung des Lokalklimas durch große Energie-erzeugungs- und Verbrauchszentren. In: Energie und Umwelt 113-116, Düsseldorf.

Fränzle, O. (1978): Die Struktur und Belastbarkeit von Ökosystemen. 41. Dtsch. Geographentag Mainz, 469-485, Steiner, Wiesbaden.

Giebel, J. (1977): Untersuchungen zur Simulation der Immissionsbelastung durch Schwefeldioxid in der Umgebung von Ballungsräumen. Schriftenr. Landesanst. Immissionssch. NRW 42: 17-31, Essen.

Giebel, J. (1978): Berücksichtigung der trockenen Ablagerung am Boden in Abhängigkeit von der effektiven Quellhöhe bei einem Gausschen Ausbreitungs-modell. Schriftenr. Landesanst. Immissionssch. NRW 43: 26-35, Essen.

Gish, C.D. and Christensen, R.E. (1973): Cadmium, Nickel, Lead and Zinc in Earthworms from Roadside Soil. Environ. Sci. Technol. 7: 1o6o-1o62.

Guderian, R. (1977): Air Pollution. Phytotoxicity of Acidic Gases and its Significance in Air Pollution Control. Ecological Stud. 22, Springer, Heidelberg.

444

Guderian, R., Krause, G. and Kaiser, H. (1977): Untersuchung zur Kombinationswirkung von Schwefeldioxid und schwermetallhaltigen Stäuben auf Pflanzen. Schriftenr. Landesanstalt für Immissionsschutz NRW 4o: 23-3o, Essen.

Hall, Ch. and Day, J. (1977): Ecosystem Modeling in Theory and Practice: An Introduction with Case Histories. Wiley,New York.

Hartkamp, H. (1975): Untersuchungen zur Immissionsstruktur einer Großstadt. Projekt "Großstadtluft". Schriftenreihe der LIB 83: 3o-38.

Hay, C.J. (1975): Arthropod stress. In: Air Pollution and Metropolitan Woody Vegetation. W.H. Smith and L.S. Dochinger (Eds.). Yale University Printing Service, New Haven, CT.

Hettche, O. (1975): Zum Problem eines Immissionsgrenzwertes für Benzo-(A)-Pyren. Umwelthygiene 2: 46-5o.

Holleman, D.F. and J.R. Luick (1975): Relationships between Potassium intake and Radiocesium retention in the Reindeer. Mineral Cycling in Southeastern Ecosystems. Springfield Virginia.

Howe, G.M. (1977): A World Geography of Human Diseases. Acad. Press, London.

Jain, S.K. (1975): Patterns of Survival and Microevolution in Plant Population. Population Genetics and Ecology.

Jefferies, D.J. and French, M.C. (1976): Mercury, Cadmium, Zinc, Copper and Organochlorine. Insecticide Levels in Small Mammals Trapped in a Wheat Field. Environm. Pollut. 1o: 175-182.

Joiris, C. and Martens, P. (1973): Teneur en pesticides organochlores d'oeufs de rapaces recoltes en Belgique en 1971. Aves 1o: 153-16o.

Jost, D. (1974): Aerological Studies on the Atmospheric Sulfur Budget. Tellus 26.

Junge, C.E. (1972): The Cycle of Atmospheric gases-Natural and Man Made. Quart. J. Royal Met. Soc. 98.

Kates. R.W. (1978): Risk Assessment of environmental Hazard. SCOPE & Preface, Salisburg.

Kellogg, W. (1977): Emissions and the Climate. In: Energie und Umwelt 117-123, Düsseldorf.

Kettlewell, H. (1973): The evolution of melanism. Oxford.

Khan, M.A. (1977): Pesticides in Aquatic Environments. Plenum Press, New York.

Khan, M., Korte, F. and Payne, J. (1977): Metabolism of Pesticides by aquatic Animals. In: Khan, Pesticides ..., p. 191-22o, Plenum Press, New York.

Koeman, J.H. et al. (1973): Effects of PCB and DDE in cormorants and evaluation of PCB residues from an experimental study. J. Reprod. Fert., Supp. 19: 353-364.

König, Ch. (1977): Energiemodelle für die Bundesrepublik Deutschland. Birkhäuser Verl., Basel.

Kutz, F.W., Murphy, R. and Strassman, S.C. (1978): Survey of Pesticide Residues and their Metabolites in Urine from the general Population. In: RAO, Pentachlorophenol, 363-369, Plenum Press, New York.

Lack, D. (1976): Island Biology, illustrated by the land birds of Jamaica. Studies in Ecology 3, pp. 445, Blackwell Scient. Publ. Oxford.

Lagerwerff, J.V. and Specht, A.W. (197o): Contamination of Roadside Soil and Vegetation with Cadmium, Nickel, Lead and Zinc. Environ. Sci. Techn. 4: 583-586.

Lamb, H.H. (1977): Climate. Present, Past and Future. Methuen, London.

Lane, D.A. and M. Katz (1977): The Photomodification of Benzo (a) Pyrene, Benzo (b) Fluoranthene, and Benzo (k) Fluoranthene under Simulated Atmospheric Conditions. In: Suffet, Fate of Pollutants... Wiley, New York.

Larson, T. et al. (1975): The influence of a Sulfur Dioxide Point Source on the Rain Chemistry of a Single Storm in the Puget Sound Region. Water Air Soil Pollut. 4.

Lees, D.R. Creed, E.R. and Duckett, J.G. (1973): Atmospheric pollution and industrial melanism. Heredity 3o: 227-232.

MacArthur, R.H. (1972): Geographical Ecology, Patterns in the Distribution of Species, Harper & Row Publ., New York.

MacArthur, R.H. and Wilson, E.O. (1971): Biogeographie der Inseln, Verl. Goldmann, München.

Mann, U. and Müller, P. (1978): Bewertungsmatrix und Lösungsstrategien für gegenwärtige ökologische und ökonomische Probleme. Ergebnisse eines Dialoges zwischen Theologen und Biogeographen in Saarbrücken; 1974-1977, Mitt. Schwerpunkt Biogeographie Univ. Saarlandes, 1o: 1-15, Saarbrücken.

Margaleff, R. (1975): Perspectives in ecological theory. Chicago, London.

Martin, M.H. and Coughtrey, P.J. (1975): Preliminary Oberservations on the Levels of Cadmium in a Contaminated Environment. Chemosphere 3: 155-16o.

Maruyama, T. (1977): Stochastic Problems in Population Genetics. Springer, Heidelberg.

Matsumura, F. (1977): Absorption, accumulation and elimination of Pesticides by aquatic organisms. In: Khan, Pesticides ..., 77-125, Plenum Press, New York.

446

Mauch, E. (1976): Leitformen der Saprobität für die biologische Gewässer-analyse. Cour. Forsch. Seneckenberg 21.

May, R.M. (1972): Will a Large Complex System be Stable? Nature 238: 413-414.

May, R.M. (1973): Stability and Complexity in Model Ecosystems. Princeton University Press, Princeton, N.Y.

May, R.M. (1977): Thresholds and breakpoints in ecosystems with a multipli-city of stable states. Nature 269: 471-477.

Metcalf, R. (1977): Modell Ecosystem Studies of Biocentration and Biodegra-dation of pesticides. In: Khan, Pesticides ..., 127-144, Plenum Press, New York.

Metcalf, R.L. (1977): Biological Fate and Transformation of Pollutants in Water. In: Suffet, Fate of Pollutants ...Wiley, New York.

Meyer, B. (1977): Sulfur, Energy, and Environment. Elseb. Publ., Amsterdam.

Miettinen, J.K. (1976): Plutonium Foodchains. Helsinki.

Moore, N.W. (1969): Sublethal effects of organochlorine insecticides in the laboratory and the field. Meded. Fakult. Landbouw.-wetenschappen Gent 34: 4o8-412.

Müller, P. (1974): La structuration de l'environnement naturel dans les regions de concentration urbaine, Bull. des Recherches agronomiques de Gembloux, Vol. extraordinaire édité à l'occasion de la semaine d'étude agriculture et environnement, p. 742-761, Gembloux.

Müller, P. (1974): Was ist Ökologie? Geoforum 18.

Müller, P. (1975): Ökologische Kriterien für die Raum- und Stadtplanung, Umwelt-Saar 1974, 6-51, Homburg.

Müller, P. (1976): Tiere als Belastungsindikatoren und ökologische Krite-rien. Daten und Dokumente zum Umweltschutz 19: 153-171, Stuttgart.

Müller, P. (1977): Biogeographie und Raumbewertung. WTB, Wiesbaden.

Müller, P. (1977): Tiergeographie, TEUBNER, Stuttgart.

Müller, P. (1978): Erfassung von Arealsystemen - eine Grundlage für die Raumbewertung. Beitrag zur Aufschlüsselung des Informationsgehaltes von Tierarealen für die Darstellung der Umweltsituation der Bundesrepublik Deutschland. In: Schriftenr. Landesanstalt für Umweltschutz BW, Karlsruhe.

Müller, P. (1978): Biogeographie. UTB, Stuttgart (im Druck).

Müller, P. (1978): Arealsysteme und Biogeographie. Ulmer. Stuttgart (im Druck).

Müller, P. and Schäfer, A. (1976): Diversitätsuntersuchungen und Expositions-tests in der mittleren Saar. Forum Umwelthygiene 2: 43-46.

Nguyen Ba Cuong, Bonsang, B. and Lambert, G. (1974): The Atmospheric Concen-tration of Sulfur Dioxide and Sulfate Aerosols over Antarctic, Subantarctic Areas and Oceans. Tellus 26.

Niehaus, F. (1977): Computersimulation langfristiger Umweltbelastung durch Energieerzeugung. Kohlendioxyd, Tritium und Radio-Kohlenstoff. Birkhäuser Verl., Basel.

Ohlendorf, H.M. (1978): Monitoring Environmental Contaminants in Wildlife and Archiving Specimens for Future Analysis. Int. Workshop on Monitoring Environmental Materials and Specimen Banking.

Park, R. (1916): The City: Suggestions for the Investigation of Human Be-havior in an Urban Environment. Amer. Journ. Sociology 2o: 577-612.

Patten, B.C. (1974): The Zero State and Ecosystems Stability. Proc. First Internat. Cong. Ecology Centre for Agricult. Publ. and Documentation, Wageningen.

Pianka, E.R. (1974): Evolutionary Ecology. Harper & Row Publ., New York.

Po-Yung, L., R.L. Metcalf, R. Furman, R. Vogel and J. Hasset (1975): Model Ecosystem Studies of Lead and Cadmium and of Urban Sewage Sludge Contai-ning this Elements. J. Environ. Qual. 4.

Prestt, J. and Ratcliffe, D.A. (1972): Effects of organochlorine insecti-cides on European birdlife. Proc. XV th intern. Ornith. Congr. 197o: 486-513.

Prinz, B. (1975): Immissionswirkungskataster in Nordrhein-Westfalen als Planungskriterium, Umwelt-Saar 1974.

Rao, K.R. (1978): Pentachlorphenol. Chemistry, Pharmacology, and Environ-mental Toxicology. Plenum Press, New York.

Rapoport, A. (1977): Human Aspects of Urban Form. Towards a Man-Environ-ment Approach to Urban Form and Design. Pergamon Press, Oxford.

Rees, P.H., Smith, A.P. and King, J.R.(1977): Population models of Cities and Regions. John Wiley, New York.

Remmert, H. (1978): Ökologie. Ein Lehrbuch. Springer, Heidelberg.

RGU = Regionale Planungsgemeinschaft Untermain (1974): Lufthygienisch-meterologische Modelluntersuchung in der Region Untermain. 5. Jahresbe-richt. Frankfurt.

Rosmanith, J., Schröder, A., Einbrodt, H.J. and Ehm, W. (1975): Untersu-chungen an Kindern aus einem mit Blei und Zink belasteten Industriegebiet. Umwelthygiene 9: 266-271.

448

Schlipköter, H.-W. (1977): Bewertung der Grenzwerte von Immissionen aus medizinischer Sicht. In: Energie und Umwelt 1oo-1o5, Düsseldorf.

Schmithüsen, J. (1976): Allgemeine Geosynergetik. Grundlagen der Landschaftskunde, De Gruyter, Berlin.

Scholl, G. (1978): Vergleich zwischen Emissionsrate und Wirkdosis von Fluorid in standardisierten Graskulturen im Bereich eines Aluminiumwerkes. Schriftenr. Landesanst. Immissionsschutz NRW 43: 75-89, Essen.

Schönbeck, H. and Van Haut, H. (1974): Methoden zur Erstellung eines Wirkungskatasters für Luftverunreinigungen durch pflanzliche Indikatoren. Verhdl. Ges. Ökologie, 435-445, Saarbrücken, Verl. Junk, The Hague.

Schönbeck, C. (1975): Der Beitrag komplexer Stadtsimulationsmodelle (vom Forrester-Typ) zur Analyse und Prognose großstädtischer Systeme. Birkhäuser Verl., Basel.

Simberloff, D.S. (1976): Trophic structure determination and equilibrium in an arthropod community. Ecology 57: 395-398.

Sorauer, P. (1911): Die makroskopische Analyse rauchgeschädigter Pflanzen. Samml. Abhdl. Abgase und Rauchschäden 7.

Steiniger, H. (1978): Genetische Variabilität bei Carabiden-Populationen inner- und außerstädtischer Standorte. Disseration, Biogeographie, Saarbrücken.

Stern, A. (1977): Air Pollution. 3. Ed., 5, Air Quality Management. Acad. Press, New York.

Steubing, L., Kirschbaum, U. and Gwinner, M. (1976): Nachweis von Fluorimmissionen durch Bioindikatoren. Angew. Botanik 5o: 169-185.

Suffet, I.H. (1977): Fate of Pollutants in the Air and Water Environments. Wiley, New York.

Sukopp, H. et al. (1974): Ökologische Charakteristik von Großstädten, besonders anthropogene Veränderungen von Klima, Boden und Vegetation. TUB 6 (4): 469-488.

Thoss, R. (1977): Möglichkeiten einer optimalen Standortverteilung von Energieversorgungsanlagen unter Berücksichtigung gesamtwirtschaftlicher Aspekte. Energie und Umwelt, 45-49, Düsseldorf.

Umplis, (1978): Verzeichnis rechnergestützter Umweltmodelle. E. Schmidt Verl., Berlin.

Vester, F. (1976): Ballungsgebiete in der Krise. Eine Anleitung zum Verstehen und Planen menschlicher Lebensräume mit Hilfe der Biokybernetik. Biering, München.

Voss, A. (1977): Ansätze zur Gesamtanalyse des Systems Mensch-Energie-Umwelt. Eine dynamische Computersimulation. Birkhäuser Verl., Basel.

Webster, J., Waide, J. and Patten, B. (1975): Nutrient recycling and the stability of Ecosystems. Mineral Cycling in Southeastern Ecosystems. ERDA Sympos. Ser., U.S. Energy Research and Development Administration, Springfield.

Wegler, R. (1977): Herbizide. In: Chemie der Pflanzenschutz- und Schädlingsbekämpfungsmittel, 5. Springer, Heidelberg.

Williams, C.H. and David, D.J. (1976): The Accumulation in Soil of Cadmium Residues from Phosphate Fertilizers and their Effect on the Cadmium Content of Plants. Soil Science 121: 86-93.

Wilson, A.G., Rees, P. and Leich, C. (1977): Models of Cities and Regions. Theoretical and Empirical Developments. John Wiley, New York.

Wilson, E. and Bossert, W. (1973): Einführung in die Populationsbiologie. Springer, Heidelberg.

CONSIDERATIONS APPLICABLE TO THE MONITORING OF ORGANO-HALO-
GENATED COMPOUNDS IN TERRESTRIAL WILDLIFE, ESPECIALLY BIRDS

Dr. R.K. Murton
Institute of Terrestrial Ecology, Monks Wood Experimental
Station, Abbots Ripton, Huntingdon, England

Introduction

In Britain, the Central Unit on Environmental Pollution was commissioned
in 1971 to prepare a report on "The Monitoring of the Environment in the
United Kingdom" (HMSO, 1974). This report defined the concept of monitoring
in both a (1) wide and (2) narrow sense.

(1) The wide interpretation implied the repeated measurement of pollutant
    concentrations to allow the following of changes over a period of time.

(2) In the restricted sense, monitoring means the regular measurement of
    pollutant levels, in relation to some standard, or in order to judge
    the effectiveness of a system of regulation and control.

Wildlife species may be used for either of these aims and the idea of
selecting appropriate indicator species (index specimen) has been broached
(Moore, 1966).
Studies which were initiated in the Nature Conservancy* in the early 1960's
were concerned with biological monitoring in the restricted sense for they
were aimed at encouraging legislation, and then of policing legislation,
designed to reduce the risks to wildlife or organochlorine insecticides.

---

* In the United Kingdom it was decided by Parliament (Nature Conservancy
Council Act, 1973) that wildlife conservation policy in Great Britain
should be the responsibility of the Nature Conservancy Council (NCC), established in November 1973, from the old Nature Conservancy, as an independent statutory body whose members are appointed by the Secretary of State
for the Environment. In consequence, the Natural Environment Research Council (NERC) decided that ecology, as an important branch of environmental
science, needed the continuing attention of a research institute. To this
end, the scientists employed by the former Nature Conservancy, who remained
with NERC, were combined with the Council's Institute of Tree Biology and
the Biology Project Group of the British Antarctic Survey to become the
Institute of Terrestrial Ecology. For practical purposes the programmes
of research into toxic chemical and wildlife which were initiated in the
old Nature Conservancy now continued in the Sub-Division of Animal Function of ITE. There has been some change of emphasis to suit present day
needs, in particular, more detailed physiological studies of mechanisms,
but great care has been taken to maintain a balance between, and to integrate, laboratory, experimental work and field, ecologically orientated
programmes. The ITE receives approximately two-thirds of its funds from
the Department of Education & Science and this money is available for fundamental research and about one-third is earned from contracts with other departments; most contract money for pollution studies presently comes from the NCC.

These programmes are now continued in the Institute of Terrestrial Ecology*,
which is a research organisation with no statutory responsibilities for
monitoring per se.However, some of the research programmes are designed
to define the biological criteria which should be the basis of any monitoring
scheme involving wildlife samples and this contribution is prepared in this
context.

The main emphasis of pollution research in ITE is on organochlorine compounds, especially the cyclodiene insecticides, DDT and the polychlorinated biphenyls, and heavy metals. Moreover, attention is focussed on the
possibility of long-term, sub-lethal effects and so any "monitoring" exercises are aimed at providing base-line information of residue levels in
wildlife species and of following spatial and temporal trends. Attention
is not confined to agricultural habitats and, although the emphasis is on
terrestrial systems, the interface between land and sea is within the re-
mit of the Institute. In contrast, scientists in the Ministry of Agriculture, Fisheries & Food (MAFF), Pest Infestation Control Laboratory (PICL),
because of their responsibilities under the Pesticides Safety Precautions
Scheme (which see below) are more concerned with the short-term effects
of agricultural chemicals and of investigating wildlife and other incidents arising from the use of these chemicals. Their efforts incline to
centre on toxicity testing with the main emphasis on organophosphorus
compounds (these having largely replaced the organochlorines as insecticides) and heavy metals occurring in agriculture. MAFF and ITE have the
largest laboratories and research effort in Britain devoted to environmental
pollution in the context of wildlife and both programmes should be considered together for a balanced appraisal. Numerous short-term, ad hoc
studies are in progress in other centres, particularly the universities,
but with the exception of the Monitoring and Assessment Research Centre
(MARC) at Chelsea College, these are of only passing relevance to this
workshop.

Monitoring schemes in Britain which do not implicate wildlife samples
are excluded from consideration here as are those applied in the marine
environment, even if wildlife samples are involved (for example, the Marine Pollution Archive which is a computer-based system developed by the
Water Data Unit for the Ministry of Agriculture, Fisheries & Food).

This contribution has been prepared in collaboration with Dr. F. Moriarty
since he and the present author both work in the same laboratory; we have
purposely avoided duplicating our efforts because, for many of the topics
to be raised in the workshop, we would have produced the same statements
(e.g. costs of analyses).

a. Review of Past and Current Programmes

The first recorded cases of mortality in birds associated with the use
of agricultural chemicals occurred in 1947, apparently caused by herbicide
use, but in the spring 1956 unprecedented numbers of deaths occurred and
such incidents, seemingly associated with cereal seed dressings were repeated each spring up to 1961; these incidents resulted in the deaths
of large numbers of graminivorous birds particularly Partridges Perdix
perdix, Pheasants Phasianus colchicus, Wood Pigeons Columba palumbus and
various finch species (Turtle et al., 1963). Widespread concern from conser-
vationists and agriculturalists encouraged extensive chemical analyses
to be performed on samples of carcases and soon it was evident that dieldrin, aldrin and heptachlor were mainly responsible for deaths. These factors led, in 1961, to a voluntary ban on the use of the cyclodiene group

of insecticides on spring grown cereals. The ban was negotiated and agreed
between government, farmers and industry. Subsequently, the Advisory
Committee on Poisonous Substances used in Agriculture and Food Storage
recommended that aldrin, dieldrin and heptachlor should only be used on
winter-sown wheat (up to the end of December) where there was a real danger of attack from wheat bulb fly. These measures substantially reduced
the incidence of direct mortality but manifestations of sub-lethal effects
continued and occasional examples of the misuse of the chemicals were reported. In 1969, a further review recommended that aldrin, dieldrin and
heptachlor seed treatments be continuously assessed and this was the pre-
lude to their complete withdrawal in 1975.
By the mid-1960's residues of organochlorine insecticides were widespread
in terrestrial, freshwater and marine wildlife throughout Britain (Walker
et al., 1967). Subsequently, Prestt & Ratcliffe (1972) could show that
organochlorine insecticide residues could be found in at least 154 different avian species representing 47 taxonomic families, i.e.over three-quar-
ters of European bird families and about one third of the European bird
species (see refs in Cramp, 1962, 1967; Moore & Walker, 1964; Moore &
Tatton, 1965; Ratcliffe, 1965; Walker & Mills, 1965; Koeman & Van Genderen,
1966; Koeman et al., 1968; Holt & Sakshaug, 1968, Jensen et al., 1969;
Koeman et al., 1969; Prestt, 1972; Prestt & Ratcliffe, 1972). In the predatory birds (Falconiformes and Strigiformes) residues were present in most
individuals even in remote regions.

It was against this background and coincident with the introduction of
the spring ban on the use of dieldrin and related compounds, that the
Nature Conservancy desided to monitor residue levels in any dead raptor
and owl specimens sent to the laboratory at Monks Wood, and national appeals
for specimens were advertised via the ornithological and conservation journals.
This project ist still in progress. Many hundred specimens of Kestrel
Falco tinnunculus, Sparrowhawk Accipiter nisus, Barn Owl Tyto alba, Heron
Ardea cinerea and lesser numbers of other species such as the Great Crested
Grebe Podiceps cristatus and Kingfisher Alcedo atthis have been received
and analysed. Prestt & Ratcliffe (1972) made a preliminary analysis of the
liver residues of 57o predatory birds, representing 18 species, which were
sent in as carcases and of these 97 % contained residues of pp'-DDE, 96 %
contained residues of dieldrin, and over two-thirds contained heptachlor
epoxide. Moreover, most individuals contained at least two different organochlorine residues, some even three or more, and we have since found that
they can also carry large loads of such heavy metals as mercury. Similarly,
266 eggs of predatory birdsall contained pp'-DDE, 95 % contained dieldrin,
55 % contained heptachlor epoxide.
The object of this terrestrial monitoring exercise has been to police the
efficacy of the various agreements introduced to limit the use of the more
toxic insecticides, and to lobby for even more effective controls so the
prime motivation has been a conservation one. Nevertheless, this scheme
is now the longest running and most comprehensive monitoring exercise involving predatory species.
Mention must also be made of the marine environment. Over 9o seabird eggs
were collected in 1963 und 1964 and all contained pp'-DDE and dieldrin
and half also contained BHC (Moore & Tatton, 1965). Since then eggs of a
wide range of marine birds have been analysed for organochlorine residues
and heavy metals and in addition these same agents are measured in the carcases of dead seabirds collected round the shores of Britain. To quote from

the report of a NERC working group on ecological research on seabirds
"Seabird eggs have been collected regularly since 1962 for analysis for
organochlorine pesticide residues; since 1967 they have also been analysed
for polychlorinated biphenyl residues; and since about 1969 for certain
trace metals - especially mercury. From the point of view of analysis,
seabirds have certain advantages over other organisms in the marine environment and over sea water itself. The most obvious is that many chemicals,
particularly those that are fat soluble, are present in much higher concentrations, and hence more easily measured. Eggs have certain advantages
over corpses, notably in that they can be obtained relatively easily,
present fewer conservation or public relations problems, represent a distinct stage in the biology and annual cycle of the individual or species,
and can be homogenised easily for analysis.
"Annual or near-annual collection and analysis of eggs over a series of
years, e.g. Shags Phalacrocorax aristotelis in north east England; Sandwich
Terns Sterna sandvicensis in north Norfolk (Parslow & Moore, 1972), have
provided information on changing (usually declining) residues of organochlorine insecticides in eggs and a check on the effectiveness of control
regulations.
"Data are also available, but probably still insufficient, to help determine whether changes are also occurring in various parts of British coastal waters in the level of contamination by PCB's and mercury, both of
which occur as significant pollutants in, for example, the Irish Sea region,
but which have been subject to voluntary pollution controls in recent years.
"Systematic collections of eggs of Guillemots Uria aalge, and a limited
range of other species have been made at colonies around the coast of Britain and Ireland to provide comparative data on levels of pollutants at
different sites. The main feature is the proportionately high levels of
all these pollutants in the Irish Sea region compared with eastern, and especially northern, colonies. This is particularly marked for mercury and
PCB's and is presumably related to the slow rate of water exchange and the
larger amounts of industrial waste and effluent it receives. In the most
contaminated British colonies, concentrations of mercury and PCB's are as
high as, or higher than, those from eggs of the same species in other parts
of its range. DDE concentrations, on the other hand, even in the Irish Sea,
are only 5 % of those in one Baltic colony and 1o-2o % of those in a colony
off the coast of the coast of California.
"In many seabird species, the pollutant residues in eggs fall within comparatively narrow limits for any one colony. This is particularly true for
the more sedentary species such as the Guillemot and those having relatively narrow food spectra. Much wider variation occurs among species having a
greater feeding range e.g. Gannets Sula bassana - also among species having
a wide variety of food, especially when individual birds specialise on particular food items - e.g. Great Black-backed Gulls Larus marinus, on
Skomer, which variously specialise on rabbits, seabirds, fish offal, gar-
bage etc. In this population of Great Black-backed Gulls, residues in eggs
appear to be related to the food preference of the pair (female) concerned,
and opportunities exist for more detailed studies on exposure/residues of
different pollutants in the same species.
"Comparison of chemical residues in the eggs of e.g. Guillemots and Kittiwakes Rissa tridactyla, from the same colony, has revealed a number of
striking differences, for example in PCB:DDE ratios. Kittiwakes contain
proportionately much more PCB and less DDE than other birds - the difference provides an important clue as to differences in the sources and pathways of these two compounds in the marine environment (or possibly to

differences in metabolism of the compounds in the birds themselves). Further work on the metabolism of toxic chemicals is required.

"Limited studies have been made of residue levels in food chain organisms and could usefully be extended for organochlorines and heavy metals.

"Some work has been undertaken to establish the relationship between pollutant residues in eggs and in the birds that laid them; between, in single egg species, the first egg and its replacement and, in species laying larger clutches, between pollutant levels in each egg in the sequence. Such studies are of potential value in determining at what stage in the annual cycle adult birds have accumulated the pollutant residues which are deposited in the egg and in the interpretation of data for monitoring purposes. Many studies have been made on the relationship between egg shell thickness and particularly DDE residues - not just in seabirds. Among British seabirds, the only species studied which show marked inverse correlations between shell thickness and DDE residues are the Gannet (Parslow & Jefferies, 1977) and Shag, There is some indication that Guillemot egg shells are marginally thinner in some Irish Sea colonies than elsewhere in Britain but the extent of the thinning is much less than the 12-13 % recorded in the same species'eggs from the Baltic and off the California coast, where much higher DDE concentrations have been recorded.

"The value of bird corpses for monitoring purposes is arguable. Different chemicals are distributed differently within the bodies of healthy birds and there are problems in choosing the tissues or organs that should be analysed. In the case of birds found dead, problems are manifold: levels of pollutant residues in different tissues can change dramatically both in vitro, for example during starvation, and post mortem. The liver is a convenient organ for analysis but the proportion of total body residues, of e.g. fat soluble substances, it contains can change substantially according to whether a bird was in good or starved condition when it died.

"Analyses of whole birds are probably best for providing data on residues for base-line and monitoring work (as well as in dosing studies) but are difficult and time-consuming to undertake. Except for birds killed at breeding colonies, a further disadvantage of corpses, in addition to those discussed above, is that there is often uncertainty as to their origin and manner of death.

'Nevertheless, the analysis of tissues from corpses has provided important clues in studies on the effects of pollutants on seabirds. For some pollutants (e.g. PCB and mercury) concentrations in the brain probably provide the best evidence of lethal effects.

"Certain heavy metals, e.g. cadmium, appear not to be transferred by the female to its eggs in easily measurable quantities. Much of the information we have on the occurrence of this trace metal in seabirds comes from studies of tissue/organ levels. Analyses of about 8oo livers of marine birds indicate that unlike mercury, which occurs in highest levels in species which feed in estuarine and inshore situations and in lowest levels in oceanic species, cadmium occurs in highest amounts in oceanic species (also in some littoral species) and in low amounts in those that feed inshore. Indications are that while mercury levels are directly related to run-off from the land, the high levels of cadmium in species such as Puffins Fratercula arctica, shearwaters and petrels occur naturally, the high levels being due to invertebrates in pelagic food chains, which concentrate this element.

"Seabirds have been relatively little used as indicators of other pollutants or potential pollutants in their environment around Britain. Such examinations as have been made (e.g. for chlorinated naphthalenes and chlorinated paraffins) have been by industry. The range of potential persistent pollutants is considerable and greater use of seabird material to search for them should be made."

Eggs of terrestrial birds have been used for monitoring in two ways:

(1) With some reservation, egg residues generally reflect those present in the adult and eggs can be sampled without the need to sacrifice adults. In addition to the marine species mentioned above, large numbers of eggs of the Peregrine Falco peregrinus, Sparrowhawk, Golden Eagle Aquila chrysaetos have been analysed for organochlorine residues. However, these species are of great conservation interest and so mostly infertile or broken eggs have been collected on an ad hoc basis (e.g. Ratcliffe, 1970). The only terrestrial species whose eggs have been taken on planned basis is the Heron, samples of all eggs laid at certain colonies in Lincolnshire and Norfolk having been procured since 1968 (Cooke, Bell & Prestt, 1976); this project continues (Cooke, Bell & Murton, in preparation; Conroy, in progress).

(2) Ratcliffe (1967, 1970), in what have become classic studies, showed that an increased incidence of egg breakage and destruction amongst Peregrines, Sparrowhawks and Golden Eagles could be correlated with a decrease in shell thickness. By examining shells from museums and private collections he was able to show that a significant decline in thickness had occurred during the period 1945-50 and implicated organochlorine insecticides. Ratcliffe devised an index:

$$\frac{\text{weight of shell (mg)}}{\text{length of shell (mm) x breadth (mm)}}$$

which allowed comparison of the thickness of whole shells without breaking them and many workers have applied his technique to show shell thinning in a wide range of species (reviewed by Cooke, 1973). Although Ratcliffe was careful not to attribute shell thinning to any one compound, field evidence strongly implicated pp'-DDE, the metabolic product of DDT (Cooke, 1973, 1975), and laboratory experiments seem to confirm this conclusion (Lincer, 1975). Thus, continuing studies of avian egg shells will help monitor the distribution of DDT.

b. Rationale for Interest or Concern

The following chemicals are of interest here:

DDT: 1,1,1-trichloro-2,2-di(chlorophenyl)ethane

DDE: 1,1-dichloro-2,2-bis(p-chlorophenyl)ethylene

DDD (TDE): 1,1-dichloro-2,2-di-(4-chlorophenyl)ethane

DDA: bis(p-chlorophenyl)acetic acid

DDT was first synthesised in 1874 although its insecticidal properties were not recognised until 1939 by Paul Müller, a Swiss chemist. It was first used extensively during the Second World War to combat lice and other body parasites, and also mosquitoes, and then became extensively used in agriculture. Problems arising from its use were insect resistance and then a long series of wildlife incidents, for example, Clear Lake, California, which was sprayed with DDD (Hunt & Bischoff, 1960).

DDT is now universally distributed and, because it has a long half-life, is likely to pose problems for the rest of the century. DDT can be degraded by soil organisms, aerobically to DDE and unaerobically to DDD, this last encouraged by flooding. The concentration of metabolites usually exceeds the concentration of residual DDT and these metabolites are more toxic to organisms. Loss occurs from soil by evaporation and is followed by global circulation and fall-out in rain. The oceans are likely to be the final sink for DDT but models attempting to define the ultimate fate of DDT and its breakdown products must be speculative (Woodwell, Craig & Johnson, 1971; Cramer, 1973).

EEC proposals have been advanced to prohibit the use of DDT, but in Britain no alternative for certain pest problems exists, e.g. caterpillars on foliage, soil pests such as cutworms, woodlice and millipedes, leaf eating weevils on top fruit, pear midge, etc., therefore, still fairly extensively used in horticulture and to some extent on certain grasslands.

HCH: Hexachlorocyclohexane - usually misnamed BHC (benzene hexachloride). Contains five isomers of which the gamma form (called lindane) mostly used as an insecticide. Residues are widespread in birds but there is no indication that it has caused significant problems. It is more soluble than most organochlorine insecticides and also more volatile.

Cyclodienes: this group of compounds was developed during the mid-1940's and introduced widely into use as insecticides during the 1950's. The main agents under consideration are aldrin, dieldrin (active product HEOD), heptachlor, chlordane, all of which are toxic to mammals. All are very fat soluble but practically insoluble in water. Although aldrin, dieldrin and heptachlor were withdrawn from general use as cereal seed dressings in 1975, dieldrin is still in use for certain seed treatments (e.g. sugar beet). Dieldrin is also used extensively as a moth-proofing agent by the woollen industry and the amount escaping into river systems needs surveillance (Central Unit of Environmental Pollution. Pollution Paper 3, HMSO, 1974). Small amounts of aldrin are used for special purposes in agriculture, for example, the control of narcissus bulb fly and the control of wireworms in potato crops.

PCB's: polychlorinated biphenyls.

First introduced in 1929 by the Monsanto Chemical Company. Their value for industrial purposes lies in a high dielectric constant, high boiling point and chemical inertness. They have been used extensively in electrical transformers, capacitors, cutting oils, hydraulic fluids, plasticizers. Estimates put the total cumulative world production at around 1 million tons. Of this total, around one half is in dumps and landfills, from which it is likely to be released slowly, while the remainder has entered the environment. Low temperature incineration of plastic waste causes PCB's to be vaporized. PCB's are degraded extremely slowly. Ultimate reservoirs appear to be river and coastal sediments. As with DDT, bioaccumulation occurs because PCB's are virtually water insoluble but highly fat soluble. During the early 1960's, when tissue samples were analysed for the Nature Conservancy by the Laboratory of the Government Chemist, unidentified peaks on the gas chromatograms were observed. These were identified as being caused by PCB's (Holmes, Simmons & Tatton, 1967). Their presence necessitated additional clean-up stages for the separation of compounds in the tissue extracts; since 1968 the method employed has involved fractional elution from a column of silica gel and this separates PCB's, hexachlorobenzene and pp'-DDE from the other commonly found organochlorine pesticide residues (Collins, Holmes & Jackson, 1972).

PCT: polychlorinated terphenyls

During 1977 a brief study of the livers of some of the terrestrial bird
samples sent to the Laboratory of the Government Chemist revealed the
presence of polychlorinated terphenyls, which, while detectable at trace
levels, were present at 1-2 orders of magnitude lower than the PCB's (Hassell
& Holmes, 1977). PCT's have been reported in the eggs and tissues of Herring
Gulls Larus argentatus (Zitko et al., 1972), in Japanese human fat (Doguchi
& Fukano, 1975), but the significance of the residues observed is unknown.
Other compounds: a tissue bank of material is kept deep frozen at Monks
Wood. Recently, a few Heron livers have been tested for the presence of
long-chain chlorinated paraffins with positive results, but details of
the analytical method have not yet been published. Similarly, polychlorinated styrene (PCS) compounds have recently been found in tissues of the
Great Blue Heron Ardea herodias in the USA (Reichel, Prouty & Gay, 1976).
In general biochemical terms, organochlorine insecticides act by increasing
the rate of transmission of neural impulses along the nerve axons and this
results in muscular spasm, convulsion and death. In birds the sub-lethal
effects of organochlorine compounds are not well understood.

c. Sample Collection and Storage

There has been no indication that the supply to Monks Wood of carcases of
predatory birds found dead might exceed demand. Obviously, the number of
bodies found and sent is a function of the number of interested observers
and their incentives. There is usually an increase in the rate of material
arriving at the laboratory following the publication of a new appeal but
the main motivation of observers appears to be a basic interest in wildlife and a curiosity to have their finds autopsied and analysed. Postage is
refunded to people sending dead bodies and later they are sent an individual report giving autopsy and analytical results.

Most material arrives at the laboratory in good condition and is stored
in deep freeze immediatley. When convenient carcases are examined; during
autopsy whole body weights and weights of individual organs are taken,
the state of the moult investigated, the likely cause of death ascertained
as far as possible and the subject allocated to one of the following categories:

1. Death through trauma
   (i) Road casualty
   (ii) All other traumas

2. Found dead
   (i) Diseased or poor condition
   (ii) Haemorrhaged
   (iii) Negative

Samples of brain, pectoral muscle, liver, kidney, and occasionally other
organs, are removed and stored in individual glass bottles before being
prepared for analysis. Freezing is satisfactory for the chemicals considered here but not for gamma HCH. Tissue banks must be prepared with knowledge of the chemicals it is intended to study.

d. Analytical Procedure

Analysis of organochlorine pesticide residues originally involved clean-up
by solvent partition (de Faubert Maunder et al., 1964) or selective solvent
extraction (Wood, 1969), followed by adsorption chromatography on a column

of alumina, final determinations being made by gas liquid chromatography. Efforts to reduce analytical time have led to a system whereby the clean-up of extracted residues is effected solely by elution from a column of alumina. As mentioned above, the discovery of PCB's necessitated additional separation stages and while this initially involved paper chromatography the current practice involves fractional elution from a column of silica gel (Collins et al., 1972).

e. Programme Design

The central problems of using wildlife species for monitoring concern sampling procedures.Species such as the raptors, which are of great conservation value, cannot be sacrificed for chemical analyses, so reliance has to be placed on the collection of dead samples. With more abundant species it is possible, and desirable, to obtain samples from the live population by shooting, trapping or other suitable means, but, even so, sampling biases must occur.

When dead carcases are sent by members of the public or a central laboratory they represent a wide range of causes of death, circumstances of recovery, geographical and spatial heterogeneity. Some specimens may never have been exposed to a particular pollutant, others may have died from a toxic dose so a wide range of residues is found on analysis. With very toxic compounds in widescale use the number of bodies sent to the laboratory would be expected to be high. However, there is no simple relationship between the number of birds dying and the number sent for analysis because the number of people interested enough to collect and send bodies seems to impose some density-related regulation.

Partly for reasons outlined in the preceding paragraph, toxic residues in wildlife species are not normally distributed, a fact well appreciated by Robinson (1967), Hazeltine (1972) and Holden (1975) but overlooked by far too many authors. Actually toxic residues are often markedly log-normally distributed and the skewness of such data makes it misleading to quote means $\pm$ S.E.M. Some kind of transformation is usually demanded unless non-parametric statistical tests are to be used and the following paragraphs set out an appropriate procedure calculated on our Merlewood computer by J.N.R. Jeffers (Murton, Bell & Jeffers, in press).

All Barn Owls Tyto alba received at Monks Wood have been pooled according to the month of collection, irrespective of the year they were received and the arithmetic means of the monthly dieldrin residues are summarised in Table 1. Peak liver residues were apparently found in April, but we need formal tests of the statistical significance of these data. Tabe 1, therefore, is extended as an analysis of variance (12 x 1 array) of these untransformed data.The "within months" variances can be seen to vary markedly, yet this analysis assumes the homogeneity of the variances for the individual months. Bartlett's test for the homogeneity of variances gives a corrected chi-square of 14o.99 with 11 degrees of freedom and this is highly significant $P < 0.001$. Thus, any test of the differences in mean monthly residues is likely to reflect differences in the variances alone. Inspection of the variances in Table 1 suggests that they might be linearly related to the means and this is confirmed in Fig. 1. This suggests a logarithmic transformation to be appropriate and so the data contributing to Table 1 were converted to logarithms (base 1o) and a second analysis of variance performed (Table 2). Now the "within months" variances show greater homogeneity and the correlated chi-square with Bartlett's

Table 1

Mean monthly residues of dieldrin, mg kg^{-1}, in livers of Barn Owl
and analysis of variance

	Arithmetic mean	degrees of freedom	Variance
January	3.14	2o	42.779
February	4.48	37	61.888
March	4.16	55	31.479
April	12.39	24	153.39o
May	6.73	11	48.933
June	1.2o	1	o.72o
July	6.16	3	67.786
August	o.67	6	1.423
September	1.43	5	1.747
October	2.o4	24	9.oo3
November	1.43	2o	7.391
December	1.32	27	2.984

Between month variance	11	223.254 F = 5.33, P<o.oo1
Pooled within month variance	233	42.898

Table 2

Mean monthly log$_{10}$ residues of dieldrin, mg kg^{-1}, in livers of Barn
Owls and analysis of variance

	Mean log$_{10}$	d.f.	Variance	Cubic regression (see text)
January	o.85	2o	o.4394	o.65
February	1.23	37	o.5169	1.52
March	1.97	55	o.3272	2.41
April	5.7o	24	o.4445	2.8o
May	3.44	11	o.364o	2.56
June	1.o4	1	o.1138	1.98
July	o.88	3	1.6469	1.39
August	o.17	6	o.6792	o.96
September	o.94	5	o.2181	o.7o
October	o.78	24	o.3719	o.58
November	o.62	2o	o.2377	o.58
December	o.69	27	o.2423	o.76

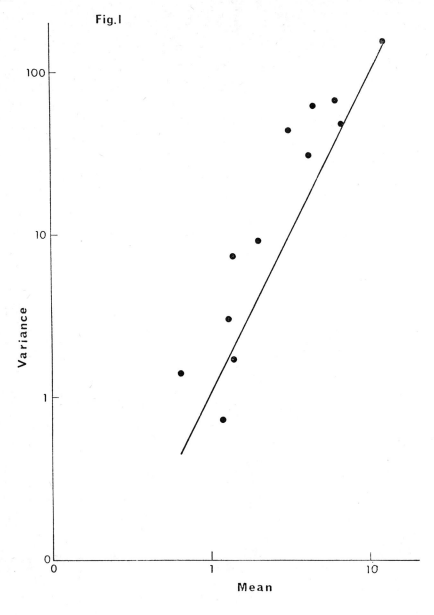

Fig.1

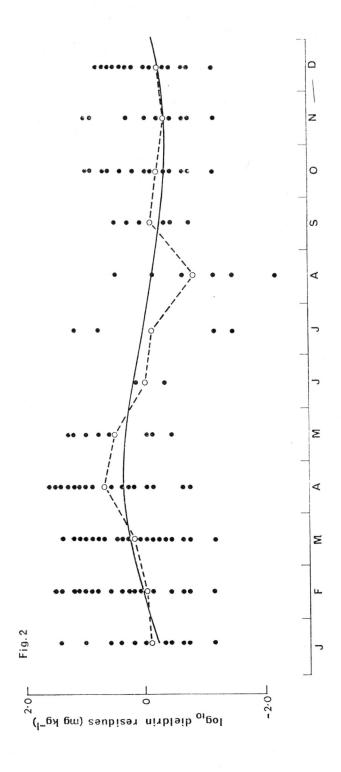

Fig. 2

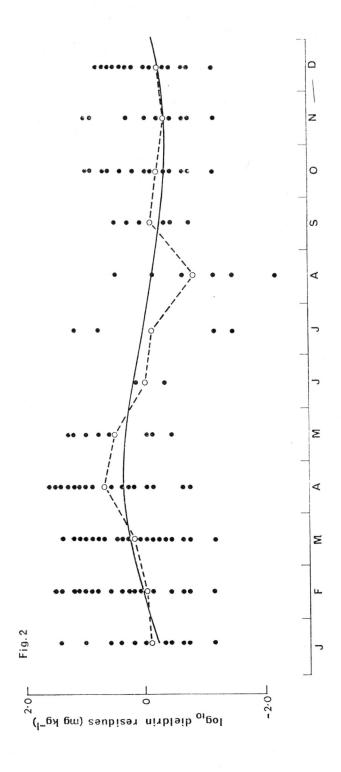

log₁₀ dieldrin residues (mg kg⁻¹)

462

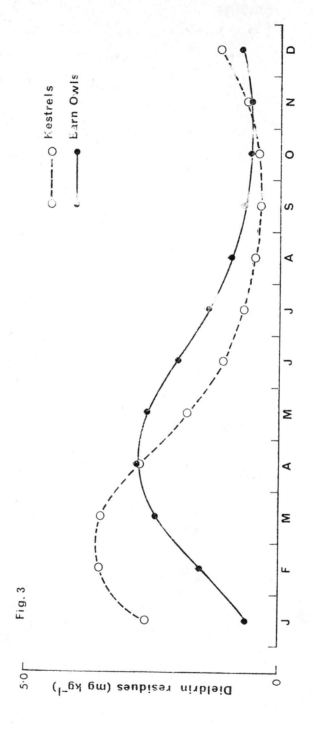

Fig. 3

Between month variance	11	2.3905	F = 6.12, P<0.001
Pooled within month variance	233	0.3907	

test gives 14.35 with 11 degrees of freedom. This value is not significant at the 0.05 level of probability so much of the heterogeneity in the data has been removed. Now the significance of differences between means of the log residues for the 12 months can be tested by the variance ratio test giving:

$$F = 2.390488/0.390663 = 6.12 \text{ with d.f. } 11 \text{ and } 233$$

for which the probability is P<0.01.

Thus, there exist significant differences in mean residues according to the month of collection and this variation needs to be considered in any monitoring scheme.

Fig. 2 plots the means of the transformed data and the mean $\log_{10}$ residue. There are grounds for believing that there could be a second peak in liver residues in some species, consequent on there being more than one period of fat mobilisation. However, there is no evidence to justify this viewpoint in Fig. 2 and it is permissable to attempt to fit regressions to the means. Using a multiple-regression programme, linear, quadratic, cubic and quartic regressions have been attempted and the deviations from these calculated. The results are as summarised:

Linear regression	1	7.077087	18.12**
Quadratic	1	4.070962	10.42**
Cubic	1	6.608811	16.92**
Quartic	1	0.003767	
Deviations	7	8.534745	1.219249	3.12**
Pooled "within months"	233	91.024469	0.390663

The calculations were complicated by the unequal numbers of observations per month. The linear, quadratic and cubic regressions were all highly significant but so were the deviations of the monthly means from the regressions. In spite of this the cubic regression has been fitted to the transformed values in Fig. 2. Obviously, the arithmetic mean is distorted by extreme values and this is largely corrected by the back-tranformation of the mean of the logarithms or by the back-transformation of the cubic regression (see Table 2).

Exactly the same procedures were applied to an analysis of residue data for 276 Kestrels; a preliminary analysis showed no significant differences between adults and juveniles (though with larger samples there would probably prove to be a temporal difference in the time peak liver residues occurred) nor between males and females. Peak liver residues occurred earlier in the year in the Kestrel and this was confirmed by an analysis of variance using Snedecor's (1967) method for an R x 2 table with unequal cell frequencies. In the case of the Kestrel a cubic regression of the transformed data was highly significant but not the deviation. In Fig. 3 the cubic regressions for the Barn Owl and Kestrel are compared having been back-transformed to give a reasonable mean residue in mg kg^{-1} which is not unduly weighted by a relatively small number of high residues.

It can be seen that for both species liver dieldrin residues are higher
in the first part of the year - presumably when fat stores are mobilised
and dieldrin is metabolised in the liver - but that Kestrels exhibit
high liver residues earlier in the season. If sample collection were temporally biased, say to the one month of February, it might be concluded
that Kestrels were prone to dieldrin poisoning, but no Barn Owls. It is
vitally important to understand the ecology and physiology of a species
before selecting it as an indicator - and again it must be emphasised that
the objective of any monitoring scheme needs careful definition. Data are
also available for the Sparrowhawk and this species shows yet another
temporal pattern in dieldrin residues. Formal comparison of three species
over 12 months (or a series of years) by an analysis of variance must involve a complicated R x 3 array with unequal cell frequencies, and the
computation involved becomes prohibitive. Yet the lack of indepence of
variances and means, lack of normality and non-orthogonality must be
countered even if transformations make the data less easy to comprehend.
An alternative is to use a distribution-free non-parametric test such
as the Kruskal-Wallis test, but this necessitates the ranking of all observations. Moreover, if significant differences between months or years
are found, these must be individually sought by paired comparisons - using
say a Mann-Whitney U-test. For practical purposes it seems simplest to perform a logarithmic transformation of residue data to produce homogeneity
and to plot the mean logs with their standard errors. Inspection of the plotted data can then reveal what statistical comparisons are needed.

Liver residues of dieldrin, DDE and PCB's peak at slightly different times
in the three raptors studied intensively, depending on their release from
fat; brain levels would probably show a similar temporal dissociation.
Dieldrin residues were almost certainly obtained from small rodents soon
after the autumn sowings were planted in October-November. In contrast,
most DDT is possibly ingested in late spring when orchards are sprayed.
We have no idea of how and when birds obtain their PCB residues. The correlation of organ residues of organochlorines has frequently been noted and
it is implied that this represents as spatial correlation in the distribution of pollutants. In fact, any correlations are probably temporal and
due to physiological factors.
Table 3 summarises the mean liver residues of three organochlorine residues
according to cause of death, as outlined on p.13. Arithmetic means and
ranges are given without details of sample size or transformation but
appropriate statistical analysis has been performed.
The important point to note is that the circumstances of recovery are
related to residue levels. Road casualties and other traumas underestimate the incidents of deaths caused by dieldrin. Birds carrying high
residues of PCB's are likely to be suffering from some disease. Biases in
sampling would probably arise, whatever method of collection was adopted.
This problem is fundamental to any monitoring exercise.
It follows from this discussion that numerous variables are involved which
complicate comparison of samples collected over a series of years. Indeed
so many variables are involved that great reservation must be placed on
any results. For this reason appropriate data are not included in this paper
but they will be made available for discussion at the workshop. It is felt
that the concept of using a convenient biological species to monitor environmental pollution is based on a false premise and that biological indicators
can only serve to answer specific questions.

Table 3

Mean liver residues of organochlorines in mg kg^{-1} according to circumstances of death in adult Kestrels

		Dieldrin	DDE	PCB's
1. Trauma				
(i)	Road casualty	o.9(o.1-4.o)	2.8(trace-15.o)	4.1(o-25.o)
(ii)	Other trauma	1.3(o.1-9.o)	3.4(o.2-21.o)	4.8(o-25.o)
2. Found dead				
(i)	Haemorrhage	2o.7(o.1-51.7)	11.3(o.4-47.o)	4.7(o-15.o)
(ii)	Disease	2.6(o.1-11.o)	8.9(o.5-55.o)	12.1(o.7-55.o)
(iii)	Negative	7.8(o.4-23.o)	7.6(o-56.o)	11.1(1.o-47.5)

f. Organisational Aspects

Toxic residues in adult birds and their eggs need not imply harmful effects on the population. Other schemes in Britain serve to keep some check on the status of bird and some other animal populations.

The Common Bird Census is a scheme, begun in 1961, run by the British Trust for Ornithology with financial support from Government, under which skilled voluntary observers throughout Britain make regular censuses of the birds of their own farmland study areas, although other habitats are also studied nowadays. The original aim was to provide an index of population fluctuations of the commoner birds, enabling the effects of agricultural change and practice, including pesticide usage, to be monitored. The drawback of this approach is that only territorial males are counted so that if there is a non-breeding surplus this is overlooked. Moreover, pesticides could kill a large proportion of the post-reproduction surplus without this affecting the number of recruits needed to maintain breeding numbers.

The British Trust for Ornithology also sponsors various other programmes, such as the nest record and bird ringing schemes and in the past attempts have been made to use the results to gauge the effects of pesticide induced mortality (Robinson, 1967); unfortunately too many false assumptions were made and the results were equivocable.

The BTO also organises a national heron census whereby either all, or in intervening years a sample of, herons' nests in England and Wales are counted (see Reynolds, 1974). Since the Heron still suffers marked egg shell thinning, around 15 % compared with the pre-1946 situation, due to DDE (Cooke et al., 1976) effects on adult numbers might be expected. In fact, there is no indication that the adult breeding population is affected by this level of breeding failure and the losses are apparently compensated for by a reduction in the juvenile mortality rate. In contrast, reductions in the breeding success of the Sparrowhawk have not been compensated for in this way and the adult population in Britain remains reduced. These examples emphasise that population dynamics of each species must be assessed independently before using bird numbers as a measure of pesticide effects. The BTO have also organised a mapping scheme whereby all breeding species have been plotted on a presence or absence basis in lo km squares throughout Britain and Ireland (Sharrock, 1976). The "Atlas of Breeding Birds in Britain and Ireland" provides a base line against which future population changes can be measured. At present the map shows very clearly the virtual absence of the Sparrowhawk form areas of intensive cereal production.

In the UK the Notification of Pesticides Scheme which became the Pesticides Safety Precautions Scheme was instituted primarily to enable government authorities to control the introduction of new pesticides which might present special risks to persons who applied them or who might consume treated crops. However, not long after the scheme was initiated a government enquiry (Zuckerman Working Party Report No.3) recommended that likely risks to wildlife should be included by the authorities among the criteria for deciding the acceptability of new pesticides and the principle was accepted by the chemical industry and included in the 1957 written description of the scheme (Turtle, 1966). At the time the Infestation Control Division (now PestInfestation Control Laboratory) was concerned with various studies of mammal and bird pests and it was possible to integrate this expertise into the general matters concerned with pesticides and wildlife. The laboratory continues to provide the scientific secretary of the PSPS scheme and through its laboratory facilities any official advice. The laboratory undertook experimental work and investigations immediately prior to the withdrawal of the more toxic seed dressings and from that time has maintained an incident investigation service. The Toxic Chemicals and Wildlife Section of the Nature Conservancy was formed in 1960 to study the ecological effects of pesticides. The Nature Conservancy provided the information on environmental contamination which contributed to the voluntary reduction of uses of aldrin and dieldrin in 1964-5.

Under the PSPS scheme agricultural chemicals are tested for their safety to wildlife before being cleared for use. Nevertheless, after the introduction of pesticides into large scale use, unforeseen hazards may come to light which affect the safety of wildlife and the environment generally. For this reason, both the Ministry of Agriculture, Fisheries & Food and the Department of Agriculture for Scotland provide a regional service under which incidents involving unusual behaviour or deaths of wildlife reported by the public, by natural history organisations or other organisations, are investigated. It was as a result of this follow-up service that the exceptional toxicity of carbophenothion, an organophosphorous compound used as a seed dressing to combat wheat bulb fly and the main replacement for cyclodiene dressings, to grey geese of the genus Anser was identified. The toxicity of this compound to black geese of the genus Branta and to ducks in considerably lower. This case provides a good example of how the most exhaustive laboratory tests and field trials may fail to identify chemical compounds that have a markedly species-specific toxicity so that any screening scheme must be backed up by field investigations. In areas where Anser geese are at risk chlorfenvinphos provides a satisfactory and safe alternative.

To conclude, new chemicals intended for agriculture or food storage use are first screened with standard laboratory tests and limited field trials. Depending on the chemical and its intended use this screening is intensified and more widespread clearance trials are authorised. Eventually, if apparently safe, the compound may be authorised for a defined use. If unforeseen problems arise these may be noticed by the "Wildlife Incident Investigation Scheme". It is at this stage that the widescale monitoring of selected species can provide a further check.

References

Collins, G.B., Holmes, D.C. & Jackson, F.J. (1972): The estimation of polychlorobiphenyls. J. Chromatography 71, 443-449.

Cooke, A.S. (1973): Shell thinning in avian eggs by environmental pollutants. Environ. Pollut. 4, 85-172.

Cooke, A.S. (1975): Pesticides and eggshell formation. Symp. zool.Soc. Lond. 35, 339-361.

Cooke, A.S., Bell, A.A. & Prestt, I. (1976): Egg shell characteristics and incidence of shell breakage for Grey Herons Ardea cinerea exposed to environmental pollutants. Environ. Pollut. 11, 59-84.

Cramer, J. (1973): Model of the circulation of DDT on earth. Atmos. Environ. 7, 241-256.

Cramp, S. (1962): The second Report of the Joint Committee of the British Trust for Ornithology and the Royal Society for the Protection of Birds on Toxic Chemicals. Royal Society for the Protection of Birds.

Cramp, S. (1967): The Sixth Report of the Joint Committee of the British Trust for Ornithology and the Royal Society for the Protection of Birds on Toxic Chemicals. Royal Society for the Protection of Birds.

Doguchi, M. & Fukano, S. (1975): Residue levels of polychlorinated terphenyls, polychlorinated biphenyls and DDT in human blood. Bull. environ. Contam. & Toxicol. 13, 57-63.

De Faubert Maunder, J.J., Egan, H., Godly, E.W., Hammond, E.W. Roburn, J. & Thomson, J. (1964): Clean up of animal fats and dairy products for the analysis of chlorinated pesticide residues. Analyst, Lond. 89, 168-174.

Hassell, K.D. & Holmes, D.C. (1977): Polychlorinated terphenyls (PCT) in some British birds. Bull. Environ. Contam. & Toxicol. 17, 618-621.

Hazeltine, W. (1972): Nature, Lond. 24o, 166.

Holden, A.V. (1975): Monitoring persistent organic pollutants. In: Organochlorine insecticides, ed. F. Moriarty, 1-27. London & New York, Academic Press.

Holmes, D.C., Simmons, J.H. & Tatton, J.O'G. (1967): Chlorinated hydrocarbons in British wildlife. Nature, Lond. 216, 227-229.

Holt, G. & Saskshaug, J. (1968): Organochlorine insecticide residues in wild birds in Norway 1965-1967. Nord. Vet.-Med. 2o, 685-695.

Hunt, E.G. & Bischoff, A.I. (196o): Inimical effects on wildlife of periodic DDD applications to Clear Lake. Calif. Fish Game 46, 91-1o6.

Jensen, S., Johnels, A.G., Olsson, M. & Otterlind, G. (1969): DDT and PCB in marine animals from Swedish waters. Nature, Lond. 224, 247-25o.

468

Koeman, J.H. & Genderen, H. Van (1966): Some preliminary notes on residues of chlorinated hydrocarbon insecticides in birds and mammals in the Netherlands. J. appl. Ecol. 3 suppl. 99-112.

Koeman, J.H., Ensink, H.J.A., Fuchs, P., Hoskam, E.G., Mörzer Bruyns, M.F. & Vos, De R. (1968): Vogelsterfte door landbouwverfigern. Landbouwkundig Tijdschrift 8o, 2o6-214.

Koeman, J.H., Vink, J.A.J. & De Goeij, J.J.M. (1969): Causes of mortality in birds of prey and owls in the Netherlands in the winter of 1968-1969. Ardea 57, 67-76.

Lincer, J.L. (1975): DDE-induced eggshell-thinning in the American Kestrel: A comparison of the field situation and laboratory results. J. appl. Ecol. 12, 781-793.

Moore, N.W. (1966): A pesticide monitoring system with special reference to the selection of indicator species. J. appl. Ecol. 3 suppl. 261-269.

Moore, N.W. & Tatton, J.O'G. (1965): Organochlorine insecticide residues in the eggs of sea birds. Nature, Lond. 2o7, 42-43.

Moore, N.W. & Walker, C.H. (1964): Organic chlorine insecticide residues in wild birds. Nature, Lond. 2o1, 1o72-1o73.

Parslow, J.L.F. & Jefferies, D.J. (1977): Gannets and toxic chemicals. Br. Birds 7o, 366-372.

Parslow, J.L.F. & Moore, N.W. (1972): Monitoring pollutants in seabird eggs. Rep. Monks Wood exp. Stn 1969-71, 2o.

Prestt, I. (1972): Wild birds and chemicals. Gerfaut 62, 127-138.

Prestt, I. & Ratcliffe, D.A. (1972): Effects of organochlorine insecticides on European birdlife. Int. orn. Congr. 15, 486-513.

Ratcliffe, D.A. (1965): Organo-chlorine residues in some raptor and corvid eggs from northern Britain. Br. Birds 58, 65-81.

Ratcliffe, D.A. (1967): Decrease in eggshell weight in certain birds of prey. Nature, Lond. 215, 2o8-21o.

Ratcliffe, D.A. (197o): Changes attributable to pesticides in eggs breakage frequency and eggshell thickness in some British birds. J. appl. Ecol. 7, 67-115.

Reichel, W.L., Prouty, R.M. & Gay, M.L. (1977): Identification of polychlorinated styrene compounds in Heron tissues by gas-liquid chromatography-mass spectrometry. Jnl Ass. Off. Anlyt. Chem. 6o, 6o-62.

Reynolds, C.M. (1974): The census of heronries 1969-73. Bird Study 21, 129-134.

Robinson, J. (1967): Residues of organochlorine insecticides in dead birds in the United Kingdom. Chemy Ind. 1967, 1974-1986.

Sharrock, J.T.R. (Ed.) (1967): The atlas of breeding birds in Britain and Ireland. Berkhamsted, Poyser for BTO and Irish Wildbird Conservancy.

Snedecor, G.W. & Cochran, W.G. (1967): Statistical Methods, 6th ed. Iowa State University Press.

Turtle, E.E. (1966): Assessing likely risk to wildlife from new uses of pesticides: the position under the pesticides safety scheme in the United Kingdom. J. appl. Ecol. 3 suppl. 283-285.

Turtle, E.E., Taylor, A., Wright, E.N.,Thearle, R.J.P., Egan, H., Evans, W.H. & Soutar, N.M. (1963): The effects on birds of certain chlorinated insecticides used as seed dressings. J. Sci. Fd Agric. 14, 567-577.

Walker, C.H. & Mills, D.H. (1965): Organic chlorine insecticide residues in Goosanders and Red-breasted Mergansers. Rep. Wildfowl Trust 16, 56-7.

Walker, C.H., Hamilton, G.A. & Harrison, R.B. (1967): Organochlorine insecticide residues in wild birds in Britain. J. Sci. Fd Agric. 18, 123-129.

Wood, N.F. (1969): Extraction and clean-up of organochlorine pesticide residues by column chromatography. Analyst, Lond. 94, 399-4o5.

Woodwell, G.M., Craig, P.P. & Johnson, H.A. (1971): DDT in the biosphere: where does it go? Science, N.Y. 174, 11o1-11o7.

Zitko, V., Hutzinger, O., Jamieson, W.D. & Choi, P.M.K. (1972): Polychlorinated terphenyls in the environment. Bull. environ. Contam. & Toxicol. 7, 2oo-2o1.

Summary

From 1962 carcases of various predatory birds found dead by members of the public have been sent, in response to advertised appeals, to Monks Wood Experimental Station, Huntingdon, England: initially the scheme was introduced by the Nature Conservancy but since 1973 it has been under the auspices of the Insitute of Terrestrial Ecology.
The scheme was initially introduced to record changes in tissue levels of various organochlorine pesticides to monitor the effects of Government legislation to limit the use of these chemicals. It now represents the longest running monitoring scheme involving birds of prey, with particularly good data refering to the Kestrel, Sparrowhawk, Barn Owl and Heron. In this contribution details of the scheme are outlined and the results discussed in terms of monitoring schemes in general. It is concluded that it is not practical to define indicator species that serve as convenient monitors of unspecified environmental pollutants. It is desirable to define in advance to objective of any programme and to select appropriate methods and species. This follows because there exist wide inter-specific variations in biological response to so-called pollutants, so that any data are most likely to reflect the pecularities of a species' physiology and ecology than trends in residue levels in the environment. This paper provides some evidence for this viewpoint, and it is hoped that the topic will be elaborated in more detail at the workshop in Berlin.

THE ROLE OF DEEP-SEA ORGANISMS IN MONITORING ENVIRONMENTAL
XENOBIOTICS

John Musick
Institute of Marine Science
Gloucester Point VA 23o62
U.S.A.

INTRODUCTION

The living space seaward of the continental margins (2oo m isobath) comprises about 9o percent of the total hydrosphere of the
planet. The oceanic or deep-sea ecosystems found in this living
space are perhaps the farthest removed from sources of human pollution. Can deep-sea organisms presently provide a relatively
unpolluted baseline source for monitoring persistent xenobiotics?
I will attempt to answer this question, and to evaluate the potential of deep sea organisms to future environmental monitoring.

DEEP-SEA ECOSYSTEMS

Pelagic deep sea living spaces have been classified by Brunn (1957),
and Marshall (1971). The most recent faunal classification of benthic deep-
sea living spaces by Menzies et al. (1973) contains much information but
suffers from overgeneralization based on limited taxonomic scope (Musick,
1976a).
I will attempt to provide a brief synoptic description of deep-sea environments. It is convenient (though obviously fallacious) to classify
deep-sea environments as pelagic or benthic. The benthic boundary layer,
that dynamic region where pelagic-benthic interactions occur, is one
of the most important and trophically complex environments in the sea.
Nonetheless, for descriptive purposes, I will describe pelagic ecosystems
first.
From the sea surface down to a depth of about 2oo m is the epipelagic
zone. This zone includes the seasonal thermocline and the euphotic
region where virtually all ecoanic primary production takes place.
Epipelagic creatures are mostly colored deep blue above and white or
silvery below, or are golden brown as the pelagic Sargassum alga which
often abounds at the sea surface. The epipelagic fish fauna includes
many large, migratory species (tunas, billfishes, sharks) which may
spend part of their lives over the continental shelves.
Proceeding deeper below the epipelagic is the mesopelagic zone which
extends down to about 1ooo m. This zone includes much of the permanent
thermocline and its upper part usually includes an oxygen minimum layer
and a high concentration of suspended particulates. This is the "twi-
light" zone where most of the bioluminescent micronektonic and planktonic inhabitants undergo diel vertical migrations, many following re-
treating isolumes toward the surface at night.
Below the mesopelagic is the bathypelagic zone, a cold ($< 4C$), sterile
zone with a very low concentration of suspended particulates and sparse
standing stocks of organisms. Most creatures here are black (fishes)or

red (crustaceans) and are characterized by reduction in anatomical systems (very low tissue density, etc.).

Deep-sea benthic environments are not so easily categorized as are the pelagic. Whereas pelagic ecosystems are mostly effected by temperature, light, depth and availability of nutrients and related primary production, benthic systems are effected by these and other interacting factors such as substrate composition, turbidity currents, nepheloid phenomena, etc.

Many schemes have been put forth to classify benthic deep-sea environments. Most of these are based on a limited taxonomic scope. Sanders and Hessler (1969) studying benthic infauna off New England noted a faunal boundary at the shelfslope break (ca. 2oo m) and a constant, gradual transition of species with depth down into the abyss. Menzies et al. (1973) proposed a rigid system of benthic faunal zonation mostly based on the distribution of isopods. Other authors (Haedrich et al., 1975) have also proposed rigid zonation of benthic faunas, particularly on the continental slope. Musick (1976b) suggested that the demersal fauna was distributed coenoclinally on the outer continental shelf, slope, and rise, and that the coenocline gradient varied bathymetrically. There was not a constant transition of species as suggested by Sanders and Hessler (1969), nor was there rigid faunal zonation as implied by Menzies et al. (1973). Further, there was a faunal mosaic with many groups of species partially overlapping and many species within groups being partially exclusive in bathymetric distribution.

Considering all that has been written recently about benthic faunal patterns in the deep sea, the following consensus emerges: There is a major faunal change at the shelf-slope break (ca. 2oo m). Faunal changes occur most frequently on the continental slope and upper rise (2oo m - ca. 2ooo m) where environmental gradients (light, temperature, available food, substrate compositon) are the steepest. Faunal transitions occur for many taxa within about the same depth regions. Thus off the Northeast coast of the U.S., faunal changes in many taxa occur between 15o-2oo m, 4oo-6oo m, 9oo-1ooo m, 14oo-16oo m, 2ooo-22oo m, and 27oo-29oo m. Beyond 3ooo m we could find little change in the fish fauna, but Menzies et al. (1973) found major changes in isopods. The region of rapid faunal change on the slope (2oo-2ooo m) has been called the bathyal zone (archibenthic of some authors). Beyond the 2ooo m isobath is the abyssal zone.

POTENTIAL XENOBIOTIC TRANSPORT ROUTES

Potential transport routes for xenobiotics into the deep sea should closely parallel energy pathways because many persistent xenobiotics become entrained and magnified in food webs, and/or may be subject to adhesion onto particulate matter which is a major mode of energy transport in the deep-sea. Sedberry and Musick (1978) have recently summarized deep-sea energy parthways thusly:

> Organic matter in the deep sea may be of continental or
> oceanic origin. Organic material of continental origin
> may enter the deep-sea through three modes:
> (1) migration of organisms from continental to oceanic
> water masses; (2) floating terrestrial and neritic plant
> material (Menzies, 1962); and (3) turbidity currents and
> related phenomena (Heezen et al., 1955). The first path-
> way may involve considerable masses of organic material, but

it would affect deep-sea ecosystems only on the upper continental slope (Musick, 1976). The second pathway is difficult to quantify, but probably becomes less important with
distance from the continental margins (Vinogradov, 1962).
The third pathway has been a subject of much conjecture
(Menzies, 1962; Sanders and Hessler, 1969, Rowe, 1972).
Menzies (1962) suggested the importance of turbidity currents as vehicles for energy transport into the deep sea
near the continental margins. However, if the nepheloid
layer is a major energy source for deep-sea communities,
as we have postulated, and if some nepheloid layers have
their origin in turbidity currents, as Eittreim et al.
(1969) have postulated, then such currents may transport
organic matter of continental origin far out onto the continental rise and even onto the abyssal plain.
Organic material of oceanic origin may enter the deep sea
through two modes: (1) settlement of decomposing particulate matter from the photic zone; (2) vertical migrations
of pelagic organisms. Direct transfer or energy by overlapping vertical migrations appears to be an important energy pathway on the continental slope. Beyond the slope,
these two pathways are probably interconnected with
vertical migrations accounting for rapid energy transfer
from the photic zone down to the bathypelagic realm (some-
where between 1ooo and 2ooo m). In deeper water, particulate
matter (of direct phytoplanktonic origin, and from fecal production, death and decomposition at higher trophic levels) slowly settles and the smaller parcels are probably cycled through
the bathypelagic food web during descent (Raymont, 197o). On-
togenetic or seasonal vertical migrations of some mesopelagic
animals down into the bathypelagic must account for periodically rapid transport of energy below the mesopelagic zone.

Organo-Halogenated Compounds

Woodwell et al. (1971) proposed a model to describe the world-wide pattern
of transport of DDT from the land through the atmosphere into the oceans
and into the oceanic abyss. Their model suggested that maximum concentrations of DDT residues occurred in air in 1966 and in the mixed layer of
the ocean in 1971. Although this model has not been without criticism
(Stewart, 1972; Edwards, 1973), Meith-Avcin et al. (1973) found evidence
to support Woodwell et al. from DDT residues in a bathyal, demersal fish,
Antimora rostrata. Specimens of A. rostrata collected at 25oo m off Cape
Hatteras U.S.A. were dissected and their livers were analyzed for residues of: dieldrin, p,p'-DDD; o,p'-DDT;p,p'DDT; aldrin, endrin; heptachlor;
heptachlor epoxide; lindane and mirex. Of these compounds the last six
were undetectable and the authors stated that their absence comprised
"a valuable baseline observation for future monitoring ... in the deep-
ocean environment". In addition Meith-Avcin et al. found an average total
DDT concentration (ppm, wet weight) in A. rostrata livers of 5.4 ppm.
This concentration is more than an order of magnitude higher than those
found in various epipelagic oceanic fishes in 1969 and 197o (Harwey et al.
1972; Duke and Wilson, 1971). Baird et al. (1975) measured DDT and its
metabolites, dieldrin and PCB's in mesopelagic fishes and zooplankton from
the Gulf of Mexico. All the mesopelagic fish species they examined fed

primarily on zooplankton, were small in size (≤ 2oo mm standard length),
and were probably short lived (≤ 3 yrs).
Short life-span does not allow pesticide accumulation in individuals over
a long period of time, but small body size permits whole body analysis of
pooled samples of large numbers of individuals of each species. Also the
tissue of most mesopelagic fishes are rich in lipids for which organochlorine residues have an affinity. Baird et al. (1975) found DDT and its
metabolites in small quantities (ool ppm wet weight) in most fishes and
in some zooplankton samples. Dieldrin occurrence was more sporadic but in
higher concentrations. PCB's were ubiquitous and were one or two orders
of magnitude higher than pesticide residues. Although Harvey et al. (1974)
found no consistent evidence of food chain magnification of PCB and total
DDT residues in pelagic deep-sea food chains, Baird et al. (1975) found
that zooplankton had organochlorine concentrations of one to two orders
of magnitude less than their mesopelagic predators captured at the same
time and depth. This finding supports the hypothesis that organochlorines
tend to accumulate at higher trophic levels in vertebrate predators through
dietary intake. Both studies (Harvey et al., 1974; Baird, et al., 1975)
found evidence that diel vertical migration of mesopelagic organisms is
a significant pathway for chlorinated hydrocarbons from the euphotic zone.
Also, both studies found much higher PCB/DDT ratios then would be postulated from production and release estimates, findings which suggest that
mechansims of uptake and movement of PCB's may be different than for
DDT in oceanic ecosystems. Harvey et al. (1974) pointed out that the lipid
stores of organisms are the major repository for chlorinated hydrocarbons.
Lipid composition may vary among species, and with season, age and body
tissue type. Also, they noted that different lipids are better hydrocarbon solvents than others regardless of the trophic level of the organisms
involved. Therefore there may be many sources of variation in organochlorine concentration in oceanic organisms. One such source of variation,
has been recently reported for zooplankton by Elder and Fowler (1977).
Their findings are significant not only in understanding variations of PCB
concentration in zooplankton but also especially in discovering an important mechanism of flox of PCB's from the epipelagic zone down to abyssal
sediments. Studying the abundant zooplankter, Meganyctiphanes norvegica
(a euphausiid shrimp) Elder and Fowler found that PCB concentrations in
the shrimp's fecal pellets were 1.5×10^6 higher than those in the surrounding ocean water and form 3.5 to 21 times higher than those in the
microplanktonic food organisms which formed the feces. Also, they noted
that fecal PCB concentrations were between 1 and 2 orders of magnitude
higher than those found in whole shrimp bodies or in shrimp molts. They
suggested that sinking zooplankton fecal pellets contribute significantly
to the downward transport of surface-introduced PCB compounds because
the rate of vertical mixing in the ocean is too slow to account for the
quantities of PCB's found in abyssal sediments, and recent studies have
shown that such fecal pellets account for much of the total sedimentation
in the open ocean.

Heavy Metals

Whereas many halogenated hydrocarbons may be transported to the open ocean
through the atmosphere, pathways for heavy metals appear to be slower and
less direct. In addition, burdens imposed by man of some heavy metals such
as mercury (Hg) have had a relatively insignificant effect on their mass
balance in the marine environment (Cross et al., 1973).

Moore (ms.) has recently studied lead (Pb), cadmium (Cd), copper (Cu), zinc (Zn) and mercury (Hg) concentrations in axial muscle tissues of the gadid fish, Phycis chesteri. This species is an ecologically dominant fish in the upper bathyal region (4oo-1ooo m) off the east coast of the U.S.A. (Wenner, 1978) where intensive industrialization has occurred. Even though heavy-metal pollution is a major problem in several riverine and estuarine systems in this area (Huggett et al., 1973; Mueller et al., 1976; Segar and Cantillo, 1976). Moore could find no detectable levels of Cd, Pb or Cu in any of the replicates of P. chesteri he examined. He found a mean Hg concentration of o.o6 ppm (wet weight). A low value within the range found in the upper abyssal fish, Halosauropsis marcrochir, by Barber et al. (1972). In addition, the Zn values Moore found were within the concentrations required for maintenance of enzymatic processes ($\bar{x}$ = 2.1 ppm). Moore found no significant correlation between the concentrations of either Hg or Zn and the length or weight of the P. chesteri he examined, probably because the size and age range of his sample was limited. Cross et al. (1973) found that the concentrations of Hg increased significantly with fish size in white muscle of the coastal pelagic fish, Pomatomus saltatrix, and the bathyal demersal fish Antimora rostrata, but that concentration of manganese (Mn), iron (Fe), copper (Cu) and zinc (Zn) remained constant or decreased. They interpreted these results to mean that these two fishes were in a steady state with the environment with respect to Mn, Fe, Cu, and Zn, but only Hg. They further suggested that the extremely high electronegativity of Hg relative to the other metals, and the high lipid solubility of methyl mercury could reduce the capacity of fishes to regulate mercury in their tissues. Consequently muscle of marine fishes may never achieve a steady state with environmental levels of Hg, and length of the life span may be an important factor in controlling absolute levels of Hg in fish muscle. Thus, older (larger) specimens should have higher concentrations than younger (smaller) specimens. Barber et al. (1975) found such a relationship in axial muscle in Antimora rostrata collected in the early 197o's and in museum specimens collected in the 18oo's (correlation coefficients = o.8o-o.9o). However, they did not find a relationship between size and Hg concentration in two other groups of upper abyssal fishes, halosaurs and macrourids of the genus Coryphaenoides (=Chalinura). Through the kindness of P.J. Whaling, I have examined the original data of Barber et al. (1975). They included several species of halosaurs in one regression analysis and at least two species of Coryphaenoides in another. Inter-specific differences in growth, maximum age, food habits, etc. may be substantial in these groups and it is not surprising that regression showed no correlation between size and Hg concentration. Barber et al. examined Hg concentrations in the liver, brain, and gill tissues of their specimens, in addition to the axial muscle. Gill tissue concentrations remained the same regardless of fish size. Brain tissue concentration showed no pattern. Concentrations in the liver increased with size (generally) in A. rostrata, but patterns were not clear in the other two groups of fishes. One surprising finding was that Hg concentration in liver tissue of halosaurs was an order of magnitude higher than in the muscle, whereas in the other fishes liver concentrations were usually about half that of muscle concentrations. Halosaurs tend to be more strictly benthic in their diets (ingesting much sediment) than are A. rostrata or the macrourids studied. Perhaps dietary or physiological differences may account for the differing distribution of Hg in the tissues.
Apparently the more usual situation for oceanic fishes is for higher Hg

concentrations to occur in the muscle than in liver. Greig and Wenzloff (1977) found this to be the case in large epipelagic sharks they studied. In contrast, Greig and Wenzloff found Cd levels to be consistently higher in shark liver tissue than in the muscles. These same authors also reported on trace metal concentrations of pooled samples of whole mesopelagic fishes and euphausid shrimps. Values of Ag, Cd, Cr, Cu, Hg, Ni, and Zn in four different species of these small short-lived fishes, and mixed samples of shrimp were low (Hg values <o.lo ppm wet weight) as would be expected.

FACTORS OF IMPORTANCE IN MONITORING TISSUES OF DEEP-SEA ANIMALS

The foregoing discussion suggests that there may be many sources of variation of xenobiotic burdens in deep-sea organisms. Among these are: trophic position, inter-specific physiological differences, tissue type, size, and age. In addition, unpublished work at the Virginia Institute of Marine Science on the halogenated hydrocarbon, Kepone suggests that body burdens in some fishes and crustaceans are sexually related. Kepone is lipid soluble and may become incorporated into the high lipid ova of certain species. Consequently, female animals may periodically purge their body burden of Kepone during spawning. This phenomenon leads to lower and more variable Kepone concentrations in females of some species than males. Whaling (personal communication) has found in bluefish (Pomatomus saltatrix) and in certain species of marlin that Hg concentrations are correlated with size but that concentrations in females are much more variable than in males. Perhaps because methyl mercury is lipid soluble this compound may be eliminated in the ova of these fishes during spawning much as some of the halogenated hydrocarbons probably are.

DEEP-SEA TISSUE BANKING - A PILOT PROGRAM

Based on existing baseline information, availability of material, and cost I recommend the following pilot program:

a. epipelagic zone:
    Liver and axial muscle tissue should continue to be sampled from the blue shark, Prionace glauca, a large oceanic predator, ubiquitous to temperate and subtropical seas.

b. mesopelagic zone:
    Whole fish samples pooled by species of common myctophids such as Ceratoscopelas sp., Myctophum sp. etc. should be continued to be sampled. These genera or their ecological equivalents are found in all seas (except perhaps in extreme polar environments). Samples should include at least 5o specimens of both sexes ranging in size form 5o to ca 15o mm standard length. Samples of euphausids pooled by species such as Meganyctiphanes norvegica should also continue to be sampled.

c. bathyal and abyssal zones:
    Liver and axial muscle tissue should continue to be sampled from Antimora rostrate, a medium-sized predator that occurs or has congeners in the major ocean basins. In addition, sampling should be begun on whole specimens of the common holuthurian genus Molpadia. These burrowing, sediment-ingesting, deposit feeders are ubiquitous and the group includes several species found at various depth ranging from the continental shelf to the abyss.

Tissue samples from medium and large animals should be collected from at least 5o specimens from a given geographic area, within a reasonably synoptic time frame (i.e., about one month maximum). Collections should include a wide range in size of individuals and both sexes. All of this information must be retained with each sample. Frequency and geographic extent of sampling should be determined within the framework of the overall pilot program.

COLLECTION, TRANSPORTATION AND STORAGE OF MATERIALS

The collection suggested above must be made from ships. Ships can be incredible sources of contamination, when attempting to sample xenobiotics. These problems and protocol by which to avoid them have been discussed by Grice et al. (1972) and Harvey and Teal (1974). It is imperative that every precaution be taken to avoid contamination of biological material with known xenobiotics (trace metals, halogenated hydrocarbons, and other hydrocarbons).
I assume that storage of materials will be in the frozen condition or perhaps by freeze-drying. Gibbs et al. (1974) have pointed out the problems in interpreting heavy metal data from biological specimens kept in traditional museum preservatives. Similar problems must exist for halogenated hydrocarbons also, because the lipids in which they are dissolved in turn may be leached out into the alcohol preservatives in which the specimens are stored.

SUMMARY

Deep-sea ecosystems can provide valuable baseline information about the extent of the world-wide distribution of xenobiotics. For some xenobiotics such as trace metals the deep-ocean may presently provide a baseline relatively uneffected by man. For other xenobiotics such as DDT and PCB's the deep-ocean can provide an index of atmospheric and oceanic processes of degradation and accumulation. Deep-ocean sediments may be the ulitmate depository for such halogenated hydrocarbons.

ACKNOWLEDGEMENT

Thanks are due to P.J. Whaling of Duke University Marine Laboratory and to K.A. Moore of the Virginia Institute of Marine Science for providing me with copies of unpublished data and manuscripts, and to R. Carney of the U.S. National Museum of Natural History, Invertebrate Division, for suggestions pertaining to the suitability of deep-sea holothurians as xenobiotics monitoring targets.

LITERATURE CITED

Baird, R.L., N.P. Thompson, T.L. Hopkins, and W.R. Weiss. 1975: Chlorinated hydrocarbons in mesopelagic fishes of the Eastern Gulf of Mexico. Bull. Mar. Sci. 25(4): 473-481.

Barber, R.T., A. Vijayakumar, F.A. Cross. 1972: Mercury concentrations in recent and ninety-year-old benthopelagic fish. Science 178: 638-639.

Barber, R.T., P.J. Whaling, and D.M. Cohen. 1975: Factors affecting mercury concentrations in recent and old bathydemersal fish. (abst.) Environ. Health Perspectives.1o: 261.

Brunn, A.F. 1957: Deep sea and abyssal depths. Geol. Soc. America, Mem. 67(1): 641-672.

Cross, F.A., L.H. Hardy, N.Y. Jones, and R.T. Barber. 1973: Relation between total body weight and concentrations of manganese, iron, copper, zinc and mercury in white muscle of bluefish (Pomatomus saltatrix) and a bathyal-demersal fish Antimora rostrata. J. Fish. Res. Bd. Can. 3o: 1287-1291.

Duke, T.W. and A.J. Wilson. 1971: Chlorinated hydrocarbons in livers of fishes from the northeastern Pacific ocean. Pesticides monitoring Journal 5(2): 228-232.

Edwards, J.G. 1973: DDT in British Rain. Science 179: 956.

Elder, D.L. and S.W. Fowler. 1977: Polychlorinated Biphenyls: Penetration into the deep ocean by zooplankton. Fecal pellet transport. Science, 197: 359-461.

Gibbs, R.H., E. Jarosewich, and H.L. Windom. 1975: Heavy metal concentrations in museum fish specimens. Effects of preservatives and time. Science 184: 475-477.

Greig, R., D. Wenzloff. 1977: Final report on heavy metals in small pelagic finfish, euphausid crustaceans and apex predators, including sharks, as well as heavy metals and hydrocarbons (C15+) in sediments collected at stations in and near Deepwater Dumsite 1o6. U.S. NOAA Dumpsite Evaluation Report, 77-1, Vol. 3: 547-564.

Grice, G.D., G.R. Harvey, V.T. Bowen, and R.H. Backus. 1972: The collection and preservations of open ocean marine organisms for pollutant analysis. Bull. Envir. Contam. and Tox., 7: 125-132.

Haedrich, R.L., G.T. Rowe, and P.T. Polloni. 1975: Zonation and faunal composition of epibenthic populations on the continental slope south of New England. J. Mar. Res. 33: 191-212.

Harvey, G.R., V.T. Bowen, R.H. Backus, and G.D. Grice. 1972: Chlorinated hydrocarbons in open-ocean Atlantic organisms. In "The Changing Chemistry of the Oceans", D. Dyrssen and D. Jaquer eds., Wiley Interscience: 177-186.

Harvey, G.R., H.P. Miklas, V.T. Bowen and W.G. Steinhauer. 1974: Observationson the distribution of chlorinated hydrocarbons in Atlantic ocean organisms.J. Mar. Res. 32 (2): 1o3-118.

Harvey, G.R. and J.M. Teal. 1973: PCB and hydrocarbon contamination of plankton by nets. Bull. Environ. Contam. and Tox. 9: 287-29o.

Hugget, R.J., M.E. Bender, and H.D. Slone. 1973: Utilizing metal concentration relationships in the eastern oyster (Crossostrea virginica) to detect heavy metal pollution. Water Res. 7: 451-46o.

Marshall, N.B. 1971: Explorations in the Life of Fishes. Harvard Un. Press. Cambridge Mass: 2o4 pp.

Meith-Avcin, N., S.W. Warlen and R.T. Barber. 1973: Organic chlorine insecticide residues in a bathyl-demersal fish from 2,5oo meters. Environmental letters. 5(4): 215-221.

Menzies, R.J., R.Y. George, and G.T. Rowe. 1973: Abyssal environment and ecology of the world oceans. John Wiley and Sons. New York: 488 pp.

Moore, K.A. (Unpubl. Ms.). Trace metal concentrations in the bathyl fish Phycis chesteri (Pisces, Gadidae) off Virginia. Va. Inst. Mar. Sci., Gloucester Point, VA: 9 pp.

Mueller, J.A., A.R. Johnson, and J.S. Jeris. 1976: Contaminants entering the New York bight: Sources, Mass loads, significance. In Middle Atlantic continental shelf and the New York bight, special symposia. Vol.2. M. Grant Gross (ed.). Amer. Soc. Lim. Ocean. :162-17o.

Musick, J.A. 1976a: Review of: Abyssal Environment and Ecology of the World Oceans, by R.J.Menzies, R.J. George and G.T. Rowe, Trans. Amer. Fish. Soc. Io5(4): 571-573.

Musick, J.A. 1976b: Community structure of fishes on the continental slope and rise off the middle Atlantic coast of the U.S. (abstr.) Joint oceanographic assembly, Edinburgh. Sec C 5/11: p 146.

Sanders, H.L. and R.R. Hessler. 1969: Ecology of the deep-sea benthos. Science. 163: 1419-1424.

Sedberry, G.R. and J.A. Musick. 1978: Feeding strategies of şome demersal fishes of the continental slope and rise off the mid-Atlantic coast of the U.S.A. Mar. Biol. 44: 357-375.

Segar, D.A. and A.Y. Cantillo. 1976: Trace metals in the New York bight. In Middle Atlantic continental shelf and the New York bight, special symposia, Vol.2. M. Grant Gross (ed.) Amer. Soc. Lim. Ocean. :171-198.

Stewart, C.A. 1972: Atmospheric circulation of DDT. Science, 177: 724-725.

Wenner, C.A. 1978: Making a living on the continental slope and in the deep sea. Life history of some dominant fishes of the Norfolk Canyon. area. Ph.D. disseration submitted to the School of Marine Science College of William and Mary: 294 pp.

Wenner, C.A. and J.A. Musick. 1977: Contribution to the ecology and life history of the morid fish, Antimora rostrata, in the western north Atlantic. J.Fish.Res.Bd. Canada. 34: 2362-2368.

Woodwell, G.M., P.P. Craig, and H.A. Johnson. 1971: DDT in the Biosphere: Where does it go? Science 174: 11o1-11o7.

THE GREY MULLET (MUGIL CEPHALUS L.) AS A MARINE BIO-INDICATOR

Colin E. Nash, Ph. D.
Kramer, Chin & Mayo, Inc.,
Seattle, Washington
U.S.A.

Abstract

The grey mullet, Mugil cephalus L, has unique qualities which make it potentially useful as a bio-indicator of the aquatic environment. This teleoste-
an fish has a worldwide geographic distribution from the temporate to the
trophic zones and is common to most coastal waters. It is a euryhaline species spending most of its life history in estuaries and brackishwater areas,
migrating annually to sea to spawn. It is a detritus and algae feeder, also
consuming particulate matter in the substrate.
Adult fish, about 1 kg in weight, are captured in many coastal fisheries.
They provide almost the only available animal protein for the subsistence
of the coastal populations of many less developed countries. It can be captured easily by gillnet. In addition to man, predators of the adults are
the higher carnivorous fishes and some marine mammals; and the juveniles
make up an important part of the diet of the wading birds and fishes in the
estuarine ecosystem.
The fish is farmed extensively because of its high tolerance to wide ranges
of temperature (3-36°C) and salinity (o-75 °/oo), and its affinity for schooling which permits intensive stocking. Its flesh is of high quality, and
the body size is appropriate for sampling. Data indicate that the tissues
are good accumulators without preconcentration for analyses.

Introduction

The grey mullet are representatives of a truly international group of fish
in the family Mugilidae (order Mugiliformes). They make up an important and
probably the most widely distributed commercial fishery in the world's coastal waters, and they are of significant importance meeting the subsistence
protein requirements of the peoples of the Pacific Basin, Southeast Asia,
India, the Mediterranean and Eastern European countries, and in many parts
of Central and South America. Mullet and mullet products contribute to small
but valuable fishery economies in many European countries, the southern
United States of America, Japan and Australia. Most of the grey mullet species
are fished to some extent, but the individual species with the greatest distribution and importance in the family is Mugil cephalus Linnaeus. Because
of its biological behavior, size and nutritional quality, M. cephalus cons-
titutes certain key continental shelf or inshore fisheries all over the world,
and its protein value is utilized immediately by the local populace. Its
life history and biological behavior place it in the key environmental
niche at the interface between fresh and saltwater.

History and Taxonomy

As the freshwater Chinese and Indian carps are part of the history of Asia, so the mullet have an established place in the archives of civilization from the area of the Mediterranean. The mullet were well known and liked by the ancient Greeks and Romans and appeared in literature and sculptured friezes. They were abundant and obtainable from the shallow coastal waters of the northern Mediterranean Sea. Mullet later appeared in the collections and compendia of Agricola in the 15th Century, and their descriptions preserved in the great natural history records of Gesner and Fuchs in the 16th Century. The common mullet were therefore repeatedly fixed into the animal phyla by the pre-evolutionary naturalists whose numbers expanded rapidly after Linnaeus produced his more orderly taxonomic system in the 18th Century. Undoubtedly mullet were used to typify a marine fish for teaching the new and exacting branch of biology called taxonomy, which was popular at the time. Overenthusiasm may therefore have been responsible for the many species of mullet which were "discovered" around the world and named in the 19th Century, and for the accusations against Linnaeus that he had confused all the Mediterranean and European species and given them one name. But, in retrospect, he was more correct in conservative recognition of new mullet species in his time.

M. cephalus is distributed abundantly throughout the subtropic regions and extends geographically approximately between the latitudes of 42° north and 42° south in all coastal waters (Figure 1). Because of this vast distribution there is still some confusion of the genera. Thomson (1966) accepted 13 genera and recorded 281 nominate species of mullets of which he recognized 7o as valid and a further 32 indeterminate for lack of better descriptions. M. cephalus alone has at least 33 scientific synonyms; and the common names, such as "grey", "striped", "silver grey", "black", "sea", and "jumping" mullet (among others) are all freely interchanged. It is therefore essential that the common name is frequently coupled with the scientific name in the literature of the Mugilidae.

The credit for first simplifying the taxonomy of a confused, largely uniform genera goes to Schultz (1946) who demonstrated that the differences between them were mostly identifiable by the diversity of the parts of the mouth and head. Microscopic examination of the tooth structure and in the patterns of dentition (Thomson, 1975), the lips, the adipose eyelids and facial morphometrics are the most commonly used features. There are, however, continual proponents for (among others) osteology (Luther, 1975), and muscle protein electrophoresis (Herzberg and Pasteur, 1975). Added to the taxonomic picture there is the evidence that races of mullet can be determined within regions by identification of the eye lens proteins (Peterson and Shehadeh, 1971).

Life history
Environment and Feeding

The environmental behavior, food preference and feeding in the nearshore waters, together place M. cephalus and other mullet species at the important environmental interface between the land and the sea. With the exception of one or two species which have adapted entirely to freshwater conditions, the mullet are euryhaline and can be found in most coastal environments. M. cephalus is probably the most oceanic of all the species and is common to most of the islands of the Pacific and Indian Oceans. But it can also tolerate freshwater conditions for prolonged periods, as well as the hypersaline lagoons of Africa. It is more commonly found and grows faster in the brackishwater areas of the subtropics, and is the preferred fish for mullet farming.

The farming of mullet has been practiced for centuries in many parts of the world. Farming probably originated in the low-saline waters of the northern Mediterranean Sea in the tradionally owned extensive "valli" of Italy. Today there are still farms in the region mixing mullet farming with eels and sea bass (de Angelis, 1969). In Taiwan mullet are reared in brackishwater with milkfish and shrimp (Tang, 1964) or in freshwater ponds with carp (Chen, 1977); in the coastal farms of the Philippines, India and Israel; and in the oceanic environments of the ancient fishponds of the Polynesians in Hawaii and other Pacific Islands.

The physiology of the adult mullet in the breeding season demands that M. cephalus and the majority of all the mullet move out into oceanic waters to spawn. Consequently, the mullet are, for the most part, recognized as catadromous migratory fish. In its breeding season, depending on locality, the large schools of M. cephalus move from the estuaries and migrate to the offshore breeding grounds. This is the time that the mullet schools are most heavily fished. Not all the adult fish migrate, and on the spawning run little or not food is consumed (Kesteven, 1942), mainly because the fish are outside the environment that contains their preferred feeds.

The food of the adult M. cephalus is predominantly a mixture of diatoms, blue-green and filamentous green algae grazed from rocks and other surfaces, together with detritus that is sucked and strained from the bottom. Some small crustaceans are also consumed. Characteristic of the mullet species the fish take particulate bottom material, such as mud and sand, into the gizzard to aid in the trituration of the high cellulose content of the plants consumed.

Emergent larvae of the grey mullet are believed to be entirely carnivorous during early development, becoming omnivorous and capable of digesting plant material sometime before metamorphosis.

The selection of the food organism by the larvae is, in all probability, made on the simple criteria of movement and size in the first instance. The ability of larvae to feed is regulated by feeding behavior and vision. As with many marine and brackishwater species, the eyes of the larvae of Mugilidae are large at hatching and become rapidly pigmented within three days. The eyes are only capable of coarse movement perception and, as with other fish species, are poorly equipped with a single type of visual cell. They have little ability to adapt to dark or light situations during the first hours after hatching.

The dearth of larval Mugilidae in plankton tows is responsible for the lack of information on their natural foods during this critical stage of development. This scarcity of knowledge during the first formative 5o days of life is to some extent compensated by the wealth of data on growth, food, and feeding habits of juveniles and adults of Mugilidae from regions throughout the world, e.g., Hiatt, 1944; Jacob and Krishnamurthi, 1948; Thomson, 1954; Sarojini, 1957; Hickling, 197o; Zismann et al., 1974; Cech and Wohlschlag, 1975; Grant and Spain, 1975; Chervinski, 1976; and Marais and Erasmus, 1977.

Young mullet develop scales in the early postlarval stages (between 8-1o mm in length) and are soon well developed (12-14 mm in length). Young mullet which first appear in small schools along the coasts and in the estuaries are fully scaled. They measure between 18-28 mm in length. Extrapolated growth data for the species indicate that young of this size are between 3o and 45 days old. The transition stage from postlarvae to juveniles does not occur until the young are between 35-45 mm in length or between 45 and 6o days old. Thomson (1963) regarded the transition complete at about 5o mm when the third anal spine formed from the anterior ray and the adipose eyelid started to form.

482

Egg and larval development

The natural spawning locations of grey mullet species which have been described or deduced by many workers throughout the world, do not indicate specific and similar environmental patterns. The picture overall is confused
both by misindentification of generic types observed and the variety of
facts on which the spawning record is being made. For example, many reports are based on the collection of adult fish with ripe gonads - usually
loose eggs: others describe small numbers of eggs or larvae in plankton
tows and make predictions about the spawning location based on tidal movement and stage of development of the samples. Some reports describe inshore
schooling and then a migration offshore, presumed to be for spawning;
others describe schooling inshore for spawning. The location of spawning
grounds for the mullet can only be described as controversial. Table 1
summarizes the spawning seasons of M. cephalus.
Environmental data on the temperature of the water during spawning of M.
cephalus indicates some adaptation from region to region, with temperatures
recorded between 12-24°C. All records show a strong preference by the fish
for oceanic water as the medium for incubation, with salinities between
32-35 °/oo.
Fertilized eggs of the Mugilidae are spherical and transparent. The surface
of the egg shell is smooth and unsculptured. The yolk appears unsegmented
and there is predominantly one large oil globule making them extremely
buoyant. The eggs are not adhesive.
Yashouv and Berner-Samsonov (197o),in an extensive contribution to the knowledge of eggs and early larval stages of Mugilidae, reviewed data of egg
and oil globule diameters in samples from M. cephalus, M. capito, M. auratus
and M. chelo at a variety of locations. They included some data from the
synopses on M. cephalus prepared by Thomson (1963 and 1966). The comprehensive data revealed a wide range of diameters reported for the same species
in different locations.
Kuo et al. (1973a)reported the mean egg diameter of fertilized eggs of M.
cephalus as 93oμ, with a range of 88o-98oμ. The single large oil globule
had a uniform diameter of 33oμ. Tung (1973) quoted a mean egg diameter
of o.89 mm for the same species, and oil globule diamter of o.39 mm. Nash
et al. (1974) specified a mean egg diameter of o.93 mm.
Bromhall (1954), Sarojini (1958), Erman (1961) and Hickling (197o) examined
the gonads of several species of mullet, including M. cephalus, and observed
that their state of development was often consistent with a seasonal production of more than one batch of eggs, possibly within a period of a month.
Kuo et al. (1973b) demonstrated that M. cephalus could be inducted to spawn
more than once a year.
Thomson (1963) reviewed a number of papers which reported the fecundity
of M. cephalus in terms of total egg numbers. He quoted estimates of between
1.2-2.8 million eggs per fish. Hickling (197o) and others listed the fecundity of several species of grey mullet as follows:

Species	Thousand eggs/Kg		Author and year
L. cunnesius	15-	57	After Sarojini (1958)
A. forsteri	126-	65o	Thomson (1955)
L. parsia	2oo-	6oo	Sarojini (1957)
C. labrosus	372-	745	Hickling (197o)
L. ramada	581-	1.243	Hickling (197o)
M. cephalus	1.2oo-	2.8oo	Thomson (1963)
M. cephalus	3.6oo-	7.2oo	Nikolskii (1954)
M. cephalus	1.572-	4.774	Grant and Spain (1975)

Kuo et al. (1973a) determined the fecundity of M. cephalus to be about
648 eggs/g body weight of three-year-old fish. Nash et al. (1974) quoted
849 eggs/g for older individuals. Liao et al. (1972) reported o.7-1.9 million per fish.

Egg development and hatching time are both temperature dependent. Tang
(1964) reported that hatching of M. cephalus took place in 59-64 hours
at temperatures ranging from 2o.o-24.5°C and salinity from 24.39-35.29 °/oo
Fertilization was low (32 percent)and the rate of hatching was below lo percent. Yashouv and Berner-Samsonov (197o) noted that, under laboratory conditions, the eggs of M. cephalus and M. capito developed and hatched within
36-44 hours at 22-32°C. Kuo et al. (1973a) stated that hatching of M. cephalus eggs was evident 36-38 hours after fertilization at 24°C, and 48-
5o hours at 22°C. Total length of the newly hatched larvae was 2,65 ± o.23
mm. Salinity was 32 °/oo.

Liao (1974) stated that hatching of M. cephalus eggs took place in 34-38
hours at 23-24.5°C, and at 49-54 hours in 22.5-23.7°C, with salinities
between 3o.1 and 33.8 °/oo. Tung (1973) described the relationships between
mean water temperature (θ) and duration of incubation period (T) as $T_e^{0.135}$
$\theta = 1,262$ in still water, and as $T_e^{0.037\theta} = 1o6$ in running water. Finally,
Sebastian and Nair (1974) recorded the incubation time of M. macrolepis
at 23 hours between 26-29°C and 29-31°/oo salinity.

Nash et al. (1974), Sylvester and Nash (1975), and Nash and Kuo (1975) report the survival of eggs of M. cephalus within broad ranges of temperature
salinity and dissolved oxygen. Their results are summarized in Figure 2.
Minimal mortalities of eggs occurred at 22°C for normal seawater (32 °/oo ,
and an effective temperature range for incubation was 11-24°C.

Some of the first descriptions on the morphology of the larvae of Mugilidae
were made by Sanzo. He observed and illustrated the early stages of M.
chelo and M. cephalus (1936), and M. labeo (1937). He considered their pro-
larvae to be poorly developed. They measured only 2.2-2.5 mm in length. The
mouth was closed and there was no trace of a branchial skeleton. Characteristic of each larvae was a voluminous yolk sac and large oil globule often accompanied by smaller oil droplets.

The first complete morphologic descriptions of larvae of Mugilidae were
made by those workers involved in the induced spawning of the adults by
hormone injection. Mostly they described the development of M. cephalus.
Among them were Tang (1964), Yashouv (1969), Yashouv and Berner-Samsonov
(197o), Liao et al. (1971), Kuo et al. (1973a), and Tung (1973).

Newly hatched larvae of M. cephalus vary in length between 2.2 and 3.5 mm.
The oil globule (and any additional small droplets) is situated in the pos-
terior part of the yolk. Tung (1973) recorded 24 myotomes. He described the
anterior half of the body bent on the yolk sac. The larvae had five or
six pairs of cupulae on the body side from eye to tail, and several pairs
on the front of the head. Feeding began three to five days after hatching.
Yashouv and Berner-Samsonov (197o) gave full descriptions of the keys to
the eggs and larvae of five mullet species: M. cephalus, M. capito, M.
saliens, M. chelo, and M. auratus.

The eggs of most marine and brackishwater species are liberated into oceanic waters and, with the emergent larvae, are adapted to develop at high
salt concentrations. However, the effect of salinity on larval survival
and development is possibly more significant than that for incubation of
the eggs. Sylvester and Nash (1975) provided tolerance levels of larvae
of M. cephalus to varying salinities (Figure 3). They showed that the larvae
could only withstand prolonged exposures to salinity between 25-34 °/oo at
2o°C during the first week of development, with an optimum at 26-28 °/oo for

96 hour exposure.
Emergent and developing larvae up to metamorphosis tolerate an ever wide-
ning temperature range and their growth rate responds accordingly. Liao
(1974) reported the successful culture of the larvae of M. cephalus over a
number of preceding years within the ambient temperature range of 19-24°C.
Sylvester and Nash (1975) recorded minimum mortality of the larvae of M.
cephalus between 18.9 and 25.3°C, although some larvae survived temperatures as low as 15.9°C and as high as 29.1°C.
Little information exists on the levels of dissolved oxygen suitable for
the larvae of the Mugilidae. Although the levels of dissolved oxygen are
measured regularly as part of many culture operations, the data are often
excluded. Sylvester and Nash (1975) determined that the survival of the
larvae of M. cephalus was significantly changed for mean oxygen concentrations below 5.4 ppm (Figure 3), Liao (1974) noted that the larvae were sensitive to light. Four-day-old larvae exhibited phototaxis and six-day-old
larvae migrated vertically according to the time of day, but fed only in
the day. Larvae avoided strong illumination but were attracted by dim light
intensity of about 6oo-1.4oo lux.
Lee et al. (1975) studied the effects of two chlorinated insecticides,
mirex and methoxychlor, on eggs, larvae juvelines and adults of the striped
mullet, Mugil cephalus L. in Hawaii. Test concentrations of both insecticides used were o.ol, o.l, 1.o and lo.o mg/l in dynamic bioassays of juveniles and adults and static bioassays of eggs and larvae. Young juveniles
standard length 2o-43 mm, were apparently more susceptible to mirex exposure than older juveniles, standard length 7o-15o mm, and adults, standard length 26o-38o mm. No mortalities occurred in older juveniles and
adults exposed to mirex for 96 hours. Young juveniles exposed to o.1 and
1.o mg/l of mirex had higher mortality rates (27 and 32 percent) than control fish, but mortalities of o.ol- and lo.o-mg/l exposed fish were not
different from controls. Significant amounts of mirex residues were accumulated in the body tissue of the test fish. Juveniles and adults exposed
to o.ol mg/l mirex were found to accumulate o.2 and o.4 µg/g respectively
during the bioassays. The concentrations in fish increased with increasing mirex concentrations in test water. The highest accumulation was found
in the adult fish exposed to lo.o mg/l (37 µg/g).
Methyoxychlor was more toxic to mullet than mirex. Mortalities were greater
than 9o percent over a 96-hour period for juvenile and adult fish at concentrations of o.1, 1.o and lo.o mg/l. Methoxychlor residues accumulated in
the tissues of test fish in samaller amounts than mirex-exposed fish. Young
adults and juveniles exposed to o.ol mg/l methoxychlor accumulated o.1
and o.2 µg/g respectively. The accumulated amounts in lo.o mg/l concentration were 1.7 µg/g for young juveniles and 11.1 µg/g for adult fish.

Predation

As an abundant predominantly herbivorous fish, the mullet play a key role
in the coastal ecosystem. In addition to extensive harvesting by man within
the coastal fisheries, most of which is used as animal protein direct for
human consumption, the mullet are part of the diet of many marine mammals.
In the tropics and subtropics the most common predators are the local
seals. Adult mullet also fall prey to many of the larger carnivorous reef
fishes, particularly the sharks. However, the sparse records indicate that
predation on the adults mostly coincides with the large migrating schools
of fish, and the congregation of schools in certain areas for spawning.

FIGURE 1
GEOGRAPHIC DISTRIBUTION OF
M. CEPHALUS

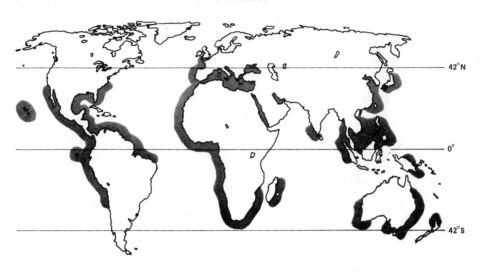

TABLE 1
SEASONAL SPAWNING OF *M. CEPHALUS*
ACCORDING TO GEOGRAPHIC REGION
(After Many Authors)

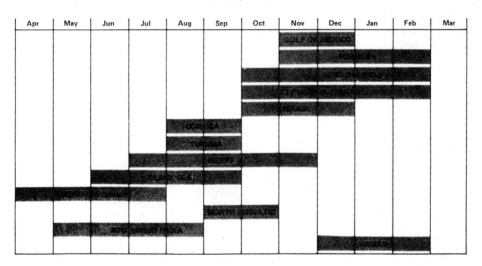

486

FIGURE 2
EGG SURVIVAL (%) AT
VARYING INCUBATION PARAMETERS
(After Nash *et. al.*, 1974; Sylvester and Nash, 1975;
Nash and Kuo, 1975)

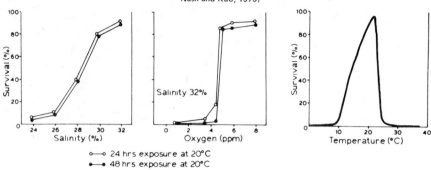

o—o 24 hrs exposure at 20°C
•—• 48 hrs exposure at 20°C

FIGURE 3
LARVAL SURVIVAL (%) AT VARYING SALINITY,
TEMPERATURE, AND OXYGEN LEVELS
(After Sylvester and Nash, 1975;
Nash and Kuo, 1975)

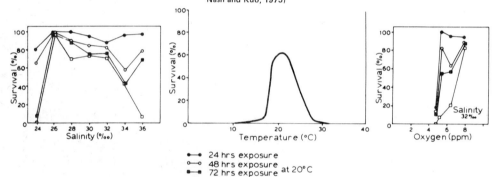

•—• 24 hrs exposure
o—o 48 hrs exposure
■—■ 72 hrs exposure   at 20°C
□—□ 96 hrs exposure

FIGURE 4
EXPLOSIVE SPAWNING OF MULLET
IN CAPTIVITY WHICH PROVIDES THE
CAPABILITY OF LABORATORY TEST ANIMALS
FOR BIOASSAY

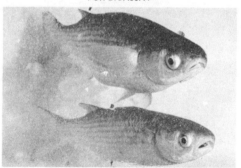

The heaviest predation occurs when the juveniles are feeding along the coastal waters. The juveniles are extremely abundant and a composite part of the diet of many carnivorous brackishwater fish, such as the sea bass, the eel, flunder and garfish. More importantly, the juveniles are a significant part of the diet of the wading birds of the world, predominantly the herons, and the kingfishers.

Summary

In summary, the mullet are a direct link between the deestritus and aquatic plants of the estuarine environment, and the higher birds and animals, including man. Throughout the critical early life stages and the first two years of growth, the mullet remain in the coastal environment, interfacing between the estuarine substrate and both salt and freshwater.
The grey mullet therefore appear to be the ideal teleost fish to use as a bio-indicator in an environmental specimen bank program.

References

Bromhall, J.D. 1954: A note on the reproduction of the grey mullet. Mugil cephalus Linnaeus. Hong Kong University Fisheries Journal 1: 19-34.

Cech, J.J. and Wohlschlag, D.E. 1975: Summer growth depression in the striped mullet, Mugil cephalus L. Marine Science, vol.19.

Chen, T.P. 1977: Aquaculture Practices in Taiwan. London: Fishing New Books Ltd.

Chervinski, J. 1976: Growth of the golden grey mullet (Liza aurata (Risso)) in saltwater ponds during 1974. Aquaculture 7(1): 51.

De Angelis, R. 1969: Mediterranean brackish water lagoons and their exploitation. Stud. Rev. Gen. Fish. Coun. Mediterr. 12: 41 pp.

Erman, F. 1961: On the biology of the thick-lipped grey mullet (M. chelo Cuv.) Repp. P.-v. Reun. Commnint. Explor. scient. Mer Mediterr. 16: 276-285.

Grant, C.J. and Spain, A.V. 1975: Reproduction, growth and size allometry of Mugil cephalus L. from North Queensland Inshore Waters. Aust. J. Zool. 23: 181-2o1.

Herzberg, A. and Pasteur, R. 1975: The identification of grey mullet species by disc electrophoresis. Aquaculture 5(1): 99-1o6.

Hiatt, R.W. 1944: Food chains and food cycle in Hawaiian fish ponds. I. The food and feeding habits of mullet (Mugil cephalus), milk fish (Chanos chanos) and the ten-pounder (Elops machnata). Transactions of the American Fisheries Society 74: 25o-261.

Hickling, C.R. 197o: A contribution to the natural history of the English grey mullets (Pisce, Mugilidae). Journal of the Marine Biological Association of the United Kingdom 5o(3): 6o9-633.

488

Jocob, P.K. and Krishnamurthi, B. 1948: Breeding and feeding habits of mullets Mugil in Ennore Creek. Journal Bombay Natural History Society 47:663-338

Kevesten, G.L. 1942: Studies in the biology of the Australian mullet. Bull. Coun. Sci. Ind. Res. Melb. 157: 98 p.

Kuo, C.M., Shehadeh, Z.H. and Milisen, K.K. 1973a: A preliminary report on the development, growth and survival of laboratory reared larvae of the grey mullet, Mugil cephalus L. Journal of Fish Biology 5: 459-47o.

Kuo, C.M., Shehadeh, Z.H. and Nash, C.E. 1973b: Induced spawning of captive grey mullet (Mugil cephalus L.) females by injection of human chorionic gonadeotropin. Aquaculture 1: 429-432.

Lee, J.H., Nash, C.E. and Sylvester, J.R. 1975: Effects of Mirex and Methoxychlor on striped mullet, Mugil cephalus L. U.S. Environmental Protection Agency Report EPA-66o/3-75-o15: 18 p.

Liao, I.C., Lu, Y.J., Huang, T.L. and Lin, M.C. 1971: Experiments on induced breeding of the grey mullet, Mugil cephalus Lennaeus. Fisheries Series Chinese-American Joint Commission on Rural Recontruction (11):1-29.

Liao, I.C., Cheng, C.S., Tseng, L.C., Lim, M.Y., Hsieh, L.S. and Chen, H.P. 1972: Preliminary report on the mass propagation of grey mullets, Mugil cephalus Linnaeus. Fisheries Series Chinese-American Joint Commission on Rural Reconstruction (12): 1-14.

Liao, I.C. 1974: The experiments on the induced breeding of the grey mullet in Taiwan from 1963-1973. Paper presented at IBP/PM International Symposium on the Grey Mullets and their Culture, Haifa, Israel. Also 1975. Aquaculture 6(1): 31.

Luther, G. 1975: New characters for consideration in the taxonomic appraisal of grey mullets. Aquaculture 5(1): 1o7 (Abstracts).

Marais, J.F.K. and Erasmus, T. 1977: Body composition of Mugil cephalus, Liza dumerili, Liza richardsoni and Liza tricuspidens caught in the Swartkops Estuary. Aquaculture 1o(1): 75.

Nash, C.E., Kuo, C.M. and McConnell, S.C. 1974: Operational procedures for rearing larvae of the grey mullet (Mugil cephalus L.). Aquaculture 3:15-24.

Nash, C.E. and Kuo, C.M. 1975: Hypotheses for problems impeding the mass propagation of grey mullet and other finfish. Aquaculture 5: 119-133.

Nikolskii, G. 1954: Specail ichthyology. Svietskaya nauka. Moscow. 2nd ed. translated from Russian, Jerusalem, 1961, 538 pp.

Peterson, G.L. and Shehadeh, Z.H. 1971: Subpopulations of the Hawaiian striped mullet, Mugil cephalus. Marine Biology 11(1(: 52-6o.

Sanzo, L. 1936: Contributi alla conoscenza dello sviluppo embrionario e postembrionario nei Mugilidi. I. Mugil cephalus Cuv., II. M. Chelo Cuv. Mem. R. Com. Talassogr. Ital. 23o: 1-11.

Sanzo, L. 1937: Uova e larve di Mugil labeo Cuv. Biol. Pesca Piscio. Hidro-biol. 13(5): 5o6-51o.

Sarojini, K.K. 1957: Biology and fisheries of the grey mullets of Gengal. 1. Biology of Mugil parsia Hamilton with notes on its fishery in Bengal. Indian Journal of Fisheries 4(1): 16o-2o7.

Sarojini, K.K. 1958: Biology and fisheries of the grey mullets of Bengal. 2. Biology of Mugil cunnesius Valenciennes. Indian Journal of Fisheries 5(1): 56-76.

Schultz, L.P. 1946: A revision of the genera of mullets, fishes of the family Mugilidae, with description of three new genera. Proc. U.S. Natl. Mus. 96(32o6): 377-395.

Sebastian, M.J. and Nair,V.A. 1974: The induced spawning of the grey mullet, Mugil macrolepis (Aguas) Smith and the large scale rearing of its larvae. Paper presented at IBP/PM International Symposium on the Grey Mullets and their Culture, Haifa,Israel.

Sylvester, J.R. and Nash, C.E. 1975: Thermal tolerance of eggs and larvae of Hawaiian striped mullet, Mugil cephalus L. Trans. Am. Fish. Soc. 1o4(1): 144-147.

Tang, Y.A. 1964: Induced spawning of striped mullet by hormone injection. Japanese Journal of Ichthyology 12(1/2): 23-28.

Thomson, J.M. 1954: The organs of feeding and the food of some Australian mullet. Australian Journal of Marine and Fresh Water Research 5(3): 469-485.

Thomson, J.M. 1955: The movements and migrations of mullet (Mugil cephalus L.). Australian Journal of Marine and Fresh Water Research 6(3): 328-347.

Thomson, J.M. 1963: Synopsis of biological data on the grey mullet Mugil cephalus Linnaeus 1758. Fish. Synop. Div. Fish. Oceanogr. C.S.I.R.O. Australia (1).

Thomson, J.M. 1966: The grey mullets. Oceanogr. Mar. Biol. Ann. Rev. 4: 3o1-335.

Thomson, J.M. 1975: The dentition of grey mullets. Aquaculture 5(1): 1o8. (Abstract).

Tung, I.H. 1973: On the egg development and larval stages of the grey mullet, Mugil cephalus Linnaeus. Report of the Institute of Fishery Biology of the Ministry of Economics Affairs and National Taiwan University 3(1): 187-215.

Yashouv, A. 1969: Preliminary report on induced spawning of Mugil cephalus L. reared in captivity in fresh water ponds. Bamidgeh 21(1): 19-24.

490

Yashouv, A. and Berner-Samsonov, E. 197o: Contribution to the knowledge of eggs and early larval stages of mullets (Mugilidae) along the Israel coast. Bamidgeh 22(3): 72-89.

Zismann, L., Berdugo, V. and Kimor, B. 1974: The food and feeding of early stages of grey mullets in the Haifa Bay region. Paper presented at IBP/PM International Symposium on the Grey Mullets and their Culture, Haifa, Israel.

ARCHIVING WILDLIFE SPECIMENS FOR FUTURE ANALYSIS

Harry M. Ohlendorf
Patuxent Wildlife Research Center
U.S. Fish and Wildlife Service
Laurel, Maryland 2o811
U.S.A.

The term"wildlife", as used here, refers primarily to birds or bird parts and occasionally their eggs, but it may logically be extended to mammals and other vertebrates. Certain fish or invertebrate species imporant in avian diets might be monitored as part of a total wildlife program; however such forms usually are considered separately.

Changes in eggshell thickness and population declines of certain wild species of birds have been associated with the widespread use of persistent organochlorine pesticides (see Stickel, L.F. 1973; Stickel, W.H., 1975; Ohlendorf et al. 1978c for review). Other environmental pollutants, particularly polychlorinated biphenyls (PCB's) and heavy metals, also are commonly found in wild birds and mammals, and they sometimes cause adverse effects. The affected species are usually terminal consumers, generally those feeding on aquatic organisms (primarily fish) or birds.

Residues of persistent compounds are being monitored in selected species of birds, and their biological effects in these and other avian species are being studied. These studies are designed to serve the U.S. Fish and Wildlife Service in its overall mission of conservation and management of fish and wildlife populations and habitats.

Review of Past and Current Programs

Duck wings from the contiguous 48 States are available for monitoring purposes as a byproduct of a nation-wide survey of waterfowl productivity. Cooperative hunters mail thousands of wings to central collection points for biological examination (Dustman et al. 1971). Of the many species whose wings are available, those of the mallard (Anas platyrhynchos) and black duck (A. rubripes) are being used in the National Pesticide Monitoring Program, because the combined range of these two species covers the contiguous United States. The mallard is relatively abundant except in the Eastern States, where the black duck predominates.

Wings of the ducks are classified according to age and sex, and grouped according to State. Wings from each State are then sorted systematically into pools of 25 wings, and pools from each State are selected randomly for chemical analysis. The number taken for each State is roughly proportional to the State's harvest. A total of about 235 samples are collected for analysis, once every third year.

Prior to selection of duck wings as the tissue for pesticide monitoring purposes, special studies were conducted to determine the relationship of pesticide residues in wings to other parts of the body (Dustman, et al. 1971). DDT residues in wings were highly correlated with those in skin, muscle, brain, liver, kidney, pancreas, adrenal, gonad, thyroid,

and uropygial gland (Dindal and Peterle 1968). A pilot study of duck-wing monitoring was made in 1964, when wings of mallards and black ducks were collected from New York and Pennsylvania (Heath and Prouty 1967). Based on the findings of that study, duck wings were considered to be appropriate for monitoring. The first nation-wide monitoring effort was conducted in the winter of 1965-1966 (Heath 1969). Since then, duck wings have been analyzed periodically for organochlorine pestici-des, and sometimes also for PCB's and heavy metals (Heath and Hill 1974; White and Heath 1976; D.H. White, unpublished manuscript).
Starlings (Sturnus vulgaris) are collected especially for use in the National Pesticide Monitoring Program (Dustman et al. 1971). The star-ling was selected for monitoring pesticide residues in the environment because it is a terrestrial species found year-round throughout most of the contiguous 48 States; it is generally regarded as expendable; and its omnivorous food habits were expected to reflect the general environ-mental presence of persistent pesticides and certain heavy metals. Sampling sites for starlings were selected when the program began. These sites are used at each sampling period unless local changes (resi-dential development, etc.) cause a need to make minor shifts in location. The 48 States were divided into blocks of 5° latitude (24° to 49°) and longitude (64° to 124°), producing 4o sampling blocks. Within each of these blocks, up to four sampling sites were selected randomly. Birds are taken either by trapping or shooting, and each sample normally consists of a pool of 1o birds collected at each site. Starlings are collected every third year at about 13o sample sites.
Monitoring of starlings began in 1967 (Martin 1969). Starlings have subsequently been analyzed for residues of organochlorines and certain heavy metals (Martin and Nickerson 1972, 1973; Nickerson and Barbehenn 1975; White 1976; White et al. 1977; D.H. White, unpublished manuscript).
Bald eagles (Haliaeetus leucocephalus) found dead throughout the Uni-ted States are sent to the U.S. Fish and Wildlife Service's National Fish and Wildlife Health Laboratory in Madison, Wisconsin. There the birds are autopsied to determine, when possible, the cause of death. Tissues are then shipped to the Patuxent Wildlife Research Center for analysis. The brain and a portion of the carcass homogenate are analy-zed separately for residues of organochlorine pesticides and PCB's. Livers and carcass homogenates are stored for future analysis for metals and other chemicals. For example, livers and carcasses of 14 eagles collected from the Virginia-Maryland Chesapeake Bay Tidewater area during 1968-1975 were found to contain Kepone when they subsequently were analyzed for this chemical (Stafford et al. 1978).
Causes of bald eagle mortality were first summarized for 196o-1975 (Coon et al. 197o), and other reports of autopsy and residue findings have been published periodically (Reichel et al. 1969; Mulhern et al. 197o; Belisle et al. 1972; Cromartie et al. 1975; Prouty et al. 1977). Following the discovery that eggshells of the brown pelican (Pelecanus occidentalis) had become significantly thinner since 1946, the effects of environmental contaminants on this species were studied intensively in the Southeastern States form 1971through 1975 (Blus 197o; Blus et al. 1971, 1974a, 1974b, 1975, 1977). An annual census was conducted of to-tal nests and fledged young in each of the two nesting colonies in South Carolina. Carcasses of pelicans found dead were saved and analyzed for organochlorines; some livers were analyzed for heavy metals. Eggs in all stages of incubation, both viable and addled, were collected throughout the nesting season. One egg was usually taken from each nest

selected for sampling. Colonies in Florida and Louisiana also were surveyed and sampled, but less intensively than those in South Carolina. Since 1975 the South Carolina pelican populations have been censused to determine trends in numbers, and specimens have been collected to determine trends in residue concentrations. Following analysis, the remaining carcass homogenates and egg contents were stored for possible further analyses in the future.

Eggs of bald eagles (Krantz et al. 197o; Wiemeyer et al. 1972), ospreys (Pandion haliaetus) (Wiemeyer et al. 1975; Wiemeyer 1977), black ducks (Reichel and Addy 1968; Longcore and Mulhern 1973), mergansers (White and Cromartie 1977), and certain wading birds (Faber and Hickey 1973; Ohlendorf et al. 1974, 1978a, 1978b) have been collected to determine geographic and temporal trends of contaminant residue concentrations in these species. Samples from most of these studies also were saved for possible future analysis.

Studies have been conducted in which archived samples were used. For example, organochlorine pesticide and PCB residues in selected fauna collected from a New Jersey salt marsh in 1973 were compared with residues in these species in 1967 (Klaas and Belisle 1977). Hurricane Doria hit the coast of New Jersey in September 1967, causing high storm tides and killing clapper rails (Rallus longirostris). Several hundred birds were found dead along causeways in Cape May County, and 43 of them from six localities were frozen and stored for analysis. Concurrently, fish and invertebrates were collected from those locations and stored. Sampling was repeated at the same localities in 1973. The two groups of samples collected 7 years apart, the first having been a year after use of DDT was discontinued in Cape May County, were then analyzed by the same procedures.

The current programs are considered valid and useful in determining geographic and temporal patterns of contaminant residues in wildlife species. Many of the species studied reflect conditions in the aquatic environment and they often represent upper trophic levels.

Residues of certain persistent pollutants can be determined accurately in field-collected specimens. However, other pollutants also may be present, soemtimes in significant quantities, but not detected because current technology is not adequate; perhaps the particular chemical has not yet been recognized as an environmental pollutant. By archiving specimens, we have often been able to re-analyze them after analytical techniques were improved or new pollutants were recognized.

Among the persistent pollutants -- those for which specimens might be analyzed after long-term storage -- organochlorines and certain heavy metals are known to cause particularly important problems for birds. Some chemicals (such as DDE, PCB's, and mercury) occur commonly in environmental specimens form ridely separated areas; mean levels may be compared on a geographic or temporal basis. However, other chemicals (such as heptachlor epoxide, endrin, and chlordane) occur less frequently, and comparisons of incidence may be more meaningful.

Rationale for Interest or Concern

Pollutants affect wild animals directly and indirectly; some chemicals are highly toxic and cause extensive mortality, but others reduce reproductive success or cause subtle effects on the ecosystem (see Stickel, L.F. 1973; Stickel, W.H. 1975; Ohlendorf et al. 1978c for review).

Determination of the effects of various chemicals is not easy, for ani-

mals of different groups vary widely in their sensitivity to different pollutants, and the effects of certain chemicals in combination may be different than would be predicted by their separate effects.
Chemical changes of pollutants within the animal body are inherent and critical parts of the kinetic process. These changes may drastically alter the toxicity, solubility, storage potential, and other characteristics of the parent compound. Despite a vast amount of research and an enormous literature, the complete series of breakdown stages of various persistent pollutants is not well known.
Organochlorines accumulate in birds from a relatively small exposure; because they are stored in adipose tissue, they may produce mortality when fat is being metabolized, long after any significant exposure to the chemicals causing death.
Many species of birds have serious degrees of eggshell thinning and impaired reproduction. The degree of shell thinning in the wild often can be correlated with the DDE content of the egg. In experimental studies shell thinning in several species has been demonstrated when DDE was administered in the diet. Other pollutants, such as dieldrin and mercury, also have been found in wild birds at levels known to impair reproduction in experimental studies.
Behavioral changes as a result of pollutant exposure have been demonstrated in birds under experimental conditions. In the field, certain observed behavioral changes were associated with elevated levels of organochlorine pesticides found in the birds.
Some avian species (especially ducks) that are being monitored for persistent pollutants are themselves eaten by humans; others may reflect human exposure because they feed on fish that also may be eaten by humans. Sometimes the pathways for human exposure are not very direct, but the fish being eaten by birds that are being studied may also be eaten by larger fish, which serve as food for humans.

Considerations for Sample Selection, Collection, Containment, Shipment, and Storage

Selection of a "best" species for monitoring is seldom a simple matter, and at least the following factors, some more obvious than others, should be considered in attempting to meet monitoring objectives (Monitoring Panel, FWGPM 1974):
1. Availability - A species must be available in numbers sufficient to provide statistically adequate sample sizes. Animals must be sufficiently abundant to insure no harm to their population as a result of the repeated sampling, expendable in that a highly disirable species is not used in lieu of a less valuable but fully suitable substitute, and sufficiently easy to collect to be practical.

2. Distribution - If the primary interest is in monitoring residue trends on a regional basis rather than in a particular species, it is highly preferable that a candidate species occur throughout that region. When an otherwise suitable species is not available throughout an entire part of the region, it may be possible to substitute an alternate species that is closely related or ecologically similar.

3. Mobility - The mobility of a species is a necessary consideration in determining if the species will serve to meet the objectives of a survey. One must consider the extent of daily and seasonal movements and, if a migratory species, the timing and pattern of migration.

4. Diet - Food habits are a primary consideration in selection of a species, since the principal route of pollutant exposure in the wild is undoubtedly through the diet. Because many persistent pollutants tend to become progressively concentrated through successive levels of food chains, a species' food habits must be representative of the segment of the environment at which the monitoring is primarily directed.

5. Habitat - The habitat preference of a species is an obvious factor, for if the intent of monitoring is to evaluate residues in a wetland ecosystem, the investigator does not select an upland species.

6. Physiology - The physiology of a species must be considered with regard to its propensity to acquire and retain residues of those pollutants to be monitored.

In addition to selecting the species, one must consider the tissues to be sampled. In general, persistent organochlorine pollutants are best determined in homogenized carcasses (after feet, beak, skin and feathers, and gastrointestinal tract have been removed) or in the brains or eggs of birds. Analysis of carcasses or eggs is considered to be most feasible and desirable in monitoring studies. The residues of organochlorines in the eggs are taken as an index of the residues that were present in the female when producing the egg.
Certain heavy metals are not readily transferred to the egg (see Ohlendorf et al. 1978c for review), and they are not concentrated in the body fat reserves. Consequently, other tissues (usually the liver or kidneys) are generally the best ones to analyze for most heavy metals. It appears that the most useful and feasible avian specimens for archiving to represent the aquatic environment would be the remainders of duck wings, following their analysis in the National Pesticide Monitoring Program. These specimens are collected regularly (every 3 years) on a nation-wide basis; supplemental collections could be made in years when they would not be done for the National Pesticide Monitoring Program. In addition, a portion of the bald eagle carcass homogenates could be stored in a central facility other than the Patuxent Wildlife Research Center. Although eagles are not collected from systematically determined locations, they are available from many regions of the Nation, feed extensively on fish, and often accumulate high levels of residues in their tissues. When the specimens (duck wings or eagle carcasses) are being prepared for analysis, a portion of the homogenate could be placed in chemically cleaned glass jars and stored.
Specimens should be skinned, dissected, and prepared as required, so that the laboratory can proceed with analysis of the materials.During preparation great care must be taken to prevent contamination. The gastrointestinal tract must be dissected out in a manner to avoid leakage or spillage of the contents onto the carcass; however, its adherent organs must remain with the carcass. Dissections should be done on clean foil or paper that can be changed frequently. Instruments should be washed with water and detergent and given a final rinse with acetone. Instruments should be acetone-rinsed frequently to avoid contamination between organs of the same or different birds.
If specimens have been frozen prior to preparation, brains should be removed before thawing to prevent leakage.
It is important to obtain weights at all stages, including original total weight, weight or organs, and weight of subsample being saved. The organ and subsample weights are determined by weighing the bottle

before and after putting the sample in it.

The notebook record should include all original data: for example, bottle alone and bottle plus sample, so that double checking can be done later.

Specimens should be placed in clean glass bottles. The bottles should be small to prevent undue evaporation. Bottle caps should be lined with teflon; aluminium foil can be used instead, but is a poorer choice because it may corrode or split.Large-mouthed squat bottles are the best, both for inserting specimens and for removing them.

Narrow-mouthed bottles with shoulders are undesirable. The specialized bottles and cap liners that are needed are not available everywhere, and must be ordered in advanced. Bottles should be cleaned by immersing them in a large glass container containing (ca. lo %) nitric acid (while wearing rubber gloves). Jars should then be rinsed separately with deionized water and frained face down on a neoprene-covered rack. Each jar should be rinsed separately with lo to 2o ml of distilled acetone (without using tongs or rubber gloves, and avoid getting these solvents on your hands) by pouring the acetone around the top of the inside of the jar so that the acetone runs down the sides; do not immerse the jar in a container filled with acetone. If the jars were still wet from the deionized water rinse, the acetone rinse should be repeated. Next, jars should be rinsed twice in distilled hexane, using the same procedure as outlined for acetone. Jars should then be permitted to air dry in an upright position and stored with aluminum foil under the screw cap.

Strips of adhesive tape around the top of the bottle provide both sealing and labeling material. Certain kinds of adhesive tape will take and retain either "magic marker" or pencil. We have found Sharpie® magic markers and Curity® wetproof adhesive tape (2.54 cm width) satisfactory for this purpose; other brands also may be satisfactory but they should first be tested for permanence of marking. A preservative-proof string tag tied firmly around the neck of each bottle can also be used. Data should be written on the tag with pencil. No type of stick-on label, magic marker or wax pencil should be used directly on the bottle, because these marks will come off.

The data on the label should be limited to information essential for identification, and it must correspond exactly to the data in the catalog. A number alone is not enough to prevent error, however. The catalog number, the name of the tissue, and the species ordinarily should suffice. The designation should be simple and clear and not subject to confusion with other specimens.

Specimens usually have been stored at temperatures of -2o°C or colder; for long-term frozen storage the temperature should not be warmer than -3o°C.

We are now experimenting with formalin preservation of specimens' and have found the method satisfactory for certain types of samples. This procedure may be more suitable and less costly than other methods of storage.

Analytical Procedures

General guidelines on analytical methodology for pesticide residues monitoring have been developed (Monitoring Panel, FWGMP 1975). These guidelines cover most of the important considerations:

1. Safety - Safety is a prime consideration in any analytical laboratory;

it is especially important in the organochlorine residue laboratory, because chemicals that may be hazardous to the health and safety of the analyst, as well as to the safety of the laboratory itself, are used extensively. Because large volumes of flammable solvents are often required in residue analysis, suitable storage vaults should be used for large containers and special fireproof storage lockers should be available for smaller amounts in or near the laboratory.

2. Solvents and reagents - Solvents and reagents should be free of substances that interfere with analysis or degrade the sample. To obtain low background levels and avoid spurious peaks arising from solvent impurities, it is usually necessary to use specially purified or distilled-in-glass solvents. Solvents should be checked for impurities and background by analyzing "solvent blank" samples. Similar precautions must be taken with reagents.

3. Dissection - Birds must be dissected prior to analysis, removing the skin and feathers, feet, beak, and gastrointestinal tract. For duck wings, most of the feathers are removed by trimming near the skin.

4. Subsampling and preparation - Representative subsamples should be taken after thorough mixing of the sample. The tissues are usually ground with sodium sulfate to bind the tissue moisture before extraction.

5. Extraction - Procedures used should yield resonably complete extraction and recovery of the desired residues. Extraction with hexane in a Soxhlet apparatus has proven most efficient for extracting wildlife tissues.

6. Cleanup - The cleanup procedures should be tested to see that they enable detection and determination of the residues being sought (a) at the desired sensitivity or limit of detection; (b) with reasonable recovery; (c) with reasonable reduction of background interferences; and (d) with adequate separation of chemicals that may interfere with each other.

7. Detection and quantitation - Electron-capture gas chromatography is the preferred method of detection. Much care is needed to assure that errors are minimized, especially because of variable response of the instrument. Quantitation is usually done by comparative measurement of area of peaks from sample and reference standards treated in the same manner.

8. Confirmation of residue identity - Identity of chemical residues should routinely be confirmed by tests in addition to the initial gas chromatography. Mass spectrometry combined with gas chromatography is recommended for this purpose, and should be used on about 1o % of the samples analyzed.

9. Reference standards - There are several sources of reference standards; they are usually available from the manufacturer or a specialized supplier, but in other instances they may be prepared in the laboratory. Whatever their source, reference standards should be used in identifying residues.

1o. Interlaboratory checks - Most analytical laboratories are not able to determine accurately the residues of organochlorine compounds in wildlife specimens, and a careful cross-check program is required.

Our Center has developed reliable techniques for analyzing environmental samples for residues of organochlorines; these are the recommended analytical procedures (Reichel, unpublished manual).
Methods also have been developed for analyzing avian tissues for heavy metals. In summary, they include:

1. Glassware preparation - All glassware is cleaned before use in 1o % nitric acid solution for an hour or more, followed by rinsing in distilled, deionized water.

2. Reagents - All reagents are analyzed reagent grade and are selected according to lowest level of heavy metal content.

3. Flame atomic absorption analysis.
   a) Wet ash methods - For lead and thallium, a 5 g sample of tissue is weighed into a round-bottom flask and a few glass beads are added. The flask is connected to a digestion apparatus, 2o ml of concentrated sulfuric-nitric acid mixture (3:1 ratio) are added, and the contents are heated to about 12o°C for 2 hr. From time to time, concentrated nitric acid may have to be added during the digestion process to clarify flask contents. After 2 hr the heat source is removed, the flask is cooled in an ice bath, and 1oo ml of deionized water and a few drops of Tymol blue indicator are added. Contents are neutralized with 5o % sodium hydroxide. The digest is transferred to a 4oo ml beaker and pH is adjusted to 5 with dilute sodium hydroxide or sulfuric acid using a pH meter. Material is then transferred to a 1,ooo ml separatory funnel and lead or thallium are chelated with 5 ml of a 1 % aqueous solution of sodium diethyldithio carbamate. The chelated lead or thallium is extracted into 1o ml of water-saturated methyl isobutyl ketone and measured by aspirating into an air-acetylene flame on an atomic absorption spectrophotometer. A reagent blank and, if possible, a clean tissue blank are treated following the same procedures as used for the sample.
   Some metals other than lead and thallium can be determined by similar chelation and extraction procedures, but using different reagents and pH conditions.
   b) Dry ash methods - For lead, copper, zinc, nickel, cadmium, and certain other metals, a 5 g sample is weighed into a Vycor crucible, and dried at 11o°C for about 3 hr in a drying oven. Lids are then put on the crucibles and they are placed in a muffle furnace where the sample chars for 2 hr at 2oo°C. The temperature is then raised at the rate of 1oo°C/hr until it reaches 5oo°C. The samples are ashed overnight at this temperature. The ash is dissolved in about 3 ml of hot nitric acid and quantitatively transferred to a 5o ml polypropylene tube. The volume is brought up to 1o ml with distilled, deionized water. Analysis is done by comparison of sample absorbence with standard absorbence after aspiration into an atomic absorption spectrophotometer.

4. Flameless atomic absorption analysis (Cold vapor atomic absorption - wet ash digestion) - For mercury, a 2-5 g sample is weighed into a 1,ooo ml round-bottom flask, which is connected to a digestion apparatus. Then 2o ml of concentrated sulfuric-nitric acid mixture (3:1 ratio) are added and the sample is digested for 2 hr with heat (up to 12o°C). Small amounts of concentrated nitric acid are added as needed to clarify the digestate, the flask is cooled with ice water,

and lo ml of hydrogen peroxide are added. The flask is then removed
from the ice bath and refluxed for another 3o min. The digest is
cooled to room temperature, and contents are transferred to a loo-ml
volumetric flask. The round-bottom flask is rinsed several times,
adding washings to the same loo-ml flask, and water is added to bring
the volume up to loo ml. A suitable aliquot of digest is transferred
to an aeration bottle and diluted to 5o ml with 15 % sulfuric acid.
Then 5 ml of lo % hydroxylamine hydrochloride solution plus 5 ml
of lo % stannous chloride solution are added. The aeration bottle
is connected to the aeration setup; mercury is liberated and measured
as it passes through a gas cell in the ultraviolet light path on
an atomic absorption spectrophotometer.

5. Graphite tube atomization - This new technique for the atomization of
   metals in a graphite tube placed in the ultraviolet light path of
   an atomic absorption spectrophotometer shows great promise. It is
   particularly recommended for analysis of very small sample sizes.
   Samples can be wet ashed, dry ashed, or injected directly into the
   furnace.

Program Design

Many considerations for program design have been incorporated into
earlier sections, particularly in the description of current programs
and considerations for sample selection.
The archiving program could include duck wing samples from all sample
sites in the National Pesticide Monitoring Program, plus subsamples
of bald eagle carcasses that are analyzed by the Patuxent Center. This
would total about 235 duck wing samples every third year, when samples
are routinely collected. About 5o - 75 eagles are analyzed each year.
It appears, however, that this number of samples would exceed the number
of wildlife specimens that would be desirable for the pilot program.
Therefore, the number should be reduced proportionally throughout the
Nation, giving the total number of samples allotted to wildlife for the
aquatic environment.
For each sample, the species, location, date, age, sex, and sample
weight should be recorded; all of this is done routinely in the current
programs.
Information on pollutant residues is published in technical journals
(usually the Pesticides Monitoring Journal) as soon as it has been
verified and interpreted; other information (sample identification,etc.)
is permanently stored in data files. Retrieval is manual and handled on
a case-by-case basis as the need arises.

Organizational Aspects

Existing programs could be used to meet the needs for archiving wildlife specimens. Although these samples could feasibly be stored in a
centralized facility, analysis of avian tissues for organochlorines
is considerably more difficult than analysis of most other environmental
samples. For this reason, routine contemporary analyses should be continued in the present manner. If there are particular problems/chemicals
to be investigated the analyses may be undertaken elsewhere, but the
work should be coordinated with the Patuxent Wildlife Research Center.
Data for the samples submitted for centralized storage would, of course,
accompany the samples.

The best procedure may be for the wildlife specimens to remain in storage at the Patuxent Center, unless it seems appropriate to have a subsample stored elsewhere to ensure against loss/spoilage of the entire sample.

A coordinated international program for measuring contaminant residues in aquatic birds and archiving samples for future analysis would be a difficult project, but perhaps a desirable one. Mallard ducks occur throughout Europe and much of Asia, so this may be a suitable species for routine sampling. In addition, eagles (Haliaeetus spp.) occur in many countries, and those found dead could be saved for analysis. This, however, would require an extensive effort because of the many problems in salvaging specimens and shipping them to a central facility.

It may be feasible to organize a system for collection of duck wings and salvage of eagles in the various participating countries. After the samples have been analyzed by the participating agency or country, a portion of the homogenized sample might be stored in a central facility. If such a system is to be developed, it would need to be organized by the various participants.

The principal value of an international program would be to help focus world-wide attention on the problems of environmental pollution. Having additonal awareness of the problems should encourage more international cooperation in solving them.

Ethical and Legal Considerations

Migratory birds may not be legally collected, transported, or stored without authorization (a Migratory Bird Scientific Collection Permit) from the U.S. Fish and Wildlife Service and the various States. In addition, an EndangeredSpecies Permit is required for work involving the bald eagle in those States where it is classified as "endangered" If archived samples are analyzed at some time in the future, information on pollutant residues should not be disseminated without first getting concurrence of the participating agency that provided the samples.

Cost Estimates

The current monitoring programs are funded by the U.S. Fish and Wildlife Service, and wildlife specimens could be archived by the Patuxent Wildlife Research Center with no substantial increase in costs. There should be no additonal cost for design of the program, because we could use one that already exists.

Current expenditures for monitoring and specimen banking activities are approximately $100,000 per year; costs for initiating an equivalent new program would be considerably greater, however, because much of the work in the current program is integrated with other research and management functons of the U.S. Fish and Wildlife Service. A lower limit of detection of o.1 ppm wet weight is usually considered satisfactory in analyzing field-collected specimens. At this level of detection, costs for organochlorine analyses are about $150 per sample. Costs for heavy metal analyses average about $15-2o per metal, but they are somewhat less if the same sample is being analyzed simultaneously for several metals. If subsamples of the wildlife specimens are to be stored elsewhere, the cost would be approximately $5,000 - 10,000 per year, depending on location and size of the facility, temperature to be maintained, and other factors. Data processing costs probably would not exceed $5,000 per year.

Summary

Duck wings and starlings are analyzed for organochlorines and selected
heavy metals in the National Pesticide Monitoring Program. In other
wildlife research projects conducted by the Patuxent Wildlife Research
Center, specimens of many other species have been analyzed to determine
geographic, species, or temporal differences in residue concentrations.
Examples include bald eagles, certain New Jersey salt marsh fauna, and
the eggs of eagles, ducks, ospreys, brown pelicans, and wading birds.
Specimens usually have been archived as frozen samples so they could
be reanalyzed when newer contaminants were discovered or analytical
procedures were improved. The procedures used in banking these specimens have been adequate for the purposes intended. Samples should be stored
at temperatures of -30°C or colder. We are now experimenting with formalin preservation of specimens and have found the method satisfactory
for certain types of samples. This procedure may be more suitable and
less costly than other methods or storage.
Samples usually have been collected to determine geographic patterns
of residue levels in the study species, or to determine which chemicals
might be associated with population declines and reproductive failure
in species of concern. In some instances, the samples constitute a nationwide collection, but more often they are taken from selected regions or
localized areas. Most samples are stored frozen, both prior to analysis
and after analyses are completed. Subsamples of duck wings and bald
eagle carcasses are the most useful and feasible avian specimens form the
aquatic environment for long-term storage in locations other than the
Patuxent Center.

References

Belisle, A.A., W.L. Reichel, L.N. Locke, T.G. Lamont, B.M. Mulhern,
R.M. Prouty, R.B. DeWolf, and E. Cromartie. 1972:
Residues of organochlorine pesticides, polychlorinated biphenyls, and
mercury and autopsy data for bald eagles, 1969 and 1970. Pestic. Monit.
J. 6 (3): 133-138.

Blus, L.J. 1970: Measurements of brown pelican eggshells from Florida
and Sotth Carolina. Bio Science 20 (15): 867-869.

Blus, L.J., A.A. Belisle, and R.M. Prouty. 1974a: Relations of the brown
pelican to certain environmental pollutants. Pestic. Monit. J. 7 (3/4):
181-194.

Blus, L.J., R.G. Heath, C.D. Gish, A.A. Belisle, and R.M. Prouty. 1971:
Eggshell thinning in the brown pelican: implication of DDE. Bio Science
21 ("4): 1213-1215.

Blus, L.J., T.Joanen, A.A. Belisle, and R.M. Prouty. 1975: The brown
pelican and certain environmental pollutants in Louisiana. Bull. Environ.
Contam. Toxicol. 13 (6): 646-655.

Blus, L.J., B.S. Neely, Jr., A.A. Belisle, and R.M. Prouty. 1974b:
Organochlorine residues in brown pelican eggs: relation to reproductive
success. Environ. Pollut. 7: 81-91.

502

Blus, L.J., B.S. Neely, Jr., T.G. Lamont, and B. Mulhern. 1977: Residues of organochlorines and heavy metals in tissues and eggs of brown pelicans, 1969-73. Pestic. Monit. J. 11 (1): 4o-53.

Coon, N.C., L.N.Locke, E. Cromartie, and W.L. Reichel. 197o: Causes of bald eagle mortality, 196o-1965. J. Wildl. Dis. 6: 72-76.

Cromartie, E., W.L. Reichel, L.N. Locke, A.A. Belisle, T.E. Kaiser, T.G. Lamont, B.M. Mulhern, R.M. Prouty, and D.M. Swineford. 1975: Residues of organochlorine pesticides and polychlorinated biphenyls and autopsy data for bald eagles, 1971-72. Pestic. Monit. J. 9 (1): 11-14.

Dindal, D.L., and T.J. Peterle. 1968: Wing and body tissue relationships of DDT and metabolite residues in mallard and lesser scaup ducks. Bull. Environ. Contam. Toxicol. 3 (1): 37-45.

Dustman, E.H., W.E. Martin, R.G. Heath, and W.L. Reichel. 1971: Monitoring pesticides in wildlife. Pestic. Monit. J. 5 (1): 5o-52.

Faber, R.A., and J.J. Hickey. 1973: Eggshell thinning, chlorinated hydrocarbons, and mercury in inland aquatic bird eggs, 1969 and 197o. Pestic. Monit. J. 7 (1): 27-36.

Heath, R.G. 1969: Nationwide residues of organochlorine pesticides in wings of mallards and black ducks. Pestic. Monit. J. 3(2): 115-123.

Heath, R.G., and S.A. Hill. 1974: Nationwide organochlorine and mercury residues in wings of adult mallards and black ducks during the 1969-7o hunting season. Pestic. Monit. J. 7 (3/4): 153-164.

Heath, R.G., and R.M. Prouty. 1967: Trial monitoring of pesticides in wings of mallards and black ducks. Bull. Environ. Contam. Toxicol. 2(2): 1o1 -11o.

Klaas, E.E., and A.A. Belisle. 1977: Organochlorine pesticide and poly-chlorinated biphenyls residues in selected fauna from a New Jersey salt marsh - 1967 vs. 1973. Pestic. Monit. J. 1o (4): 149-158.

Krantz, W.C., B.M. Mulhern, G.E. Bagley, A. Sprunt, IV, F.J. Ligas, and W.B. Robertson, Jr. 197o:
Organochlorine and heavy metal residues in bald eagle eggs. Pestic. Monit. J. 3 (3): 136-14o.

Longcore, J.R., and B.M. Mulhern. 1973: Organochlorine pesticides and polychlorinated biphenyls in black duck eggs from the United States and Canada - 1971. Pestic. Monit. J. 7 (1): 62-66.

Martin, W.E. 1969: Organochlorine insecticide residues in starlings. Pestic. Monit. J. 3 (2): 1o2-114.

Martin, W.E., and P.R.Nickerson. 1972: Organochlorine residues in star-lings - 197o. Pestic. Monit. J. 6 (1): 33-4o.

Martin, W.E., and P.R. Nickerson. 1973: Mercury. lead, cadmium, and arsenic residues in starlings - 1971. Pestic. Monit. J. 7(1): 67-72.

Monitoring Panel, FWGPM. 1974: Guidelines on sampling and statistical methodologies for ambient pesticide monitoring. Federal Working Group on Pest Management, Washington, D.C.

Monitoring Panel, FWGPM. 1975: Guidelines on analytical methodology for pesticide residue monitoring. Federal Working Group on Pest Management, Washington, D.C.

Mulhern, B.M., W.L. Reichel, L.N. Locke, T.G. Lamont, A. Belisle, E. Cromartie, G.E. Bagley, and R.M. Prouty. 197o: Organochlorine residues and autopsy data from bald eagles 1966-68. Pestic. Monit. J. 4 (3): 141-144.

Nickerson,P.R., and K.R. Barbehenn. 1975: Organochlorine residues in starlings, 1972. Pestic. Monit. J. 8 (4): 247-254.

Ohlendorf, H.M., E.E. Klaas, and T.E. Kaiser. 1974: Environmental pollution in relation to estuarine birds. Pp. 53-81 in M.A.Q. Khan and J.P. Bederka, Jr., eds. Survival in toxic environments. Academic Press, Inc. New York.

Ohlendorf, H.M., E.E. Klaas, and T.E. Kaiser. 1978a: Environmental pollutants and eggshell thinning in the black-crowned night heron. Pp. 63-82 in A. Sprunt, IV, J.C.Ogden, and S. Winckler, eds. Wading birds. National Audubon Society Research Report No. 7.

Ohlendorf. H.M., E.E. Klaas, and T.E. Kaiser, 1978b: Organochlorine residues and eggshell thinning in anhingas and waders. Pp. 185-195 in Proceedings of 1977 Conference of the Colonial Waterbird Group. DeKalb, Illinois.

Ohlendorf, H.M., R.W. Risebrough, and K. Vermeer. 1978c: Exposure of marine birds to environmental pollutants. Wildlife Research Report No. 9. U.S. Fish and Wildlife Service.

Prouty, R.M., W.L. Reichel, L.N.Locke, A.A. Belisle, E. Cromartie, T.E. Kaiser, T.G. Lamont, B.M. Mulhern, andD.M. Swineford. 1977: Residues of organochlorine pesticides and polychlorinated biphenyls and autopsy data for bald eagles, 1973-74. Pestic. Monit. J. 11 (3): 134-137.

Reichel, W.L. (compiler). Patuxent analytical manual for organochlorine compounds. U.S. Department of the Interior, Fish and Wildlife Service, Patuxent Wildlife Research Center, Laurel MD (mimeo).

Reichel, W.L., and C.E. Addy. 1968a: A survey of chlorinated pesticide residues in black duck eggs. Bull. Environ. Contam. Toxicol. 3 (3): 174-179.

Reichel, W.L., E. Cromartie, T.G. Lamont, B.M. Mulhern, and R.M. Prouty. 1969: Pesticide residues in eagles. Pestic. Monit. J. 3(3): 142-144.

Stafford, C.J., W.L. Reichel, D.M. Swineford, R.M.Prouty, and M.L. Cay. 1978: Gas-liquid chromatographic determination of Kepone in field-collected avian tissues and eggs. J. Assoc. Off. Anal. Chem. 6(1): 8-14.

504

Stickel, L.F. 1973: Pesticide residues in birds and mammals. Pp. 254-312 in C.A. Edwards, ed.:Environmental pollution by pesticides. Plenum Press. New York.

Stickel, W.H. 1975: Some effects of pollutants in terrestrial ecosystems. Pp. 25-74 in A.D. McIntyre and C.F. Mills, eds. Ecological toxicology research. Plenum Press. New York.

White, D.H. 1976: Nationwide residues of organochlorines in starlings, 1974. Pestic. Monit. J. 1o (1): 1o-17.

White, D.H. 1978: Nationwide residues or organochlorines in starlings, 1976. Submitted to Pesticides Monitoring Journal.

White, D.H. 1978: Nationwide residues of organochlorines in wings of adult mallards and black ducks, 1976-77. In review.

White, D.H., J.R. Bean, and J.R. Longcore. 1977: Nationwide residues of mercury, lead, cadmium, arsenic, and selenium in starlings, 1973. Pestic. Monit. J. 11 (1): 35-39.

White, D.H., and E. Crormartie. 1977: Residues of environmental pollutants and shell thinning in merganser eggs. Wilson Bull. 89 (4): 532-542.

White, D.H., and R.G. Heath. 1976: Nationwide residues of organochlorines in wings of adult mallards and black ducks, 1972-73. Pestic. Monit. J. 9 (4): 176-185.

Wiemeyer, S.N. 1977: Reproductive success of Potomac River ospreys, 1971. Pp. 115-119 in J.C. Ogden, ed. Transactions North American Osprey Research Conference. U.S. National Park Service, Transaction and Proceedings Series, No. 2.

Wiemeyer, S.N., B.M. Mulhern, F.J. Ligas, R.J. Hensel, J.E. Mathisen, F.C. Robards, and S. Postupalsky. 1972: Residues of organochlorine pesticides, polychlorinated biphenyls, and mercury in bald eagle eggs and changes in shell thickness -- 1969-197o. Pestic. Monit. J. 6 (1): 5o-55.

Wiemeyer, S.N., P.R. Spitzer, W.C. Krantz, T.G. Lamont, and E. Cromartie. 1975: Effects of environmental pollutants on Connecticut and Maryland ospreys. J. Wildl. Manage. 39 (1): 124-139.

TRACE METALS IN LIVING MARINE RESOURCES TAKEN FROM NORTH ATLANTIC WATERS

John B. Pearce
U.S. Department of Commerce
National Oceanic and Atmospheric Administration
National Marine Fisheries Service
Northeast Fisheries Center
Sandy Hook Laboratory
Highlands, New Jersey o7732

For some years public officials have been concerned with the presence of toxic substances in foods used for human consumption. It was not until the past decade, however, that public health personnel became aware of problems of toxic substances in living marine resources. The first indication that was brought to the general public's attention was the report by McDuffy (19) that tuna used for human consumption might contain dangerous levels of mercury; however, Westöö (1966,1967) and others had reported upon this phenomena earlier.

Following the findings of McDuffy, a growing concern for toxic substances in living marine resources developed. An immediate response was to collect fish, that might be used for human consumption, in a more or less standard fashion so that the tissues could be analyzed for the presence of mercury and other toxic heavy metals.

Public health officials also were alerted to the possibility that PCB's, other halogenated hydrocarbons, and other organic materials might also be found in fish tissues in amounts that could be hazardous to individuals consuming such fish flesh.

Because of the possibility of toxic substances used in fish for human consumption, large numbers of fish were collected by the National Marine Fisheries Service for analysis in order to determine if, indeed, fish did contain heavy metals such as mercury, cadmium, silver, copper, zinc, nickel, manganese, lead, and chromium in amounts that might be deleterious. The Southeast Utilization Research Center at College Park, Maryland, examined some 1o,ooo samples of over 2oo commercial and recreational fish species to garner preliminary data on certain heavy metals. The results of their studies of heavy metals in marine organisms were released in an interim report entitled "First Interim Report on Microconstituent Resource Survey" (1975). This report was not widely circulated since it was deemed to be a preliminary report based on incomplete data.

While there was a great concern for the public health aspects of heavy metals in marine organisms, relatively little information existed in regard to how these heavy metals were distributed in fish taken over broad geographic areas and within a diversity of organisms which comprise marine food chains culminating in fish and shellfish used for human consumption. The Environmental Chemistry Investigation, Division of Environmental Assessment, Northeast Fisheries Center, began to study distributions of heavy metals in a wide range of marine organisms collected from waters off the New England and Middle Atlantic States of the United States in the early 197o's. This Investigation also concerned itself with relative amounts of

heavy metals to be found in sediments and waters of the same general geographic area. Intensive collections of sediments and waters were made in
order to show the general distributions of heavy metals in estuaries, coastal and oceanic waters. The results of these studies have been published
in serveral papers which will be discussed in the following paragraphs.

Heavy Metals in the Physical Environment

Because of the work of Bryan (1976) it is now well-known that many organisms
can take up significant quantities of heavy metals from sediments contaminated by naturally occurring metals as well as by metals having an anthropogenic source. Other studies have indicated that marine animals are capable of taking up metals from the water or through ingesting plant and animal life previously contaminated by heavy metals. For this reason it is
important to have an understanding of the distribution of heavy metals in
marine sediments, especially those in polluted or contaminated estuarine
and coastal waters. Carmody, Pearce and Yasso (1973) showed the distribution of heavy metals in sediments in the New York Bight apex which have
been contaminated through ocean dumping of sewage sludge and dredging
spoils, and riverine run off from the heavily polluted Hudson River drainage system. Later, Greig and McGrath (1977) showed that the sediments in
Raritan Bay have extremely high levels of heavy metals. Much of the dredged material dumped in the New York Bight apex has its origins in Raritan
Bay and the lower Hudson River. In a recent paper by Multer and Nadeau
(1978) it was indicated that many heavy metals exist in extremely high
levels in tributaries feeding into the Hudson River - Raritan Bay drainage
systems. Their studies in the Passiac River showed that very high levels
of heavy metals exist in the river, especially in urbanized/industrialized
areas of the lower river. There seems little doubt that these metals have
their origin in the discharge of industrial wastes.
In a study of heavy metals by Greig, Reid and Wenzloff (1977) it was found
that, again, in Long Island Sound embayment adjunct to the New York Bight,
there are far greater amounts of heavy metals in the western portion of the
Sound, which is in close proximity to the urbanized/industrialized metropolitan New York complex. Studies done in other parts of the world such as
the Southern California Bight would also suggest that those marine sediments
in proximity to highly urbanized/industrialized areas are likely to have
elevated values of sediment metals (Eganhouse, 1976).
Multer and Nadeau (1978) indicate that there are significant variations
in heavy metals occuring over time in Raritan Bay, and suggest that these
fluctuations may be natural. Recent studies in the New York Bight also indicate that there are variations in the amounts of heavy metals in sediments
there. It is not presently known whether these variations are natural, resulting from changes in the actual amounts of heavy metals (due to resus-
pension during storms), or whether the variations are due simply to additional inputs of less contaminated sediments or organic materials, with
reduced amounts of heavy metals.
In addition to heavy metals in sediments there is a continuing interest of
heavy metals in marine waters. Because of the greater difficulty in analyzing waters for heavy metals and other contaminants, our data base is far
less complete. Waldhauer, Matte and Tucker (1978) have recently found very
high levels of heavy metals in waters of the Raritan Bay - Hudson River
area. They report values for copper that are as high as those measured in
any marine waters of the world. The same authors have also found unusually
high values for lead. It is assumed that other metals which are discharged

from industrial and domestic sources into riverine and estuarine waters
culminating in the New York Bight apex may also occur in unusually high
amounts.
In addition to collecting sediments and waters for analyses, personnel
of the Division of Environmental Assessment have in recent months been collecting samples of phytoplankton and zooplankton for heavy metal analyses.
Selected samples have been analyzed and are reported in Greig, Adams and
Wenzloff (1977). As part of the developing Ocean Pulse program (Pearce,
1977a) personnel of the Northeast Fisheries Center are attempting to selectively collect inorganic materials that are suspended in the water for
analyses separate from the plankton and organic materials found in marine
waters. It is important to understand how heavy metals are bound to colloidal matrices as well as to the finer clays, silts and sands which may be
in suspension in the water column.

Methodologies for Analysis of Physical Environmental Samples.

The procedures used for chemical analyses of sediments differed depending
on whether atomic absorption analysis or neutron activation analysis was
used. In the case of atomic absorption analysis, two separate procedures
were employed: (a) for Hg, and (b) for Cd, Cu, Mn, Ni, Pb, and Zn.
Procedure (a) was taken from a procedure by Anon.(1972) as follows:
up to o.5 g dry sediment was weighed into 125 ml Erlenmeyer flasks. Ten
ml distilled water and lo ml aqua regia were added to each sample. Samples
were heated at 9o-95oC for two min and cooled. Fifteen ml 6 % potassium
permanganate were added and the samples heated at 9o-95oC for 3o min. The
samples were left at room temperature overnight and then analyzed by a
"cold vapour" atomic absorption technique. This latter technique was as
follows: using 2o % sulphuric acid, the sample was transferred to a gas
washing bottle equipped with a fritted end on the stem. Twenty ml of re-
ductant, consisting of about 6oo ml of distilled water, loo ml of concentrated sulphuric acid, 15 g of sodium chloride, 3o g of hydroxylamine sulphate, and 6o g of stannous sulphate, were added to the sample and
stirred for one min. Air, at about looo ml per min. was introduced and the
mercury swept through a 2.5 x 15 cm cell mounted in the light path of the
instrument. Peak heights of recorder response of samples were compared to
those of standards for quantitation.
Procedure (b) was adapted from a procedure of Carmody (1972): up to 5 g
of dry sediment was mixed with 2o ml of 1:1 conc. HNO_3- distilled water.
The sample-acid mixture was shaken vigorously for 2 h at room temperature on a mechanical shaker, then filtered through Whatman No. 2 filter
paper and diluted to loo ml with distilled water. Acid extracts were analyzed directly, using an atomic absorption spectrophotometer (Perkin-
Elmer, Model 4o3).
Neutron activation analysis -- The following procedure was used for Ag,
Co, Cr, Sb, Sc, and Se: up to 1 g of dried sediment and standard solutions
was sealed in quartz tubes. Two samples and one standard were wired together to provide comparable geometries during neutron bombardment for
lo h. The tubes were set aside for 5 weeks after irradiation to allow interfering, short-lived radioisotopes to decay. The tubes were cut and the
samples transferred via 1 M H_2SO_4 into counting vials. Analysis of the
samples and standards was accomplished by gamma ray spectrometry employing a lithium drifted (germanium) gamma ray detector coupled to a pulse
height analyzer system (Nuclear Data Model 44oo). Calculations of the
element concentrations were accomplished via computer programming, utilizing the built-in memory capability of the pulse height analyzer system.

The precision of the sediment metal analyses was measured by relative standard deviations for replicate determinations on a number of typical sediment samples. The mean and confidence limits $(x + ts\sqrt{n})$ for the relative standard deviations for the metals are presented in Table 1. Precision data could not be obtained for the selenium analyses.

The data show that the precision of the analyses of these sediments was quite good with the exceptions of the Ag, Ni, and Pb analyses. For purposes of this study, where relatively large differences in metal concentrations are of primary concern, the precision of the analyses for these three metals was acceptable.

The chemical analyses used for seawater were as follows: Waters from the Raritan Bay, Lower New York Bay system were sampled at 28 locations. Duplicate samples from single casts at surface and bottom were collected at each station in a Niskin sampling bottle modified by replacing the standard O-ring gaskets with those of viton rubber and using silicon tubing in place of the gum rubber supplied by the manufacturer. These modifications eliminated introduction of extraneous metals, primarily zinc, during sampling.

Upon collection, one sample was filtered within 6 h through a o.45 um Millipore filter then acidified with HNO_3 to approximately pH 2, to prevent deposition and loss of metal to container walls. This sample was denoted as the soluble fraction. The other sample, called the acidified fraction, was immediately acidified to pH 2. The soluble fraction was analyzed first thereby allowing approximately a differential of 3 months for leaching the particulate material in the second group. Prior to polarographic analysis (ASV), the second group was also filtered. Ultra pure HNO_3 (Aristar) was used for the acidification, and purified reagents were used throughout the subsequent analysis. Metal concentrations were determined on a 5 ml aliquot using a Princeton Applied Research Model 174 Polarograph coupled with an Environmental Science Associates composite mercury graphite electrode and cell, following the procedures described by Matson (1968) and Fitzgerald (197o). Before each determination, the pH of the sample was raised to 5.3 with purified 1 M sodium acetate-o.2 M sodium chloride buffer. A plating time of lo min was used, and measurements were made on at least three aliquots from each sample. Error associated with the analytical method is estimated to range between $\pm$ o.2 ug $1.^{-1}$ while error introduced by sampling and storage may be as great as $\pm$ lo % at low metal concentrations.

Handling of Samples

In most instances sediment samples were collected using a Smith McIntyre bottom grab from which subsamples were taken with 3.5 cm i.d. plastic (Polybutyrate) coring tubes inserted into the sediment. The tubes were capped and stored frozen until prepared for analysis.

The top 4 cm of sediment were removed from the tubes, placed in a plastic weigh boat and any visible organisms, large stones, and shells were removed from the sample. The sample was dried at 6o°C for 48 h and ground in a glass mortar and pestle.

In most instances the sediment and water samples collected have been frozen prior to analysis. The samples were held in commercial freezers (-2o°C) until such time as the chemical analyses were performed. In several instances, however, samples are being retained for longer periods of time. In these instances we wish to be able to hold sediment core samples for analysis of heavy metal species which might not have been considered in the earlier chemical analyses. Moreover, selected samples from different por-

ions of the New York Bight estuarine system and coastal waters from
Cape Hatteras to Canada are being retained so that in the future samples
can be analyzed and compared with core samples from similar stations taken
some months, years or decades later. Obviously these cores will also be
of importance for comparing the content of certain organic contaminants
against amounts found in cores which might be taken for the same purpose
at a later date. Finally, it is anticipated that as industrialization continues there will be other, as yet unidentified, contaminants which have
some environmental significance. In these instances environmental chemists
would want to have samples collected some years or decades earlier so that
the amounts of an as yet unidentified contaminant can be measured and compared with the values for the same contaminant in marine sediments or
waters collected years or decades earlier.

Heavy Metals in Biota

As was mentioned earlier, scientists of the National Marine Fisheries Service have been interested in the amounts of heavy metals to be found in
living marine resources used for human consumption. These scientists have
also been interested in measuring amounts of heavy metals in various biota
which form part of the complex food chain or food web which culminates
in larger marine fish, frequently designated as apex predators. Measurements
using atomic absorption and neutron activation analyses have been carried
on for several years (Greig, 1975; Greig, Wenzloff and Shelpuk, 1975;
Greig and Jones, 1976; Greig et al., 1977a; Greig et al., 1977b, Greig,
et al., 1978, Pearce, 1977b; and Greig, Wenzloff, and Pearce, 1978;
Greig and Wenzloff, 1977a). The results of these analyses have indicated
that the finfish most often used for human consumption are, generally relatively free from exceptionally large amounts of heavy metals. Apex predators such as the blue and mako sharks have been found, however, to have
large amounts of heavy metals, especially mercury, in both their muscula-
ture and liver tissues (Greig and Wenzloff, 1977b).
In regard to mercury, analysis of 41 species of fish (Greig, Wenzloff,
and Shelpuk, 1975), as well as invertebrate samples, collected from North
Atlantic offshore waters in 1971 indicated that the average mercury concentration in fish muscle was o.154 ppm with a standard deviation of o.124.
Invertebrate samples had mercury concentrations usually less than o.1 ppm;
a single lobster sample, however, had o.31 ppm mercury in the tail muscle
and o.6o ppm in the liver.
In a later special series of analyses for mercury in three species of
fish from the North Atlantic offshore waters (Greig et al., 1977a), spiny
dogfish were obtained from five areas. No significant difference in mercury levels was found in the muscle tissue as related to geographic area.
Mercury levels ranged from o.21 to o.62 ppm. These values approached the
mercury values which were found in blue and mako sharks. It should be
emphasized that at the present time very few sharks or dogfish are sold
for human consumption in the United States. The voluminous amount of data
which have resulted from analyses for heavy metals by scientists attached
to the Division of Environmental Assessment has recently been compiled in
a report to the International Council for the Exploration of the Sea
(ICES) (Pearce, 1977b). Additional findings on heavy metals in fish collected from the New York Bight apex in 1978 have recently been submitted
to the ICES Working Group on Pollution Baseline and Monitoring Studies
in the North Atlantic (Greig, Wenzloff, and Pearce, 1978). Both of these
studies indicated that there were no unusual amounts of heavy metals in

finfish collected from the New York Bight apex or other waters of the
Middle Atlantic Bight. This evaluation was based on comparison of these
data with those provided on heavy metals in finfish from Scottish
waters (Topping, 1973) as well as other European areas (Portmann, 1972).
One of the major problems has been to determine,however, what consti-
tutes unacceptable levels of heavy metals in marine fish. The United
States has established recommended guidelines for mercury and cadmium. Other countries have done the same. Unfortunately, there is at the
present time no sound set of data which would indicate the significance
of slightly elevated or even unusually high amounts of heavy metals in
body tissues of fish in terms of the fishes' well-being.
The data which resulted from the preliminary studies of the College Park
Laboratory, Southeast Utilization Research Center, were very similar to
those produced by the chemical analyses conducted by the Northeast Fisheries Center. Ninety-four percent, or 2,265 of the samples analyzed by the
College Park Laboratory were below the FDA interim guideline of o.5 ppm
of mercury. Over one half of the samples analyzed for their report had
mean mercury values below   ppm. Likewise, the mean cadmium levels were
below o.3 ppm except for certain species of mulluscs. They found that the
majority of the muscle samples from finfish fell between o.1 and o.6 ppm
copper; 2.o and 24.o ppm zinc; o.1 and o.3 ppm of nickel and o.1 and o.2 ppm
of manganese.
Atlantic oysters that had been collected from a contaminated river leading
into Long Island Sound had higher amounts than the mean of other samples of
the Atlantic oysters in regard to cadmium, silver, copper, zinc, nickel and
manganese.
Recently, Wenzloff, Greig, Merrill and Ropes (1978) reported that heavy
metals in two bivalve molluscs, the surf clam and ocean quahog, collected
from offshore waters of the Middle Atlantic coast of the United States,
had an interesting pattern of heavy metal distribution. Clams taken from
the southern portions of their ranges had relatively low levels of heavy
metals; in the northern portions of their ranges the amounts of heavy metals increased (Figures 1 and 2). Both of these clam species are found
offshore and would normally be regarded as forms not likely to be impinged
upon by heavy metals having their origin in polluted estuaries. It is significant that there is a linear relationship between increasing heavy metals and latitude. It has been suggested that the clams taken from the
more northern portions of their ranges may be exposed to heavy metals
which are emanating from the Hudson River estuary and Raritan Bay complex.
Further research will be required to document this relationship. Nevertheless, this is one of the few instances where a sedentary species collected
simultaneously over a wide range of latitude does show increases in heavy
metals when it is found in waters which have been shown to be contaminated
with heavy metals.
The samples collected for the foregoing studies were selected on the basis
of several criteria. First, samples were collected to yield species of
interest. In both the College Park and the Northeast Fisheries Center studies, it was desirable to obtain fish from several trophic levels including
apex predators, herbivorous forms , and fish intermediate within the food
chain. Also, it was deemed important to collect certain species of sedan-
tary shellfish such as the ocean quahog, surf clam, and oyster. The
latter forms have little mobility and are exposed continuously to sources
of heavy metals; unlike the motile fish and certain of the natatory
crustaceans, the bivalve molluscs cannot avoid the presence of heavy metals
or other contaminant stress by swimming away. The samples were collected
in a consistent fashion and shipboard preparation involved avoidance of

sources of metals that might be introduced through mishandling or contact with metal surfaces or instruments.The fish and shellfish tissues were usually preserved in metal-free containers and frozen until such time as the chemical analyses could be performed. The methods used for chemical analyses have been given in several papers prepared by chemists for the Northeast Fisheries Center (Greig, 1975; Wenzloff and Shelpuk, 1975; Greig and Jones, 1976; Greig et al., 1977a; Greig et al., 1977b; Greig, et al., 1978; Pearce, 1977b; and Greig, Wenzloff, and Pearce, 1978; Greig and Wenzloff, 1977a).

Two different procedures were used for heavy metal analyses of biota at the Milford Laboratory, one for mercury and one for the other seven metals. For mercury the method of Greig et al. (1975) was used and the method for the other metals was Ten-g samples were placed in Pyrex beakers and charred over a bunsen burner or on a hot plate until smoke evolvement subsided. Samples were then placed in a cool muffle furnace and brought slowly to 250°C for 1 hr, then removed and cooled. The ash was moistened with concentrated nitric acid and the beakers were placed on hot plates to evaporate the acid to dryness. Dried samples were returned to a cool muffle furnace and slowly brought to 4oo°C. The process of adding acid to dryness and heating at 4oo°C was repeated 3 to 5 times until the material was reduced to a nearly white residue. Samples were then taken up in several small portions of 1o % nitric acid and filtered through Whatman No. 2 filter paper, then brought to 1o or 25 ml with 1o % nitric acid. Acid solutions were analyzed directly with an atomic absorption spectrophotometer (Perkin Elmer Model 4o3). Data from this and other laboratories were calculated as ppm, wet weight.

Per cent recoveries were determined for metals added to fish. Results show that all but silver in fish produced mean recoveries greater than 9o % which is very satisfactory. The mean silver recovery in fish for the atomic absorption method was 74.7 %; however, as stated earlier Greig (1975) showed that this atomic absorption technique gave data that compared very well with that of a neutron activation procedure. In addition to percent recovery data, information was obtained on a National Bureau of Standards (NBS)reference material - on orchard leaf. The results show that very favorable comparative data were obtained with the methods described here as compared to the NBS certified values.

It should be noted that the chemical analyses conducted on fish and shellfish tissues by both the College Park Laboratory and the Environmental Chemistry Investigation, Northeast Fisheries Center, involved the same techniques as have been used in intercalibration exercises sponsored by the International Council for the Exploration of the Sea (ICES). The results of these analyses have recently been the subject of a report by Topping (1978). In addition to the ICES- sponsored intercalibration exercises, samples have been analyzed using both atomic absorption and neutron activation in order to compare the results for the determination of silver, chromium, and zinc in various marine organisms (Greig, 1975). Greig and Jones (1976) also discussed the analysis of marine organisms using nondestructive neutron activation techniques. Again, the results compare favorably with results obtained from atomic absorption spectrophotometry.

During the development of the new Ocean Pulse environmental assessment program (Pearce, 1977a), increased attention is being given to program design, especially in regard to developing future baseline and monitoring studies in regard to the distribution and abundance of metals in the marine ecosystem. Furthermore, program design also emphasizes the development of techniques which will allow the modeling of heavy metal flow within estuaries and within marine food webs. The research concerned with heavy metal distributions in the physical environment and biota that is being organized in the Northeast Fisheries Center emphasizes interactions with other federal agencies such as the U.S. Environmental Protection Agency and various state environmental protection administrations or groups. The research also anticipates participation of scientists from the academic community. Part of the program design includes the development of tissue banks which will be used to retain tissues collected from representative types of organisms, including microorganisms, as well as examples of the various trophic levels found within marine food webs. Samples of bivalve tissue from several estuaries, as well as from coastal and offshore waters, are presently processed and being retained for future examination. Four key species of finfish including the oceanpout, cunner, winter flounder, and silver hake, which are characteristic of the Middle Atlantic Bight, are being retained in the tissue bank. Samples of apex predators such as the blue and mako sharks as well as tuna and species such as bluefish are also being retained. The bivalves have particular importance since, as previously mentioned, they are sedentary and may provide the best diagnosis for increased metals within the physical environment. Apex predators are important inasmuch as they have been shown to consistently have increased metal values relative to other finfish. The four species of fish from the Middle Atlantic Bight and other species, are being held in our tissue bank since they occupy niches within several ecosystems likely to be impacted by heavy metals. For instance, the winter flounder is a bottom-dwelling fish which spends the majoritiy of its life within a reasonably circumscribed area in more or less constant contact with bottom sediments, many of which may be polluted. The ocean pout and cunner are fish which are often associated with artificial and natural reefs in the New York Bight apex and thus are exposed to waters some distance removed from the bottom sediment.

Finally, sediment samples from many portions of the New York Bight as well as the larger Middle Atlantic Bight have been retained in a frozen condition. As earlier mentioned these samples will provide a reference for assessing possible changes in heavy metals distributions and abundance. They may also be used in the future for comparison for contaminants that have not yet been identified as having particular significance. We have also partitioned sediment samples collected from certain key areas so that they can be examined on a vertical basis. Some preliminary evidence would suggest that sediments that are closest to the surface layers may contain more heavy metals than deeper sediments.

It is assumed that tissue banks as well as other facilities for the retention of physical samples, including both water and sediments, will become increasingly important as mankind releases additional contaminants to the marine environment. It is obvious that considerable forethought should be given so that limited storage space can be most effectively used. Personnel within the Northeast Fisheries Center have anticipated that it would be impossible to retain samples of each species and circumscribed geographic area. It is important, however, to provide storage for long-term holdings of certain key species as well as physical samples from key environments. It is hoped that the results of the workshop on tissue banks will bring to the attention of the world the need for tissue banks as well, as provide information on the most appropriate ways for handling and storing tissues for long periods of time. Techniques such as freeze drying should be examined. Also, collection and storage procedures should be evaluated and recommendations made in regard to the most efficient way to hold tissues

without contamination.For many of the contaminants now of interest to mankind the analyses must be performed at the parts per billion level. Certain contaminants may only exist at the parts per trillion level in certain
instances and yet some limited information indicates that such contaminants
may have an effect at these low levels.

LITERATURE CITED

Anonymous. 1972: Provisional method. Analytical Quality Control, Laboratory
1o14 Broadway, Cincinnati, Ohio.

Bryan, G.W. 1976: Some aspects of heavy metal tolerance in aquatic organisms.
Pages 7-34 in A.P.M. Lockwood, ed. Effects of pollutants on aquatic orga-
nisms, Vol 2. Society for Experimental Biology Seminar Series, Cambridge
University Press.

Carmody, D.J. 1972: The distribution of five heavy metals in the sediments
of the New York Bight. Ph.D. dissertation.Columbia University Teachers
College. University Microfilms, Ann Arbor, Mich.

Carmody, D.J., J.P. Pearce, and W.E. Yasso. 1973: Trace metals in sediments of the New York Bight. Mar. Poll. Bull 4(9): 132-135.

Eganhouse, R.P., Jr. 1976: Mercury in sediments. Pages 83-89 in Coastal
water research project annual report for the year ended 3o June 1976.
(Southern California Coastal Water Research Project, El Segundo, Calif.)

First Interim Report on Microconstituent Resource Survey. 1975: A preli-
minary report of incomplete research. National Marine Fisheries Service,
Southeast Utilization Research Center, February 19, 1975. (College Park,
Md.).

Fitzgerald, W.F. 197o: A study of certain trace metals in seawater using
anoidic stripping voltammetry. Ph.D. Thesis. M.I.T. and Woods Hole Oceanogr. Inst.

Greig, R.A. 1975: Comparison of atomic absorption and neutron activation
analyses for the determination of silver, chromium, and zinc in various
marine organisms. Anal. Chem. 47(9): 1682-1684.

Greig, R.A., A. Adams, and D.R. Wenzloff. 1977: Trace metal content of
plankton and zooplankton collected from the New York Bight and Long Island
Sound. Bull. Environ. Contam. & Toxicol. 18(1): 3-8.

Greig, R.A., and J. Jones. 1976: Nondestructive neutron activation analysis
of marine organisms collected from ocean dump sites of the middle eastern
United States. Archives Environ. Contam. & Toxicol. 4(4): 42o-434.

Greig, R.A., and R.A. McGrath. 1977: Trace metals in sediments of Raritan
Bay. Mar. Poll. Bull 8(8): 188-192.

Greig, R.A., R.N. Reid, and D.R. Wenzloff. 1977: Trace metal concentrations
in sediments from Long Island Sound. Mar. Poll. Bull. 8(8): 183-188.

514

Greig, R.A., and D.R. Wenzloff. 1977a: Trace metals in finfish from the New York Bight and Long Island Sound. Mar. Poll. Bull 8(9): 198-2oo.

Greig, R.A., and D.R. Wenzloff. 1977b: Final report on heavy metals in small pelagic finfish, euphausid crustaceans and apex predators, including sharks, as well as on heavy metals and hydrocarbons (C_{15+}) in sediments collected at stations in and near deepwater dumpsite 1o6. Pages 547-564 in Baseline report of environmental conditions in Deepwater Dumpsite 1o6. NOAA Dumpsite Evaluation Report 77-1, June 1977, Vol. III. Rockville, Md.

Greig, R.A., D.R. Wenzloff, and J.B. Pearce. 1978: Report to the Working Group on Pollution Baseline and Monitoring Studies in the North Atlantic on heavy metals in selected finfish and shellfish from the New York Bight. Report to International Council for the Exploration of the Sea. 12 pp.

Greig, R.A., D.R. Wenzloff, and C. Shelpuk. 1975: Mercury concentrations in fish, North Atlantic offshore waters - 1971. Pesticides Monit. J. 9 (1): 15-19.

Greig, R.A., D.R. Wenzloff, A. Adams, B. Nelson, and C. Shelpuk. 1977a: Trace metals in organisms from ocean disposal sites of the middle eastern United States. Archives Environ. Contam. & Toxicol. 6: 395-4o9.

Greig, R.A., D. Wenzloff, C. Shelpuk, and A. Adams. 1977b: Mercury concentrations in three species of fish from North Atlantic offshore waters. Archives Environ. Contam. & Toxicol. 5: 315-323.

Greig, R.A., D.R. Wenzloff, C.L. MacKenzie, Jr., A.S. Merrill, and V.S. Zdanowicz. 1978: Trace metals in sea scallops, Placopecten magellanicus, from eastern United States. Bull. Environ. Contam. & Toxicol. ooo7-4861/ 78/oo19-o326: 326-334.

Matson, W.R. 1968: Trace metals, equilibrium and kinetics of trace metal complexes in natural media. Ph.D. Thesis. Dept. of Chem., M.I.T.

Pearce, J. 1977a: A report on a new environmental assessment and monitoring program, Ocean Pulse. C.M. 1977/E: 65, Fisheries Improvement Commitee International Council for the Exploration of the Sea. 12 pp. 1977b: Report to the Working Group on Pollution Baseline and Monitoring Studies in the OSLO Commission and ICNAF areas on heavy metals in selected finfish and shellfish from the Northwest Atlantic. C.M.1977/E:34, Fisheries Improvement Committee. International Council for the Exploration of the Sea. 98 pp.

Topping, G. 1978: Preliminary report on the fourth ICES trace metal intercomparison exercise. Poll.78Ag.7.3. ICES Working Group on Marine Pollution Baseline and Monitoring Studies in the North Atlantic. International Council for the Exploration of the Sea. 1o pp.

Waldhauer, R., A. Matte, and R. Tucker. 1978: Lead and copper in the waters of Raritan and Lower New York Bight. Mar. Poll. Bull. 9(2): 38-42.

Wenzloff, D.R., R.A. Greig, A.S. Merrill, and J.W. Ropes. 1978: A survey of heavy metals in two bivalve molluscs of the mid-Atlantic coast of the United States. Fish.Bull. In press.

Westöö, G. 1966: Determining of methylmercury compounds in foodstuffs. 1. Methylmercury compounds in fish,identification and determination. Acta chem. scand. 2o: 2131-2137.
1967: Mercury in fish. Var Föda 19: 1-7 (in Swedish).

SOME U.S. LEGAL CONCERNS IN OBTAINING, ARCHIVING, AND USING NON-HUMAN TISSUE SAMPLES

Jan C. Prager, Ph.D., and David A. Flemer, Ph.D.
U.S. Environmental Protection Agency
Narragansett, Rhode Island o2882 and Washington, D.C. 2o46o
and Richard C. Browne, J.D., Washington,D.C.

Abstract

Current U.S. law at municipal, state, and federal governmental levels relates directly and indirectly to obtaining non-human tissue samples, transporting them, maintaining them, utilizing them in studies, and releasing information obtained from such studies. The text discussed various premitting authorities involved in obtaining samples; chain of custody procedures required to maintain scientific and legal integrity, human safety constraints, and procedures required to protect samples, processors, archivists, and investigators; proprietary information, privacy and the "Freedom of Information Act".

Introduction

Most of the scientific community seldom think about legal aspects of the conduct or communication of science. Aside from issues of patent or publication rights, only the occasional scientist, even in a regulatory agency, becomes familiar with water law, conservation law, administrative law, or courtroom procedures pertaining to the uses and limits of science in formulating public policy. Yet, all humanity and human endeavour exist and function subject to governance by the law.

The law is a creature of its community, a creature of man-made protocols, and is itself quite admittedly unable to reach conclusions in any area other than law per se. Therefore, in the interaction of science and the law it is of paramount importance to understand that at any time and under any circumstances, science remains science -- with all of its own community standards of self evaluation and judgement -- and the law too remains a system unto itself. Thus law can not make good science bad, nor bad science good. Therefore, the scientist need not fear it and, in fact, need only look to the law for governance in non-scientific aspects of scientific work.

We in science from time to time have had to consider the legal aspects of our field and laboratory studies as they have been used for regulatory purposes. The information that we offer here represents not legal counsel but rather relates to the experiences of scientists helping to formulate public policy or to enforce existing law, and offers some afterthoughts about them. As a scientist, if you find that the law is used as an impediment to the free conduct of your work rather than as an aid, we only can advise you to consult an attorney. If you do this to the same extent that your would have scientists consulted in the wise formulation of public policy, we may broaden an all too narrow channel of communication.

LAWS AFFECTING VARIOUS STAGES OF SAMPLING AND ARCHIVING

Access to Samples:

Amost always, the material that you want to sample belongs to someone else. Before you proceed to take it, you need to consider (1) who it belongs to, (2) what is its value to the owner, (3) who will be helped by your taking it, (4) who will be hurt by your taking it, and (5) what are the rights of the persons and things involved. Except in rare instances[1] you safely may assume that you have no rights to the materials that you want to sample unless they are granted to you specifically by the owner.

Non-human tissue samples can become very controversial subjects of adversary proceedings and therefore the sampler should be assured that sampling itself is performed under legal circumstances. Materials sampled will be owned privately or by municipal, state, or federal government. The sampler must assure a right to enter the sampling area as well as permission to sample. Ideally both permissions should be obtained in some written form from the person, corporation, or governmental body involved. In addition, certain species are protected under law to varying extents, and appropriate licensing may be required to take them.[2] Both state and federal government concern themselves with licensing the taking of finfish, shellfish, and wildlife. No species listed on the U.S. Endangered Species list[3] may be taken for any purposes by any U.S. Department of the Interior. In general, federal involvement in various hunting and fishing licensure is indirect, regulating water quality and chemical contamination of flesh, whereas state governments issue licenses regulating amount of material which may be taken, locations and means of taking, and times during which takings are permitted. Most states will issue special collecting permits for taking plant and animal material in normally prohibited times, amounts, or places, if the material is to be used exclusively for purposes of research or monitoring. Ordinarily such licenses are issued by the state's Department of Fish and Game or its nominal equivalent.

Sampling Methods:

Two concerns arise in regard to method. First, the method of obtaining samples must not be prohibited by law. For example, certain states prohibit taking of specific shellfishes by SCUBA divers. Poisoning and blasting also are usually prohibited methods of sampling -- although in special circumstances where such non-discriminatory methods can be justified, state exemptions may be obtained. Other methodological prohibitions concern use of specified (or non-prohibited) firearms, net-types, gear-types, or means of transportation while sampling. Again, reasonable and justifiable exemptions from such laws or regulations may be obtained from appropriate state

---

1/eg. (1) You own the material, (2) You are acting as an agent of a duly empowered governmental agency rightfully using its police power, or (3) no one owns the material and it is outside any governmental jurisdiction.

2/eg. The National Marine Fisheries Service in the U.S. Department of Commerce administers regulations and issues permits required by the Marine Mammal Protection Act of 1972 (16 U.S.C. 1361) and the Endangered Species Act of 1973 (16 U.S.C. 1531).

3/The Endangered Species List is updated and republished annually by the U.S. Fish and Wildlife Service in the Department of the Interior. The most recent list appeared in the Federal Register for December 11, 1978.

authorities. Such laws and regulations commonly apply to organisms of commercial or recreational importance, leaving the samplers of viruses, bacteria, protozoa, lichens, and many non-flowering plants much to their own devices. In the U.S., information gained by government agents by illegal means can not be used in a court of law in a proceeding against a person from whom the data or information was taken.[4]

Second, sampling methods should be scientifically sound and thoroughly documented. This is particularly important in tissue banking because the materials archived probably will be investigated well after sampling and not by the original sampler. Thus information on sampling time, place, circumstances and method must be exact and complete for the sake of highly reliable information. Reliability is extremely important if the data obtained from banked tissues are used in formulation of public policy (laws, regulations, standards, or criteria); and doubly so if they become the subject of adversary proceedings.

Transport of Samples:

Transport of non-human tissue samples is usually subject to question only at international borders. National concerns about importation of disease or disease vectors and exportation of commercially valuable, rare, or endangered species are reflected in federal laws concerning transfer of animal species or agricultural materials across a national border. Such prohibitions are not always obvious to the scientist, who may well understand the problems of transporting venomous reptiles or virulent microorganisms but need think twice about the impact of certain plant imports upon agricultural economy. Arrangements for international transport of even tissues samples should be made with appropriate customs and consular officials well in advance if the speedy transport and integrity of the materials is to be assured.

Within the U.S. transport of materials also poses certain legal problems. Federal transportation regulations closely regulate shipments of materials containing potentially hazardous elements such as dry ice or liquid nitrogen.[5] Materials possessing dangerous properties such as flammability, radioactivity, virulence, toxicity, and perishability usually need be transported by road or rail and here too are subject to federal and state regulation concerning mode of transport, containment, and warning markings. Although most tissue materials do not fall into the dangerous category, their media or preservative may and such matters need to be thought through well before samples are taken and shipped.

Legal Integrity of Samples:

If data derived from archived samples are to be useful in public policy formulation, they must be able to withstand attack in an adversary proceeding. The "chain of custody" from sampler to archivist to investigator must be unbroken in the sense that the materials can be guaranteed by all concerned to be as they are represented -- in kind, amount, identity, mar-

---

4/The U.S. Supreme Court recently discussed the development of the rule governing use of illegally obtained evidence in U.S. v JANIS, 96S.C. 3o21(1976).

5/Regulations governing shipment of hazardous materials are administered by the Materials Transportation Bureau in the U.S. Department of Transportation and are published in the Code of Federal Regulations (49 CFR §§17o-189).

kings, and condition. Thus, the sampler must be able to testify that a
sample was taken as recorded (time, place, circumstances, method, etc.),
marked as found, and transported by some tamper-proof method by reliable means to the archivist. The archivist in turn must be able to
testify that the materials were received in sealed and unadulterated condition, were permanently marked, and were maintained intact, so were given
to the investigator. So for the investigator. Although all of this may
seem a bit overly legalistic, upon reflection it may be recognized as
nothing more than the prudent and cautions scientist would require of
materials upon which one may stake a reputation among ones' peers. The
only real difference between normal scientific prudence and legalistic
practice is an added stress upon written accountability. To extend an
introductory remark, the law can not make good science bad, nor bad
science good, but it can help to make good science better -- and perhaps
conversely, to make bad science obvious.

LAWS AFFECTING STAGES OF INVESTIGATION AND COMMUNICATION

Worker Protection:

Laboratories, and therefore tissue archives, really are dangerous places.
They abound with sharp adged glassware, poisonous chemicals, flammables,
dangerous gases and persons who, no matter how well trained, may be subject to lapses in judgement. The Occupational Safety and Health Act
(OSHA) is a recent U.S. attempt to improve the safety of the workplace
and its healthfulness for the worker. OSHA publishes guidelines for chemically and biologically hazardous situations which, if followed,
should reduce danger to persons working in potentially hazardous situations.
Occupational safety regulations cover new laboratory building construction
and operation, laboratory chemical and electrical equipment standards, and
many other features of importance to tissue banking and scientific investigation. Although the bench scientist may not perceive him or herself as a supervisor of personnel, this incorrect perception can be corrected quickly and unpleasantly by a lawsuit resulting from an employee
grievance or, far worse, a hurt employee. A conscientious program of OSHA
standards checks and worker training would not be out of place in a
tissue archive laboratory.

Communication and Confidentiality:

Collegial communications common among pure research personnel become a
problem the moment that data or information communicated cross the translucent and fuzzy border from pure science into the realms of proprietary
information or adversary evidence. Unless you are employed in a federal
laboratory, you are not required to provide information to persons whom
you may not know or trust without legal process such as a subpoena. If
you are employed in a federal laboratory, files and data are subject
to the "Freedom of Information Act" which, with certain exceptions
(such as draft and working papers, personnel records, or confidential
trade secret data), make them public information which must be offered
up to the requestor within a legally set time limit. Faced with a request
for data or information from an unknown, suspect, or non-research source,
you should run rather than walk to your laboratory or institutional legal
counsel for assistance. Unverified data or written opinions based upon
preliminary or incomplete data sets never should be communicated unless
they are so identified in writing -- and it is good practice to traffic
only in published reports when answering written requests for information.
Again, upon reflection this may be recognized as the prudent method of the

520

cautions and conservative scientist avoiding conclusions unsupported by fact.

Confidentiality is less of an issue in non-human tissue sample archiving, research, and monitoring than it is in regard to human tissues -- but there are situations in which it may arise. In matters under litigation or in dealing with samples the analysis of which could disclose proprietary information, or secrets of national security importance, the rights of other parties may supercede the right of scientific disclosure. Again, should issues of confidentiality occur spontaneously to you or be brought to your attention, seek legal counsel immediately. Such situations are highly unlikely to happen to more than one in a thousand of us -- even including those of us in federal and state regulatory agencies -- but in spite of the odds against an occurrence, its possibility requires some consideration.

Disposal of Samples and Process Wastes:

All laboratory wastes are subject to the same federal and state clean air and clean water laws as are any other wastes from any other sources. Therefore, appropriate permits for discharges must be obtained from federal and state authorities. The content of tissue bank process wastes can be determined either by measurement of flows and their chemical constituents or by performing mass budget calculations on the amount of preservatives and other toxics purchased per unit time and the concentrations discharged per batch, its dilution, etc. Such information is required if waste streams are discharged from the facility into publicly owned wastewater treatment works or navigable waters of the U.S.

SUMMARY

Both science and law are evolving, independent systems unto themselves. They do not change each other in their practice, but only in their evolution of thought. Thus, the sampling, archiving, and utilization of non-human tissues never shall affect the practice of law, but they well may influence the development of present and future legislation concerning environmental protection, natural resource management, conservation, preservation, and other human benefits. Similarly, passage of human law can not affect the laws of nature, but it can influence the activities of science and scientists by providing positive and negative incentives to investigate selected subjects. We believe that the working histological archivist should understand these relationships, become conversant with those aspects of the law which govern the non-scientific aspects of this science, and pursue scientific investigation secure in the knowledge that when law impinges upon science, it only can make good science better and poor science abvious.

POLLUTION EFFECTS IN FRESHWATER
COMMUNITIES

O. Ravera
Department of Physical and Natural Sciences
Commissione delle Comunità Europee
Centro Comune di Ricerca
21o2o Ispra (Varese) Italy

Introduction

The protection of man against pollution is exercised both at the individual
and at the population level. The same criterion cannot be used for the
protection of animals and plants and, consequently, the value of a single
specimen varies with the size and turnover-rate of the population to which
it belongs. Hence, knowledge of the effects of pollution at population and
community level is the fundamental background for protecting the biota.

Because there is a certain confusion about the word "pollution", it seems
opportune to clarify the meaning adopted for this paper. Pollution is the
immission into an aquatic environment of substances or calories deriving
from man and his activities in such amounts as to produce noxious effects
at population level and community level. This definition is in a good
agreement with that proposed by Margalef (1975). "We can consider pollution as essentially being something "out of place" usually as a consequence
of interference by man". The degree of pollution cannot be evaluated on
the basis of the use made by man of the environment; this criterion must
be adopted for planning interventions to improve the environmental situation.
The dramatic consequences of the nuclear explosions in Japan during the
Second World War and the following 336 nuclear tests causing a sudden increase of the natural level of the environmental radioactivity, have made
the public and the authorities afraid of radioactive pollution. These were
the first facts showing the need to control and reduce pollution on a world
scale. Successively, the widespread distribution of lead, DDT and PCB has
become a classical example of pollution involving the whole biosphere.

For no type of pollution has so much research been done, so many precautions adopted and such precise rules laid down at the national and international level as for radioactive contamination. As a consequence, it
seems desirable that some criteria developed for radioprotection (e.g.
critical pathway, critical group, concentration factor) be adopted for
protecting man and ecosystem against non-radioactive pollution (Ravera,
1972).

Another recent aspect of the pollution problem is the damage deriving from
waste water treatment, for example, the pollutants produced by chlorination and ozonation of organic compounds existing in the effluents (Carlson et al., 1975).

Pollutant categories

It is usual to group the pollutants into categories on the basis of their
very evident chemical or physical characteristics or their use (e.g. radionuclides, heavy metals, hydrocarbons, pesticides, detergents and fertilizers) or according to their degradability (e.g. persistent, easily decomposed pollutants). These groupings have a certain advantage for describing
the type of pollution charge into a water body, but they have less meaning
for evaluating pollutant toxicity. In fact, the noxious effects of a substance introduced into an ecosystem vary in relation with its physical and
chemical form the characteristics of the physical environment and those
of the biota living in it. For example, several pesticides are very toxic
for Arthropods, but not for Molluscs and a herbicide may kill the larger
aquatic plants of a river, but may have no influence on fish. For the same
taxonomical group (e.g. Chlorophycaea) some heavy metals (e.g. Cu, Cd) have
a high toxicity, others very low (e.g. Zn, Pb). Large differences of toxicity have been observed within the category of the hydrocarbons and within
detergents. The toxicity of non-ionized ammonia is very high for fish, but
if temperature and pH of the water are low, ammonia changes to the ionized
form, which has a very low toxicity.

The degree of persistence of a pollutant is obviously a very important property; for example, Kimerle et al. (1975) demonstrated that the first step
of biodegradation of LAS (alkyl benzene sulfonate) decreases its toxicity
by an order of magnitude. It is evident that some detergents, pesticides
and hydrocarbons are persistent pollutants; while other pollutants classified in the same categories are less persistent.

Radioactive decay may be considered a process of degradation, because of
this process the hazard of radioactive material decreases with time. The
radioactive decay is independent of the characteristics of the environment,
while the degradability is an effect of the microbial activity or of chemical and physical processes. In other words, the half-life of the radioisotopes is constant, that of the non-radioactive organic substances is strictly related to the environmental characteristics. In conclusion, if the persistent radioisotopes with half-life of days or years may be separated, in
an arbitrary way, from those with half-life of minutes or seconds; it is
often difficult the degradation rate of certain non-radioactive pollutants
discharged in natural environment.

A classification of the pollutants by their ability to be accumulated in
the organism cannot be done, because bioaccumulation is controlled, in
addition to the characteristics of the pollutant, by the behaviour, physiology and biochemistry of the organism. For example, ionic iron is easily incorporated in the algal cell, but some Diatoms (e.g. Asterionella
japonica) have a preferential uptake for iron in colloidal form. Bioaccumulation is a result of two processes: uptake and elimination. Because the
rates of these processes vary with the species and the physiological stage,
different accumulation for the same substance in different species and
stages may be expected.

In addition, it is important to take into account the variation of the toxicity of a pollutant for synergism and antagonism; two widely diffused
phenomena creating difficulties for any classification. These phenomena

need additional research because it is not completely clear what are the basis mechanisms of action involved in these processes. In addition, the organism is able to reduce, at least partly, the noxious effects of the pollutants introduced in its body be means of physiological and biochemical mechanisms (e.g. break-down of the pollutant, excretion, storage of toxic lipophilic molecules in fat depots).

These considerations make evident the difficulty of clasifying pollutants by their biological effects.

Attempts have been made to group organic pollutants (e.g. hydrocarbons, pesticides, detergents) according to the relation between their structure and the biological effects produced by them. To predict the effects on biota of a compound from knowledge of its structure and physical and chemical properties is an attractive idea and would be of great benefit in evaluating the toxicity of new chemicals. So far little work has been done on this subject, but the difficulties in putting this idea into practice are evident, because of the great variability of the biota and the influence of the physical environment. In addition one of the most important limitations to generalizing the relationship between structure and effect is the choice of appropriate type of biological reaction. Anyway, several interesting results in this research area have been obtained.

According to Zitko (1975) the toxicity of some organophosphate pesticides is related to their water solubility and, generally, but not always, the acute toxicity increases with decreasing solubility of the compounds. There is a good correlation between the inhibition of acetylcholinesterase and toxicity from organophosphate pesticides. This is very evident for insects but not for molluscs. In freshwater snails a correlation between sulphydryl-group blocking activity and toxicity of alkylvinyl sulfones has been found (Bond et al., 1971). Zitko (1974) demonstrated that the molecular weight of certain organic pollutants has no influence on their uptake by fish. The toxicity of linear LAS is related to alkyl chain length and phenyl isomer position (Marchetti, 1965, Divo, 1974). Longer chains and terminal isomers are more toxic, but they are also the first components to be degraded. On the other hand, it seems that this detergent is easily metabolized by fish independent of its partition coefficient, which may vary by up to an order of magnitude in relation with its concentration in the water and some environmental characteristics.

Pharmacologists commonly use the partition coefficient between octanol and water to measure the biological activity of serveral compounds. Neely et al. (1974) correlated the bioaccumulation in fish with the partition coefficients of some organic compounds. Because surfactants have both hydrophilic and lipophilic groups in the same molecule, their partition coefficient may vary with the electrical conductivity hardness and pH of the water. As a consequence, the toxicity of a surfactant is also related to the properties of the water body in which it is discharged.

In conclusion, up to today there exist no classification of the pollutants completely satisfying from the point of view of toxicity. Consequently the actual effects of a pollutant must be evaluated in relation with its characteristics and those of the ecosystem (physical environment plus biota) in which it is immitted. On the other hand, to know the relation between the structure and physico-chemical properties of pollutants and

biological effects is so important that research in this area should be
encouraged.

Biological effects

Biological effects of pollution range from sublethal and genetical alterations to the death of some individuals (weaker or more exposed) as the
extinction of the whole population. Some pollutants are indirectly dangerous in decreasing the resistance of the organism to microbial and viral
diseases. An example of this effect is given by Giussani et al. (1976)
for the mass mortality of fish in eutrophicated lakes of Northern Italy
and Southern Switzerland. During some periods of the year the ammonia
concentration in the water is rather high and in the same time an epidemic
of Saprolegnaceae kills a large number of fish. According to this Author
the high concentration of ammonia increases fish susceptibility to parasitical diseases.

For the most pollutants the relationship between their concentration in
the natural environment and their biological effects is not known. This
knowledge seems to be still beyond our capability, there being an absence,
or at least a deficiency, of guiding concepts (Vollenweider and Ravera,
in press) and systems being extremely complex.

Because of their simplicity laboratory experiments may show clear relations between concentration of apollutant and one or more reactions of
the organism. On the other hand, the results obtained from laboratory
experiments may not be easily extrapolated to natural populations.

The choice of the biological reaction to measure the toxicity of a given
substance gives rise to an additional difficulty. Indeed, it is not easy
to estimate how important to the survival of an organism are the behavioural
physiological and biochemical reactions chosen and it is more difficult to
predict the importance of these reactions at population level. Mortality
of a given number of individuals is the parameter more commonly used,
whereas other demographical characteristics (e.g. fertility) not less important, are generally neglected.

The choice of species is a fundamental problem in testing the toxicity of
pollutants. At present the number of species used to this aim (commonly
used are some species of fish and Daphnia) is too low to reach valuable
conclusions on the possible effects of pollutants on the whole community.
Indeed, the sensitivity of a given pollutant varies with the taxonomical
group; for example, the sensitivity of algae to cadmium salts is greater
than that of fish, and snails are much more resistant to organophosphate
pesticides than Crustaceans and Insects. In addition to test the actual
sensitivity of a given species to a given pollutant, experiments must
be carried out on adult specimens as well as on the other developmental
stages, which are sometimes the more sensitive ones.

According to the duration of the experiment, the responses may be diveded
into two types: those that deal with acute effects (short-term effects,
that is those effects accurring after a few hours or days) and those involving chronic effects (long-term effects, over more than a week). Short-
term experiments are more easy to carry out, but they often provide inadequate information on the toxicity of pollutants. Long-term experiments

are more difficult but they provide more realistic information. Certain
pollutants, at low concentrations, produce sublethal effects which reduce the mean lifespan of the organism. To record this effect, the duration
of the experiment must be of the same order of magnitude as that of the
lifespan of the species considered. As a consequence, more attention must
be payed to the sublethal effects produced by substances supposed nontoxic on the basis of short-term experiments.

To compare the responses of different species by means of experiments of
the same duration, we must take into consideration that the unit of time
may have a different meaning for species with very different physiological
lives. For example, the period of 48 hours represents about 3o % of the
lifespan of organisms that live one week, but about 1 % of those with a
mean lifespan of six month.

The influence of the chemical and physical characteristics of the water
on the toxicity has been clearly demonstrated forseveral pollutants (e.g.
Steeman-Nielsen et al., 1969; 197o; Erickson et al., 197o; Ravera, 1972;
Greene et al., 1975; Premazzi et al. in press). Theoretical and practical
difficulties regarding experimentation and the treatment of results are
discussed in greater detail in the literature (e.g. Sprague, 1969, 197o,
1971; Ravera, 1975).

From the pollution effects on individuals, physiological functions, enzymatic systems and chromosomes it is very difficult to predict the ultimate
consequences on the population to which the material tested belongs. Indeed,
research at the individual level does not take into account the possibility of adaptation to the pollution in successive generations and the
effects on population dynamics produced by concentrations which have no
effect on individual survival. Information concerning the effects on populations in aquatic environments are very few. Unfortunately, there is very
little information about the mechanisms regulating population-size in nonpolluted environments and a lack of results in polluted ones. Very few
investigations have been made on experimental populations of aquatic organisms exposed to pollutants (e.g. Hoppenheit et al., 1977). A compromise
between experiments under laboratory conditions and field research, could
be the studies carried out on populations living in semi-natural micro-
enviroments (plastic enclosures) artificially polluted.

The study of pollution effects on natural populations is a very difficult
task. For example, since populations are submitted to several natural
stresses, producing large numerical fluctuations and permanent modifications, the effects of low pollutant concentrations may be easily masked.

Modifications of the environmental characteristics, by means of natural causes, may reduce the population size, but a certain number of resistant individuals generally survive. If the numerical reduction is not too severe,
the population, after a certain time, may attain and surpass its initial
density. A similar reaction by the population living in a polluted environment may be expected. The survival of a part of the population, despite the
stress from pollution, is an important point of discussion and "a priori"
it is impossible to predict the probability and the time of numerical recovery if the fecundity of the population is unknown. We must suppose that
some populations live in the same environment and they have the same sensi-

tivity to certain pollutants. Populations with a high fecundity and vaibility have more probabilities to recover than others with a lower biotic potential. Some taxa (e.g. Pulmonate snails, Cladocerans, Fish, Insects) have a so great biotic potential that they may survive even if the size of their population is yearly reduced until 7o %. In other species with a low biotic potential a far lower reduction of the population size may strongly decrease its survival probability. More detailed information on this subject has been collected in Technical Report No. 172, LAEA, Wien 1976. Applying these considerations to the pollution problem we may foresee that those populations with a demographical recovery smaller than the aliquot of individuals eliminated by pollution will be eliminated and other populations with the same sensitivity but with a greater biotic potential will recover in a more or less long time.

Different demographical characteristics of the populations and different resistence of the taxa to the same pollutants combine to modify more or less strongly the community structure in the polluted environments. This biological reaction at community level is the crucial problem in evaluating the real damage from pollution in natural environments and in protecting the biota.

The community properties play an important role in amplifying or reducing the damage deriving from a given pollution charge. As an example, in a community with very complex food-web the pollution effects seem to be reduces. In fact in a community with high diversity, on substitution of one or few species, less resistant to pollution, with others, more resistant the interactions between the species are less modified than those of a community with a lower degreee of diversity. In addition, a community able to maintain its structure not too modified, after having been exposed to a certain level of pollution, is probably more stable than before. This stability is the effect of the elimination, by selective processes, operated by pollution on the more sensitive species.

Another important aspect of the pollution problem is the genetical damage at population level. Population is a store of genetic variability and a population with a high degree of variability is more adapted to environmental variations, may extend its distribution area and has an advantage in its competition with other populations with lower variability. The degree of population variability is the result of the mutation rate, the population size and the selection operated by the environment. Several pollutants (e.g.pesticides, radionuclides) induce mutations but, frequently, these are unfavorable. Natural selection protects populations against these detrimental genetic characteristics by reducing the number of individuals bearing noxious mutations. If detrimental effects are evident on a single generation, they are called short term genetical effects, responsible for the sterility and death of the individuals. In this way the accumulation of unfavourable genetic characteristics within the population is prevented. The long term effects are more noxious to the population, because they occur in successive generations giving rise to anomalies and "genetic diseases".

Information on this important aspect of the problem is very limited. It must be considered that from laboratory experiments, at individual level, on mutagenic effects induced by pollutants, it is impossible to predict the actual effects produced on populations by the same pollutants.

Pollution problems also concern those non-toxic substances which, if discharged into an environment significantly alterate the water quality and the community structure. For example, phosphorus and nitrogen compounds, above a certain concentration, are the most important cause of eutrophication. The effects of eutrophication are well known, but there is no information, or extremely little, on the effects produced by the interaction between the concentration of algal nutrients (e.g. phosphorus and nitrogen)and that of toxic pollutants. Because several lakes and rivers receive a mixed charge of toxic pollutants and nutrient, the knowledge of their combined effects on the biota seems of great importance.

Biological monitoring

Monitoring of a water body based on its physical and chemical characteristics is very expensive. This problem has grown up very rapidly in the last decades for the great number of pollutants descharged into aquatic environments. Several pollutants (e.g. pesticides, heavy metals) require well equipped laboratories and expert technicians. Although these analyses are indispensable, there is a growing interest in developing biological methods for monitoring and controlling freshwaters and particularly running water. Assuming that the biological methods are acceptable the sampling frequency for chemical analyses and the number of these latter could be reduced, without decreasing the information on the state of the surface waters.

The use of biological monitoring shows some advantages; the most important of which are the following:

1. The answer obtained is related to a given situation and not to a single parameter. The biological answer is the result of the antagonistic effects as well as of the synergic and additive ones. In other words, the modification of the structure of the community, or a part of it, is the effect produced by all the pollutants existing in the environment.

2. Chemical analyses are related to the time at which the sample is collected, while the biological answer is the result of the pollution stress occurring over a time more or less long.

3. Biological monitoring seems to have a lower cost than chemical monitoring, if the number of pollutants to be analyzed is high.

4. The toxicity of a pollutant is actually judged on its biological effects and not on its concentration in the water. As a consequence, biological monitoring represents the direct evaluation of the pollution level.

5. The result obtained is expressed by a number, a very simple figure easily understood also by a lawer or administrator.

In conclusion, biological monitoring may be considered as supplying an answer which is synthetic, direct and integrated on the time of the pollution degree of the environment.

Biological monitoring has also some disadvantages:

1. The commonly used methods (e.g. saproby, biotic indices) have been developed principally, or exclusively, for sewage pollution, that is for

easily degradable organic material. At present, because in several areas industrial wastes assume great importance there is a need for biological methods also to include this type of pollution.

2. The best results obtained by means of biological methods are those concerning environments well studied before pollution; unfortunately, these environments are rather few.

3. The most simple methods are the least sensitive.

4. Effects deriving from natural stress may often mask those produced by pollution.

5. The more practical methods (e.g. biotic indices) are difficult to apply to deep water courses. The results concerning the river sides cannot reflect the situation of the whole river. In addition, some difficulties are met for the zone of the river with muddy sediments. Up to today there is no practical method for monitoring lakes and reservoirs.

Standardization of the biological methods should permit an easier comparison of the results. On the other hand, standardization has its limits basically given by the variability of the environments. In addition, there are several reasons (some valid, some less) that prevent standardization being accepted by different countries. There are several approaches (for example, those done during the last years by C.E.C.) to implement at least an armonization of the methods, that is to establish a scale permitting comparison between the results obtained by different methods. This target has not yet been reached.

There are several methods proposed for biological monitoring and controlling of freshwater. The most common are the following:

Saprobic systems

Several methods, more or less complex, are called by this name. They have been developed principlaay for domestic and municipal wastes. The analyses required by this method need a relatively long time and a very expert technician.

Vernaux and Tuffery method

Its theoretical basis is acceptable, but, according to some experts, its general validity is not yet demonstrated. These methods require several expert to identify the taxa.

Fish zonation

Valuable method for rivers rich in fish, sometimes it is difficult to apply to polluted water courses.

Macroinvertebrate zonation

From this method good results may be obtained if several specialists are involved and the river is rather shallow.

Artificial substrate

The biota structure settled on the substrate may differ considerably from

that of the river bottom. The method needs expert technicians. If microscopic organisms are considered additional speciality are required.

Diversity indices

These are more or less simple to be applied. The best one (Shannon and
Weaver, 1963) is the most sophisticated. Diversity indices have a broad
application, that is, may be used for both domestic and for industrial
pollution. On the other hand this method involves such laborious techniques and requires such high qualified personal that it is very seldom
correctly used.

Biotic indices

This is a very practical method, because it does not require qualified
staff, but its sensitivity is rather small. One of the more popular is
that proposed by Woodiwiss (1964). The method used in Ireland consists
in a slight modification of that by Woodiwiss, with the additional analyses of few parameters. "Mapos" is the name of the method adopted in
Switzerland which is rather similar to that used in Ireland.

In addition, techniques for a continuous biological control of water courses have been developed as well as for domestic and industrial pollutants.
In several cases an aliquot of the river water to be controlled is drawn
into tanks, or artificial ponds, in which live one or few species of fish.
Their behaviour and the state of their health is the answer chosen for
evaluating the degreee of pollution of the river water (e.g. Cairns et
al., 1973; Besch et al., 1974).

In conclusion, it seems that the best method for monitoring and controlling the freshwater environment is the study carried out in different
seasons on one or more compartments of the community (e.g. macroinvertebrates). Data obtained should be treated according to the Shannon and Weaver index. On the other hand, this technique may be hard to apply practically. In my opinion, a less sophisticated method such as "biotic indices"
may be adopted to provide at least a rough idea of the state of the water
body. This method principally concerns shallow water courses with hard
bottoms and domestical and municipal pollution. For a broad application
of this method additional research is needed.

In several situations the information obtained by the biological monitoring mentioned above is not satisfying (e.g. radioactive pollution). In
these cases it is essential to choose the best strategy to obtain a satisfactory knowledge of the environment considered and prevent a too heavy
programme of chemical and/or biological analyses.

A preliminary study of the water body, including its water-shed, must be
carried out to identify the "critical points" to be considered. "Critical
points" mean the zone to be controlled as well as the organism, the season
and the pollutant. On this basis a monitoring programme will be planned.
For example, in a water course the "critical points" generally are: sediments and macrophytes, that is the components of the ecosystem which accumulate the greatest part of the pollutants. A study of plankton is far
less important, but it may be considered a good material for standing
water (lakes and reservoirs). Organisms which are able to accumulate some

pollutants even from very dilute solutions may be analyzed to detect the degree of pollution of the environment and to map the distribution of the same noxious substances in it. This method has been succesfully applied for pesticides and radionuclides (e.g. Ravera, 1964; Ravera, 1966; Schreiber, 1967; Calapaj, 1967; Gaglione et al., 1967) and heavy metals (e.g. Manly et al., 1977).

Risk

The concept of "acceptable risk" and the criteria for evaluating it have been developed for radioactive pollution. To transfer this experience to the field of non-radioactive pollution is not easy. Indeed, to evaluate the risk of non-radioactive pollution there is no common basis, while the radioactive risk has one common concept, the dose, independent of its emitter, that is the radionuclide.

Anyway some criteria of radioprotection may also be applied to the non-radioactive field. For example, for reducing the charge of pollution into water bodies the concept of the maximal acceptable concentration of pollutants in the effluent has been adopted. This is a very rough concept because it is independent of the total amount of pollutants and the dilution capacity of the water body in which the toxic substances are discharged. This practice may be considered a first step of environmental protection, but other criteria must be developed. In radioprotection the concept of "radiological capacity" has been adopted from some years (Commission of the European Communities, 197o).

"Radiological capacity" is the maximum amount of radioactive material that may be discharged into a water body without its becoming noxious for man who uses the water body for drinking, fishing, bathing, etc. This evaluation of the risk may also applied for non-radioactive pollution. Some examples of the risk evaluation are given by studies on lake eutrophication coordinated by O.E.C.D.

Scientists agree that the "critical concentration" of phosphorus in lake water is 2o μg/l. Higher concentrations produce an increasing eutrophication of the environment. This evaluation of the risk is very useful in planning the type and the importance of the interventions to decrease the trophic level of a lake. An approach has been developed by Vollenweider and Dillon (1974) to classify lakes according to their trophic level; oligotrophic, mesotrophic and eutrophic. This classification is based on the charge of phosphorus and the ratio between the mean depth of the lake and the turnover time of its waters. The mesotrophic stage, but not the eutrophic, has been judged acceptable. As a consequence, if the mean depth of a mesotrophic lake and its turnover time are known, the risk that this environment will become eutrophic for a given increase of phosphorus charge may be quantified. On the contrary, the decrease of phosphorus charge for transforming a eutrophic lake into mesotrophic one may be predicted. There are several studies on the transfer of radionuclides through food-chains, radionuclide concentration in food and the quantity and quality of food taken in daily by man in some countries (e.g. Essig et al., 1973).

From the results of these studies the risk of contamination for the inhabitants from these countries has been quantified. There exists some information on this problem concerning a very few non-radioactive pollutants

(e.g. DDT, Mercury, Lead); therefore, research on this subject must be encouraged. There are three main types of risk deriving from pollution:
a) the accumulation by resistent organisms of toxic substances which are
transferred to other organisms less resistent; b) the decrease of the
diversity in a community produced by elimination of the less resistent
species or species with a low biotic potential; c) the diffusion of long-
term genetic effects (malformation and genetic diseases).

Because studies, monitoring and control of the pollution and the counter-
actions should be planned in relation to the risk for man and his environment, considerable effort must be concentrated on its evaluation.

Summary

The advantages and disadvantages of grouping pollutants into categories
has been discussed and the relationship between the structure of a toxic
substance and its biological effects illustrated. In spite of the difficulty of generalizing this relationship, its importance is evident because
on this basis it is possible to predict the biological effects of new substances before they are tested.

Because communities and populations of animals and plants are protected
against pollution, but not the single individual, the effects at the community and population level have been illustrated. The importance of genetic damage has also been evaluated. The value of laboratory experiments
and the difficulties involved in extrapolating their results to the natural
environment have been discussed.

Some methods of biological control and their advantages and disadvantages
have been listed. The need for a strategy for obtaining satisfactory information on polluted environments without adopting too heavy programme
of chemical and biological analyses has been emphasized.

A comparison between the evaluation of the risk in the radioprotection
field and in that for non-radioactive pollutants has been made. Some
examples of the evaluation of risk concerning lake eutrophication have
been given to illustrate the practical advantages of applying this fundamental concept. The most important types of risk from pollution have
been listed.

References

Besch, W.K., Loserier, H.G., Meyer Waarden, K. and W. Schmitz, 1974:
Warntest zum Nachweis akut toxischer Konzentrationen von Wasserinhalts-
stoffen. Arch. Hydrobiol., 74: 551-565.

Bond, H.W. and G.C. Fuller, 1971: Correlation of structure versus activity of pollutants of freshwater. Dept. of Commerce (U.S.) NTIS, PB 205-
6o6, 11p.

Cairns, J., Sparks, R.E. and T. Waller, 1973: The use of fish as sensor
in industrial waste lines to prevent fish kills. Hydrobiologia, 41: 151-
167.

532

Calapaj, G.C., 1967: Ricerche su alcuni concentratori biologici del ^{54}Mn nell'ambiente marino. Gion. Fis. San. Radioprot., 11: 3-19.

Carlson, R.M., Kopperman, H.L., Caple, R. and R.E. Carlson, 1975: Structure-activity relationship applied. In: Structure-activity correlations in studies of toxicity and bioconcentration with aquatic organism. (Proc. Symp., Burlington, March 11-13, 1975) Ed. Gilman D. Veith and Dennis E. Konasewich, 1975, Windsor, Ontario.

Commission of the European Communities, Principles and general methods of establishing the limiting radiological capacity of a hydrobiological system. C.E.C., Directorate for Health and Safety, Luxembourg, 197o.

Divo, C., 1974: A survey on fish toxicity and biodegradability of linear sodium alkylbenzene sulphonates. In: Proc. 12th Congress of the International Society for Fat Research, Milano, September 2-7, 1974.

Erickson, S.J., Maloney, T.E. and H.H. Gentile, 197o: Effect of nitrilotriacetic acid on the growth and metabolism of estuarin phytoplankton. J. Water Poll. Control. Fed., 42: 229-235.

Essig, T.H., Endres, G.W.R., Soldat, J.K. and J.F. Honstead, 1973: Concentrations of ^{65} Zn in marine foodstuffs and Pacific coastal residents. Radioactive contamination of the marine environment, Wien 1973: 651-67o.

Gaglione, P. and O. Ravera, 1964: ^{54}Mn concentration in fall-out, water and Unio mussels of Lake Maggiore, 196o-1963. Nature, 2o4: 1215-1216.

Giussani, G., Borroni, I. and E. Grimaldi, 1976: Role of un-ionized ammonia in predisposing gill apparatus of Alburnus alburnus alborella to fungal and bacterial diseases. Mem. Ist. ital. Idrobiol., 33: 161-176.

Greene, J.C., Miller, W.E., Shiroyama, T. and E. Marvin, 1975: Toxicity of zinc to the green algae Selenastrum capricornutum as a function of phosphorus or ionic strength. In: Proc. Biostimulation Nutrient Assessment Workshop, EPA 66o/3-75-o34: 28-43.

Hoppenheit, M. and K.R. Sperling, 1977: On the dynamics of exploited populations of Tisbe holothuriae (Copepoda, Harpacticoida). IV The toxicity of cadmium: response to lethal exposure. Helgolander wiss. Meeresunters., 29: 328-336.

International Atomic Energy Agency, Effects of ionizing radiation on aquatic ecosystems. I.A.E.A. Technical Report Series No. 172, Wien, 131 pp.

Kimerle, R.A. Swisher, R.D. and R.M. Schroeder-Comotto, 1975: Surfactant structure and aquatic toxicology. In: Structure-activity correlations in studies of toxicity and bioconcentration with aquatic organisms, (Proc. Symp. Burlington, March 11-13, 1975) Ed. Gilman D. Veith and Dennis E. Konasewich, 1975, Windsor, Ontario.

Manly, R. and W.O. George, 1977: The occurrence of some heavy metals in populations of the freshwater mussel Anodonta anatina (L.) from the river Thames, Environ. Pollut., 14: 139-154.

Marchetti, R., 1965: Critical review of the effects of synthetic detergents on aquatic like. Stud. Rev. Gen. Fish Com. Medit., No. 26, FAO, Rome.

Margalef, R., 1975: External factors and ecosystem stability. Schweiz. Zeitsch. Hydrol., 37: 1o2-117.

Neely, W.B., Branson, D.R. and G.E. Blau, 1974: Partition coefficient to measure bioconcentration potential of organic chemicals to fish. Environmental Science and Technology, 8: 1113-1115.

Premazzi, G., Bertone, R., Freddi, A. and O. Ravera, 1977: Combined effects of heavy metals and chelating substances on Selenastrum cultures. In: Ecological tests relevant to the implmentation of proposed regulations concerning environmental chemicals: evaluation and research needs. (Proc. Seminar, Berlin, Dec. 7-9, 1977) C.E.C. and Umweltbundesamt, Berlin (in press).

Ravera, O., 1964: Distribution of ^{54}Mn from fall-out in population of freshwater Lamellibranchs (Unio mancus var. elongatulus, Pfeiffer) Verh. Internat. Verein. Limnol., 15: 885-892.

Ravera, O. 1966: L'utilizzazione delle piante acquatiche nello studio delle contaminazioni radioattive di bacini lcustri. Minerva Fisico-nucleare, 1o: 162-165.

Ravera, O. 1972: Aspetti comuni degli inquinamenti convenzionale e radioattivo. Inquinamento, acqua, aria e suolo, No. 7: 27-32.

Ravera, O. 1972: What is the nature of the damage caused by the pollution load of water due to its content of substances that can be decomposed only with difficulty, as regards the biology of water? Bull. F.E.P.E., No. 19: 28-3o.

Ravera, O., 1975: Critique of concepts and techniques regarding biological indicators. Boll. Zool., 42, 111-121.

Schreiber, B., 1967: Ecology of Acantharia in relation of Sr circulation in the see. Final Report I.A.E.A., Contract US/62 (1-9o).

Shannon, C.E. and W. Weaver: The mathematical theory of communication. Univ. Illinois Press, 1963.

Sprague, J.B., 1969: Measurement of pollutant toxicity to fish. I. Bioassay methods for acute toxicity. Water Research, 3: 793-821.

Sprague, J.B., 197o: Measurement of pollutant toxicity to fish. II. Utilizing and applying bioassay results. Water Research, 4: 3-32.

Sprague, J.B., 1971: Measurement of pollutant toxicity to fish. III. Sublethal effects and "safe" concentrations. ibid. 5: 245-266.

Steeman-Nielsen, E., Kamp-Nielson, L. and S. Wium-Anderson, 1969: The effects of deleterious concentrations of copper on the photosynthesis of Chlorella pyrenoidosa. Physiol. Plant., 22: 1121-1133.

534

Vollenweider, R.A. and P.J. Dillon, 1974: The application of the phosphorus loading concept to eutrophication research. Bull. NRCC No. 13690, National Research Council of Canada.

Vollenweider, R.A. and O. Ravera, Sources, pathways, exposure and risk of environmental pollutants (in press).

Woodiwiss, F.S., 1964: The biological system of stream classification used by the Trent River Board. Chemistry and Industry, March 1964.

Zitko, V., 1974: Uptake of chlorinated paraffins and PCB from suspended solids and food by juvenile Atlantic salmon. Bull. Environ. Contam. Toxicol., 12: 4o6.

Zitko, V., 1975: Structure activity relationship in fish toxicology. In: Structure-activity correlations in studies of toxicity and bioconcentration with aquatic organisms (Proc. Symp. Burlington, March 11-13, 1975). Ed. Gilman D. Veith and Dennis E. Konasewich, 1975, Windsor, Ontario.

Annex I

Remarks on the biological methodology for monitoring and controlling streams and rivers

a) Shallow and stony streams

Because the aim is the monitoring and controlling the pollution level of the water body and the answer obtained by "biotic indices"[1] is rather rough, the sampling must be simple and reproducible. It is more important to adopt the same sampling method, also if it is not the best, than to improve it in successive times. One of the commonly used methods may be adopted; for example, surber method, hand collection for the unit surface of bottom, or for time unit.

Soon after the collection, material must be preserved, with alcohol or formalin solution, in large mouth bottles labelled with information on time and place of the sampling.

To identify the organisms collected, books with figures, reporting the most evident taxonomical characteristics of the species, should be used (for example, the Scientific Publication by Freshwater Biological Association, U.K.).

b) Deep rivers and streams with muddy and silty sediments

Basket containing a certain number of stones (1o-2o cm size) are placed on the bottom at different sections of the river. One end of a strong rope is tied to the basket and the other to a floating body. The basket may be recovered at given intervals of time and the macroinvertebrates living on the stones collected and studied according to the method of the "biotic indices".

---

[1] In my opinion these methods are the most practical ones for our aim.

In addition, these environments may be controlled by using small artificial substrates (e.g. glass slides) suspended in the water at different sections of the river. Examination of the small organisms (e.g. bacteria, algae, nematods, protozoa) living on these slides is consuming time, tedious and needs of an expert. As a consequence, most practical testing methods should be developed.

c) Continuous control of a stream or river

This control may be exerted by pumping river water to fill a series of tanks inhabited by one or more species of fish. The reaction of these organisms (e.g. mortality, behaviour) is used to test the pollution level of the river waters. The organisms chosen must come from environments very similar for all the most important characteristics, except pollution, to the river to be monitored.

For laboratory experiment methodology see, for example, Sprague, 1969: Ravera, 1975.

Sprague, J.B., 1969: Measurement of pollution toxicity for fish. I. Bioassay methods for acute toxicity. Water Research, 3: 793-821.

Ravera, O., 1975: Critique of concepts and techniques regarding biological indicators. Boll. Zool., 42: 111-121.

536

THE USE OF FISHES IN THE MONITORING ENVIRONMENTAL MATERIALS AND SPECIMEN BANKING

H.-H. Reichenbach-Klinke
Institut für Zoologie und Hydrobiologie
Fachbereich Tiermedizin
Universität München
Federal Republic of Germany

The fish is one of the most important parts in our food chain and a non missible indicator in the environment water. He is passaged resp. reached by nearly all substances existing in the circle of the biosphere. The fish is a vertebrate like man with related anatomical and physiological features; we therefore cannot overlook it when it is necessary to test any substance touching man or probably touching him.

The fish is very useful for a longer monitoring banking previously being tested in view of its conservation proprieties. The accumulation of heavy metals primarily takes place in kidney and liver; these organs therefore are to be prefered for banking. Before conservation all objects must be handled in standardized methods.

The following items are to be fulfilled:

The chosen species of fish should be if possible an indigenous species, i.e. adapted to local circumstances. The species on the other hand should be distributed over a wide area that it could be used in an area as extended as possible. If the ecological factors are extremely different in a great area it should be discussed to chose more than one species of fish, f.i. in Germany the carp as an animal living in warm water and withstanding oxigen deficiencies, and the rainbow trout living in cold water and needing high oxigen content. In certain cases it must be considered to research fish embryos of a certain species.

The fish to be tested should have lived under nearly similar environmental conditions. This is concerning the trophical situation as well as the food itself. A short time before the fixation every food consumption should be prohibited.

The trophic situation is beneath other factors expressed by the so-called corpulence factor, which also should be standardized.

The fixation, conservation resp. frosting of the objects should if possible be done exactly after the fish's catching. The mechanical killing should be prefered in fishes of medium and greater size, little fish should be narcotisized. The choice of examples concerns before all kidney, liver, muscles and skin. After Müller & Prosi f.i. zinc and cadmium are accumulasing in maximal intensity in the kidney whereas

copper is enriching preferably in the liver. These organs therefore
are demonstrating the source the most secure for the accumulation of
heavy metals.

The water in which the examined fishes were living must present of
course equal conditions. Extreme qualities of water are to be evitated.
On the other hand it is recommended to take fishes from differently
polluted waters and from ecologically different situated hatcheries.

Summary

The role of fish in the monitoring banking of environmental materials
is characterized as member of the food chain beginning in water and
ending in man. On the other hand fish gives a picture of the present
ecological situation in water. If we are comparing the fish with
other materials in our environment several factors must be acknowledged: the fish must be taken from a water with special quality, it
must be conserved or fixed after standardized methods and it must be
a species comparable to related forms. Experiences have shown that
kidney and liver are those fish organs with the greatest accumulation
of heavy metals. It therefore seems best for the banking to use these
organs.

MONITORING SERIAL INORGANIC POLLUTANTS
BY PLANT INDICATOR SPECIMENS

Prof. Dr. L. Steubing
Institut für Pflanzenökologie
Heinrich-Buff-Ring 38
63oo Lahn-Giessen
Federal Republic of Germany

1. Introduction

Regional air pollution containing inorganic particulate matter such as Al, Co, Cd, Cr, Cu, Fe, Hg, Mn, Mo, Ni, Pb, Sn, U, V and Zn is an old problem beginning with the smelting of ores. But now - caused by human activity - the worldwide increase of trace elements in our environment is of general interest. The most important sources of these emissions are mining, refining, metal smelting, combustion engines, high tension lines and also sources associated with the complexities of urban living. The consequence of this type of air pollution is the contamination of soil, water and organisms with heavy metals.

Additional to the particular air pollution there are gaseous contaminants all over the world, especially SO_2. On the other hand HF, HCl or NO_x and the components which are responsible for the photochemical smog have a more local distribution. Normally the immission load of an ecosystem does not only result from one immission type but from the whole complex of air pollutants whereby special components may cause synergistic or antogonistic effects.

In comparison to gaseous immissions (Guderian 1977) there are relatively few reports on effects of air pollutants by heavy metals on the vegetation. Therefore in this paper will be dealt with reactions of plants which have been used for recognition and effects monitoring particularly of aerial heavy metal pollutants in terrestrial ecosystems. Basing on this description of results will be proposed a short list of plant specimens which seem to be particularly suitable for monitoring and banking.

2. Methods of effects monitoring by plants

Plant organisms have been successfully used for effects monitoring of air pollution, for trend analyses and for demarcation of burdening areas. An advantage of these bioindicators is, that they - contrary to animals - are stationary. Commonly they are available in large numbers and give relatively equal reactions. Normally their requirement on substrate and climate conditions is $\pm$ well known or can be easily examined by laboratory experiments. The response to the pollutants may be to evolve specific tolerance (see 3.1) or to suffer under the immission load showing visible injuries (3.2) or only "hidden" injuries i.g. changes in the metabolism. If the species are too sensitive they are eliminated while less sensitive or resistent plants show high accumulation of the pollutant (Steubing 1978).

There are two methods to obtain informations on the distribution pattern of heavy metal (and also of other pollutants) in terrestrial ecosystems:

2.1. Effects monitoring by wildliving species

a) Mapping plant associations or the occurence of special plants (indicator plants) the change of the distribution and abundance indicates an alteration of environmental conditions for instance the penetration of pollutants in the ecosystem. Typical plant associations which refer to a high concentration of heavy metals in the soil exist on all continents.

Lichens react very sensitive to the whole phytotoxic immission complex of an area. In our urban ecosystems we find a characteristic change in the spectrum of species and the number of species according to the degree of pollutants. In the urban-industrial region of North Rhine-Westphalia was determined that the death rate of lichens was correlated to burdening with SO_2, HF and Pb (Prinz and Scholl 1978). Mapping the natural lichen growth on the bark of trees in the small town of Giessen (figure 1) we find also a typical zonation which gives a good relation in the same way to the complex of SO_2 load and the traffic situation (measured on the lead content of test plants). On the figure can be seen a small dark spot in the southeast, which indicates by the change in the lichen zone, that in this region must be a higher burdening of air pollution. The reason for it are the immissions of an HF emittant factory.

b) Visible injuries on plants (wildliving and agricultural plants) caused by heavy metal pollutions have been observed generally only in the direct vicinity of smelting industries.

To confirm field observations but also to evaluate the risk by immissions containing heavy metals (or other contaminants) residue analyses of the supposed immission types are indispensable. Table 1 indicates the chemical analyses of plants or parts of them such as the annual rings of trees give good information on the trend of pollution concentrations in relation to the time.

Tabel 1: Concentration of lead in annual rings of spruce trees along traffic routs (Keller and Preis 1967).

period of growth	concentration of lead
1943 - 1951	o,3 - o,4 ppm
1951 - 1954	o,4 ppm
1954 - 1957	o,9 ppm
1957 - 196o	1,2 ppm
196o - 1962	2,4 ppm

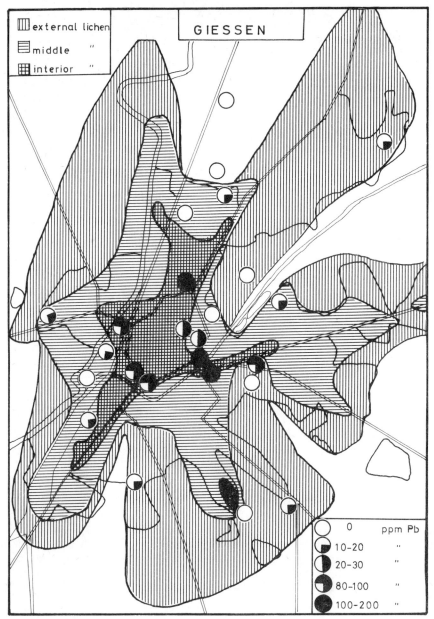

Fig. 1

2.2 Exposure of test plants ("standardized" plants)

The test plant method is the best technique to determine the rate of heavy
metal sediments and its absorption by the plants (it is also suitable for
effects monitoring of other pollutants which enter in the ecosystem, respectively will be accumulated in the organism): it is a standardized method
for the elimination of a lot of factors which complicate evaluations on the
natural vegetation in the field. The test plants are cultivated in special
containers filled with standardized soil (if possible genetic uniform material). At a defined growth state the plants will be exposed at various
monitoring stations both inside and outside the polluted area. By means
of chemical analyses the accumulation of aerial pollutants by heavy metals in plant and soil can be measured. The comparison of the pollutant
concentrations of the same plant species grown in the natural soil and as
test plant in the standardized soil allow e.g. the evaluation if these
wildliving plants or vegetables are dangerous as food for animals or man
(table 2).

Table 2: Indicator values for lead, cadmium, zinc and fluorine in food
plants for man and animals (Prinz and Scholl 1978)

component	concentration ug/g dry weight	object	remarks
lead	1o	grazing animals	tolerance limit in the food
	5	man	recommended indicator value for limitation of contents in food
cadmium	5 (5o)	grazing animals	tolerance limit
	1	man	recommended indicator value for limitation of contents in food
zinc	25o	grazing animals	tolerance limit
	6oo	man	upper limitation of daily absorption
fluorine	3o	grazing animals	tolerance limit
	2oo	man	tolerance limit for daily oral absorption

Figure 2 demonstrates that there have been significant differences in the
accumulation of lead, cadmium and zinc by standardized and by wildliving
plants, which grew in the same ambient and were harvested at the same time.

Moreover test plants are suitable to recognize immission injuries in an
early stage by monitoring changes of physiological and biochemical processes
in the organism such as enzyme activity, photosynthesis, respiration, trans-
piration caused by immission load.

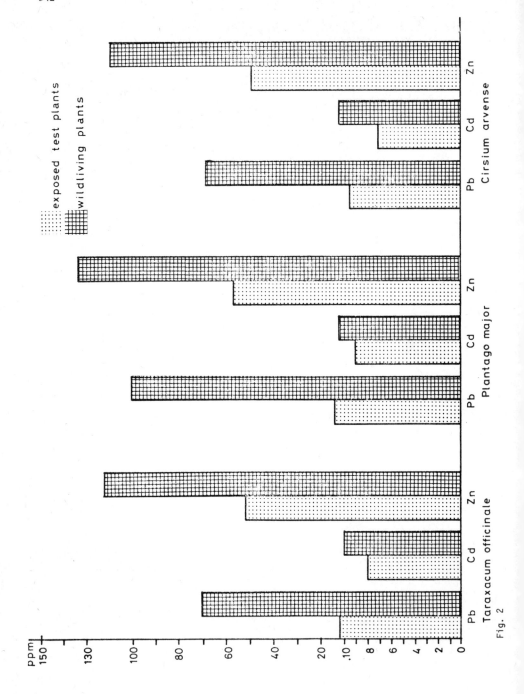

Fig. 2

Lichen exposure method (see 4.3) and grass culture technique (see 4.4) belong to the most frequently used test plant methods.

2.3 Laboratory experiments

To analyse visible (acute) and "hidden" (chronical) injuries on plants caused by pollutants and to understand the mechanisms of responses, physiological and biochemical laboratory experiments are necessary. In the same way as fumigation chambers for fumigation experiments, a dusting chamber has been built and described in detail by Krause (1977). By dusting, by sprinkling with heavy metal containing solutions or by contaminating the soil with different concentrations of trace elements may be investigated the specific reaction and sensitivity of plant species to particular pollutants. Such lab experiments include the possibility to obtain informations on the concentration-time relation and on synergistic effects of certain heavy metal immissions on plants. For early diagnosis of plant injury which could be expected with the period,are often such ecophysiological and biochemical experiments very helpful.

3. Phytotoxicity of heavy metals

3.1 Heavy metal tolerant plants

Most of the research data are available on plants growing in metalliferous soils. Well known are plant indicator associations which have been used for prospecting. Elements for which exist special indicator plants in various parts of the world are: Co, Cu, Fe, Mn,Mo, Ni, Se, Zn (Cannon 1971, Brooks 1972, Ernst 1974). These tolerant plants have been found frequently also in mine areas. Metalliferous soils have evolved specific tolerance in those heavy metals which are abundant. Industrial immissions of cadmium, copper, zinc, nickel and lead can stimulate the process of evolution to tolerant ecotypes by this new selection pressure (Bradshaw 1975, Ernst, Mathys and Janiesch 1975). According to Ernst (1974) are long-lived plants, such as shrubs and trees, unable to evolve metal-tolerant ecotypes, whereas grasses and a lot of dicotyledons are succesful. Kovalskij (1977) dealt with results of the variability in resistance to heavy metal pollution of soil microorganisms and the occurrence of resistant ecotypes in contaminated areas.

The significant feature of metal tolerance is the prevention of heavy metals from exerting disturbance in the metabolic system of the cells. According to Ernst (1976) in roots of some heavy metal tolerant plants the cell wall is important in acting as a heavy metal accumulator. In leaves and stems, however, the cell vacuole system is the main place for heavy metal deposition. Some microorganisms excepted, angiospermous plants, have not developed heavy metal resistant enzymes or specific heavy metal rich metabolites. The physiological basis of tolerance seems to be the increase in the production of malate and oxalate in zinc tolerant plants and of phenolic compounds in copper tolerant populations.

3.2 Sensitive plants to aerial heavy metal pollutants

Phytotoxicity of trace elements containing immissions has been found only in the direct vicinity of smelting processes industries, where the accumulation of heavy metals settleable dust on leaves and in the soil overloaded the mechanisms of metabolism. Visible injuries and $\pm$ reduction of the production caused by an excess of this type of immission are according to Cannon (196o) and Malyuga (1964):

Al : leaf scorch, mottling
Co : white dead spots on leaves
Cd : yellow-white chlorotic spots between the veins which change
     with the age to red-brown
Cr : yellow leaves with green veins and dried dead patches on
     lower leaves frequently beginning on the tip, purple stem
Fe : stunted tops, thin or sometimes stubby roots
Mn : chlorotic leaves, curling and dead areas on leaf margin;
     reddish coloration and lesions of stem
Mo : stunting development, yellow-orange coloration
Ni : white dead spots on leaves or chlorotic leaves, abnormal forms
Zn : chlorotic leaves with green veins; white dwarfed forms;
     dead areas on leaf tips
U : stalked-leaf rosette; unusually shaped fruits

If there is dust deposit by heavy metals only on the foliage and there is no contamination of soil, also the described injuries can take place but with retardation. The listened visible injuries show that it is e.g. impossible to recognize exactly only by optical evaluation the special type of heavy metal immission which has affected the plant. Therefore it is necessary, to confirm the occurrence of a supposed pollutant by chemical analyses.

From soil absorbed trace elements are not uniformly distributed throughout the plant, so that different organs may vary in their ability to concentrate heavy metals. Particular in the roots have been found high quantities of Pb, Zn, Cd, Cu, Cr, (Kloke 1972, Denaeyer-De-Smet 1974, Maschmeyer 1976, Ohki 1977, Van de Geijn 1978). But there is also the possibility of foliar uptake of superficial deposit (Krause 1977, Guderian et al. 1977). Heavy metal absorption by leaves depends - besides the physical state of the trace element and the climatic conditions - largely on the morphology of the leaf surface. 25 - 3o % of the total zinc and cadmium, but only 3 % of total lead may be absorbed by leaf surface. Cell wall and vacuoles are discussed to serve as sink to inactivate excess heavy metals (Timperley et al. 1973, Polar 1976). Therefore it is no absolutely necessary that anomal high accumulation of heavy metal is accompanied by visible injuries. There is a certain danger, because it includes the possibility that grazing animals feed on plants, which seem to be without injury. The hidden accumulation of heavy metals in the plant may cause animal disease (Vetter et al. 1971). If polluted plants serve for nutrition of animals and man, it is of interest, to know the percentage of absorbed and the percentage of only externally adsorbed heavy metal dust.

Generally only a part of the external dust is adsorbed removable by washing, for instance: the data dealt with for removable lead are between 9o - 3o %. With the length of time during which plants grow in such polluted area, the rate of washing off declines. Steenken (1973) could remove 65 - 75 % of lead dust from his test plants, which were contaminated for 3 days with lead containing immissions, but this part was reduced to 35 - 4o % after 21 days.

The toxicity of the elements Cd, Pb, Zn is excess declines from cadmium

to zinc (Cd:Pb:Zn = 1oo:1o:1). The degree of toxicity, that can be developed is relative and depends on many factors such as the age of plant organs, the concentration of ions in the growth substrate and the interactions with the polluting toxic ion (Lepp 1977). Beckett and Davis
(1978) examined the interactions between Cu, Ni and Zn in young barley
and they found that these results are very similar to those of similar
studies on the toxicity of mixed solutions to fish. Generally the toxicity of heavy metals can be modified also by organic compounds.

At last it must be considered that the microorganisms, which are responsible for the mineralisation processes in the soil and therefor a great
importance for higher plants, may be injured by the increasing accumulation
of aerial pollutants in the substrate. Sometimes the soil may be additionally contaminated by the use of metal-rich sewage sludge as fertilizer
in agriculture.

4. Review on indicator specimens used for effects monitoring

Heavy metal dust can effect the plant by the deposited particulate matter
on the surface and by contamination of the soil. In consequence it is necessary to obtain information on the sensitivity of plants to this type of
pollutants but there are also required data of the sinsitivity of soil microorganisms.

4.1. Soil microflora

Not much is known of the tolerance levels of the different species of soil
organisms for individual metals, but the ability to evolve tolerance on
the basis of the genetic variability may be especially developed by these
microorganisms (Kovalskij 1977). Sadler and Trudinger (1967) stated the
tolerance of yeast to heavy metals. Tornabene et al. (1972) and Den Doren
de Jong (1971) proved Azotobacter on its persistance in lead polluted substrates. While the last mentioned author found morphological change in the
bacterium, the other ascertained no influence of lead on the vitality of
Azotobacter. Babich et al. (1977) tested a variety of microorganisms for
their sensitivity to cadmium: the actinomycetes were more tolerant to
cadmium than were the eubacteria; gram-negative eubacteria have been more
tolerant than gram-positiv. The toxicity of Cd to eubacteria, actinomycetes
and fungi appears to be pH dependent. Fungal sporulation was more sensitive
to cadmium than mycelial growth.

Of interest are the few data available regarding the relations between
heavy metals in the soil and soil activity. Tyler (1974, 1975) contested
that litter decomposition, soil enzymatic activity surrounding metal processing industries are influenced by high concentrations of heavy metal
deposits. Beginning with a concentration of 5o ppm Cu in the soil the
ammonification rate declined. Lipman et al. (1914) stated that leadsulfate
up to 5o ppm had a toxic effect on the ammonification, while the nitrification was easily stimulated by low and retarded by high lead contamination. Increasing concentration of lead in the soil causes reduction of the
CO_2-production and dehydrogenase-activity; fungi, bacteria and actinomycetes are influenced in the rate of growth only by high concentration of this
trace element; more sensitive are those microorganisms, which are responsible for the decomposition of cellulose and protein (Korn 1975).

Basing on literature may be recommended as indicator specimen the investigation of soil activity, especially mineralisation processes (ammonification, nitrification, decomposition of cellulose) and soil respiration.

4.2. Mosses

Mosses are very suitable as indicator specimens for heavy metal or radionuclide fallout, because they have the ability to adsorb settleable dusts very well and to absorb the different components whereby the cation exchange capacity and ability of forming organo-metallic complexes may be of special importance (Rump et al. 1977). Ophus et al. (1974) found within the leaves of Rhytidiadelphus, which were collected from roadsides exposed to lead pollution from traffic, accumulation of this trace element in the cell wall and also in the plasmalemma, vacuoles and in the nucleus. Simola (1977) reported, that the peat moss Sphagnum nemorum could in a nutrient medium with added o,1 mM lead while the same concentration of added cadmium was lethal.

Peat mosses seem to be particularly appropriate for monitoring immissions because they receive their nutrients only from the aerial deposits and the precipitation. Pakarinen et al. (1976) used Sphagnum to gain a survey of aerial pollutants of lead, cadmium, mercury, iron, zinc, nickel, chromium and copper in Finland. The concentration of mercury was the lowest, always less than o,1 ppm, while the content of iron was the highest (5o6 ppm). The level of the studied metals was generally lower than the data given for Sphagnum collected from a peat-bog in the Rhön in Germany with a content of 63o ppm Fe, 21o ppm Zn, 332 ppm Pb, 19 ppm Cu and 12 ppm Cd (Rump et al. 1977). Lötschert et al. (1975) demonstrated in moss samples collected in the city of Frankfurt the rising level of Pb and Cd with increasing age of the moss and a higher content in the stem than in the leaves. Similar to other authors they found increasing values of heavy metals near highway traffic and industrial or general urban areas (Rühling et al. 197o, Wittenberger 1975).According to Lötschert (1975) the lead content in the moss Bryum argenteum declined from 1222 ppm next to the roadside to 777 ppm in 2 m distance. Briggs (1972) reported that aerial lead pollution from combustion engines has selected metal-tolerant individuals of the livermoss Marchantia polymorpha. Monitoring a distinct region it is not absolutely necessary to analyse mosses which are collected from their natural environment. Keller (1974) transplanted with succes moss samples from unpolluted areas into cities to study the heavy metal fallout in a definite time.

Of particular interest are the copper-mosses which grow on mineral rich mine spoil heaps. Species such as Mielichhoferia possess a very large resistence to copper and chromium.

Indicator specimens which have been used are: Sphagnum spec., Hylocomium splendens, Rhytidiadelphus spec., Bryum argenteum, Hypnum cupressiforme, Torula muralis, Grimmia pulvinata, Brachythecium rutabulum.

4.3 Lichens

Terricolous and epiphytic lichens were often analysed for the detection of a wide spectrum of aerial pollutants by heavy metals (James 1973). Most detailed information is available on the accumulation of radionuclide fallout. Similar to the mosses the lichens have a preposition for cation uptake from the atmosphere and from the substrate which exceeds their biological requirement. Lichens, generally characterized by very slow growth rates and great longevity, contain frequently larger values of heavy metals than mosses and higher plants. Many of the investigators emphasize the role of substrate in supplying the excess of metals. Noeske et al. (1970) show that iron and copper were accumulated in the crust and on the upper face and sides of the areoles of Acarospora sinoptica, while the maximum concentration of zinc was found in the lower zone of the cortex. Nieboer et al. (1972) stated also the accumulation of nickel, copper, zinc and iron in the cortex of the squamules in Cladonia deformis, and here outside the hyphae. These results agree with those of Rühling et al. (1970) and Brown and Slingsby (1972), who found lead bound in an exchangeable form located in the hyphal walls. According to Nieboer et al.(1972) the exchangeable metals vary from metal to metal. In lichen samples collected from the immediate vicinity of a nickel smelter were exchangeable 12 % for Fe, 2o % for Ni, 53 % for Cu and 83 % for Zn, Puckett (1976) studied the effect of rising concentrations of heavy metals on phtosynthesis, chlorophyll and membrane integrity. The relative toxicities of these metals on photosynthesis changed somewhat for short-term exposures in the series Ag, Hg, Co, Cu, Cd, Pb, Ni and extended exposures Ag, Hg, Cu Pb, Co Ni. It appears that lichens - especially the species of Umbilicaria, Cladonia and Stereocaulon - are selective in the uptake of heavy metals (with a preference sequence of Fe Pb Cu Ni, Zn Co. Kershaw (1963) believes that the increasing of Stereocaulon nanodes nearby the roads, polluted by the traffic may be promoted by their affinity for lead.

In the immediate vicinity of smelting industries the accumulation mechanisms of the lichens can be overloaded by settleable heavy metal dust and the concentration of these trace elements may exceed toxic levels. Such observations are described by Nash (1976). Mapping the lichen vegetation he stated in the area of a nickel smelter a reduction of the lichen diversity and abundance of 9o %. The zone of extreme lichen community impoverishment extended 6 km W and 15 km E of the smelter. In this area concentrations as high as 135 ppm Zn and 1,7 ppm Cd in the litter have been analysed. He could ascertain that zinc was the primary cause of lichen impverishment in this area. He cited data from other authors who found also high concentrations of heavy metals in lichens nearby special industries such as 9o ooo ppm Fe, 5 ooo ppm Ni and 45 ooo ppm Pb in the area of a steel mill in England. Seawart (1974), Schönbeck (1974) and Prinz et al. (1975) used the accumulation of heavy metals in transplanted lichens for monitoring. They could correlate immission load with the occurance of observed injury and concentration of the trace elements in the thalli (Lichen exposure method).
Lichens which have been used particularly as indicator specimens are the following species: Peltigera rufescens, Cladonia rangiformis, Stereocaulon nanodes, Umbilicaria spec., Lecanora spec., Hypogymnia physodes, Evernia prunastri, Parmelia furfuracea.

For monitoring may be used chemical analyses of lichens samples collected from the natural environment, but there have been obtained also interesting informations on distribution pattern of trace element deposits by lichen exposure technique.

548

4.4 Higher plants

There is a lot of publications concerning the accumulation of heavy metals in higher plants which are growing as indicator specimens in metalliferous soils (Cannon 196o, Brooks 1972, Denayer-De smet et al. 1974, Ernst 1974, Simon 1975). There are also results of heavy metal distribution pattern in certain regions basing on observations and analyses of the natural vegetation and test plants (Lagerwerf 1971, Van Haut 1974, Schönbeck 1974, Prinz et al. 1975, Beavington 1975, Collet 1977, Crant et al. 1977).Visible injuries related to high concentrations of trace elements in the vegetation have been found in the immediate vicinity of sources of heavy metal pollution, but they are rarely detected in urban atmosphere. Of special interest may be tables with data of normal value, limit value and toxicity and maximum value of heavy metals in different plant species, whereby trace element concentration in food plants play an important role (Michels et al. 1974, Ohki 1975, von Hodenberg 1975, Sommer et al. 1976, Crössmann 1978).

Contrary to the data of trace element level in lichens and mosses the analyses of heavy metal concentration in higher plants have been made separately on special organs. In the rough bark of trees can be accumulated a lot of different pollutants. Keller et al. (1967) gave a survey on lead pollution in a distinct area by chemical analyses of the annual rings of trees. He found a good correlation between increasing lead content in the annual rings of different age and increase of road traffic density (table 1). The relation between motorcar exhaust and lead contamination also have been studied by Little et al. (1972), Fidora (1972), Davies et al. (1974), Lerche et al (1974), Keller (1974), Steubing et al. (1976). Needles of conifers and leaves of different plant species have been used for effects monitoring in the field and for programs with standardized exposure (test plant method). The structure and the extend of the leafarea influence the possiblity to catch and absorb a maximum of serial pollutants. Therefore have been often selected trees, bushes and herbs with leaves of large extend; e.g. 1) wildliving plants: Aesculus hippocastanum, Tilia spec., Acer spec., Sambucus nigra, Carpinus betulus, Solidago spec., Taraxacum officinale, Plantago major. (Some trees have specific selectivity of absorption of heavy metals contaminated soils, e.g. archs are specialysed to accumulate zinc, while oaks and beeches accumulate more mangane.);
2) agricultural plants: Beta vulgaris, Lactuca sativa, Solanum tuberosum, Solanum lycopersicum, Brassica spec.;
3) test plants for exposure: Brassica oleracea, Spinacia oleracea, Phaseolus vulgaris, Petunia hybrida, Solanum lycopersicum.

On the other hand causes the dense growth of grasses which have small leaf areas nevertheless a very good accumulation of aerial contaminants in the shoots. Grass is easy to cultivate and the so called grass culture technique with Lolium multiflorum as test plant is used for trend monitoring in Europe, USA and Japan.

5. Plant species for effects and trend monitoring and banking

To evaluate the risk of possible immission injury on the vegetation with which the food web begins and at the end of which there is the human being, Plant species must be selected according to a list of criteria (see

P. Müller

- The species must be representative for an appropriate environmental area and indicate the immission load by accumulation of the pollutants in the organs so that residue analyses will be possible.
- The position in the food web and the relations to endagered species should be clear.
- They must have a large geographic distribution and are available in sufficient number; genetic uniformity is desirable.
- The physiology, ecology and sensitivity to pollutants should be known.

The following plant species comply these criteria to a high extend:

Table 3: List of plants for effects monitoring and banking.

species	remarks
I Monitoring effects on population in the natural ambient	
a) wildliving plants	
lichens: Hypogymnia physodes	best sensors and integrators of widely dispersed pollutants: Effects monitoring of ecosystems
peat mosses: Sphagnum spec.	longtime accumulators of heavy metals (and hydrocarbons) effects and trend monitoring
Sambucus nigra Picea spec.	sensitive accumulators of widely dispersed pollutants; effects and trend monitoring
Plantago major Taraxacum officinale Lolium multiflorum	accumulators of a lot of pollutants; important significance in the food web; effects and trend monitoring
b) culture plants	
Tobacco Bel W3	integrators of a broad spectrum of pollutants; sensor of photochemical smog: effects monitoring
Brassica oleracea Phaseolus vulgaris Spinacia oleracea Triticum sativum	world-wide distributed integrators of a broad spectrum of pollutants; direct significance for man: effects and trend monitoring
II. Exposure of test plants	
Brassica oleracea Lolium multiflorum	significance in the food chain: effects and trend monitoring
Hypogymnia physodes	indirect significance for man: effects and trend monitoring

Literature

Babich, H. and G. Stotzky: Sensitivity of various bacteria, including actinomycetes and fungi to cadmium and the influence of pH on sensitivity. Appl. and Environm. Microbiol. 33, 681-695 (1977).

Beckett, P.H. and R.D. Davis: The additivity of the toxic effects of Cu, Ni and Zn in young barley. New Phytol. 81, 155-173 (1978).

Briggs, G.E.: Population differention in Marchantia polymorpha L. in various lead pollution levels. Nature 238, 16o-167 (1972).

Beavington, F.: Heavy metal contamination and vegetables and soil in domestic gardens around a smelting complex. Environm. Pollution 9, 221-217 (1975).

Bown, J.E.: Absorption of copper, zinc and manganese by surgarcane leaf tissue. Plant Physiol. 44, 255-261 (1969).

Bradshaw, A.D.,; T.S. McNeilly and R.P. Gregory: Industrialization, evolution and the development of heavy metal tolerance. In: plant Ecology and the industrial society. British Ecol. Soc. Symp. 5, 327-343, Oxford.

Brooks, R.: Geobotany and biochemistry in mineral exploration. New York 1972.

Cannon, H.L.: The development of botanical methods of prospecting for uranium on the Colorado Plateau. U.S. Geol. Survey, Bull. 1o85-A,1-5o (196o).

Cannon, H.L.: The use of plant indicators in ground water surveys, geological mapping and mineral prospecting. Taxon 2o, 227-256 (1971).

Collet, P.: Über den Gehalt von Blei, Cadmium und Kupfer in Speisepilzen. Dt. Lebensm. Rundsch. 73, 75-82 (1977).

Crössmann, G.: Schwermetalle in handels- und wirtschaftseigenen Futtermitteln. Ber. Landwirtschaft 55, 785-795 (1977/78).

Davies, B.E. and P.E. Holmes: Lead contamination of roadside soil and grass in Birmingham, England, in relation to naturally occurring levels. J. agr. Sci., Camb. 79, 479-484 (1972).

Denayer-De Smet, S.: Premier apercu de la distribution du cadmium dans divers écosystêmes terrestres non polluês et polluês.Oecol. Plant. 9, 169-182 (1974).

Denaeyer-De Smet, S. and P. Duvigneaud: Accumulation de metaux lourds toxiques dans divers ecosystemes terrestres pollues par des retombees d'origine industrielle. Bull. Soc. Roy. Belg. 1o7, 147-156 (1974).

Den Doren de Jong, L.E.: Tolerance of Azotobacter for metallic and non-metallic ions. Antonie van Leuwenhoek 37, 119-124 (1971).

Ernst, W.: Schwermetallvegetation der Erde. Stuttgart 1974.

Ernst, W., Salaske, S. and P. Janiesch: Aspekte von Schwermetallbelastungen in Westfalen. Abhandl. Landesmuseum Naturkd. Münster, Westf. 36, 1-3o (1974).

Ernst, W.: Physiological and biochemical aspects of metal tolerance. In: Effects of air pollutants on plants. Cambridge, 115-133 (1976).

Fidora, B.: Der Bleigehalt von Pflanzen verkehrsnaher Standorte in Abhängigkeit von der Vegetationsperiode. Ber. Dt. Bot. Ges. 85, 219-227 (1972).

Geijn, van de S.C.: In vivo measurement of cadmium ($^{115\ m}$Cd) transport and accumulation in the stems of intact tomato plants Lycopersicon esculentum Mill.). Planta 138, 137-151 (1978).

Grant, C. and A.J. Dobbs: The growth and metal content of plants grown in soil contaminated by a copper/chrome/arsenic wood preservative. Environm. Pollution 14, 214-226 (1977).

Guderian, G., Krause, H.M. and H. Kaiser: Untersuchungen zur Kombinationswirkung von Schwefeldioxid und schwermetallhaltigen Stäuben auf Pflanzen. Schr. Reihe Landesanst. Immissionsschutz Heft 4o, 23 (1977).

Guderian, R.: Air Pollution, Phytotoxicity of acid gases and its significance in air pollution control; Ecological Studies 22, Springer Verlag, Berlin, Heidelberg, New York (1977).

Haut van, H.: Nachweis mehrerer Luftverunreinigungskomponenten mit Hilfe von Blätterkohl (Brassica oleracea acephala) als Indikatorpflanze. Staub-Reinhaltg. Luft, 32, 1o9-111 (1974).

Hodenberg von A. and A. Fink: Ermittlung von Toxizitäts-Grenzwerten für Zink, Kupfer und Blei in Hafer und Rotklee. Z. Pflanzenern., Düng. und Bodenk. 118, 489-5o3 (1975).

James, P.W.: The effect of air pollutants other than hydrogen fluorid and sulphur dioxide on lichens. In: Air pollution and lichens. 143-175 (1973).

Keller, Th.: Verkehrsbedingte Luftverunreinigungen und Vegetation. Garten und Landsch. 1o, 547-551 (1974).

Keller, Th. and H. Preis: Der Bleigehalt von Fichtennadeln als Indikator einer verkehrsbedingten Luftverunreinigung. Schweiz. Z. f. Forstwesen, 3, 143-162 (1967).

Kershaw, K.A.: Lichens, Endeavour 22, 65-9o (1963).

Kloke, A.: Blei,Zink, Cadmium-Anreicherung in Böden und Pflanzen. Staub Reinhaltg. Luft 34, 18-21 (1974).

Korn, S.: Bleibelastung des Bodens und ihre Wirkung auf die Aktivität der Bodenorganismen. Unveröff. Diplomarbeit, Gießen, 1975.

Krause, G.H.M.: Aufbau und Funktion eines Bestaubungsapparates für biologische Experimente. Staub-Reinhaltg. Luft 37, 234 (1977).

Kowalski, V.V.M.: Geochemische Ökologie, Biogeochemie. Berlin 1977.

Lagerwerf, J.V.: Uptake of cadmium, lead and zinc by radish from soil and air. Soil Sci. 3, 129-133 (1971).

Lepp, N.W.: Interactions between acmium and other heavy metals in affecting the growth of lettuce (Lactuca sativa L.c.v. Webbs Wonderful) seedlings. Z. Pflanzenphysiol. 84, 363-367 (1977).

Lerche, H. and S.W. Breckle: Untersuchungen zum Bleigehalt von Baumblättern im Bonner Raum. Angew. Bot. 48, 3o9-33o (1974).

Lipman, C.B. and P.S. Burgess: The effect of copper, zinc and lead salts on ammonification and nitrification in soils. Publ. Agric. Sci. 1, 127-139 (1914).

Little, P.: A study of heavy metal contamination of leaf surfaces. Environm. Pollution 5, 159-172 (1972).

Lötschert, W., Wandtner, R. and H. Hiller: Schwermetallanreicherung bei Bodenmoosen in Immissionsgebieten. Ber. Dt. Bot. Ges. 88, 419-431 (1975).

Malyuga, D.P.: Biogeochemical methods of prospecting. Consultants Bureau, New York 1964.

Maschmeyer, J.P. and J.A. Quinn: Copper tolerance in New Jersey populations of Agrostis stolonifera and Paronychia fastigiata. Bull. Torrey Bot. Club 1o3, 244-252 (1976).

Michels, S., Crössmann, G. and G. Scholl: Über die Kontamination von Nahrungsmitteln mit Schwermetallen. Staub-Reinhaltg. Luft 34, (1974).

Nash, Th.H.: Lichens as indicators of air pollution. Naturw. 63, 364-367 (1976).

Nieboer, E., H.M. Ahmed, Puckett, K.J. and D.H. Richardson: Heavy metal content of lichens in relation to distance from a nickel smelter in Sudbury, Ontario. Lichenologist 52, 292-3o4 (1972).

Noeske, Lächli, A., Lange, O.L., Vieweg, G.H. and H.Ziegler: Konzentration und Lokalisierung von Schwermetallen in Flechten der Erzschlackenhalden des Harzes. Dt. Bot. Ges. N.F. 4, 67-79 (197o).

Ohki, K.: Lower and upper critical zinc levels in relation to cotton growth and development. Physiol. Plant. 35, 96-1oo (1975).

Ophus, E.M. and B.M. Hullvag: Localisation of lead within leaf cells of Thytidiadelphus squarrosus (Hedw.) Warnst. by means of transmission eletron microscopy and Y-ray microanalysis. Cytobios 1o, 45-58 (1974).

Pakarinen, P. and K. Tolonen: Regional survey of heavy metals in peat mosses (Sphagnum). Ambio 5, 38-4o (1976).

Prinz, B. and G. Scholl: Erhebungen über die Aufnahme und Wirkung gas- und partikelförmiger Luftverunreinigungen im Rahmen eines Wirkungska- tasters. Schr. Landesanst. f. Immissions- und Bodennutzungsschutz des Landes NRW. 36, 62-86 (1975).

Puckett, K.J.: The effect of heavy metals on some aspects of lichen phy- siology. Canad. Journ. of Bot. 54, 2695-27o3 (1976).

Purves, D.: Contamination of urban garden soils with copper, boron and lead. Plant and Soil 26, 38o-382 (1967).

Rump, H.H., van Werden, K. and R. Hermann: Über die vertikale Änderung von Metallkonzentrationen in einem Hochmoor. Catena 4, 149-164 (1977).

Rühling, F. and G. Tyler: Sorption and retention of heavy metals in the woodland moss Hylocomium splendens (Hedw.) Br. et Sch. Oikos 21, 92-97 (197o).

Polar, E.: Variations in zinc content of subcellular fractions from young and old roots, stems and leaves of broad beans (Vicia faba) Physiol. Plant. 38, 159 (1976).

Sadler, W.E. and P.A. Trudinger: The inhibition of microorganisms by heavy metals. Mineralium Deposita 2, 158-168 (19767).

Schönbeck, H.: Nachweis schwermetallhaltiger Immissionen durch ausgewählte pflanzliche Indikatoren. VDI Ber. 2o3, 75-85 (1974).

Simola, L.K.: The tolerance of Sphagnum fimbriatum towards lead and cadmium. Ann. Bot. Fenn. 14, 1-5 (1977).

Simon, E.: La dynamique de la végetation de quelques sites metalliferes dans les régions d'Eupen et d'Aix-La Chapelle en realtion avec les fac- teurs édaphiques. Bull. Soc. Roy. Belg. 1o8, 273-286 (1975).

Sommer, G. and A. Stritesky: Gefäßversuche zur Ermittlung von Schadgrenzen von Cd, Cu and Pb sowie Zn im Hinblick auf den Einsatz von Abfallstoffen in der Landwirtschaft. Land. Forschg. 29 (1976).

Sommer, G., Rosopulo and J. Klee: Die Bleikontamination von Pflanzen und Böden durch Kraftfahrzeugabgase. Z. Pflanzenerh. und Bodenkd. 13o, 193- 2o5 (1971).

Steenken, F.: Begasungen von Nutzpflanzen mit bleihaltigen und bleifreien Autoabgasen. Z. Pflanzenkrankh. u. Pflanzenschutz 8o, 513-527 (1973).

Steubing, L.: Wirkungen von Luftverunreinigungen auf Pflanzen; Pflanzen als Bioindikatoren. In: Buchwald/Engelhardt: Handbuch für Planung, Ge- staltung und Schutz der Umwelt. BLV Verl. 166-175 (1978).

554

Steubing, L. and U. Kirschbaum: Immissionsbelastung der Straßenrandvegetation. Natur und Landschaft 51, 239-244 (1976).

Timperley, M.H., R.P. Brooks and P.J. Peterson: The distribution of nickel, copper, zinc and iron in tree leaves. J. Exp. Bot. 24, 889 (1973).

Tornabene, T.G. and H.W. Edwards: Microbial uptake of lead. Sci. 176, 1334-1335 (1972).

Tyler, G.: The effect of cadmium, lead and sodium salts on nitrification in a mull soil. Plant and Soil 4o, 237-242 (1974).

Tyler, G.: Heavy metal pollution and mineralisation of nitrogen in forst soils. Nature 255, 7o1-7o2 (1975).

Vetter, H. and R. Mähleop: Untersuchungen über Blei, Zink und Fluor-Immissionen und dadurch verursachte Schäden an Pflanzen und Tieren. Landw. Forschg. 24, 294-315 (1971).

Wittenberer, G.: Moose als mögliche Bioindikatoren für Luftverschmutzung, dargestellt am Beispiel von Offenbach a. M. Natur u. Landsch. 5o, 143-145 (1975).

CHOICE OF SPECIES, SAMPLING AND SAMPLE PRETREATMENT FOR SUBSEQUENT ANALYSIS AND BANKING OF MARINE ORGANISMS USEFUL FOR Hg, Pb AND Cd MONITORING

M. Stoeppler
Institute of Chemistry
Institute 4 Applied Physical Chemistry
Nuclear Research Centre, (KFA), Jülich
Federal Republic of Germany

Summary

The continuous transport of man made and natural amounts of toxic heavy metals and its compounds into the aquatic and marine environment makes real time monitoring and also banking of selected species necessary.
Since the total aquatic and marine load of Hg and Cd is much higher than man's contributions, for Cd only regional problems exist. For Hg also general health risks have to be considered. They are due to the biotransformation of less toxic Hg compounds into the highly toxic methylmercury, predominantly accumulated in the aquatic and marine food chain. Production and wasting of Pb by far exceeds natural sources. Though this seems only moderately reflected in the marine food chain, data from Pb accumulating tissue may contribute to a better understanding of biogeochemical phenomena.
In order to monitor particular as well as general impacts on marine and estuarine ecosystems, a balanced selection of accumulating species is recommended. Thus, to distinguish between contributions of toxic metal levels from the dissolved state, from particulate matter and from the food chain a bivalve, a macroalga and a teleost, non migratory fish should be used, with a probable later extension to a cephalopod and a pelagic prey fish.
Sampling and sample preparation for marine species needs proper procedures. Dissecting, homogenizing, deep freezing down to 77 K, and packaging for subsequent analysis and/or banking should be performed in mobile units having all the necessary equipment to reduce the contamination level drastically. For data normalization a meaningful weight basis is unavoidable and may be realized by e.g. the simultaneous use of an actual weight and a dry weight after freeze or oven drying.
The preparation of composite and single samples after shock freezing should result in sample aliquots of about 2 g fresh weight adding to a total sample amount of about 1 kg for subsequent trace analysis and banking.
Within the frame of the whole program very sophisticated and also independent analytical methods are required. For that purpose further detailed methodological evaluation and optimization is necessary.

1. Introductory part

1.1. General Remarks

An enormous load of soluble and suspended matter of natural and man made origin is continuously transported from the continents to an stored in the marine environment.

These fluxes are in the first place attributed to rivers, but also sub-
marine vulcanism and the input from the atmosphere, the latter including
an appreciable amount of man made materials, play a significant role.
Though the mixing with the giant water mass of the sea seems to result in
an extreme dilution and also further cleaning processes due to adsorption
phenomena at particulate matter and sediments are to be expected, the real
situation is different. Highly soluble compounds of e.g. man made origin
accumulate due to the slow exchange rates with deeper waters to some extent in the upper mixed oceanic layer (depth around loo m) in which biological activity is predominant and bioaccumulation as well as biotransformation occur. On the other hand less soluble materials and those with
a tendency to be adsorbed on particulate matter may be continuously transported into deeper zones and finally to deep sea sediments, thus relatively fast disappearing from equilibrium. Further, estuaries with shallow
waters and tidal influences reflect very strongly also in their biomass
the load of rivers and contain, compared with deep sea regions, rather
highly mobile amounts of pollutants.
This situation makes the use of particular marine oroganisms with accumulation properties for global, regional or local monitoring possible and
desirable.
But, due to different mechanisms for different substances a meaningful
selection and analysis of species is rather difficult.
Therefore in a condensed manner some aspects of heavy metal monitoring
and banking are discussed from the viewpoint of own experiences gained
during several extended baseline studies.

1.2. Global and regional situation for Hg, Cd and Pb

With the exception of artifical organic substances, not to be discussed
here, toxic metals introduced into the marine environment contribute regularly to the normal biogeochemical cycle and finally to the total load.
In the case of Hg the mean (decreasing) annual world production accounts
to about 10^4 tons/year. Cd shows a mean, increasing annual world production
of 2.10^4 tons. That leads to quite high concentrations in some environmental compartments as rivers, estuaries and particularly for Hg in the Mediterranean Sea, and may also rise regional and local risks but will not
contribute substantially to the global marine biogeochemistry which is
very different for both these elements. Cd plays actually only a regional
- but sometimes a very important - role due to relatively low concentrations in the edible part of pelagic organisms. Hg is predominantly in the
Mediterranean Sea in some stages of the marine food chain, e.g. in pelagic prey and other fishes, as e.g. Thunnus thynnus and Xyphias gladius
etc., highly enriched well above the recommended safe threshold /1-6/.
This accumulation ability through the aquatic and marine food chain is
mainly due to organomercurials, by far predominantly methylmercury, produced by biotransformation of inorganic and phenylmercury in simpler organisms /7-8/. Despite the assumption of a prohibitive effect of Se on
Hg toxicity, as Se is always present together with Hg in a rather distinct
relation /9a,9b/, the further investigation of unexpected high levels
of Hg in fishes from particular coastal and pelagic zones of e.g. the
Mediterranean Sea is an urgent challenge and should be tackled by further
intensified research on this topic.
The production of Pb followed by the release of its compounds (including
the at present decreasing use of Pb alkyl compounds as antiknock agents)
by far exceeds the natural contributions: The estimated man made input
into the oceans is > 10^5 tons/year /1o/. The total industrial world production of Pb and Pb compounds amounts to about 3.10^6 tons/year compared

with a natural input of $\geq 10^4$ tons/year. This should have markedly rised also the global marine concentration of dissolved Pb in the upper oceanic layer although a continuous regulation and sedimentation via biological debris and adsorption on particulate matter takes place. These facts may also stimulate Pb monitoring using some marine organisms to assess increasing global as well as regional levels in the marine biosphere as will be discussed below.

2. Choice of Marine Organisms as Biological Monitors for Trace Metals

2.1. Typical Trace Metal Levels in Marine Species

Pb and Cd concentrations are extremely low in the edible part of fishes as tuna /11/ and others /12,13/. From Pattersons studies for Pb /11/ and a recently carried out preliminary study in our laboratory for Pb, Cd and Cu in a group of selected marine organisms it seems that numerous hitherto reported values on Pb contents in fish muscle are highly based by contamination from laboratory environment etc. Thus, the real concentrations are at the low ng/g or even picogram/g level. The results or our mentioned study are summarized in table 1 and demonstrate that higher Pb and also Cd concentrations could only be detected in benthic organisms at lower trophic levels of the marine food chain, e.g. copepods, mussels and crustaceans. Also algae show a remarkable accumulation of Pb and Cd /14,15/. Of particular interest for monitoring purposes may be that in the cephalopod Sepia officinalis appreciable Cd levels were found in contrast to low Pb values which may be explained by a different metabolic behaviour in organisms like sepiae.

TABLE 1

LEAD, CADMIUM AND COPPER CONTENT IN DIFFERENT MARINE SPECIES (31 SPECIMEN) FROM MEDITERRANEAN SEA AND NORTH SEA (values in ng/g fresh weight)

Species	(n)	$\bar{x}$ Lead range	$\bar{x}$ Cadmium range	$\bar{x}$ Copper range
Solea solea Clupea harengus Gadus morhua Mullus barbatus	17	N.D.[+)]	≥ 2	28o,1oo-55o
Sepia officinalis	4	N.D.[+)]	45,35-55	3ooo,22oo-46oo
Portunus spec.	5	23o,15o-42o	48,32-74	12ooo,67oo-194oo
Mytilus spec.	5	11oo,22o-25oo	35o,15o-57o	14oo,63o-24oo

[+)] not detectable, determination limit during this preliminary study ≤2o ng/g using electrothermal atomic absorption spectrometry (HGA 74/PE 4oo) after nitric acid pressure decomposition /41/.

558

TABLE 2

TYPICAL MERCURY LEVELS OF SOME MARINE SPECIES (TOTAL MERCURY)
Values in ng/g fresh weight

Species	Origin	(specimen number) (n)	$\bar{x}$	range
Solea vulgaris	Atlantic	3o	45	14 — 116
Solea solea	North Sea	11	12o	63 — 28o
Clupea harengus	North Sea	25	41	2o — 75
Gadus morhua	North Sea	35	11o	4o — 26o
Mullus barbatus	Atlantic	15	26o	5o — 62o
Mullus barbatus	Med. Sea	86	16o	2o — 8oo
Scomber scombrus	Med. Sea	15	343	13o — 51o
Scomber scombrus	North Sea	18	278	45 — 548
Scomber japonicus	Atlantic	9	76	43 — 96
Sepia officinalis	Med. Sea	54	385	6o —11oo
Sepia officinalis	Atlantic	15	12o	6o — 29o
Sepia officinalis	North Sea	13	8o	5o — 12o
Portunus spec.	Med. Sea	15	4o	2o — 65
Mytilus spec.	Med. Sea	8o	7o	15 — 23o
Mytilus spec.	Med. Sea	96	85	25 — 2o6

Table 2 summarizes Hg values in the same and a few additional species
as in table 1. These data (all species from the Mediterranean Sea were
caught off the Western Italian coast /4,6/ demonstrate the above mentioned different Hg concentrations in the same species collected in different regionsof the oceans.
Thus, with the aid of these tables and further facts to be discussed below
a few additional species useful for monitoring purposes shall advocated
for careful consideration in the introductory phase of the environmental
specimen bank program.

2.2. Proposed Selection of Species

In studies of the abundance of toxic metals a biological monitor should
be an organism which may be used to quantify levels of pollution by the
measurement of the concentration of the toxic substance in its tissues
/15/. Either the entire organism or a particular part or tissue of it may
be used. Such a biological monitor should be:

- Sedentary or at least non-migrating in order to be representative of
  the collecting area
- Abundant in all regions to be monitored (if possible)
- Of reasonable size, giving adequate tissue for analysis
- Easy to collect
- A good accumulator allowing direct analysis without preconcentra-
  tion
- Able to give a simple correlation between the metal content of the
  accumulator and the average metal concentration in its surroundings.

Since mussels were strongly recommended for marine monitoring purposes
within the specimen bank program, on the basis of the above given outline
it seems doubtful whether it is possible to obtain all necessary informations from a single type of species. Besides the obvious advantages of bivalves - e.g. high accumulation rates for at least Pb and Cd with a good

reflection of the local surrounding - there are also disadvantages or
at least limitations: Since they are filter feeders, obtaining trace metals not only from food and from the solution but also from the ingestion
of inorganic particulate material /15,16/ the exact proportions of their
body trace metal value due to each of these three routes are still uncertain. Further from hitherto not yet confirmed assumptions the amount of
organomercurials seems to be relatively poor in this species, possibly
due to the competing action of inorganic particulates. Another disadvantage is,that single specimens are rather small. Thus, a separation of
e.g. the muscle tissue from organs is practically impossible yielding
a rather high inhomogeneity within each single specimen. Finally it is
also very difficult to define a relatively correct fresh or even actual
weight, (see 3.4.) because of problems in standardizing the moisture
content. This particular point, respresenting a central problem for reliable analytical data will be discussed below.
Thus, from the authors experience the additional consideration of a few
promising possible species would be very helpful for the specimen bank
program:
- First, an excellent additional species would be a macroalga. Algae reach
- at least partly - the above listed properties, they are excellent accumulators of heavy metals, they show due to their simple structure, homogeneous metal distribution and reflect very sensitively the soluble fraction of these metals, while they do not reflect total metal loads (practically no uptake of metals associated to organic or inorganic particulate
matter). The time integration of ambient metal concentrations is rather
high, due to the extremely long biological half-lifes of bound trace metals /15/. Thus, it is to be expected that data from a distinct alga with
wide spread distribution and good adaptability to different environmental factors (e.g. Ulva lactuca) may supplement the results obtained with
the non-differentiating bivalves. This is, of course, only the case if
all species considered are collected from the same area.
- Second, a teleost fish should also taken as a monitoring species, since
fishes reflect very sensitive the trace metal content both from food and
solution. This is the fact at least for Hg, predominantly in the form of
methyl-Hg which seems not to be accumulated to a very high extent in algae
and bivalves. To obtain in the view of the above mentioned strategy comparable data, a non migratory species (flat fishes: pleuronectidae, e.g.
solea spec. etc.) is wanted. Possibly also juvenile organisms, non-migrating for a distinct time span, may be useful. Moreover, although the Pb
content in the muscle of marine fishes is very low, it is also known, that
this metal accumulates, e.g. in bones, bony parts and to some extent also
in the spleen /15,17/. Cd is reported to accumulate in gills, liver, etc.
/18,19/. Thus, the preparation of various accumulating tissues from fish
seems also very promising for monitoring and banking purposes.
- Third, also the introduction of other more or less migratory, organisms
(e.g. prey fishes) note the very high Hg values in Thunnus thynnus and
Xyphias gladius /1,2/ and the accumulation ability of molluscs as sepiae
for Cd and Hg (table 1) at a later stage may be useful in particular cases, but should not be discussed at present since the now performed monitoring programs in marine ecosystems (see 3.1.) should give more insight
in problems of that kind.
Considering these facts a nearly comprehensive real time monitoring and
banking program seems possible in the marine environment if only a few
additional organisms were collected. This may also cover, if the supplementary monitoring of particular tissues of teleost fishes is settled,
the requirements of monitoring programs for artificial and (relatively)
persistent organic substances.

Further, such a combined program may also make use of the large and comprehensive potentialities offered by the sea: The monitoring of fluxes of dissolved, particulate bond (mainly inorganic and debris) and bioaccumulated (food chain) trace metals in more or less polluted regions (i.e. reflections of local and regional sources) in comparison to selected sampling sites without direct man made impacts. These data may also substantially contribute to a better knowledge of the global inventory for e.g. Pb and persistent organic pollutants. This shall further provide reliable data for the hitherto to some extent still uncertain value of the global Pb increase in the upper layer of the oceans within, from the geological point of view, a relatively short period of time.

3. Technical and Analytical Aspects

3.1. Introduction

In 1975, under the Mediterranean Action plan, developed by the United Nations Environmental Program (UNEP) and endorsed by the Intergovernmental Meeting on the Protection of the Mediterranean, a Coordinated Mediterranean Pollution Monitoring and Research Program was established. As part of this program an FAO (GFCM)/UNEP Joint Coordinated Project on "Pollution in the Mediterranean" was initiated. The project, among other subjects, aims at organizing baseline studies and the monitoring of metals, particularly Hg, and of DDT,PCB's and other chlorinated hydrocarbons, in marine organisms. Our Institute - continously performing since1975 physicochemical and analytical studies in aquatic and marine ecosystems in the frame of a Bilateral Scientific Cooperation with Yugoslavia (Project title: Environmental Research in Aquatic Systems) also joined 1976 the mentioned FAO/UNEP project. This is performed based on our marine station at Fiascherino in Cooperation with the CNEN (Comitato Nazionale per l'Energia Nucleare), Environmental Research Division, Laboratory for Marine Contamination, Fiascherino, Italy. Since 1977 an additional marine project on "Comparative Studies on Heavy Metal Pollution and Balance in Selected Regions of European Seas" +) under contract No 173-77-ENVD in the frame of the 2nd Environmental Research Program of the European Communities was started. Hitherto published results in the course of these extended research and monitoring programs contribute to basic marine and aquatic trace chemistry and physicochemistry as well as to baseline studies in seawater, inland waters and in biological materials /2o-34/.
For investigations only concerned with marine organisms, FAO Fisheries Technical Publications, particularly Technical Paper No. 158 /35/ and Identification Sheet for Fisheries Purposes /36/ were invaluable for identification, sampling and sample preparation of the collected marine species. A minor part of the up to date obtained results in shown in Tables 1 and 2 /4,6/.
Technical and analytical contributions to the methodological evaluation of sampling and sample pretreatment techniques followed by the automated trace metal determination in biological and environmental materials and aqueous samples were further additionally supported in particular research programs sponsored by the German Federal Ministry of Research and Technology. The achieved methodological developments offer now fast and reliable, to

---

+) Project Leader: Prof. Dr.H.W. Nürnberg, Director, Institute of Chemistry, Institute 4 Applied Physical Chemistry, Nuclear Research Centre (KFA), Juelich

a certain extent already automated, methods for trace metals with determination ranges from the µg/g down to the ng/g- and in some cases even
the pg/g-level /22,27,29,37-42/.
Based on hitherto gained experience and also encountered difficulties at
particular technical stages in the following paragraphs an outline shall
be given of possible future tasks in the frame of a pilot study for an
environmental specimen bank considering all the above mentioned marine
species.

3.2. Sampling and Sample Preparation

From the viewpoint of the analysis of trace elements and methylmercury
in the considered organisms, there are usually no sampling problems
concerning identification, availability of species and contamination
during collection to be expected if the sampling area is clearly defined
as a whole, the staff is well trained and experienced and the sites
of sampled mussels and algae are known or installed, e.g. the use of
cages for mussel monitoring is recommendable. Fish catching should always be done by fishermen experienced and trained to perform their duty
very carefully under particular contract for the program.
All organisms to be taken for real time monitoring and banking purpose
should be prepared either for direct analysis or short, medium or long
term storage in the bank and subsequent analysis immediately after sampling. This is extremely important at least for fishes or their muscle
meat and for molluscs to obtain proper conditions e.g.
homogenization, portioning and weight determination. If samples were
frozen shortly after sampling a later portioning is difficult if no
prior homogenization step had been included. The preservation ability
of e.g. shock freezing techniques must therefore be studied separately
and carefully.
Preparations in the described manner have to be performed with the aid of
very sophisticated technical equipments for weighing, dissection, portioning, package, shock and deep freezing at ≥ 77 K. Also dust minimali-
zation by the use of laminar flow systems and contamination control
mats and sheets for wall protection has to be assured.
Since these requirements can only be reached in well equipped analytical
laboratories, the need for mobile units of corresponding performance is
obvious. In the frame of our environmental research programs a mobile
laboratory on a diesel powered truck was designed, constructed, and subsequently and successfully tested during field missions from 1976 to 1978
/43/. It offers a space of about 13 m³, regularly provided with two clean
benches and the necessary furniture. Additional equipment may contain
devices for trace analysis usually for electrothermal and cold vapor AAS
and for voltammetry, an outside tent, deep freezing (77 K) homogenizing
and freezer mill systems, freeze driers, digestion apparatus, electronic
balances etc. A diesel power generator on a trailer provides the power
supply in the field.

3.3. Contamination Precautions

The trace metal levels of all till now recommended materials for banking
and real time monitoring vary significantly from the µg/g down to the
ng/g range. Thus, frequently a separate preparation of collected materials
shall be performed to avoid cross-contamination. In the case of the mentioned marine species the simultaneous preparation at least of bivalves
and algae is possible without problems, since the expected concentrations
for Hg, Cd and Pb are roughly of the same order of magnitude with comparatively low Hg levels.

If e.g. a teleost fish and a mollusc have to be prepared care must be
taken, because as it can be seen from table 1, the Pb and Cd concentration in muscle is extremely low, but even concentrations in organs and
bony parts are much lower than the normal levels in algae, bivalves,
and dust particles. To avoid contamination as far as possible, besides
the continuous use of clean benches, contamination control mats etc.,
the use of carefully cleaned plastic foils (polyethylene, teflon) on
the dissecting boards, precleaned quartz knives and plastic pincettes
is mandatory, also always the wearing of gloves. Prior to use these
parts of equipment have to be scrupulously cleaned with diluted ultra-
pure acids or complexing agents.
The same applies to all other instruments, devices and containers necessary for dissecting, portioning, homogenizing, packaging and for intermediate or final storage. All these gear has to be very carefully pre-
cleaned and the cleaning and washing solutions have to be continuously
checked for their trace metal content. Also of great importance is the
control of acids and chelating agents used for cleaning purposes. If
necessary, they have to be precleaned, e.g. by subboiling distillation
(acids) or solvent extraction (aqueous solutions of chelates).
The tolerable contamination level should be, as a rule, as far as possible
controlled and always kept well below lo %of the concentration of the respective trace element in the respective banking material. This includes
all treatments necessary from sampling via homogenization to storage.

3.4. Weight Standardization

Of paramount importance for reliable data but hitherto not satisfactory
is the standardization of sample weight. Numerous scientists report the
weight as fresh weight, others determine a dry weight predominantly
after oven drying rather than after e.g. freeze drying. Both these stan-
dardizations show advantages and disadvantages. An advantage of fresh
weight, often favoured by biologists during food and environmental
surveillance, is its direct relation to the reality, i.e. the consumption figures of e.g. the food basket expressed in weight units. A disadvantage is that due to a continuous loss of moisture, even during short
term storage, the reported fresh weight varies considerably and represents
therefore rather a rough approach to the initial weight than a really
exact figure.
The oven drying procedures normally achieving a "constant weight", earlier
introduced by analytical chemists, are excellent for technical and ro-
bust materials and therefore also absolutely necessary in classical analytical chemistry. Doubtless this approach seems generally to be more exact
due to its rigid regulations. Unfortunately it is not always applicable.
Biological and hence very often extremely sensitive materials show
during thermal treatment frequently a disintegration tendency and therefore no constant weight due to the loss of volatile decay products. The
standardization of the time span for the drying procedure may result
in a more or less constant weight, but this is merely a random than a biologically significant factor.
Thus, frequently the use of internal standards in biological materials as
additional parameters were advocated. Examples are carbon, sulfur, nitrogen, or zink contents of biological materials. Though this may be
helpful in some particular materials and may become in the future also
valuable for an environmental specimen bank, for the pilot stage and
marine samples a provisionally approach seems more feasible. It consists
of the determination of an actual weight, which should be as close as possible to the fresh weight, i.e. the weight determined during or immediately

after sampling together with dry weight data. The latter should be determined by taking sufficient amounts of the homogenized material for subsequent drying procedures including freeze and oven drying and in some cases also the mild treatment in a desiccator. This strategy should give for the moment sufficient informations for an arbitrary content/weight relationship and the later discussion of weight standardization by means of additonal independent and relatively precise methods.

3.5. Sample Pretreatment for Banking and Real Time Monitoring

Under the above discussed precautions (see 3.3.) and if rather homogeneous marine material, showing no extremely low trace metal contents, is considered, usually it seems possible to obtain also representative composite samples for long term banking. For this purpose from each particular species (except bivalves, as discussed below) and sampling site a sufficient number of specimens or tissues with the necessary excess weight must be taken and carefully prepared in the described manner. Immediately after finishing the dissection the fresh samples should be carefully homogenized or milled, if necessary divided, weighed,and filled into clean containers. Appropriate materials are: teflon, polyethylene, quartz. Subsequently follows deep or shock freezing (temperatures 226 - 77 K). The efficiency of the choosen milling or homogenization technique must be scrupulously checked in series of experiments using single, oligo- and multielement methods to ensure an absolute minimum of contamination and a representative and statistically satisfactory final sample. For real time monitoring also single samples must be taken and adequately prepared to find out the range of trace element values for each sampling area and series of analyzed specimens.
Since the present analytical methods are very sensitive and the concentrations at least of Cd and Hg, in some samples (mussels, algae, selected organ tissues, bones) also of Pb, are in the higher ng/g or even the lower µg/g range, the subsample weights must not exceed 2 g actual weight (i.e. less than 1 g dry weight), if the samples are sufficient homogeneous at this trace element level.
For bivalves, e.g. mytilus spec. there may arise problems, since the presence of particulate matter in each specimen can lead to a considerable inhomogeneity in the final (composite) sample even if powerful milling and grinding procedures are applied. This should be studied very carefully in the pilot phase. Possibly it is more advisable not to homogenize or to grind and to determine single specimens separately. This may certainly lead to the need of higher sample amounts for bivalves.
At present it is still unknown if methylmercury decomposes during long-term storage. For this reason a detailed research program is necessary. This program has to include also the feasibility of freeze drying, perhaps of advantage at least for species as algae and terrestrial materials with relatively high contents of trace elements, if only the analysis of these elements, also in a retrospective manner is of interest.

3.6. Analysis

3.6.1. Introductory Remarks

General problems and the state of-the-art of todays analytical and trace analytical chemistry are amply and critically discussed elsewhere /16,44-47/. Thus, finally some particular analytical tasks in connection with banking and real time monitoring will be outlined.

To obtain today as reliable as ever possible informations on the true trace
element concentration in the considered materials great efforts will be
necessary. This includes series of careful investigations about matrix
adapted particular pretreatment procedures (digestion-dilution, digestion-
dilution-solvent extraction etc.) for the subsequent determination, applying r .adiotracers and at least two independent analytical methods of high
selectivity and sensitivity (dual principle of independent method application /21,22,25,33,46,47/).
At the moment advanced atomic absorption spectrophotometry (e.g. electrothermal and cold vapor techniques) and voltammetry (e.g. differential
pulse stripping voltammetry with mercury film or solid electrodes) together with isotope dilution mass spectrometry offer the best possibilities
for the mentioned elements in this concentration range. At higher concentrations also atomic absorption with the flame and voltammetry at the
dropping and stationary mercury electrode show good results with an excellent within-run and day-to-day precision.
The question of long-term storage behaviour of methylmercury must be tackled by methods as gas chromatography with electron capture or voltammetric
detectors, voltammetry with solid electrodes and automated cold vapor
atomic absorption spectroscopy. Since during storage only weak alterations
per storage time interval have to be expected, the hitherto used methods
for the quantitiative determiantion of this compound have to be substantially improved with respect to better sensitivity, precision and accuracy. This will need time and staff with particular expertise and will
therefore have not a low cost factor.

3.6.2. Description of Analytical Procedures

Mercury

As the working horse for the analysis of <u>total mercury</u> in tissues cold
vapor AAS is at present due to its practically freedom from matrix
interferences successfully applied.
Usually the procedure starts with either a wet (reflux) or a pressurized
decomposition of subsamples with wet (fresh) weights from o.2 to 2.5 g
depending on mercury levels.
Pressurized decomposition may be performed in routine analysis because of
its simplicity and low vulnerability to contamination or elemental losses preferably with multisample units (41) also carefully investigated
for pressure evaluation and carbon balance (48).
The subsequent mercury determination in the digests may be carried out
with semi-automated commercial systems using either $SnCl_2$ or $NaBH_4$
(35,49) and also, in a fully automated manner, by coupling a modified
Technicon Auto Analyzer $^®$-II-System with a conventional AAS-instrument
and a quartz tube, containing silver wool for the occasionally necessary
preconcentration of mercury. This combination enables to perform up to
2o mercury determinations/h due to its flexibility in a rather large
concentration range without prior dilution with an absolute determination
limit of $\geq$ o.5 ng and an accuracy $\geq$ 3o % for single samples starting at
a concentration of about 2o ng/g. For series n $\geq$ lo samples the error
of the mean was shown to be usually $\geq$ lo % for p = o.o5 (6,4o).
Alternative and checking methods are instrumental and radiochemical neutron activation analysis with a quite good accuracy and precision (5o,51).
Also a new electrochemical method is very promising. This method, developed in our laboratory, consists of differential pulse anodic stripping
in the subtractive mode (DPASV-S) at a twin disc rotating gold electrode

and offers an outstanding sensitivity and precision (26).
The determination of <u>methyl mercury</u> in fish tissue is feasible after
a thoroughly performed clean-up. The method is based either on the
use of a hydrochloric or hydrobromic acid treatment modification of
a former WESTØØ procedure (35) or alkali hydroxide treatment (52).
Methylmercury determination is performed by gas-chromatorgraphy and
and ^{63}Ni-electron capture detector with an absolute detection limit
≤ o.o5 ng (53). Atomic absorption and DPASV-S are useful as well to
determine the Hg present in solution from liquid extraction. These
techniques seem also very promising for a future application in routine
analysis, possibly in combination with high performance liquid chromatography (HPLC).

Lead

The determination of lead in the above advocated tissues and bony parts
has to cope with levels from about 1oo to a few thousand ng/g. These levels provide the application of AAS, DPASV, and also as an ultimate and
checking method, isotope dilution mass spectrometry. The problems concerning the application of AAS for the determination of lead in biological
materials are recently amply and critically discussed (54).
In general, the sample preparation may be performed, due to the volatilization properties of lead either by wet (55,56), also in the particular
pressurized decomposition version (41,48), or alternatively by dry ashing
techniques including low temperature ashing in a microwave induced oxygen plasma, recently very carefully investigated and optimized in our
laboratory (27).
Since lead determinations with AAS sometimes suffer from a relatively
low sensitivity and matrix interferences only to be completely overcome
by solvent extraction,the at present obtainable accuracy and precision
is only satisfactory for the demands of an Environmental Specimen Bank
and thus, also for a pilot study, if marine samples are considered, when
the flame is applicable, reaching total errors ≤ 1o %. Since the use of
flame AAS is limited in the mentioned materials only to samples with
concentrations ≤2 µg/g, the working horse, at least for precision analysis,
is DPASV, very sensitive over the whole range and also offering an excellent precision and accuracy with often a total error around or even below
1o % (21,22,23,25,29,33). The sample pretreatment may be carried out for
these methods either by improved wet or low temperature ashing. For
checking purposes and the characterization of standard materials or working standards isotope dilution mass spectrometry (IDMS) offers a further
improvement with total errors ≤ 5 %, if all precautions, also against
contamination, are taken. The main disadvantages of this analytical principle are its high costs and the very low number of analysis/day. In relation to flame AAS (if a first class instrument with all necessary technical equipment, also including automated sample introduction and data
evaluation, is used, up to 15o measurements/h are possible) compared
to IDMS the ratio of total expenses/analysis exceed a factor of 15o. In
relation to automated electrothermal AAS and DPASV the factor is still
5o, with the advantage of DPASV, that the latter method is more precise
and more accurate, particularly for lead determinations at lower levels,
if compared with electrothermal AAS (54).

Cadmium

In principle the situation is similar to that discussed for lead. But AAS
offers for cadmium an about a factor of 2o higher sensitivity with an
absolute detection limit around 1o^{-13} g, hence the application of flame AAS

reaches a broader field of application if the species discussed here
were considered. Further, the relatively easy volatilization of cadmium
makes a temperature programming in electrothermal AAS possible which
circumvents frequently most of the matrix problems encountered.
Thus, besides the recommended continuous application of DPASV/HMDE,AAS,
either in the flame or electrothermal version, may substantially contribute to routine analysis after wet or low temperature ashing. The application of IDMS also for Cd is now in the introductory stage. From hitherto
gained experience this method will contribute, as it is also discussed
under lead, to the characterization of reference materials and working
standards.·

4. Program Design and Statistics

It is intended to propose and subsequently to perform the sampling of
three species in the pilot phase: a mussel, an alga (e.g. ulva lactuca)
and a widespread fish (e.g. solea spec.) at about six different places
and also to carry out some preliminary investigations on a prey fish and
sepiae (cephalopods) also found in several European seas. The latter is
at present the case in the mentioned FAO (GFCM)/WHO and EC programs.
The obtained results will be made available also in the form of preliminary reports as particular contributions to the pilot specimen bank project.
Also to the fundamental items to be very carefully considered belong
statistical investigations on the usefulness of the data of the proposed
species. At present only some general remarks are possible. From the
hitherto obtained results of studies performed on the Hg level in numerous
specimens from the Mediterranean Sea, the Atlantic and also from the North
Sea and the Baltic, rather differing results were obtained, including
also the view of a statistical reliable judgement. Since the evaluation
of thousands of individual measurements is at present not completed only
a few main points may be made to show the line to be followed upon for
a useful and reliable inclusion of statistical aspects in the program
design.
The hitherto obtained data for mussels (mytilus galloprovincialis) show,
that the statistical distribution is quite different if different locations are observed. In the case of e.g. uniform environmental conditions
(i.e. low local fluctuations) the shape seems quite simple, showing a
nearly regular gaussian distribution. If strong fluctuations occur, e.g.
in some estuaries of the North and the Mediterranean Sea, in samples taken within a distinct region rather strong differences were observed.
This makes the use of a particular sampling technique highly recommendable. For mussels the best approach may be the use of the before mentioned
cages to monitor the water close to algae accumulations also used as a
sedentary biological monitoring species. Regrettably for algae at present
no statistical reliable data were at hand from our before mentioned marine
studies.
Concerning the at present attainable statistical uncertainty (mean error
of the mean) of less than 1o % (p = 0.05) of analytical data, at least
for Hg, Pb, and Cd, only differences above this level may be recognized.
For this purpose and considering a mussel watch ≥ 1oo single samples (i.e.
a total amount of ≥ 15o g fresh weight) either for mussels or algae
should be analyzed at this stage of the project and the data statistically
evaluated if it is possible also to use lower sample numbers.
The same is valid for the analysis of subsamples from e.g. solea solea,
since only fishes from a distinct and very limited area promise comparable
values. These organisms, collected in our program in the Atlantic as well

as in the North Sea showed a rather acceptable and narrow Hg range (e.g. from 6o - 28o ng/g for one area in the North Sea and 14 - 116 for three Atlantic areas) and also general differences in mean values far below analytical errors (mean from the North Sea 11o ng/g and from the Atlantic 45 ng/g) promising at least to recognize significant regional differences and, later, also local and regional trends if the collecting conditions are carefully defined and maintained by a well trained and experienced staff.

5. Organizational Aspects and Cost Estimation

The last sentence of the prior chapter is the introductory sentence here: the project as a whole must be carried out by a well trained and experienced staff from sampling to sample preparation, analysis and banking. Also clear instructions in a written form, supplied by several selected and simple drawings and tables together with the demand of a scrupulous documentation of all data needed in easily understandable and computer accessible forms are mandatory. Also it is clearly understood, that detailed procedures for all the above mentioned working steps must be developed carefully by experts from different scientific branches as e.g. marine biology, ecology, analytical and/or physical chemistry and bio-chemistry, statistics, electronics and deep freezetechnology.

A preliminary cost estimation was recently prepared for the BMFT (German Federal Ministry of Research and Technology) on the basis of the present available instrumentation and personnel in our institute and for the possible operation of a part of the Pilot Environmental Specimen Bank. Since, here special aspects will be addressed and a cost estimation given, this is mainly calculated for the purpose of the sampling of marine species followed by the necessary pretreatment up to a real time analysis, if feasible, and banking techniques. The real expenses are at present covered in our programme predominantly by EC contracts and the regular KFA budget.

Estimation of expenses for a sub-program "marine species" in the frame of a pilot specimen bank:

1.) Personnel costs:

- Fishermen under contract for theprogram together with appropriate vessels. Sampling four times a year in six selected areas, including also one in the Mediterranean Sea DM 2o.ooo

- Staff, two man years, also included contributions from different scientists and contracts with e.g. biological experts etc. DM 22o.ooo

- (This number comprises the total running personnel expenses including the continuous use of the KFA infrastructure, workshops, reactors, ect.)
- Traveling costs, Europe including Med. Sea DM 2o.ooo

2.) Other running costs. Here only the proportion of the particular costs for the mentioned marine subprogram is given as deductive costs per annum.

- Rent of rooms for intermediate sample storage, storage of supplementary instruments, etc. DM 5.ooo

- Chemicals, laboratory ware, storage vessels,
  and the proportion of running costs for the mobile
  laboratory (fuel, repair etc.), cages for the
  mussel watch etc.   DM 25.ooo

- Mobile laboratory, deductive costs for the whole
  unit including a special equipment with a power
  generator, an outside tent, deep freeze and shock
  freeze installation, deep freezer mills, laminar
  flow boxes etc.   DM 1o.ooo

- Storage capacity (liquid nitrogen cooling) for
  intermediate and long term storage at $\geq$ 77 K
  including also control and data acquisition
  systems, the proportion of the pilot bank building and laboratory use (increasing costs due to
  increasing sample number in the bank must be calculated)   DM 3o.ooo

- Deductive Costs for analytical instruments (AAS,
  DPASV, digestion systems, balances, freeze driers,
  etc.)   DM 2o.ooo
                                                       ─────────────
  Total estimated costs per annum   DM 35o.ooo

From these rather roughly calculated expenses for three marine species
it may be seen, that by far the dominant part is manpower. Thus, it
is obvious, that even the most sophisticated cooling system for the
bank, here liquid nitrogen was assumed as coolant, will not markedly
increase the total costs as much as the steady increase of personnel
costs, with an estimated total annual increase around 5 %. Another
reason for the relatively high personnel costs is also that the staff
has to be very carefully selected to guarantee the best possible performance of the project as a whole. If the pilot specimen bank is considered, the ratio mentioned here is practically the same, with the
exception that the initial sampling step is less expensive for some
sample types as e.g. sewage sludge, grasses, wheat etc.

References

1. Y. Thibaud
   Teneur en mercure dans quelques poissons de consommation courante.
   Sci. Peche 2o8,1, (1971).

2. G. Cumont, et al.
   Contamination des poissons de mer par la mercure.
   Rev. Int. Océanogr. Med. 28, 95 (1972).

3. A. Renzoni, E. Bacci and L. Falciai
   Mercury Concentration in the Water, Sediments and Fauna of an Area
   of the Tyrrhenian Coast. Rev. Int. Océanogr. Med. 36/37, 17 (1973).

4. M. Stoeppler, M. Bernhard, F. Backhaus, and E. Schulte
   Mercury in Marine Organisms of the Mediterranean and other European
   Seas. Rapp. Comm. Int. Mer. Médit., 24, 8; 39 (1977).

5. M. Bernhard, A. Renzoni
   Mercury Concentration in Mediterranean Marine Organisms and their
   Environment: Natural or Anthropogenic Origin. Thalassia Jugoslavica,
   in press (1978).

6. M. Stoeppler, M. Bernhard, F. Backhaus, E. Schulte
   Mercury in Marine Organisms from Central and Western Mediterranean
   Sea and the Strait of Gibraltar. Mar. Poll. Bull., to appear.

7. S. Jensen, A. Jernelöv
   Behaviour of Mercury in the Environment. In: Mercury Contamination
   in Man and his Environment, Techn. Rep. Ser. 137, IAEA, Vienna,
   1972, p. 43.

8. A. Jernelöv
   Microbial Alkylation of Metals. In: International Converence on
   Heavy Metals in the Environment, Symposium proceedings, Vol. II,
   Part 2, Toronto, Ontario, October 27-31, 1975, p. 845.

9a J.H. Koeman, W.S.M. van de Ven, J.J.M. de Goeij, P.S. Tjioe and
   J.L. van Haaften
   Mercury and Selenium in Marine Mammals and Birds, The Science of
   the Total Environment, 3, 279 (1975).

9b L. Kosta et al.
   Some Trace Elements in the Waters, Marine Organisms and Sediments
   of the Adriatic by Neutron Activation Analysis.
   J. Radioanal. Chem., in press.

1o. C. Patterson, P. Settle, B. Schaule, M. Burnett
    Transport of Pollutant Lead to the Oceans and within Ocean Eco-
    systems. In: Marine Pollutant Transfer, Lexington Books, Lex. Mass.,
    1976, p. 23.

11. T.J. Chow, C.C. Patterson, D. Settle
    Occurrence of Lead in Tuna, Nature, 251, 159 (1974).

12. E. Bacci, A. Renzoni
    Personal Communication

13. U. Harms
    The Levels of Heavy Metals (Mn, Fe, Co, Ni, Cu, Zn, Cd, Pb, Hg)
    in Fish from Onshore and Offshore Waters of the German Bight.
    Z. Lebensm. Unters.-Forsch. 157, 125 (1975).

14. M. Bernhard, A. Zattera
    Major Pollutants in the Marine Environment. In: Marine Pollution
    & Marine Waste Disposal, Pearson and Frangipane, Eds., Pergamon
    Press, 1975, p. 195.

15. D.J.H. Philipps
    The Use of Biological Indicator Organisms to Monitor Trace Metal
    Pollution in Marine and Estuarine Environments - A Review
    Environ. Pollut. 13, 281 (1977).

16. E.I. Hamilton
    Review of the Chemical Elements and Environmental Chemistry - Stra-
    tegies and Tactics. The Science of the Total Environment 5, 1 (1976).

17. G.N. Somero et al.
    Lead Accumulation Rates in Tissues of the Estuarine Teleost Fish
    Gillichthys mirabilis
    Arch. Environm. Contam. Toxicol. 6, 337 (1977).

18. R. Eisler
    Cadmium Poisoning in Fundulus heteroclitus and other Marine Organisms.
    J. Fish. Res. Bd. Can. 28, 1225 (1971).

570

19. R. Eisler et al.
    Cadmium Uptake by Marine Organisms. J. Fish Res. Bd. Can. 29, 1367
    (1972).

2o. H.W. Nürnberg, P. Valenta
    Polarography and Voltammetry in Marine Chemistry. In: The Nature
    of Sea Water. E.D. Goldberg, edit., Dahlem Konferenzen, Berlin
    1975, p. 87.

21. H.W. Nürnberg, M. Stoeppler, P. Valenta
    On the Accuracy and Reliability of Trace Metal Determinations in
    Environmental Matrix Types by Advanced Polarographic and Spectros-
    copic Techniques. Thalassia Jugoslavica, 11, 85 (1975).

22. M. Stoeppler et al.
    Zur Blei- und Cadmiumanalytik in biologischen Matrices. Proc. Int.
    Symp. Recent Advances in the Assessment of Health Effects of Environ-
    mental Pollution, Luxembourg (1975), p. 2231.

23. H.W. Nürnberg, P. Valenta, L.Mart, B. Raspor, L. Sipos
    Applications of Polarography and Voltammetry to Marine and Aquatic
    Chemistry. II. The Polarographic Approach to the Determination and
    Speciation of Toxic Metals in the Marine Environment. Z. Anal. Chem.
    282, 357 (1976).

24. H.W.Nürnberg, L. Mart, P. Valenta
    Concentrations of Cd, Pb and Cu in Ligurian and Tyrrhenian Coastal
    Waters. Rapp. Comm. Int. Mer. Médit. 24, 8; 25 (1977).

25. H.W. Nürnberg
    Potentialities and Applications of Advanced Polarographic and Vol-
    tammetric Methods in Environmental Research and Surveillance of
    Toxic Metals. Electrochimica Acta, 22, 935 (1977).

26. L. Sipos, P. Valenta, H.W. Nürnberg, M. Branica
    A New Voltammetric Method for the Study of Mercury Traces in Sea
    Water and Inland Waters. J. Electroanal. Chem. 77, 263 (1977).

27. P. Valenta, H. Rützel, H.W. Nürnberg, M. Stoeppler
    Trace Chemistry of Toxic Metals in Biomatrices. II. Voltammetric
    Determination of the Trace Content of Cadmium and other Toxic
    Metals in Human Whole Blood. Z. Anal. Chem. 285, 25 (1977).

28. P. Valenta, L. Mart, H.W. Nürnberg, M. Stoeppler
    Voltammetrische simultane Spurenanalyse toxischer Metalle in Meer-
    wasser, Binnengewässern, Trink- und Brauchwasser. "Vom Wasser",
    48, 89 (1977).

29. P. Valenta, L. Mart, H. Rützel
    New Potentialities in Ultra Trace Analysis with Differential Pulse
    Anodic Stripping Voltammetry. J. Electroanal. Chem. 82, 327 (1977).

3o. B. Raspor, P. Valenta, H.W. Nürnberg, M. Branica
    The Chelation of Cadmium with NTA in Sea Water as a Model for the
    Typical Behaviour of Trace Heavy Metal Chelates in Natural Waters.
    The Science of the Total Environment, 9, 87 (1977).

31. M. Stoeppler, W. Matthes
    Storage Behaviour of Inorganic Mercury and Methyl Mercury Chloride
    in Sea Water. Anal. Chim. Acta, 98, 389 (1978).

32. H.W. Nürnberg, L. Mart, P. Valenta, M. Stoeppler
    Applications of Polarography and Voltammetry to Marine and Aquatic
    Chemistry. III. Determination of Levels of Toxic Trace Metals
    Dissolved in Sea Water and Inland Waters by Differential Pulse
    Anodic Stripping Voltammetry. Thalassia Jugoslavica, in press.

33. H.W. Nürnberg
    Polarography and Voltammetry in Studies of Toxic Metals in Man and
    His Environment. Pure Applied Chem., in press.

34. B. Raspor, P. Valenta, H.W. Nürnberg, M. Branica
    Applications of Polarography and Voltammetry to Speciation of Trace
    Metals in Natural Waters. II. Polarographic Studies on the Kine-
    tics and Mechanism of Cd (II) - Chelate Formation with EDTA in Sea
    Water. Thalassia Jugoslavica, in press.

35. M. Bernhard
    FAO Fisheries Technical Paper No. 158. Naual of Methods in Aquatic
    Environment Research. Part 3 - Sampling and Analysis of Biological
    Materials, FAO, Rome, 1976.

36. FAO Species Indentification Sheets for Fisheries Purposes, Mediter-
    ranean and Black Sea. FAO, Rome, 1973.

37. R. Dahl, M. Stoeppler
    Studien zu automatischen Probenaufgabe bei der flammenlosen AAS mit
    der Perkin-Elmer Graphitküvette HGA 72. Ber. KFA Jülich, (1975)
    Jül-1254.

38. H. Hagedorn-Götz, M. Stoeppler
    Bestimmung anorganischer Schad- und Spurenelement in Biomatrices
    mit Zweikanal-AAS und flammenloser Atomisierung. Jül-Conf. 11 (III)
    (1974) 13-2o.

39. M. Stoeppler, M. Kampel, B. Welz
    Contributions to Automated Trace Analysis. I. Studies on Automated
    Flameless Atomic Absorption Spectrometry. Z. Anal. Chem. 282, 369
    (1976).

4o. W. Matthes, R. Flucht, M. Stoeppler
    Beiträge zur automatisierten Spurenanalyse, III. Eine empfindliche
    automatisierte Methode zur Quecksilberbestimmung in biologischen
    und Umweltproben. Fresenius Z. Anal. Chem., 291, 2o (1978).

41. M. Stoeppler, F. Backhaus
    Pretreatment Studies with Biological and Environmental Materials.
    I. Systems for Pressurized Multisample Decomposition. Fresenius
    Z. Anal. Chem., 291, 116 (1978).

42. M. Stoeppler, K. Brandt, T.C. Rains
    Contribution to Automated Trace Analysis. II. Rapid Method for the
    Automated Determination of Lead in Whole Blood by Electrothermal
    Atomic Absorption Spectrometry. Analyst, 1o3, 714 (1978).

43. M. Stoeppler, F. Backhaus
    Entwicklung, Bau und Betrieb eines mobilen Spurenmeßlabors für
    Umweltforschung und Umweltüberwachung, Ber. KFA Jülich, (1978)
    in press.

44. D.J. Lisk
    Recent Developments in the Analysis of Toxic Elements. Science,
    184, 1137 (1974).

572

45. G. Tölg
Zur Analytik von Spurenelementen in biologischem Material.
Z. Anal. Chem. 283, 257 (1977).

46. M. Stoeppler, H.W. Nürnberg
Critical Review of Analytical Methods for the Determination of
Trace Elements in Biological Materials. Int. Workshop on Biological Specimen Collection, Luxembourg, 18-22 April 1977, to appear
(1978).

47. M. Stoeppler
Analyses of Toxic Metals in Biological Materials. In: Clinical
Chemistry and Chemical Toxicology of Metals, S.S. Brown, ed.,
Elsevier/North-Holland Biomedical Press, 1977, p. 3o7.

48. M. Stoeppler, K.P. Müller, F. Backhaus
Pretreatment Studies with Biological and Environmental Materials.
III. Pressure Evaluation and Carbon Balance During Pressurized
Decomposition with Nitric Acid, Fresenius, Z. Anal. Chem.,
in preparation.

49. R. Breder, H.W. Nürnberg, M. Stoeppler, to be published.

5o. G. Erdtmann, H.W. Nürnberg
Activation Analysis of Organic Substances and Materials in:
Methodum Chimicum, F. Korte, Ed., Academic Press, New York,
San Francisco, London, 1974.

51. J.F. Diehl and R. Schelenz
Neutron Activation Analysis for Multielement Determination in
Foodstuffs and in other Biological Samples, Lebensm.-Wiss. u.
Technol., 8, 154 (1975).

52. Analytical Methods Committee
Determination of Mercury and Methylmercury in Fish,
Analyst, 1o2, 769 (1977).

53. R. Ahmed, H.W. Dürbeck, M. Stoeppler, to be published.

54. M. Stoeppler, Present Potentialities and Limitations of Atomic
Absorption Spectroscopy in Environmental and Biological Materials
with Particular Reference to Lead Determinations,
Proc. International Experts Discussion on Lead-Occurence, Fate
and Pollution in the Marine Environment, Rovinj
Pergamon Press, Oxford, in preparation.

55. J. Colimowski, P. Valenta, M. Stoeppler and H.W.Nürnberg
Ein Verfahren zur raschen voltammetrischen Simultanbestimmung
der toxischen Spurenmetalle Cd und Pb im Harn,
Fresenius Z. Anal. Chem., 29o, 1o7 (1978).

56. K. May, M. Stoeppler
Pretreatment Studies with Biological and Environmental Materials,
II. Complete Wet Digestion of Carbonic and Environmental Materials
by Perchloric Acid Mixtures, Fresenius Z. Anal. Chem., in press
(1978).

SPECIMEN BANKING OF FOOD SAMPLES FOR LONG TERM MONITORING OF NUTRIENT TRACE ELEMENTS

Wayne R. Wolf
Nutrient Composition Laboratory
Science and Education Administration
Agricultural Research, U.S.D.A.
Beltsville, Maryland 2o7o5

Abstract

Specimen Banking of Food Samples for Long Term Monitoring of Nutrient Trace Elements.
Wayne R. Wolf, Nutrient Composition Laboratory, Nutrition Institute, Science and Education Administration, Agricultural Research, U.S.A. Department of Agriculture, Beltsville,Maryland 2o7o5.

There is a growing need for more accurate and precise assessment and long term monitoring of the nutrient content of the U.S. diet. The American dietary has changed markedly and continues to change. In order to assess the magnitude, extent and trend of these changes in the nutrient content of the diet, a long term monitoring system should be established and maintained. Of necessity in this monitoring system would be the collection and storage of representative samples for use as a base line for future comparison. Establishment of programs for monitoring environmental materials and specimen banking of samples for assessment of pollutants and environmental materials is compatible with the needs for long term nutrient monitoring. The recognition of beneficial aspects of certain of the trace elements at low levels of intake and the harmful effects of these same element at higher levels requires precise definition of the actual levels in the diet. Available technologies for analysis and storage of samples make the monitoring of trace elements in U.S. diets feasible. Cooperative programs in long term monitoring of trace elements as nutrients and pollutants would enhance the benefits of both programs.

Introduction

Recent interest and advances in nutrition and nutrition research have led to an awareness of potential public health problems regarding optimum nutrient intake of the U.S. population (1). There is a growing need to much more accurately and precisely assess and monitor the nutrient content of the U.S. diet. Changes in food production practices, processing storage and handling times, consumer demand,increasingly wider spread distribution of foods outside of production areas, and changes in costs of certain foods have significantly changed the dietary of the U.S. population. Study of the effects of these changes on the nutrient content of the U.S. diet has been limited (2).
For assessment of the magnitude, extent and trend of these changes in the nutrient composition of foods, a long term monitoring system should be established and maintained. The task of monitoring the U.S. food supply would be of great magnitude and no single laboratory or group

could assume the responsibility for the long term assessment of the composition of all food items that are available to consumers. Therefore, this task should be shared by the entire scientific nutritional community. For any valid comparison of data among laboratories or over a period of time a well defined, validated, accurate and precise measurement system must be set up. The key to this system is the collection and storage of a set of well characterized, well documented representative samples of known nutrient content, for use as a base line for future comparisons. Each sample must be representative of the food under study, and must be handled, homogenized and stored under extremely well documented conditions that would,insure the long term stability and integrity of the sample and its nutrient content. These samples must be well characterized by the most advanced analytical techniques and be available for base line comparison when new "state of the art" techniques are developed. As new nutrients of interest appear and the need for trend data becomes apparent, these base line samples would be available for retrospective analysis and comparison to the "now" samples. The requirements for collection, storage and analysis of these base line samples of food for long term nutrient monitoring, are very compatible with the requirements of the environmental monitoring system proposed in this International Workshop.

Although this Workshop was first conceived to discuss monitoring systems for pollutants in our environment, the needs for a monitoring system for nutrients in our food supply are so compatible, that an expansion of the role of these monitoring systems to include nutrients in foods would benefit both areas. The elimination of duplication of effort in "specimen banking" is self evident. The awareness and knowledge of interactions between pollutant burden and the nutritional status of populations who are recipients of that burden are greatly increasing.A joint program to simultaneously monitor the trends of both factors would facilitate valid assessments of the consequences of each factor. Awareness and knowledge are increasing of the importance of defining the consequences of different levels of intake of substances that are known to be harmful at high levels. The beneficial aspect of certain of the trace elements at low levels of intake and the harmful effects of these same trace elements at high levels of intake require precise definition of the actual levels in diets. An effective program for sampling foods is essential in any program for monitoring the environment if the ultimate concern is the effect of these substances on active body burden to humans. For many of these substances food consumption is the major route of human exposure. This is true for many of the harmful substances as well as obviously for the nutrients.

The area of greatest overlap between harmful and beneficial effects is for the trace elements. The trace elements of interest in nutrition are listed in Table I. Of the 17 environmental inorganic pollutants of interest listed in the information note (October 1977) describing the objective, structure and plan for this Workshop, 11 (As, Co, Cr, F, Mo, Mn, Ni, Se, Sn, V and Zn) are in this table of "essential" trace elements. These elements comprise an area of specific concern because the actual levels of human exposure must be accurately defined to ensure that the population is getting neither too much nor too little of these trace elements. Our present technology is probably adequate to determine feasible conditions to determine and preserve the trace element content of foods for extended storage. I believe it is both feasible and necessary in environmental monitoring programs to include selected food samples to be maintained, stored, and analyzed for nutrient trace element content.

Table I. Trace Elements in Nutrition (3)

Element	Discovery of Requirement	RDA Established (b)	Human Subadequate Intakes Identified	Fortification Recommendations
Iron	17th Century	Yes	Yes	Yes
Iodine	1850	Yes	Yes	Yes
Copper	1928	Pending	?	More Data Needed
Manganese	1931	No	No	No
Zinc	1934	Yes	Yes	Yes
Cobalt	1935	No (B_{12})	No (B_{12} Yes)	No
Molybdenum	1953	Pending	No (animals)	No
Selenium	1957	Pending	Yes	More Data Needed
Chromium	1959	Pending	Yes	More Data Needed
Tin	1970	No	Experimental	Unknown
Vanadium	1971	No	Experimental	Unknown
Fluorine	1972	Pending	Experimental	Unknown
Silicon	1972	No	Experimental	Unknown
Nickel	1973	No	Experimental	Unknown
Arsenic	1975	No	Experimental	Unknown

The prospect for specimen banking of food samples for analysis of additional nutrients particularly trace organic nutrients, is at present less certain because of our more limited knowledge of proper analyses and proper storage conditions for these less stable nutrients. Further basic research is necessary on analysis and storage of the pure organic nutrient compounds before we can proceed to food mixtures containing these compounds. Such research could be an important adjunct to environmental monitoring programs.

Need for Base Line Samples

Attempted correlations between older published data and modern data usually have no basis for valid comparison, due to the lack of well characterized samples referencing the sets of data to a common base. Changes in the nutrient content of the food supply that are observed in long term monitoring studies must to be referenced to a constant set of well characterized, well documented samples in order to ascertain whether apparent changes in nutrients are real or only reflect changes in analytical procedures. The interlaboratory analytical variations can far out-weigh and confuse the actual differences among data collected at different times.

The content of the essential trace element, copper, in the U.S. diet is a good illustration of this point. At present there is no Recommended Dietary Allowance for copper set by the NAS/NRC Food and Nutrition Board (4). In best estimates of the required intake based upon published and recent balance studies, the requirement was determined to be about 2.o mg/day for an ddult (4). Previous estimates of the actual Cu intake were accepted to be well above this level, in the range of 2.o to 5.omg/day (4). However, in recent studies, dietary intake of Cu was only 1.o to 1.3 mg/day (5). Those data suggested that intake of copper is marginal and the question of adequate copper intake became important. Another question arise in assessing the consequences of this marginal intake.

For any kind of long term real time monitoring, the analytical procedure should be consistant, and well defined, well characterized, properly stored samples should be available to serve as a base line for comparison with samples to be collected in the future. Because of the increasing development and refinement of analytical techniques, a "sample bank" is imperative. The amounts of these samples must be sufficient to that subsamples could be periodically withdrawn for comparison of procedures and data. This type of interaction between the retrospective analysis of stored samples and real time monitoring is necessary for optimum functioning of the system. Then long term real time monitoring would show actual trends and serve as a guide line for action or inaction on nutrient intake.

Defined Measurement System

For any type oflong term monitoring system of our food supply, whether it be for nutrient or pollutant content, the measurement system must be well defined, and stable over the time frame of the monitoring. When dealing with a matrix as complex as foods, the analytical methodology is not at the present time fully under control and definitive for every individual nutrient.

For some nutrient trace elements, we do have analytical methodology that is considered definitive. The best example is stable isotope dilution mass spectrometry (6). In this method a known amount of a stable isotope, different from the most abundant natural isotope, is added to a sample. The sample is generally acid digested to destroy its chemical history and to insure complete exchange with the added isotope spike, which is critical to obtaining correct results by this technique. Upon equilibration, an aliquot of the solution is analyzed by mass spectrometry for the isotopic ratio of the metal of interest. The change in this ratio from the naturally occuring ratio depends upon the unknown amount of metal originally in the sample and the known amount of stable isotope spike added. Because isotopic ratios can be measured very precisely with todays mass spectrometers, the unknown original concentration can be accurately and precisely determined. With adequate precaution to insure equilibration of added isotope spike and sample and avoidance of contamination during analysis, this method can be definitive and stable over a period of time. Use of this definitive procedure and confirmation with other highly sensitive techniques for total metal analysis such as NAA or AAS, can give precise analytical data that have a high assurance of accuracy. For such high assurance of accuracy and precision, analysis of a single sample can be relatively time consuming and costly. For long term monitoring, analysis of many samples would be required for required surveys of the distribution of nutrients or pollutants. Thus, this type of analytical work on every single sample is not feasible in real-life constraints of resources and time. For large scale surveys, such as monitoring nutrient content of the U.S. food supply, it is necessary to have procedures with sufficient precision to determine the effects under study. Such procedures must be capable of rapid, economic, automated analyses of a large number of samples in a short time. To ensure accuracy of these procedures proper quality control techniques must be carried out. The best way to ensure this quality control is the routine analysis of a standard working sample of the same matrix as the unknown samples -- such as the biological Standard Reference Materials issued by the National Bureau of Standards. Due to the extremely high cost in time, money, and research effort to obtain, homogenize, certify, store, and distribute sufficient amounts of a single SRM it is not feasible to develop appropriate SRM's for all the different food items. Maintenance of a "sample bank" of highly characterized samples of different matrices which could be used as primary standards materials for calibration of secondary working standards is the only feasible way to maintain the accuracy of the measurement system throughout various laboratories and projects. By use of these "sample bank" specimens to establish base line comparison for large studies, benefits of the support, time and effort expended for the highest degree of accuracy in "sample bank" specimen could be significantly magnified. The high level accuracy of the"sample bank" system could be transferred to the entire nutrient composition measurement system.

Choice of Food Samples for Specimen Banking

Several criteria must be met for choice of food samples for a specimen banking system for long term nutrient monitoring. Because the initial discussions concerned a pilot banking system for study of the feasibility of long term storage, the samples should be:

1. Representative of foods consumed in significant amounts by a large portion of the population.
2. Suitable for long term storage
3. Available from a variety of geographical and marketing areas.

Two types of foods that would be suitable for pilot studies for specimen banking are a cereal grain and a dairy product. For a significant portion of the population cereal grain represents a large portion of the dietary intake, has a known potential for long term storage, and is grown, processed and marketed in many geographical areas. In the United States wheat is the predominant grain for human consumption. Milk samples would be of interest to an environmental monitoring program The technology for storage and handling of dried milk is known and feasible. Milk is a food of significant consumption by a large percentage of the U.S. population. Dairy products are also one of the few foods in the U.S. that are not widely distributed. They are produced and sold locally and would be more reflective of local conditions. Milk might be an integrator of the plant and soil conditions where the animals have grazed.

The choice of individual samples for banking depends upon the objective of the initial pilot environmental monitoring programs. If the main objective of the pilot programs is to study, find and document standard protocols for collection, sampling and storage of the specimen samples to insure long term integrity, the choice of samples would not be severely restrictive. If the main objective of the program is to commence actual environmental monitoring, the effort and resources devoted to sample selection become a very major concern. The food samples selected must then be representative of the total growing, production, marketing, and consumption system for that food. This approach involves very complex, detailed statistical modeling to properly choose numbers and types of samples that would be representative and would give significant answers to the questions asked.

The second objective can not be accomplished as an initial pilot program. The standard protocols must be developed and the analytical procedures defined with known error limits before the statistical modeling can be done. Thus the initial task must be to define the sampling protocols, the protocols must be tested on the types of food to be collected and banked, and the facilities and mechanism set up to carry out these protocols. This will require extensive basic study on the problems of storage and maintaining the samples.

The initial samples chosen should be from only a few areas and should be ofsufficient quantitiy to allow adequate numbers of subsamples in order to properly study a variety of storage and handling conditions. For foods, adequate quantities of available sample are very seldom a serious problem, as might be the case for human tissue samples. The collection of a large amount of sample (several kilograms), the homogenization of this sample and the handling and storage of sufficient aliquots by several different techniques would allow the needed basic data to be accumulated. The choices of wheat and milk as initial samples would be suitable for this scheme. For the wheat, choice of the grain from a given supply source, or better, the fine grinding and blending of wheat from several sources would give a sufficient amount of a homogenous sample. Fluid milk chosen from several sources could be readily blended. The choice of whole milk would be prefered to skim or de-fatted milk because the knowledge of proper storage conditions for fat containing foods is very critical for extension to other types of food such as meat.

Sample Collection, Storage and Preservation

The proper handling of the samples to prevent spoilage and loss or contamination of the nutrient of interest is critical to the purpose of long

term specimen banking. Amounts of inorganic elements are not markedly
affected by storage, but bioavailability of some of the trace element
nutrients might be affected. Of particular concern is iron, which
exists in some foods in the highly utilizable biologic form of heme
iron. Different forms of nutrients should be identified and measured.
For most trace elements, the biologically available form has not been
identified structurally and quantitative methods for their analysis
have not been developed. Interest is increasing in these areas and new
methods are being developed. As these analytical procedures are verified, the existance of good retrospective samples would be of great
benefit.

For the organic nutrients, levels, and/or bioavailability, are generally
reduced in foods following harvest, collection or slaughter. Many of
the vitamins are subject to loss and isomerization to a biologically
less active form. Loss of carbohydrates may occur. Control of loss or
gain of moisture or water content is a very serious problem in storage
or banking of food samples. These changes in moisture, must be rigidly
defined to enable analytical results on the stored samples to be related
to similar items reaching the consumer in the market place. Protein
content may not be markedly changed upon storage, but protein availability may be much reduced. The problems with storing samples containing
lipids or fatty materials are well known. Even storage at -4o°C does
not prevent lipid decomposition that apparently occurs through a free
radical process which can be stabilized at low temperatures. The changes
due to microbial or enzymatic activity on "spoilage" is a large area
of concern in storage of foods or any biological material.

Although changes in the organic nutrients may not affect the inorganic
nutrients, samples that had undergone any significant changes in composition would have little value for a specimen banking system. Organic
nutrients are of considerable future concern for any specimen banking
program and the problems associated with storage of samples would require
extensive basic research.

Scrupulous care is necessary to prevent trace element contamination during
collection, handling and storage of samples. The benefits of sensitive,
precise sophisticated methods and equipment for analysis would be canceled
if the integrity of the samples were not preserved. Sampling equipment
must be designed to be as metal free as possible, and procedures must
prevent exposure to airborne particulate matter, and to other materials
or reagents that might introduce trace amounts of metal to the sample.
The levels of trace elements in foods ar quite low. For example, the
chromium content in foods is in the low parts per billion range, being
1o-3o ppb in wheat. Any blending or homogenization of the sample must
be done in a system that does not introduce the metal of interest. For
example, most food handling devices are made of corosion resistant stainless steel. Depending upon the type, stainless steel can contain 12
- 26 % chromium, 3 to 22 % Ni or 1 to 1o % Mn as major constituents. Those
metals are of nutrient interest and occur in foods at low ppm or ppb
levels. Therefore, the chance of significant contamination upon contact
with stainless steel equipment is great. Plastics are a better material for
handling food samples to prevent trace element contamination. For applications involving cutting, grinding, etc. that require a hard material, instruments should be specifically designed or fabricated from known materials
such as titanium, which do not contain metals of nutrient interest. Glass
materials and containers are not usually indicated for storage or handling of food samples for trace element analysis because of the extreme
difficulty of properly cleaning the inside of the containers.

Glass can be cleaned, adequately, but it is a laborious, time consuming task. Sometimes glass containers must be used to store samples at very low temperatures where plastics will not hold up. However, rigorously cleaned glas containers can adsorb metal from fluid samples and cause significant loss of trace amounts of metals from the samples.
The frozen storage of food samples in the dried state is feasible, but loss or contamination of the metal must be prevented during the drying process. The technology of freeze drying is sufficiently advanced for treatment of samples for trace element analysis.

Analytical Methods

For characterizing the samples in the specimen bank for trace element content, the analytical methodology must be sufficiently sensitive to determine extremely low levels with good precision and potential for definitive accuracy. Any uncertainty in the methods must be well known and defined. Trace element content should be determined by at least two different methods that agree within defined error limits to ensure that the methods have no systematic bias. If possible, all analyses should be referenced by calibration or simultaneous analyses to a certified primary Standard Reference Material. For the Wheat, SRM-1567 Wheat Flour is available from the National Bureau of Standards and should be of mandatory use in analyzing banked wheat samples for trace element content.
For trace element analyses, the analytical techniques of most probable use would be Neutron Activation Analysis (NAA), Isotope Dilution Mass Spectrometry (IDMS) and Atomic Spectroscopy (AS) including atomic absorption and emission. With appropriate facilities the first two techniques can be very sensitive, precise and accurate. NAA requires a source of neutrons, appropriate facilities for handling radioactive samples and some aspects of "clean" laboratory speace for handling samples before irradiation. IDMS (discussed previously) requires extensive "clean" laboratory space to prevent contamination and blank problems and extensive sophisticated mass spectrometric equipment. In both NAA and IDMS, precision and accuracy are high, but the trade offs are a low number of samples at high cost in time, expense and resources.

Number of Samples

The number of samples to be stored in a specimen bank raises important questions. If the number is small, each sample can be analyzed by the more sophisticated techniques and highest accuracy and precision can be obtained for each sample. If the number becomes large, which is likely in any environmental monitoring system, it is no longer feasible to expend the optimum resources on each and every sample. For trace element analysis, several atomic spectroscopic techniques such as atomic absorption, flame atomic emission, plasma emission, and others are rugged, economic and fast. The expenditure of optimum effort on a few priority samples and routine quality controlled effort on the remainder should be a feasible way to gain maximum benefit from the monitoring system. A small number of priority samples would be representative of the large number of additional samples and would serve as quality control standards for the additional samples. Atomic absorption methods and procedures could be developed, calibrated, and documented using these priority samples. Thus the analytical measurement accuracy obtained on these priority samples could be transferred to the whole of the

specimens in the bank.
For long term or trend monitoring of a particular trace element in food,
collection of many samples from a variety of areas would be necessary
to statistically describe the dietary system being studied. For any
such studies a central bank of specimens would be essential to the collection of base line data.

References

1. Senate Select Committee on Nutrition and Human Needs, 1977:
   Dietary Goals for the United States, 2nd Ed. U.S. Government Printing Office, Washington, D.C. 2o4o2, Stock No. o52-o7o-o4376-8.

2. K.K. Stewart
   Hearings Before the Senate Select Committee on Nutrition and Human
   Needs on Food Quality in Federal Food Programs, Part 2, September
   3o, 1977, U.S. Government Printing Office, Washington,D.C. 2o4o2.

3. W.R. Wolf
   "Nutrient Trace Element Composition of Foods: Analytical Needs and
   Problems" Anal. Chem. 5o (2), 19oA-194A, 1978.

4. Food and Nutrition Board
   "Recommended Dietary Allowances" National Academy of Sciences/Na-
   tional Research Council, Eighth Ed., 1974.

5. Holden, J., Wolf, W. and Mertz, M.
   "Levels of Zinc and Copper in Self Selected Diets" J. Am. Diet Assoc.,
   In Press.

6. P.J. Paulson
   "Spark Source Mass Spectrometric Isotope Dilution", in Procedures
   Used at the National Bureau of Standards to Determine Selected
   Trace Elements in Biological and Botanical Materials; NBS Special
   Publication 492, R. Mavrodineanu, Ed., November 1977.

ANNEX III

List of Contributors and Participants

R. AMAVIS
Commissison of the European Communities
E. C. P. S.
200, Rue de la Loi
1049 Brussels
Belgium

K. H. BALLSCHMITER
Universität Ulm
Abt. Analytische Chemie
Oberer Eselsberg
7900 Ulm/Donau
Federal Republic of Germany

D. BARTH
University of Nevada, Las Vegas
College of Science, Mathematics and Engineering
4505 Maryland Parkway
Las Vegas, Nevada 89154
U. S. A.

K. BAUER
Bundesministerium für Forschung und Technologie
Postfach 120370
5300 Bonn 2
Federal Republic of Germany

H. BECK
Bundesgesundheitsamt
Postfach
1000 Berlin 33
Federal Republic of Germany

A. BERLIN
Commission of the European Communities
bat. j. monnet
Luxembourg

H. P. BERTRAM
Institut für Pharmakologie und Toxikologie
der Westfälischen Wilhelms-Universität
Westring 12
4400 Münster
Federal Republic of Germany

M. CARPENTIER
Director – General
Environmental and Consumer Protection Service
Commission of the European Communities
200, Rue de la Loi
1049 Brussels
Belgium

P. L. CHAMBERS
Environmental Sciences Committee
National Board for Sciences and Technology
c/o Trinity College
Dublin 2
United Kingdom

B. CLAUSEN
State Veterinary Serum Laboratory
Bülowsvej 27
1870 Copenhagen V
Denmark

D. C. COLEMAN
Natural Resource Ecology Laboratory
Colorade State University
Ft. Collins, Colorado 80523
U. S. A.

B. W. CORNABY
Ecology and Ecosystems Analysis Section
Battelle Columbus Laboratories
505 King Avenue
Columbus, Ohio 43021
U. S. A.

B. COLLETTE
NOAA/NMFS National Systematics Laboratory
National Museum of Natural History
10th & Constitution Avenues, N. W.
Washington, D. C. 20560
U. S. A.

G. CRÖSSMANN
Landwirtschaftskammer Westfalen-Lippe
Landwirtschaftliche Untersuchungs- und
Forschungsanstalt
– Joseph-König-Institut –
Kanalstraße 240, Postfach 5929
4400 Münster
Federal Republic of Germany

J. BOUQUIAUX
Service Environment
Institut d'Hygiene et d'Epidemiologie
14, Rue Juliette Wytsman
1050 Bruxelles
Belgium

P. BOURDEAU
Commission of the European Communities
E. C. P. S.
200, Rue de la Loi
1049 Brussels
Belgium

D. L. BRITT
Ecological Programs
Flow Resources Corp.
7655 Old Springhouse Road
McLean, Virginia 22102
U. S. A.

J. J. BROMENSHENK
Department of Botany
University of Montana
Missoula, Montana 59812
U. S. A.

F. BRO-RASMUSSEN
Technical University of Denmark
Environmental Science and Ecology
Building 224
2800 Lyngby
Denmark

A. BUTLER
Branch of Ecological Monitoring
U. S. Environmental Protection Agency
Sabine Island, Gulf Breeze
Florida
U. S. A.

R. CABRIDENC
I. R. C. H. A.
Charge de Mission au Ministere
de la Culture et de l'Environment
Paris
France

M. F. CUTHBERT
Dept. of Health and Social Security
Hannibal House, Elephant and Castle
London SE 16 TE
United Kingdom

T. DICK
Nedeco
Instituto de Biociencias
Universidado Federal do Rio G. Do Sul
90.000 Porto Alegre
Brazil

U. DRESCHER - KADEN
Institut für Physiologie, Physiologische Chemie
und Ernährungsphysiologie
Fachbereich Tiermedizin
Universität München
Veterinärstraße 13
8000 München
Federal Republic of Germany

H.-W. DÜRBECK
Institute for Chemistry
Inst. 4: Applied Physical Chemistry
Nuclear Research Center (KFA)
Postfach 1913
5170 Jülich
Federal Republic of Germany

R. A. DURST
Center for Analytical Chemistry
U. S. Dept. of Commerce, NBS
Gaithersburg, MD 20234
U. S. A.

K. W. EBING
Biologische Bundesanstalt für Land- und
Forstwirtschaft
Institut für Pflanzenschutzmittelforschung
Königin-Luise-Straße 19
1000 Berlin 33 (Dahlem)
Federal Republic of Germany

R. ECKARD
Institut für Pharmakologie und Toxikologie
der Westfälischen Wilhelms-Universität
Westring 12
4400 Münster
Federal Republic of Germany

H. EGAN
Laboratory of the Government Chemist
Cornwall House, Stamford Street
London, SE 1 9NQ
United Kingdom

R. ENGEL
U. S. Department of Agriculture
Romm 402, Annex
RSQF 12th & C Street, S. W.
Washington, D. C. 20250
U. S. A.

A. FLEMER
Ecological Effects Division
U. S. EPA, Office of Research and Development
(RD - 683)
401 M Street S. W.
Washington, D. C. 10460
U. S. A.

S. W. FOWLER
International Atomic Energy Agency
International Laboratory of Marine Radioactivity
Oceanographic Museum
Monaco Ville
Principaliy of Monaco

C. FRANCIS
Environmental Science Division
OAK Ridge, Tennessee 37830
U. S. A.

P. F. GHETTI
Laboratorio di Ecologia
dell'Universita'di Parma
Borgo Carissimi 10
43100 Parma
Italy

T. GILLS
NBS, National Bureau of Standards
BLDG, 235, Room B - 108
Gaithersburg, MD 921 - 2166
U. S. A.

G. GOLDSTEIN
Clinical Pathology Branch
U. S. Environmental Protection Agency
Research Triangle Park NC 27711
U. S. A.

M. GOTO
Department of Chemistry
Gakushuin University
Toshima-Ku
Tokyo, 171
Japan

P. A. GREVE
Unit for Residue Analysis
National Institute of Public Health
Postbus 1
2660 Bilthoven
Netherlands

G. GRIMMER
Biochemisches Institut für Umweltcarcinogene
Sieker Landstraße 19
2070 Ahrensburg
Federal Republic of Germany

T. HAMA
Fac. Pharmaceutical Science
Kobe Gakuin University
Arise, Igawadaninmachi
Taruminku, Kobe 673
Hyogo-Ken
Japan

H.-J. HAPKE
Abteilung für Toxikologie
Institut für Pharmakologie der Tierärztlichen
Hochschule
Bischofsholer Damm 15
3000 Hannover
Federal Republic of Germany

D. HEESCHEN
Bundesanstalt für Milchforschung
Institut für Hygiene
Hermann-Weigand-Str. 1 - 27
2300 Kiel
Federal Republic of Germany

H. HERTZ
Trace Organic Division
U. S. Department of Commerce
NBS
Gaithersburg, MD 20234
U. S. A.

E. HIEKE
Max-von-Pettenkofer-Institut,
Bundesgesundheitsamt
Postfach
1000 Berlin 33
Federal Republic of Germany

T. HINDS
Terrestrial Ecology
Pacific Northwest Laboratory
P. O. Box 999
Richland, Washinton 99352
U. S. A.

A. V. HOLDEN
Department of Agriculture and Fisheries for
Scotland
Freshwater Fisheries Lab.
Faskally Pitlochry
Perthshire PH 16 5LB
United Kingdom

J. W. HUCKABEE
Oak Ridge National Laboratory
Oak Ridge, Tennessee 37830
U. S. A.

J. M. HUSHEON
Mitre Corp. Metrek Div.
1820 Dolley Madison Boulevard
McLean, Virginia 22101
U. S. A.

W. KAEFERSTEIN
Bundesgesundheitsamt
Postfach
1000 Berlin 33
Federal Republic of Germany

M. O. KARLOG
Odense University − Campusvej 75
Institute of Biology
5230 Odense M
Denmark

D. KAYSER
Umweltbundesamt
Bismarckplatz 1
1000 Berlin 33
Federal Republic of Germany

F. H. KEMPER
Institut für Pharmakologie und Toxikologie
der Westfälischen Wilhelms-Universität
Westring 12
4400 Münster
Federal Republic of Germany

M. D. KERN
Biology Department
College of Wooster
Wooster, Ohio 44691
U. S. A.

W. KLEIN
Gesellschaft für Strahlen- und
Umweltforschung mbH
München
Institut für Ökologische Chemie
Ingolstädter Landstraße 2
8042 Neuherberg, Post Oberschleißheim
Federal Republic of Germany

M. KONDO
Fac. Pharmaceutical Science
Osaka University
Kamiyamada Suita
Osaka 565
Japan

W. KORANSKY
Philipps-Universität
Institut für Toxikologie und Pharmakologie
Pilgrimsteig 2
3550 Marburg
Federal Republic of Germany

F. KORTE
Lehrstuhl für Ökologische Chemie
der TU München und
Institut für Ökologische Chemie der GSF
Ingolstädter Landstraße 2
8042 Neuherberg, Post Oberschleißheim
Federal Republic of Germany

P. LEFLEUR
Center for Analytical Chemistry
U. S. Department of Commerce, NBS
Gaithersburg, MD 20234
U. S. A.

H. VON LERSNER
Präsident
Umweltbundesamt
Bismarckplatz 1
1000 Berlin 33
Federal Republic of Germany

R. A. LEWIS
Office of the Assistant Secretary for Environment
Mail Stop E - 201
U. S. Department of Energy
Washinton, D. C. 20545
U. S. A.

B. LIGHTHART
TSD/CERL / U. S. EPA
Corvallis, Oregon 97330
U. S. A.

G. LOWMAN
U. S. Environmental Protection Agency
Environmental Research Laboratory
South Ferry Road
Narragansett, Rhode Island
U. S. A.

N.-P. LUEPKE
Institut für Pharmakologie und Toxikologie
der Westfälischen Wilhelms-Universität
Westring 12
4400 Münster
Federal Republic of Germany

J. L. LUDKE
Columbia National Fisheries Research Laboratory
U. S. Fish & Wildlife Service,
Rt. 1, New Haven School Road
Columbia, Missouri 65201
U. S. A.

R. MARTY
Laboratory of Animal Ecology and Ecophysiology
Bordeaux I University
33405 Bordeaux − Talence
France

M. MOLITOR
Administration des Eaux et Forêts
Porte Neuve
Luxemborg

F. MORIARTY
Institute of Terrestrial Ecology
Monks Wood Experimental Station I. T. E.
Monks Wood Experimental Research Council
Abbots Ripton
Huntingdon, England PE 17 2 LS
United Kingdom

M. MOSSELMANS
Commission of the European Communities
E. C. P. S.
200, Rue de la Loi
1049 Brussels
Belgium

R. K. MURTON
Institute of Terrestrial Ecology
Monks Wood Experimental Station
Abbots Ripton
Huntingdon, PE 17 2 LS
United Kingdom

P. MUELLER
Schwerpunkt für Biogeographie
Fachbereich 6 Geographie
Universität des Saarlandes
6600 Saarbrücken
Federal Republic of Germany

J. MUSICK
Institute of Marine Science
Cloucester Point VA 23062
U. S. A.

C. NASH
Kramer, Chin and Mayo, Inc.
1917 1st Avenue
Seattle, Washington 98101
U. S. A.

H. W. NUERNBERG
Institute for Chemistry
Nuclear Research Center (KFA)
Postfach 1913
5170 Jülich
Federal Republic of Germany

H. M. OHLENDORF
U. S. Fish & Wildlife Service
Patuxent Wildlife Research Center
Laurel, MD 20811
U. S. A.

J. B. PEARCE
U. S. Department of Commerce
National Oceanic and Atmospheric Administration
National Marine Fisheries Service
Northeast Fisheries Center
Sandy Hood Laboratory
Highlands, New Jersey 07732
U. S. A.

D. K. PHELPS
EPA — Environmental Research Lab.
South Ferry Road
Narragansett, Rhode Island 02882
U. S. A.

I. M. PRICE
Advice and Support Section
Wildlife Toxicology Division
Canadian Wildlife Service
Ottawa, Ontario
Canada

C. PRIES
Department of Analytical Chemistry
Maatschappelijke Technologie
Nijverheidsorganisatie TNO
Postbus 217
2600 AE Delft
Netherlands

L. C. RANIERE
Terrestrial Ecology Branch
Corvallis Environmental Research Laboratory
200 S. W. 35th Street
Corvallis, Oregon 97330
U. S. A.

O. RAVERA
Department of Physical and Natural Sciences
C. C. R. — EURATOM
21020 Ispra (Varese)
Italy

H. H. REICHENBACH-KLINKE
Institut für Zoologie und Hydrobiologie
Kaulbachstr. 37
8000 München 22
Federal Republic of Germany

C. RICHIR
Université de Bordeaux II
146, Rue les Saignat
33076 Bordeaux
France

D. ROEMER-MAEHLER
Bundesministerium für Forschung und
Technologie
Postfach 120370
5300 Bonn 2
Federal Republic of Germany

H. ROOK
Center for Analytical Chemistry
U. S. Department of Commerce, NBS
Gaithersburg, MD 20234
U. S. A.

W. ROSEN
Office of Toxic Substances
U. S. EPA
401 M Street, SW
Washington, D. C. 20460
U. S. A.

R. W. SCHREIBER
Natural History Museum
900 Exposition Boulevard
Los Angeles, California 90007
U. S. A.

J. W. SKELLY
Department of Plant Pathology and Physiology
Virginia State University
Blacksburg, Birginia 24060
U. S. A.

W. SPIESS
Bundesforschungsanstalt für Ernährung
Engesser Str. 20
7500 Karlsruhe
Federal Republic of Germany

J. SMEETS
Commission of the European Communities
E. C. P. S.
200, Rue de la Loi
1049 Brussels
Belgium

H. D. SCHENKE
Umweltbundesamt
Werner-Voss-Damm 62
1000 Berlin 42
Federal Republic of Germany

F. SCHMIDT – BLEEK
Umweltbundesamt
Bismarckplatz 1
1000 Berlin 33
Federal Republic of Germany

J. B. STATES
Battelle Northwest Laboratories
Battelle Avenue
Richland, Washington 99352
U. S. A.

L. STEUBING
Institut für Pflanzenökologie
Heinrich-Buff-Ring 38
6300 Lahn-Giessen
Federal Republic of Germany

M. STOEPPLER
Institut für Chemie der Kernforschungsanlage
Jülich GmbH
Inst. 4: Angewandte Physikalische Chemie
Postfach 1913
5170 Jülich
Federal Republic of Germany

J. SWINEBROAD
Office of Health and Environmentlal Research
U. S. Department of Energy
Washington, D. C. 20545
U. S. A.

W. TALBOT
Health Effects Division
Office of Research and Development
U. S. Environmental Protection Agency
Washington, D. C. 20460
U. S. A.

G. TENDRON
Service de Conservation de la Nature
Museum National d'Histoire Naturelle
36 Rue Geoffrey St.-Hilaire
75231 Paris Cedex 05
France

M. UPPENBRINK
Umweltbundesamt
Bismarckplatz 1
1000 Berlin 33
Federal Republic of Germany

A. P. WATSON
Health and Safety Research Division
Oak Ridge, Tennessee 37830
U. S. A.

M. WESSELS-BOER
Ministerie voor de Volksgezondheit
en Milieuhygiëne
Dokter Reijerstraat 10
Leidschendam
Netherlands

P. WISSMATH
Bereich für Hygiene und Technologie
Veterinärstr. 13
8000 München
Federal Republic of Germany

A. WOLF
Bundesforschungsanstalt für Ernährung
Engesser Straße 20
7500 Karlsruhe
Federal Republic of Germany

W. R. WOLF
Science and Education Administration
Federal Research, U. S. D. A.
Beltsville, Maryland 20705
U. S. A.

C.WOTEKI
OTA
United States Congress
Food Group
Washington, D. C. 20510
U. S. A.

The Use of Biological Specimens for the Assessment of Human Exposure to Environmental Pollutants

edited by
A. BERLIN
Commission of European Communities

A. H. WOLFF
University of Illinois, U.S.A.

Y. HASEGAWA
World Health Organisation, New York, U.S.A.

These are the proceedings of the international Workshop on the Use of Biological Specimens for the Assessment of Human Exposure to Environmental Pollutants, held in Luxemburg, 18-22 April 1977.
The main objectives of the workshop were:
 - to assess the types of environmental pollutants and human specimens most suitable for 'biological monitoring', and to evaluate the probable usefulness of biological specimen banking.
 - to examine the state of the art and the technical feasibility of programmes designed to collect, analyse and store samples relative to biological monitoring and biological specimen banking.
 - to develop guidelines for sampling, sample preparation, analytical requirements and storage.
 - to draw up recommendations for further research and development.

1979, x, 368 pp., cloth   ISBN 90-247-2168-7

Martinus Nijhoff Publishers

P.O. Box 566, The Hague, The Netherlands
160 Old Derby Street, Hingham, MA 02043, USA